The Central Nervous System: Clinical Research and Advances

The Central Nervous System: Clinical Research and Advances

Edited by Scarlett Santos

AMERICAN
MEDICAL PUBLISHERS
www.americanmedicalpublishers.com

American Medical Publishers,
41 Flatbush Avenue,
1st Floor, New York,
NY 11217, USA

Visit us on the World Wide Web at:
www.americanmedicalpublishers.com

ISBN: 978-1-63927-332-4

Cataloging-in-Publication Data

The central nervous system : clinical research and advances / edited by Scarlett Santos.
p. cm.
Includes bibliographical references and index.
ISBN 978-1-63927-332-4
1. Central nervous system. 2. Central nervous system--Diseases--Treatment.
3. Nervous system. 4. Neurosciences. I. Santos, Scarlett.
RC361 .C46 2022
616.8--dc23

Table of Contents

Preface

Over the recent decade, advancements and applications have progressed exponentially. This has led to the increased interest in this field and projects are being conducted to enhance knowledge. The main objective of this book is to present some of the critical challenges and provide insights into possible solutions. This book will answer the varied questions that arise in the field and also provide an increased scope for furthering studies.

The central nervous system (CNS) refers to that part of the nervous system that consists of the brain and spinal cord. It is responsible for the integration of information and coordination of the activities of all the parts of the body. Retina, optic nerve, cranial nerves and olfactory epithelium are also considered as a part of the CNS. The brain is covered and protected by the skull and the vertebrae protect the spinal cord. Brain and spinal cord are enclosed in membranes known as meninges. There are many diseases and conditions associated with CNS. These include alzheimer's disease, parkinson's disease, autoimmune diseases, Krabbe's disease, multiple sclerosis, etc. The brain disorders can be diagnosed through neurological imaging. This book outlines the processes of the central nervous system in detail. It presents researches and studies performed by experts across the globe. The extensive content of this book provides the readers with a thorough understanding of the subject.

I hope that this book, with its visionary approach, will be a valuable addition and will promote interest among readers. Each of the authors has provided their extraordinary competence in their specific fields by providing different perspectives as they come from diverse nations and regions. I thank them for their contributions.

Editor

1

Chemokine and cytokine levels in the lumbar cerebrospinal fluid of preterm infants with post-hemorrhagic hydrocephalus

Gakwaya Habiyaremye[1†], Diego M. Morales[1*†], Clinton D. Morgan[2], James P. McAllister[1], Travis S. CreveCoeur[1], Rowland H. Han[1], Mohamed Gabir[1], Brandon Baksh[1], Deanna Mercer[1] and David D. Limbrick Jr.[3]

Abstract

Background: Neuroinflammation has been implicated in the pathophysiology of post-hemorrhagic hydrocephalus (PHH) of prematurity, but no comprehensive analysis of signaling molecules has been performed using human cerebrospinal fluid (CSF).

Methods: Lumbar CSF levels of key cytokines (IL-1α, IL-1β, IL-4, IL-6, IL-8, IL-10, IL-12, TNF-α, TGF-β1, IFN-γ) and chemokines (XCL-1, CCL-2, CCL-3, CCL-19, CXCL-10, CXCL-11, CXCL-12) were measured using conventional and multiplexed Enzyme-linked Immunosorbent Assays and compared between preterm infants with PHH and those with no known neurological injury. The relationships between individual biomarker levels and specific CSF cell counts were examined.

Results: Total protein (TP) CSF levels were elevated in the PHH subjects compared to controls. CSF levels of IL-1α, IL-4, IL-6, IL-12, TNF-α, CCL-3, CCL-19, and CXCL-10 were significantly increased in PHH whereas XCL-1 was significantly decreased in PHH. When normalizing by TP, IL-1α, IL-1β, IL-10, IL-12, CCL-3, and CCL-19 levels were significantly elevated compared to controls, while XCL-1 levels remained significantly decreased. Among those with significantly different levels in both absolute and normalized levels, only absolute CCL-19 levels showed a significant correlation with CSF nucleated cells, neutrophils, and lymphocytes. IL-1β and CXCL-10 also were correlated with total cell count, nucleated cells, red blood cells, and neutrophils.

Conclusions: Neuroinflammation is likely to be an important process in the pathophysiology of PHH. To our knowledge, this is the first study to investigate CSF levels of chemokines in PHH as well as the only one to show XCL-1 selectively decreased in a diseased state. Additionally, CCL-19 was the only analyte studied that showed significant differences between groups and had significant correlation with cell count analysis. The selectivity of CCL-19 and XCL-1 should be further investigated. Future studies will further delineate the role of these cytokines and chemokines in PHH.

Keywords: Cytokines, Chemokines, Post-hemorrhagic, Hydrocephalus, CSF, Cerebrospinal fluid, Preterm, Prematurity

Background

Post-hemorrhagic hydrocephalus (PHH) develops in up to 25% of preterm infants with intraventricular hemorrhage (IVH) and is a leading cause of infant hydrocephalus in North America [1, 2]. While the association between IVH and PHH is well established [3], the pathophysiological mechanisms linking these two conditions remain unclear. Data from experimental studies and limited clinical series have implicated neuroinflammation in the pathogenesis of PHH [4–7]. IVH-related blood or blood breakdown products may trigger inflammatory fibrosis or arachnoiditis with gliosis that may contribute to an imbalance in cerebrospinal fluid (CSF) production, absorption, or transit [4, 8].

*Correspondence: d.morales@wustl.edu

†Gakwaya Habiyaremye and Diego M. Morales contributed equally to this work

[1] Department of Neurological Surgery, Washington University in St. Louis School of Medicine, One Children's Way, 4S20, St. Louis, MO 63110, USA

A number of reports have detailed changes in the CSF levels of IL-1β, IL-6, IL-8, TNF-α, IFN-γ, TGF-β1, and TGF-β2 in the setting of experimental or human PHH [1, 9–13]. Indeed, there is experimental evidence that inhibition of TGF-β or lysophosphatidic acid may prevent the development of PHH [9, 14]. To date, human studies into the neuroinflammatory basis of PHH have largely targeted select proteins and, to our knowledge, have not considered the role of chemokines. Informed by our previous work in CSF proteomics [15], we decided to take a broad approach to survey neuro-inflammatory processes at play in the CSF of human infants with PHH. Commercially available multiplex assays offer the advantage of simultaneously measuring proteins from multiple pathways involved in inflammatory modulation while using very little CSF volume. In the current study, we used multiplex analyses investigate the CSF levels of key inflammatory cytokines (IL-1α, IL-1β, IL-4, IL-6, IL-8, IL-10, IL-12, TNF-α, TGF-β1, IFN-γ) and chemokines (XCL-1, CCL-2, CCL-3, CCL-19, CXCL-10, CXCL-11, CXCL-12) in the setting of human infant PHH.

These and related proteins have been evaluated in various clinical contexts previously and have been reviewed in detail by Turner et al. 2014 [16]. IL-1α, IL-1β, IL-6, IL-8, TNF-α, and IFN-γ, among other functions, provide pro-inflammatory signaling for bone marrow cell proliferation, IgG production, chemotaxis, phagocyte cell activation, and anti-viral, macrophage activation. IL-10 and IL-12 are anti-inflammatory signaling molecules and inhibit cytokine production and activate natural killer cells. TGF-β1 has been shown to inhibit T and B cell proliferation. Chemokines also function in inflammatory and immunological responses. XCL-1 provides chemotactic activity specific for lymphocytes while contributing to regulatory T cell development. CCL-2, CCL-3, and CCL-19 among other functions serve to recruit monocytes to inflammation sites and regulate proliferation of progenitor cells. CXCL-10, -11, and -12 are chemotactic for monocytes and T-lymphocytes and with the exception of CXCL-11, have been upregulated in post-traumatic brain injury studies [16–23].

As these studies suggest, neuroinflammation is likely to be an important process in the pathophysiology of PHH and its associated neurological injury. In the current study, we used multiplex analyses to broadly investigate proteins involved in inflammatory modulation and their relationship to CSF cell counts. Based on the results presented herein, future studies will delineate the role of specific cytokines and chemokines in the pathophysiology of PHH.

Methods

Research subjects

Washington University Human Research Protection Office (WU-HRPO) approval was obtained prior to beginning this study (WU-HRPO #201101887). Research subjects comprised two study groups: control and PHH. Control CSF samples were acquired from 31 infants born $\leq$ 35 weeks post-menstrual age (PMA) without known neurological injury via lumbar puncture (LP) performed as part of routine sepsis/meningitis evaluation. Final microbiological cultures were verified as sterile in all controls. PHH CSF samples were acquired from infants born $\leq$ 30 weeks PMA with PHH as described previously via clinically-indicated LP [24]. Prior to LP, all PHH subjects demonstrated progressive increase in occipital-frontal circumference, full fontanel, splaying of the sagittal suture $\geq$ 2 mm [25] and a frontal-occipital horn ratio (FOR) $\geq$ 0.55 [26]. Thirteen of the 14 PHH infants included in this report required ventriculo-peritoneal (VP) shunts between 34 and 59 weeks PMA (Table 1).

Cerebrospinal fluid processing

CSF samples were acquired via LP under sterile conditions for clinical purposes and transferred to the St. Louis Children's Hospital clinical laboratory. The clinical laboratory performed cell counts of the PHH CSF including total cell count, nucleated cells, and red blood cells (all measured as cells/μL). They also performed a differential analysis including neutrophils, lymphocytes, and monocytes (measured as percentages). The laboratory then stored the samples at – 80 °C. At the time of experimental analysis, samples were thawed and centrifuged at 2500 rpm for 6 min. The supernatant was aliquoted and used for biomarker assays.

Total protein measurements

The Pierce Bicinchoninic Acid protein assay kit (Thermo Scientific; Waltham, Massachusetts) was used to estimate total protein (TP) concentration in each CSF sample. Serum albumin standards as well as CSF samples were placed in microplate wells in duplicate. After addition of the working reagent, the plate was incubated at 37 °C for 30 min. The plate was then cooled to room temperature and absorbance at 562 nm was measured on a plate reader. Total protein concentrations were determined with a 4-parameter logistic standard curve.

Chemokine and cytokine analysis

Enzyme-linked Immunosorbent Assays (ELISAs) were used to measure concentrations of TGF-β1 and the chemokine CXCL-12 in both control and PHH CSF samples (R&D systems, catalog # DY240 and DY350 respectively, Minneapolis, MN). Sigma-Aldrich ELISA kits (Sigma, catalog #RAB0073 and RAB0515) were used for the measurement of CCL-3 and XCL-1 concentrations. All ELISA samples were run in duplicate and the

Table 1 Characteristics of study subjects with post-hemorrhagic hydrocephalus

Subject ID	Sex	PMA at birth (weeks)	TP (μg/ml)	PMA at CSF sample (weeks)	Temporizing neuro-surgical procedure	PMA at temporizing procedure (weeks)	VP shunt surgery PMA (weeks)
1	M	24.00	2369	26.86	RES	27.00	37.57
2	F	29.57	1745	30.29	RES	31.29	36.57
3	F	24.00	6072	26.86	RES	27.86	34.71
4	M	29.00	4564	31.14	RES	31.57	40.86
5	M	26.00	9596	27.43	RES	28.14	38.14
6	M	28.14	2606	28.71	RES	30.14	37.14
7	F	24.57	1270	28.00	RES	30.57	39.29
8	M	24.71	1869	30.57	RES	34.14	59.29
9	M	25.43	1420	27.57	NA[a]	NA	NA
10	M	25.43	2620	28.71	RES	31.00	53.57
11	M	25.86	1902	27.71	RES	28.14	NA[b]
12	M	25.29	3735	27.71	RES	28.00	40.00
13	F	29.57	2331	30.00	RES	31.29	36.57
14	F	24.00	4300	26.43	RES	27.00	37.57

PMA post-menstrual age, *TP* total protein, *CSF* cerebrospinal fluid, *VP* ventriculo-peritoneal, *RES* ventricular reservoir, *NA* not available

[a] Subject 9 expired after withdrawal of care by family

[b] Subject 11 developed a *S. capitis* RES infection 12 weeks after RES implantation and device tapping for cerebrospinal fluid removal (CSF). CSF samples prior to the 12-week sample were sterile on culture. After infection, the RES was removed and replaced with an external ventricular drain, which was later successfully weaned, and no shunt was implanted. Subject 10 underwent endoscopic third ventriculostomy with choroid plexus cauterization prior to VP shunt placement. Subject 1 had a shunt malfunction within 6 months of VP shunt implantation

absorbance at 450 nm was measured on a Versamax plate reader (Molecular Devices, Sunnyvale, CA). Chemokine and cytokine concentrations were determined using a 4 parameter logistic standard curve. Aushon (Billerica, MA) human cytokine array #2 and human chemokine array #2 multiplexes were used to measure concentrations of IL-1α, IL-1β, IL-4, IL-6, IL-8, IL-10, IL-12, TNF-α, IFN-γ, CCL-2, CCL-19, CXCL-10, and CXCL-11. Prefabricated assays for these analytes were run according to the manufacturer's instructions. Multiplex samples were also run in duplicate and analyzed on the Aushon Ciraplex® Assays system.

Due to differences in TP between samples, we normalized analyte measurements by dividing absolute levels by their corresponding TP. Where specified, statistical comparisons were conducted using these normalized measurements.

Statistical analysis

CSF analyte levels were reported as mean ± standard deviation (SD), and mean difference between groups with a 95% confidence interval. Comparisons between control and PHH groups were conducted using two-tailed independent samples *t* tests assuming unequal variances in Prism 5.0 (GraphPad Software, La Jolla, CA). Linear regressions between CSF cell count parameters and absolute levels of PHH CSF cytokines and chemokines were performed using Spearman correlation coefficients in SAS 9.3 (SAS Institute, Cary NC). A predetermined significance level of 0.05 was used for all statistical tests.

Results

Subject characteristics

Fourteen preterm infants with PHH (Table 1) were included in this study. Ventricular reservoirs (RES) were placed in all infants except one, where the family opted for withdrawal of care. Of the 13 remaining subjects, all except one required a VP shunt. The subject not requiring a VP shunt developed a *S. capitis* infection 12 weeks after RES implantation (after weeks of sterile cultures) and underwent device removal and replacement with an external ventricular drain, which was later weaned and removed. Subject 10 had endoscopic third ventriculostomy with choroid plexus cauterization prior to VP shunt placement. Subject 1 underwent VP shunt revision within 6 months of VP shunt implantation. The control group presented with a broad array of clinical reasons for LP, but the primary reason was for sepsis diagnosis. For both groups, the CSF sampled cultures were monitored for 3.68 ± 0.13 days and remained negative.

Seven out of the 31 control subjects were female, while 5 out of the 15 PHH subjects were female. The mean birth PMA for the PHH group was 25.75 ± 2.19 weeks and for the control group was 30.12 ± 3.23 weeks ($p < 0.0001$). The CSF sample PMA was also significantly different between the groups (31.86 ± 2.83 for control,

28.88 ± 2.97 for PHH; p = 0.003). Ventricular size measurements were only available for 7 out of the 31 control subjects due to a lack of cranial images. Of the 7, 3 of them had ventricular sizes too small to be accurately measured and the other 4 had an FOR of 0.40 ± 0.05. PHH subjects demonstrated much higher FOR measurements (0.62 ± 0.07) for imaging performed within 24 h of CSF sample collection (p < 0.0001).

Cerebrospinal fluid total protein, cytokines and chemokines

CSF TP, cytokine, and chemokine concentrations were measured and compared between control and PHH subjects (Fig. 1a; Tables 2, 3). TP was significantly elevated in PHH versus control (3285 ± 2266 μg/ml vs 1540 ± 985.6 μg/ml, respectively, p = 0.0008). CSF levels of IL-1α, IL-4, IL-6, IL-12, TNF-α, CCL-3, CCL-19, and CXCL-10 were significantly elevated in PHH versus control while IL-1β, IL-8, IL-10, TGFβ1, IFN-γ, CCL-2, CXCL-11, and CXCL-12 were not (Tables 2 and 3). After normalizing by total protein, IL-1α, IL-1β, IL-10, IL-12, CCL-3, and CCL-19 were significantly elevated compared with control, while IL-4, IL-6, IL-8, TNF-α, TGFβ1, IFN-γ, CCL-2, CXCL-10, CXCL-11, and CXCL-12 were not significantly different (Tables 2 and 3). XCL-1 was the only analyte that was significantly decreased in PHH, even when normalized by TP (Table 3). The most robust candidate neuroinflammatory CSF biomarkers—those that retained statistical significance irrespective of normalization by TP levels—included IL-1α (increased), IL-12 (increased), CCL-3 (increased), CCL-19 (increased), and XCL-1 (decreased) (Fig. 1b–d).

Cerebrospinal fluid cytokines and chemokines correlation with cell counts

Total cell count measurements for PHH CSF were 72964.86 ± 114192 cells/μL, nucleated cells were 4057.2 ± 13319 cells/μL, and red blood cells were 68907.64 ± 103612 cells/μL. Neutrophils, lymphocytes, and monocytes within the 14 PHH CSF samples were 48.15 ± 33.60, 19.54 ± 21.96, and 21.79 ± 17.32%, respectively. The individual data points for these cell counts were analyzed for a correlation with absolute cytokine and chemokine levels within PHH CSF (Tables 4 and 5). IL-1α correlated with neutrophils with a Spearman r value of 0.73 and a p value of 0.0246. IL-1β correlated with total cell count (r: 0.64; p = 0.0479), red blood cells (r: 0.64; p = 0.0479), neutrophils (r: 0.88; p = 0.0016),

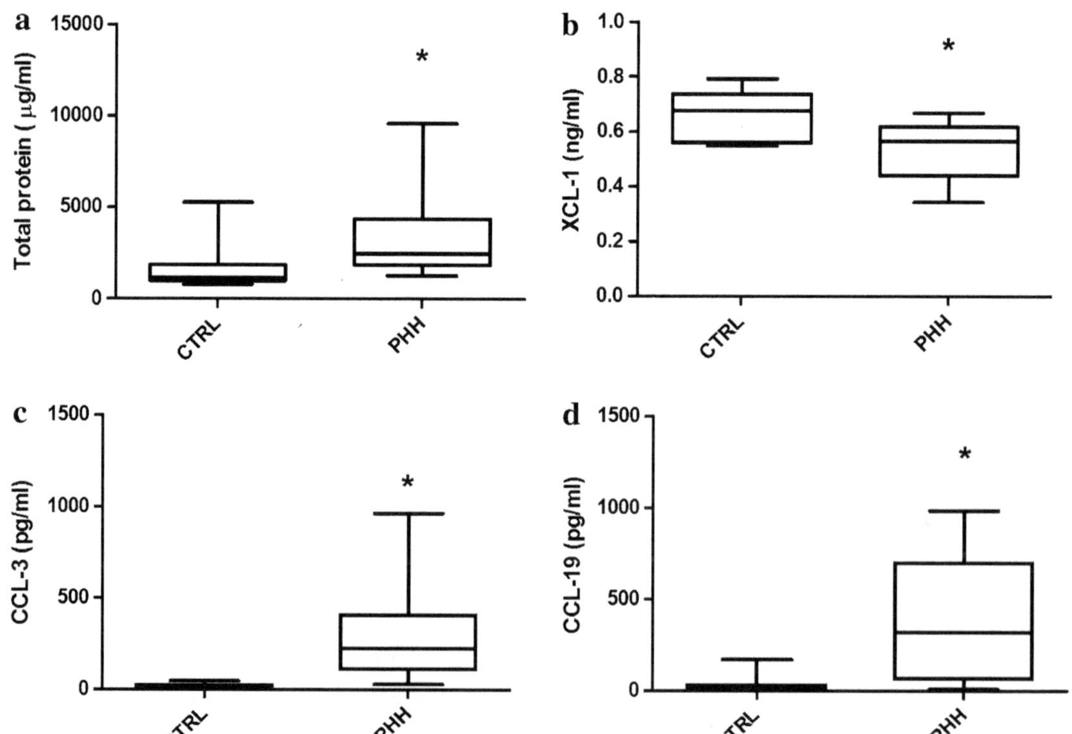

Fig. 1 Lumbar cerebrospinal fluid levels of total protein (**a**), XCL-1 (**b**), CCL-3 (**c**), and CCL-19 (**d**) in human preterm infants without (control) or with post-hemorrhagic hydrocephalus. Boxes represent the median with 25th and 75th percentiles and the whiskers show interquartile range multiplied by 1. Levels of Total protein, CCL-3 and CCL-19 were significantly increased in PHH. The levels of XCL-1 were decreased in PHH subjects. *Denotes significance at p ≤ 0.05. *CTRL* control, *PHH* post-hemorrhagic hydrocephalus

Table 2 Comparison of cerebrospinal fluid absolute and normalized concentrations of common cytokines in control and post-hemorrhagic hydrocephalus subjects

	Control mean (SD)	PHH mean (SD)	Mean difference	95% confidence interval	p value
Total protein (μg/ml)	1540 (985.6)	3285 (2265.9)	1745.0	2714–775.3	0.0008
IL-1α (pg/ml)	2.385 (3.758)	13.51 (11.03)	11.13	17.67–4.577	0.0019
Normalized IL-1α	1.58E−7 (2.72E−7)	4.89E−7 (4.56E−7)	3.31E−7	6.40E−7 to 2.31E−8	0.0363
IL-1β (pg/ml)	4.600 (15.05)	79.89 (146.3)	75.29	156.2 to − 5.664	n.s.
Normalized IL-1β	1.27E−7 (2.93E−7)	1.90E−6 (2.2E−6)	1.78E−6	3.02E−6 to 5.31E−7	0.0072
IL-4 (pg/ml)	0.266 (0.4465)	1.010 (0.5653)	0.7444	− 1.173 to − 0.3164	0.0016
Normalized IL-4	1.64E−9 (2.53E−9)	4.20E-9 (3.55E−9)	2.56E−9	5.13E−9 to − 1.11E−11	n.s.
IL-6 (pg/ml)	268.2 (667.8)	981.3 (932.6)	713.1	1389–37.32	0.0395
Normalized IL-6	1.8E−5 (5.6E−5)	4.27E−5 (5.82E−5)	2.49E−5	7.38E−5 to − 2.40E−5	n.s.
IL-8 (pg/ml)	522.5 (528)	1958 (3158)	1436	3205 to − 333.3	n.s.
Normalized IL-8	4.4E−5 (5.3E−5)	1.04E−4 (1.95E−4)	6.0E−5	1.9E−4 to − 6.7E−5	n.s.
IL-10 (pg/ml)	5.154 (14.59)	128 (274.8)	122.8	274.1 to − 28.38	n.s.
Normalized IL-10	1.81E−7 (3.13E−7)	2.53E−6 (3.75E−6)	2.35E−6	4.42E−6 to 2.84E−7	0.0277
IL-12 (pg/ml)	1.763 (2.446)	11.58 (9.234)	9.819	15.14 to 4.497	0.0009
Normalized IL-12	1.3E−7 (2.2E−7)	3.75E−7 (3.12E−7)	2.45E−7	4.70E−7 to 2.043E−8	0.0339
TNF-α (pg/ml)	2.147 (3.337)	9.71 (7.384)	7.566	12.18–2.951	0.0026
Normalized TNF-α	1.61E−7 (3.0E−7)	3.42E−7 (2.97E−7)	1.81E−7	4.38E−7 to − 7.55E−8	n.s.
TGF-β1 (ng/ml)	0.4504 (0.8607)	1.161 (2.270)	0.7103	2.278 to − 0.857	n.s.
Normalized TGF-β1	1.9E−5 (2.0E−5)	2.4E−5 (2.1E−5)	4.55E−6	2.02E−5 to − 1.5E−5	n.s.
IFN-γ (pg/ml)	0.6463 (1.552)	1.191 (1.357)	0.5446	1.812 to − 0.7226	n.s.
Normalized IFN-γ	2.93E−8 (5.65E−8)	3.42E−8 (2.35E−8)	4.91E−9	4.44E−8 to − 3.45E−8	n.s.

SD standard deviation, *PHH*: post-hemorrhagic hydrocephalus

Table 3 Comparison of cerebrospinal fluid absolute and normalized concentrations of common chemokines in control and post-hemorrhagic hydrocephalus subjects

	Control mean (SD)	PHH mean (SD)	Mean difference	95% confidence interval	p value
XCL-1 (ng/ml)	0.6680 (0.0833)	0.5528 (0.1121)	− 0.1152	− 0.0224 to − 0.2079	0.0176
Normalized XCL-1	5.4E−5 (1.6E−5)	2.19E−5 (1.1E−5)	− 3.3E−5	− 1.76E−5 to − 4.8E−5	0.0002
CCL-2 (pg/ml)	9436 (5117)	9535 (5089)	99.45	− 4622 to 4821	n.s.
Normalized CCL-2	7.79E−4 (5.76E−4)	4.16E−4 (4.08E−4)	− 3.62E−4	− 8.47E−4 to 1.21E−4	n.s.
CCL-3 (pg/ml)	16.50 (11.02)	360.0 (327.7)	343.5	537.9–149.1	0.0018
Normalized CCL-3	0.015 (0.0092)	1.2E−5 (9.9E−6)	− 0.0146	− 0.00658 to − 0.0227	0.0014
CCL-19 (pg/ml)	28.46 (45.15)	410.8 (377.9)	382.4	591.8–173.0	0.0011
Normalized CCL-19	1.73E−6 (2.14E−6)	1.41E−5(2.1E−5)	1.23E−5	2.36E−5 to 9.96E−7	0.0345
CXCL-10 (pg/ml)	809.6 (776.6)	1480 (742.6)	670	1325–15.09	0.0454
Normalized CXCL-10	5.9E−5 (5.8E−5)	5.72E−5 (4.42E−5)	− 2.14E−6	4.32E-5 to − 4.75E-5	n.s.
CXCL-11 (pg/ml)	5.162 (10.68)	5.15 (4.58)	− 8.7E−3	7.869 to − 7.886	n.s.
Normalized CXCL-11	4.08E−7 (1.01E−6)	1.38E−7 (8.01E−8)	− 2.71E−7	4.39E−7 to − 9.80E−7	n.s.
CXCL-12 (ng/ml)	0.5187 (0.5528)	0.9930 (1.0002)	0.4743	1.052 to − 0.1033	n.s.
Normalized CXCL-12	4.5E−5 (5.3E−5)	1.4E−5 (9.6E−6)	− 3.01E−5	2.01E-5 to − 7.5E−5	n.s.

SD standard deviation, *PHH* post-hemorrhagic hydrocephalus

and lymphocytes (r: − 0.75; p = 0.0199). IL-6 and IL-10 were significantly correlated with neutrophils (r: 0.67; p = 0.0499 and r: 0.78; p = 0.0075 respectively). TGF-β1 was significantly correlated with nucleated cells (r: 0.83; p = 0.0102). CCL-19 showed significant and strong correlation with nucleated cells (r: 0.71; p = 0.0465),

Table 4 Post-hemorrhagic hydrocephalus cerebrospinal fluid absolute cytokine Spearman correlations with cell counts

	IL-1α r p value	IL-1β r p value	IL-4 r p value	IL-6 r p value	IL-8 r p value	IL-10 r p value	IL-12 r p value	TNF-α r p value	TGF-β1 r p value	IFN-γ r p value
Total cell count	0.52727 n.s.	0.63636 0.0479	0.29697 n.s.	0.26061 n.s.	0.16387 n.s.	0.49091 n.s.	0.26061 n.s.	0.06667 n.s.	0.69048 n.s.	0.23636 n.s.
Nucleated cells	0.49091 n.s.	0.57576 n.s.	0.15152 n.s.	0.20000 n.s.	0.16387 n.s.	0.50303 n.s.	0.24848 n.s.	0.06667 n.s.	0.83333 0.0102	0.21212 n.s.
Red blood cells	0.52727 n.s.	0.63636 0.0479	0.29697 n.s.	0.26061 n.s.	0.16387 n.s.	0.49091 n.s.	0.26061 n.s.	0.06667 n.s.	0.69048 n.s.	0.23636 n.s.
Neutrophils	0.73333 0.0246	0.88333 0.0016	0.61667 n.s.	0.66667 0.0499	0.12780 n.s.	0.78333 0.0125	0.31667 n.s.	0.05000 n.s.	0.45238 n.s.	0.41667 n.s.
Lymphocytes	− 0.61667 n.s.	− 0.75000 0.0199	− 0.28333 n.s.	− 0.16667 n.s.	− 0.20083 n.s.	− 0.56667 n.s.	− 0.30000 n.s.	− 0.13333 n.s.	− 0.38095 n.s.	− 0.26667 n.s.
Monocytes	− 0.40122 n.s.	− 0.46201 n.s.	− 0.14590 n.s.	− 0.16413 n.s.	0.03424 n.s.	− 0.46201 n.s.	− 0.14590 n.s.	0.09726 n.s.	− 0.35714 n.s.	− 0.19453 n.s.

r Spearman correlation coefficient

Table 5 Post-hemorrhagic hydrocephalus cerebrospinal fluid absolute chemokine Spearman correlations with cell counts

	XCL-1 r p value	CCL-2 r p value	CCL-3 r p value	CCL-19 r p value	CXCL-10 r p value	CXCL-11 r p value	CXCL-12 r p value
Total cell count	− 0.37143 n.s.	0.09524 n.s.	0.48571 n.s.	0.64286 n.s.	0.63222 0.0498	0.48333 n.s.	0.37126 n.s.
Nucleated cells	− 0.20000 n.s.	0.30952 n.s.	0.08571 n.s.	0.71429 0.0465	0.58967 n.s.	0.63333 n.s.	0.46707 n.s.
Red blood cells	− 0.37143 n.s.	0.09524 n.s.	0.48571 n.s.	0.64286 n.s.	0.63222 0.0498	0.48333 n.s.	0.37126 n.s.
Neutrophils	− 0.25714 n.s.	0.21429 n.s.	0.70000 n.s.	0.78571 0.0208	0.87867 0.0018	0.66667 0.0499	0.70660 n.s.
Lymphocytes	0.31429 n.s.	− 0.09524 n.s.	− 0.54286 n.s.	− 0.73810 0.0366	− 0.78333 0.0125	− 0.58333 n.s.	− 0.73055 0.0396
Monocytes	− 0.25714 n.s.	− 0.30952 n.s.	− 0.55078 n.s.	− 0.54762 n.s.	− 0.46951 n.s.	− 0.53333 n.s.	− 0.80241 0.0165

r Spearman correlation coefficient

neutrophils (r: 0.78; $p = 0.0208$), and lymphocytes (r: − 0.74; $p = 0.0366$). CXCL-10 was significantly correlated with total cell counts (r: 0.63; $p = 0.0498$), red blood cells (r: 0.63; $p = 0.0498$), neutrophils (r: 0.88; $p = 0.0018$), and lymphocytes (r: 0.78; $p = 0.0125$). CXCL-11 showed correlation with neutrophils (r: 0.67; $p = 0.0499$), while CXCL-12 showed correlation with lymphocytes (r: − 0.73; $p = 0.0396$) and monocytes (r: − 0.80; $p = 0.0165$). XCL-1 and CCL-3 levels did not correlate significantly with any cell counts.

Discussion

This study aimed to advance the current understanding of neuroinflammation in PHH by measuring key inflammatory cytokines and chemokines in the CSF. Among 17 CSF biomarkers, 8 were significantly increased (IL-1α, IL-4, IL-6, IL-12, TNF-α, CCL-3, CCL-19, and CXCL-10) and one was significantly decreased (XCL-1) in PHH. Of note, CSF in the clinical setting of PHH contains high levels of protein related to the IVH itself (e.g. albumin); in order to account for any potential effect of CSF protein on CSF biomarker levels, we also report the level of each cytokine and chemokine after normalization by total CSF protein (TP). When normalized by TP, IL-1α, IL-1β, IL-10, IL-12, CCL-3, CCL-19 were elevated, while XCL-1 remained decreased. The most robust candidate CSF biomarkers were significantly altered in PHH irrespective of normalization by TP, which included IL-1α, IL-12, CCL-3, and CCL-19 as increased, and XCL1 as decreased. Of those 5, only absolute levels of CCL-19 correlated with CSF nucleated cells, neutrophils, and lymphocytes, strongly implicating this chemokine in the neuroinflammatory processes of PHH pathophysiology. Neuroinflammatory profile specificity may have important implications in the pathophysiology of PHH and could shape future pharmacological studies in treating PHH.

Neuroinflammation accompanying IVH and PHH is complex and hypothesized to be initiated by blood and its breakdown products in the ventricular system prompting ventriculitis, gliosis and arachnoiditis. Past studies demonstrate that infants with PHH and periventricular white matter injury have increased CSF concentrations of IL-1β, IL-6, IL-8, and TGF-β1 [10, 12, 13, 27, 28]. Although increased levels of TGF-β1 have been implicated in white matter injury in the setting of IVH and PHH, Heep et al. [11] contrarily found no significant difference. A recent review by Szpecht et al. [29] on the role of cytokines in the pathogenesis of IVH suggested an association between IL-1β, IL-6, IL-8, and TNF-α with increased risk of PHH [12, 13, 30].

The current report demonstrates that CSF levels of the cytokines TNF-α, IL-1α, IL-4, IL-6, and IL-12 are significantly increased in PHH. TNF-α and IL-1α findings are consistent with previous studies of their association with acute phase reactions and pro-inflammatory responses to pathogen or tissue injury [31, 32]. Astrocytes, microglia, and neurons typically produce basal levels of TNF-α and maintain homeostasis in normal central nervous system (CNS) physiology; however, just microglia and astrocytes are assumed to be responsible for elevated levels during neuroinflammation [33–37]. IL-1α is constitutively secreted by many cell types, but its expression surges in response to pathogens or brain tissue injury [38]. IL-1α behaves as an upstream signal for multiple proinflammatory cytokines, chemokines, and prostaglandins [31]. Di Paolo et al. demonstrated that IL-1α was the only cytokine to show absolute differences between the two groups with a significant Spearman correlation in the cell count analysis. IL-1α and TNF-α may be associated with acute phase reactions as well as pro-inflammatory states that occur in PHH pathophysiology. Increased levels of TNF-α and IL-6 are also consistent with Savman et al. [12]. Mainly secreted by T-cells, macrophages, and endothelial cells, IL-6 also increases in PHH, which is consistent with previous studies which showed its involvement in neuronal and glial function as well as neuroinflammation pathways in the CNS [39, 40].

IL-4 is a regulatory cytokine that assumes a myriad of immune and non-immune functions. In extravascular tissues, it is involved in alternative activation of macrophages into M2 cells (repair macrophages) and inhibits activation of M1 cells (inflammatory macrophages) resulting in decreased pathological inflammation [41]. It is plausible that increased CSF levels of IL-4 in PHH could be associated with decreased M1 macrophage activity to contain secondary injury from inflammatory cells. Zundler and Neurath [42] describe the main sources of IL-12 as macrophages, monocytes, dendritic cells, granulocytes and B cells; it induces production of IFN-γ to foster both innate and adaptive cell-mediated immune responses. Increased levels of IL-12 in PHH could be caused by microglial activation during neuroinflammation to enhance the innate immune response for phagocytosis of extravascular blood, blood-breakdown products, and cell debris resulting from IVH.

Normalization to TP significantly altered the results such that we found selective and significant increases in CSF IL-1α, IL-1β, IL-10, and IL-12 levels in PHH. Furthermore, absolute IL-1β levels significantly correlated with total cell count, red blood cells, neutrophils, and lymphocytes. IL-1β is a potent pro-inflammatory cytokine that initiates and amplifies innate immunity and host responses to microbial and tissue injury [43]. A previous study by Savman et al. [12] showed that IL-1β is significantly elevated in the CSF of premature infants with PHH. Innate responses from phagocytic immune cells, such as macrophages and neutrophils, may be associated with increased IL-1β levels in PHH. We also found a significant correlation between IL-6 and IL-10 levels with neutrophil counts. IL-10 functions in the activation, inhibition, growth, and migration of hematopoietic cells. In the context of tissue injury, whether by infectious or sterile inflammation, IL-10 downregulates and terminates inflammation [44]. Increased IL-10 levels may be associated with down-regulation of neuroinflammation in the setting of IVH or PHH. Contrary to past studies, we did not observe increased TGF-β1 levels in the CSF of PHH subjects [10, 11, 28]. This may have been due to differences between studies such as location of CSF (LP versus ventricular), methods and timing of CSF sample acquisition, or methods of detection. However, there was a significant correlation between absolute TGF-β1 levels and nucleated cells.

To our knowledge, this is the first study investigating CSF chemokine levels in PHH. CSF levels of seven chemokines (XCL-1, CCL-2, CCL-3, CCL-19, CXCL-10, CXCL-11, and CXCL-12) were measured and compared between PHH and control groups. Absolute levels of CCL-3, CCL-19, and CXCL-10 were significantly elevated in the CSF of PHH subjects; CCL-3 and CCL-19 levels remained elevated after normalization with TP. CCL-3, also known as Macrophage Inflammatory Protein 1-α, is primarily secreted by astrocytes, microglia, endothelial cells, and neurons [45–49] and has been found to be upregulated in the CSF of patients after traumatic brain injury [50–53]. CCL-3 is believed to be a potent chemo-attractant of polymorphonuclear leukocytes (PMNLs; neutrophils) in humans and mice [54] and induces peroxide production in PMNLs [55, 56]. In

IVH and PHH, reactive oxygen species produced by activated PMNLs may cause local tissue injury, ventriculitis, ependymal layer scarring, and denudation. Chui et al. [48] reported that CCL-3 is a critical early inflammatory chemokine that is greatly upregulated in active Schwann cells and infiltrating macrophages in areas of brain tissue injury. In our CSF samples, CCL-3 is several-fold higher in PHH than controls, thus suggesting that it may have an important role in neuroinflammation.

CCL-19 and CXCL-10 correlated with cell counts, either total, nucleated cells, red blood cells, neutrophils, and lymphocytes. CCL-19, is also known as Macrophage Inflammatory Protein-3β, is involved in immune surveillance of the CNS by lymphocytes. Its ectopic expression may also trigger activation and/or recruitment of infiltrating leukocytes in response to specific offending stimuli [57]. Since CCL-19 is primarily expressed in cerebrovascular endothelium and choroid plexus [57–61], it is readily available to potentially promote neuroinflammation in IVH and PHH. Absolute concentration of CXCL-10 was significantly increased in PHH but there was no difference after normalization by CSF TP. We also found correlations between CXCL10 and total cell count, red blood cells, neutrophils, and lymphocytes, suggesting a possible role in PHH neuroinflammation. CXCL-10 has been reported to be upregulated in post-traumatic brain injury in some studies, but others found absent mRNA expression of CXCL-10 after head injury [21, 50, 62, 63]. Interestingly, both absolute and normalized levels of XCL-1 were decreased in PHH, but absolute levels did not correlate significantly with any cell counts. XCL-1, also known as Lymphotactin, is a chemokine of the –C– class that is expressed by T Cells (Natural Killer Cells, Natural Killer T Cells) in response to pathogenic or injurious stimuli [64]. It is expressed in various infectious and autoimmune diseases, suggesting its predominant role in protective and pathological immune responses [65].

There are a number of limitations in this study. Small sample sizes and inherent clinical heterogeneity were present within both our control and PHH groups. Indeed, non-neurological challenges or conditions could affect CSF levels of neuro-inflammatory markers in both groups. Further, there were also differences between groups in terms of birth and sample PMA (4 and 3 weeks, respectively), raising the possibility of age-dependent variability in CSF flow rate and maturity of arachnoid villi, though in theory, the effect of arachnoid villi maturity would be expected to be minor, since their development is limited until term equivalent age [66–68]. In the PHH group, heterogeneity was inevitably compounded by the complex and dynamic neuro-inflammatory response to IVH and the timing of acquisition of CSF samples, particularly since small molecules, such as those measured in this study, may be metabolized or undergo reuptake into cells in the interstitial fluids and along the CSF pathways. Any combination of these factors could impact cytokine and chemokine levels to such a degree that changes in levels can occur simultaneous with, prior to, or after CSF sampling. Finally, the data for CSF cell types and cell counts reported here were all taken from clinical laboratory reports. Thus, we were reliant on existing institutional clinical laboratory methods and were unable to measure or subtype many cell types (e.g. Th2 cells, CD8 cells) that could provide insight into the immune response itself (protein elaboration, cellular recruitment). These analyses and additional validation studies must be conducted through multi-institutional collaboration and experimental models.

Conclusion

In summary, the neuroinflammatory processes associated with PHH pathophysiology are complex and remain incompletely understood. In our current study, we measured the levels of CSF cytokines and chemokines in PHH relative to control. CSF levels of IL-1α, IL-4, IL-6, IL-12, TNF-α, CCL-3, CCL-19, CXCL-10, and TP were significantly increased in PHH, whereas XCL-1 was significantly decreased. However, only the cytokines IL-1α and IL-12, and the chemokines CCL-3, CCL-19, and XCL-1 retained their statistical significance for PHH when normalized to CSF TP levels. Furthermore, CCL-19 was the only analyte studied that also had a significant correlation with CSF cell counts. To our knowledge, this is the first study to investigate CSF levels of chemokines in PHH as well as the only one to show that XCL-1 selectively decreased in a diseased state, whether absolute or normalized levels are considered. The selectivity of CCL-19 and XCL-1 should be further investigated. These findings provide novel insights into the neuro-inflammatory processes at play in IVH and PHH, and may help inform future studies of pharmacological treatments for PHH.

Abbreviations

CCL: CC chemokine ligands; CNS: central nervous system; CSF: cerebrospinal fluid; CXCL: CXC chemokine ligands; ELISA: enzyme-linked immunosorbent assay; FOR: frontal-occipital horn ratio; IFN: interferon gamma; IL: interleukins; IVH: intraventricular hemorrhage; LP: lumbar puncture; PHH: post-hemorrhagic hydrocephalus; PMA: post-menstrual age; PMNL: polymorphonuclear leukocytes; RES: ventricular reservoir; SD: standard deviation; TGF: transforming growth factor; TNF: tumor necrosis factor; TP: total protein; VP: ventriculo-peritoneal; HRPO: Human Research Protection Office; XCL: XC chemokine ligand.

Authors' contributions

GH made substantial contributions to conception and design, analysis and interpretation of data, drafting the manuscript. DMM made substantial contribution to acquisition of data, analysis and interpretation of data, and revising the manuscript. CDM made substantial contribution to analysis and interpretation of data, and revising the manuscript. JPM made substantial contribution to analysis and interpretation of data, and revising the manuscript. TSC made substantial contribution to cell count analysis and re-interpretation of data, and revising the manuscript. RHH made substantial contribution to statistical analysis and revising the manuscript. MG made substantial contribution to interpretation of data, and revising the manuscript. BB made substantial contribution to data acquisition and maintenance. DM made substantial contribution to data acquisition and maintenance. DDL made substantial contributions to general supervision of the research group, acquisition of funding, conception and design, acquisition of data, analysis and interpretation of data, drafting and revising the manuscript. All authors read and approved the final manuscript.

Author details
[1] Department of Neurological Surgery, Washington University in St. Louis School of Medicine, One Children's Way, 4S20, St. Louis, MO 63110, USA. [2] Barrow Neurological Institute, 350 West Thomas Road, Phoenix, AZ 85013, USA. [3] Department of Neurological Surgery and Pediatrics, Washington University in St. Louis School of Medicine, One Children's Way, 4S20, St. Louis, MO 63110, USA.

Acknowledgements
We would like to thank Dr. David Gibson and his staff at the Immunoassay Core at Washington University in St. Louis for their technical assistance in running the multiplex analysis. We would also like to thank Dr. Yan Yan at Washington University in St. Louis, for his statistical assistance throughout the manuscript.

Competing interests
Drs. DDL and JPM have received research, educational, and philanthropic support for unrelated research through Medtronic, Inc. and Karl Storz, Inc.

Funding
This project was supported by NIH/NINDS K23 NS075151, ICTS UL1 TR000448, CTSA UL1 RR024992, TL1 TR000449, and a grant from the Children's Surgical Sciences Institute, St. Louis Children's Hospital (D.L.). JPM received support from a Hydrocephalus Association Innovator Award, a Seed Grant from the Washington University Hope Center for Neurological Disorders, the Rudi Schulte Research Institute, and STARS-kids.

References

1. Merhar S. Biomarkers in neonatal posthemorrhagic hydrocephalus. Neonatology. 2012;101:1–7.
2. Murphy BP, Inder TE, Rooks V, Taylor GA, Anderson NJ, Mogridge N, Horwood LJ, Volpe JJ. Posthaemorrhagic ventricular dilatation in the premature infant: natural history and predictors of outcome. Arch Dis Child Fetal Neonatal Ed. 2002;87:F37–41.
3. Tsitouras V, Sgouros S. Infantile posthemorrhagic hydrocephalus. Child's Nerv Syst. 2011;27:1595–608.
4. Cherian S, Whitelaw A, Thoresen M, Love S. The pathogenesis of neonatal post-hemorrhagic hydrocephalus. Brain Pathol. 2004;14:305–11.
5. Lekic T, Manaenko A, Rolland W, Krafft PR, Peters R, Hartman RE, Altay O, Tang J, Zhang JH. Rodent neonatal germinal matrix hemorrhage mimics the human brain injury, neurological consequences, and post-hemorrhagic hydrocephalus. Exp Neurol. 2012;236:69–78.
6. Strahle J, Garton HJ, Maher CO, Muraszko KM, Keep RF, Xi G. Mechanisms of hydrocephalus after neonatal and adult intraventricular hemorrhage. Transl Stroke Res. 2012;3:25–38.
7. Takizawa T, Tada T, Kitazawa K, Tanaka Y, Hongo K, Kameko M, Uemura KI. Inflammatory cytokine cascade released by leukocytes in cerebrospinal fluid after subarachnoid hemorrhage. Neurol Res. 2001;23:724–30.
8. Robinson S. Neonatal posthemorrhagic hydrocephalus from prematurity: pathophysiology and current treatment concepts. J Neurosurg Pediatr. 2012;9:242–58.
9. Botfield H, Gonzalez AM, Abdullah O, Skjolding AD, Berry M, McAllister JP 2nd, Logan A. Decorin prevents the development of juvenile communicating hydrocephalus. Brain. 2013;136:2842–58.
10. Chow LC, Soliman A, Zandian M, Danielpour M, Krueger RC Jr. Accumulation of transforming growth factor-beta2 and nitrated chondroitin sulfate proteoglycans in cerebrospinal fluid correlates with poor neurologic outcome in preterm hydrocephalus. Biol Neonate. 2005;88:1–11.
11. Heep A, Stoffel-Wagner B, Bartmann P, Benseler S, Schaller C, Groneck P, Obladen M, Felderhoff-Mueser U. Vascular endothelial growth factor and transforming growth factor-beta1 are highly expressed in the cerebrospinal fluid of premature infants with posthemorrhagic hydrocephalus. Pediatr Res. 2004;56:768–74.
12. Savman K, Blennow M, Hagberg H, Tarkowski E, Thoresen M, Whitelaw A. Cytokine response in cerebrospinal fluid from preterm infants with posthaemorrhagic ventricular dilatation. Acta Paediatr. 2002;91:1357–63.
13. Schmitz T, Heep A, Groenendaal F, Huseman D, Kie S, Bartmann P, Obladen M, Felderhoff-Muser U. Interleukin-1beta, interleukin-18, and interferon-gamma expression in the cerebrospinal fluid of premature infants with posthemorrhagic hydrocephalus—markers of white matter damage? Pediatr Res. 2007;61:722–6.
14. Yung YC, Mutoh T, Lin ME, Noguchi K, Rivera RR, Choi JW, Kingsbury MA, Chun J. Lysophosphatidic acid signaling may initiate fetal hydrocephalus. Sci Transl Med. 2011;3:99ra87.
15. Morales DM, Townsend RR, Malone JP, Ewersmann CA, Macy EM, Inder TE, Limbrick DD Jr. Alterations in protein regulators of neurodevelopment in the cerebrospinal fluid of infants with posthemorrhagic hydrocephalus of prematurity. Mol Cell Proteom. 2012;11(M111):011973.
16. Turner MD, Nedjai B, Hurst T, Pennington DJ. Cytokines and chemokines: at the crossroads of cell signalling and inflammatory disease. Biochim Biophys Acta. 2014;1843:2563–82.
17. Trifilo MJ, Lane TE. Adenovirus-mediated expression of CXCL10 in the central nervous system results in T-cell recruitment and limited neuropathology. J Neurovirol. 2003;9:315–24.
18. Trifilo MJ, Lane TE. The CC chemokine ligand 3 regulates CD11c+ CD11b+ CD8alpha− dendritic cell maturation and activation following viral infection of the central nervous system: implications for a role in T cell activation. Virology. 2004;327:8–15.
19. Klein RS. Regulation of neuroinflammation: the role of CXCL10 in lymphocyte infiltration during autoimmune encephalomyelitis. J Cell Biochem. 2004;92:213–22.
20. Karman J, Chu HH, Co DO, Seroogy CM, Sandor M, Fabry Z. Dendritic cells amplify T cell-mediated immune responses in the central nervous system. J Immunol. 2006;177:7750–60.
21. Israelsson C, Bengtsson H, Kylberg A, Kullander K, Lewen A, Hillered L, Ebendal T. Distinct cellular patterns of upregulated chemokine expression supporting a prominent inflammatory role in traumatic brain injury. J Neurotrauma. 2008;25:959–74.
22. Itoh T, Satou T, Ishida H, Nishida S, Tsubaki M, Hashimoto S, Ito H. The relationship between SDF-1alpha/CXCR4 and neural stem cells appearing in damaged area after traumatic brain injury in rats. Neurol Res. 2009;31:90–102.
23. Schutt RC, Burdick MD, Strieter RM, Mehrad B, Keeley EC. Plasma CXCL12 levels as a predictor of future stroke. Stroke. 2012;43:3382–6.
24. Morales DM, Silver SA, Morgan CD, Mercer D, Inder TE, Holtzman DM, Wallendorf MJ, Rao R, McAllister JP, Limbrick DD Jr. Lumbar cerebrospinal fluid biomarkers of posthemorrhagic hydrocephalus of prematurity: amyloid precursor protein, soluble amyloid precursor protein alpha, and L1 cell adhesion molecule. Neurosurgery. 2016;80(1):82–90.
25. Wellons JC 3rd, Holubkov R, Browd SR, Riva-Cambrin J, Whitehead W, Kestle J, Kulkarni AV. Hydrocephalus Clinical Research N: the assessment of bulging fontanel and splitting of sutures in premature infants: an interrater reliability study by the Hydrocephalus Clinical Research Network. J Neurosurg Pediatr. 2013;11:12–4.
26. O'Hayon BB, Drake JM, Ossip MG, Tuli S, Clarke M. Frontal and occipital horn ratio: a linear estimate of ventricular size for multiple imaging modalities in pediatric hydrocephalus. Pediatr Neurosurg. 1998;29:245–9.
27. Baumeister FA, Pohl-Koppe A, Hofer M, Kim JO, Weiss M. IL-6 in CSF during ventriculitis in preterm infants with posthemorrhagic hydrocephalus. Infection. 2000;28:234–6.
28. Whitelaw A, Christie S, Pople I. Transforming growth factor-beta1: a possible signal molecule for posthemorrhagic hydrocephalus? Pediatr Res. 1999;46:576–80.

29. Szpecht D, Wiak K, Braszak A, Szymankiewicz M, Gadzinowski J. Role of selected cytokines in the etiopathogenesis of intraventricular hemorrhage in preterm newborns. Childs Nerv Syst. 2016;32:2097–103.
30. Viscardi RM, Muhumuza CK, Rodriguez A, Fairchild KD, Sun CC, Gross GW, Campbell AB, Wilson PD, Hester L, Hasday JD. Inflammatory markers in intrauterine and fetal blood and cerebrospinal fluid compartments are associated with adverse pulmonary and neurologic outcomes in preterm infants. Pediatr Res. 2004;55:1009–17.
31. Di Paolo NC, Shayakhmetov DM. Interleukin 1alpha and the inflammatory process. Nat Immunol. 2016;17:906–13.
32. Rochfort KD, Collins LE, McLoughlin A, Cummins PM. Tumour necrosis factor-alpha-mediated disruption of cerebrovascular endothelial barrier integrity in vitro involves the production of proinflammatory interleukin-6. J Neurochem. 2016;136:564–72.
33. Chung IY, Benveniste EN. Tumor necrosis factor-alpha production by astrocytes. Induction by lipopolysaccharide, IFN-gamma, and IL-1 beta. J Immunol. 1990;144:2999–3007.
34. Breder CD, Tsujimoto M, Terano Y, Scott DW, Saper CB. Distribution and characterization of tumor necrosis factor-alpha-like immunoreactivity in the murine central nervous system. J Comp Neurol. 1993;337:543–67.
35. Welser-Alves JV, Milner R. Microglia are the major source of TNF-alpha and TGF-beta1 in postnatal glial cultures; regulation by cytokines, lipopolysaccharide, and vitronectin. Neurochem Int. 2013;63:47–53.
36. Gahring LC, Carlson NG, Kulmar RA, Rogers SW. Neuronal expression of tumor necrosis factor alpha in the murine brain. Neuroimmunomodulation. 1996;3:289–303.
37. Montgomery SL, Bowers WJ. Tumor necrosis factor-alpha and the roles it plays in homeostatic and degenerative processes within the central nervous system. J Neuroimmune Pharmacol. 2012;7:42–59.
38. Basu A, Krady JK, Levison SW. Interleukin-1: a master regulator of neuroinflammation. J Neurosci Res. 2004;78:151–6.
39. Rochfort KD, Cummins PM. The blood-brain barrier endothelium: a target for pro-inflammatory cytokines. Biochem Soc Trans. 2015;43:702–6.
40. Rothaug M, Becker-Pauly C, Rose-John S. The role of interleukin-6 signaling in nervous tissue. Biochem Biophys Acta. 2016;1863:1218–27.
41. Seder RA, Paul WE, Davis MM. Fazekas de St Groth B: the presence of interleukin 4 during in vitro priming determines the lymphokine-producing potential of CD4+ T cells from T cell receptor transgenic mice. J Exp Med. 1992;176:1091–8.
42. Zundler S, Neurath MF. Interleukin-12: functional activities and implications for disease. Cytokine Growth Factor Rev. 2015;26:559–68.
43. Eder C. Mechanisms of interleukin-1beta release. Immunobiology. 2009;214:543–53.
44. Moore KW, de Waal Malefyt R, Coffman RL, O'Garra A. Interleukin-10 and the interleukin-10 receptor. Annu Rev Immunol. 2001;19:683–765.
45. Ambrosini E, Remoli ME, Giacomini E, Rosicarelli B, Serafini B, Lande R, Aloisi F, Coccia EM. Astrocytes produce dendritic cell-attracting chemokines in vitro and in multiple sclerosis lesions. J Neuropathol Exp Neurol. 2005;64:706–15.
46. Hayashi M, Luo Y, Laning J, Strieter RM, Dorf ME. Production and function of monocyte chemoattractant protein-1 and other beta-chemokines in murine glial cells. J Neuroimmunol. 1995;60:143–50.
47. Okamura T, Katayama T, Obinata C, Iso Y, Chiba Y, Kobayashi H, Yamada Y, Harashima H, Minami M. Neuronal injury induces microglial production of macrophage inflammatory protein-1alpha in rat corticostriatal slice cultures. J Neurosci Res. 2012;90:2127–33.
48. Chui R, Dorovini-Zis K. Regulation of CCL2 and CCL3 expression in human brain endothelial cells by cytokines and lipopolysaccharide. J Neuroinflammation. 2010;7:1.
49. Xia MQ, Qin SX, Wu LJ, Mackay CR, Hyman BT. Immunohistochemical study of the beta-chemokine receptors CCR3 and CCR5 and their ligands in normal and Alzheimer's disease brains. Am J Pathol. 1998;153:31–7.
50. Stefini R, Catenacci E, Piva S, Sozzani S, Valerio A, Bergomi R, Cenzato M, Mortini P, Latronico N. Chemokine detection in the cerebral tissue of patients with posttraumatic brain contusions. J Neurosurg. 2008;108:958–62.
51. Helmy A, De Simoni MG, Guilfoyle MR, Carpenter KL, Hutchinson PJ. Cytokines and innate inflammation in the pathogenesis of human traumatic brain injury. Prog Neurobiol. 2011;95:352–72.
52. Helmy A, Carpenter KL, Menon DK, Pickard JD, Hutchinson PJ. The cytokine response to human traumatic brain injury: temporal profiles and evidence for cerebral parenchymal production. J Cereb Blood Flow Metab. 2011;31:658–70.
53. Holmin S, Hojeberg B. In situ detection of intracerebral cytokine expression after human brain contusion. Neurosci Lett. 2004;369:108–14.
54. Jaerve A, Muller HW. Chemokines in CNS injury and repair. Cell Tissue Res. 2012;349:229–48.
55. Sherry B, Tekamp-Olson P, Gallegos C, Bauer D, Davatelis G, Wolpe SD, Masiarz F, Coit D, Cerami A. Resolution of the two components of macrophage inflammatory protein 1, and cloning and characterization of one of those components, macrophage inflammatory protein 1 beta. J Exp Med. 1988;168:2251–9.
56. Wolpe SD, Davatelis G, Sherry B, Beutler B, Hesse DG, Nguyen HT, Moldawer LL, Nathan CF, Lowry SF, Cerami A. Macrophages secrete a novel heparin-binding protein with inflammatory and neutrophil chemokinetic properties. J Exp Med. 1988;167:570–81.
57. Lalor SJ, Segal BM. Lymphoid chemokines in the CNS. J Neuroimmunol. 2010;224:56–61.
58. Alt C, Laschinger M, Engelhardt B. Functional expression of the lymphoid chemokines CCL19 (ELC) and CCL 21 (SLC) at the blood-brain barrier suggests their involvement in G-protein-dependent lymphocyte recruitment into the central nervous system during experimental autoimmune encephalomyelitis. Eur J Immunol. 2002;32:2133–44.
59. Kivisakk P, Mahad DJ, Callahan MK, Sikora K, Trebst C, Tucky B, Wujek J, Ravid R, Staugaitis SM, Lassmann H, Ransohoff RM. Expression of CCR7 in multiple sclerosis: implications for CNS immunity. Ann Neurol. 2004;55:627–38.
60. Williams JL, Holman DW, Klein RS. Chemokines in the balance: maintenance of homeostasis and protection at CNS barriers. Front Cell Neurosci. 2014;8:154.
61. Krumbholz M, Theil D, Steinmeyer F, Cepok S, Hemmer B, Hofbauer M, Farina C, Derfuss T, Junker A, Arzberger T, Sinicina I, Hartle C, Newcombe J, Hohlfeld R, Meinl E. CCL19 is constitutively expressed in the CNS, up-regulated in neuroinflammation, active and also inactive multiple sclerosis lesions. J Neuroimmunol. 2007;190:72–9.
62. Israelsson C, Bengtsson H, Lobell A, Nilsson LN, Kylberg A, Isaksson M, Wootz H, Lannfelt L, Kullander K, Hillered L, Ebendal T. Appearance of Cxcl10-expressing cell clusters is common for traumatic brain injury and neurodegenerative disorders. Eur J Neurosci. 2010;31:852–63.
63. Helmy A, Antoniades CA, Guilfoyle MR, Carpenter KL, Hutchinson PJ. Principal component analysis of the cytokine and chemokine response to human traumatic brain injury. PLoS ONE. 2012;7:e39677.
64. Dorner BG, Dorner MB, Zhou X, Opitz C, Mora A, Guttler S, Hutloff A, Mages HW, Ranke K, Schaefer M, Jack RS, Henn V, Kroczek RA. Selective expression of the chemokine receptor XCR1 on cross-presenting dendritic cells determines cooperation with CD8+ T cells. Immunity. 2009;31:823–33.
65. Lei Y, Takahama Y. XCL1 and XCR1 in the immune system. Microbes Infect. 2012;14:262–7.
66. Gomez DG, DiBenedetto AT, Pavese AM, Firpo A, Hershan DB, Potts DG. Development of arachnoid villi and granulations in man. Acta Anat (Basel). 1982;111:247–58.
67. Chazal J, Tanguy A, Irthum B, Janny P, Vanneuville G. Dilatation of the subarachnoid pericerebral space and absorption of cerebrospinal fluid in the infant. Anat Clin. 1985;7:61–6.
68. Sakka L, Coll G, Chazal J. Anatomy and physiology of cerebrospinal fluid. Eur Ann Otorhinolaryngol Head Neck Dis. 2011;128:309–16.

2

Accelerated differentiation of human induced pluripotent stem cells to blood–brain barrier endothelial cells

Emma K. Hollmann[1], Amanda K. Bailey[1], Archit V. Potharazu[1], M. Diana Neely[3], Aaron B. Bowman[2,3,4] and Ethan S. Lippmann[1*]

Abstract

Background: Due to their ability to limitlessly proliferate and specialize into almost any cell type, human induced pluripotent stem cells (iPSCs) offer an unprecedented opportunity to generate human brain microvascular endothelial cells (BMECs), which compose the blood–brain barrier (BBB), for research purposes. Unfortunately, the time, expense, and expertise required to differentiate iPSCs to purified BMECs precludes their widespread use. Here, we report the use of a defined medium that accelerates the differentiation of iPSCs to BMECs while achieving comparable performance to BMECs produced by established methods.

Methods: Induced pluripotent stem cells were seeded at defined densities and differentiated to BMECs using defined medium termed E6. Resultant purified BMEC phenotypes were assessed through trans-endothelial electrical resistance (TEER), fluorescein permeability, and P-glycoprotein and MRP family efflux transporter activity. Expression of endothelial markers and their signature tight junction proteins were confirmed using immunocytochemistry. The influence of co-culture with astrocytes and pericytes on purified BMECs was assessed via TEER measurements. The robustness of the differentiation method was confirmed across independent iPSC lines.

Results: The use of E6 medium, coupled with updated culture methods, reduced the differentiation time of iPSCs to BMECs from thirteen to 8 days. E6-derived BMECs expressed GLUT-1, claudin-5, occludin, PECAM-1, and VE-cadherin and consistently achieved TEER values exceeding 2500 $\Omega \times cm^2$ across multiple iPSC lines, with a maximum TEER value of $4678 \pm 49\ \Omega \times cm^2$ and fluorescein permeability below 1.95×10^{-7} cm/s. E6-derived BMECs maintained TEER above 1000 $\Omega \times cm^2$ for a minimum of 8 days and showed no statistical difference in efflux transporter activity compared to BMECs differentiated by conventional means. The method was also found to support long-term stability of BMECs harboring biallelic *PARK2* mutations associated with Parkinson's Disease. Finally, BMECs differentiated using E6 medium responded to inductive cues from astrocytes and pericytes and achieved a maximum TEER value of $6635 \pm 315\ \Omega \times cm^2$, which to our knowledge is the highest reported in vitro TEER value to date.

Conclusions: Given the accelerated differentiation, equivalent performance, and reduced cost to produce BMECs, our updated methods should make iPSC-derived in vitro BBB models more accessible for a wide variety of applications.

Keywords: Induced pluripotent stem cells (iPSCs), In vitro blood–brain barrier (BBB) model, Brain microvascular endothelial cells (BMECs), Defined differentiation medium

*Correspondence: ethan.s.lippmann@vanderbilt.edu
[1] Department of Chemical and Biomolecular Engineering, Vanderbilt University, 2201 West End Ave, Nashville, TN 37235, USA

Background

The blood–brain barrier (BBB) is composed of brain microvascular endothelial cells (BMECs), which strictly regulate molecular transport between the bloodstream and the brain to ensure proper function of neuronal circuits, synaptic transmission, and other essential processes that depend upon a tightly controlled neurovascular environment [1]. BMECs are characterized by specialized tight junctions [2, 3] that limit paracellular flux of biologics, hydrophilic small molecules, and ions, which results in a characteristically high trans-endothelial electrical resistance (TEER) across the barrier not observed in other capillary beds in the body [4, 5]. For import and export of molecules, BMECs express multiple transporters, such as GLUT-1 [6], and active efflux transporters [6], including P-glycoprotein and multidrug resistance related protein (MRP) family transporters [7], that confer protection. BBB disruption is implicated in many chronic neurodegenerative diseases, such as multiple sclerosis [8], traumatic brain injury [9], ischemic stroke [10–13], and in natural aging of the neurovascular unit [14]. Moreover, the BBB often hinders delivery of therapeutics to diseased tissue when the barrier remains intact [15]. The time, expense, difficulty, and limited throughput of all in vivo research often precludes widespread use of such techniques, necessitating in vitro platforms to investigate certain biological phenomena. Therefore, in vitro BBB models are often employed to study BBB mechanisms, neurovascular cell–cell interactions, and to perform screens for BBB-permeant therapeutics.

In vitro BBB models have most often been constructed using primary BMECs isolated from rat, bovine, and porcine sources [16–21]. Such models extended to BMECs in co-culture with astrocytes, pericytes, and neurons, cell types known to enhance the BBB phenotype and thereby more accurately recapitulate the in vivo neurovascular environment [17, 18]. These models can be used to study BBB development, regulation, and disease, as well as assay potential drug candidates for permeability [19, 20]. However, due to species' differences in transporter sequences/structures, activities, and expression levels [21], a robust fully-human BBB model is preferred to investigate BBB function and disease in a human context and to perform drug screens that yield the most promising pharmacological compounds for clinical applications.

Human in vitro BBB models have most often utilized either BMECs isolated from primary tissue [22] or immortalized BMEC cell lines [23]. Primary BMECs demonstrate moderate barrier properties, but difficult isolation procedures and low yields hinder their widespread use. Immortalized BMECs provide a readily scalable source of cells for in vitro models, but these cells do not recapitulate the impermeable character of the BBB. Due to their ability to limitlessly proliferate and specialize into any cell type, human induced pluripotent stem cells (iPSCs) offer an unprecedented opportunity to provide human BMECs for research purposes. iPSCs were recently shown to be capable of differentiating to endothelial cells with BBB properties [24]. Though the first-generation differentiation procedure yielded BMECs with passive barrier properties that remained below measurements in animals [4], the addition of retinoic acid (RA) during the differentiation process substantially improved the BBB phenotype, and RA-treated BMECs exhibited TEER reaching near in vivo levels after co-culture with other cell types of the neurovascular unit [25]. Unfortunately, full differentiation from the iPSC state to purified BMECs is a protracted multi-week process and uses complex, expensive maintenance and differentiation medium. The time and cost associated with iPSC culture and this differentiation method are detrimental to widespread use of these BMECs, and an expedited and less costly differentiation process yielding cells of equal performance with significantly less associated expense would alleviate some of these hurdles.

Induced pluripotent stem cell maintenance and differentiation procedures are rapidly evolving towards fully defined compositions [26–29]. In this study, we sought to adopt these procedures in an effort to streamline the BBB differentiation process. We transitioned to recently-described E8 medium for iPSC maintenance [27], as utilized by others for BBB differentiation [30], with no discernible issues. A derivative of E8 medium composition, collectively termed E6 medium (Dulbecco's modified Eagle's medium [DMEM]/F-12, ascorbic acid, sodium bicarbonate, selenium, human transferrin, and human insulin) has recently been used for efficient conversion of iPSCs to neuroectoderm [28], and we decided to explore its use in place of unconditioned medium (UM) in the BBB differentiation process. Intriguingly, we discovered that E6 medium, compared to UM, shortens the differentiation timeline without compromising BMEC performance as measured by TEER, sodium fluorescein permeability, and efflux transporter activity [24, 25]. The E6 differentiation procedure was reproducible across several iPSC lines, and upon co-culture with iPSC-derived astrocytes and primary human brain pericytes, BMECs achieved maximum TEER of $6635 \pm 315\ \Omega \times cm^2$, which to our knowledge is the highest value ever recorded in any BBB model, and stability of the barrier above 1000 $\Omega \times cm^2$ was observed for 22 days. Overall, we have shortened the differentiation procedure to 8 days with no discernible loss of BBB character. Given that defined medias can be prepared in-house at greatly reduced costs, we suggest that the methods described herein will better enable widespread use of iPSC-derived BMECs.

Methods

Media preparation

E4 medium

E4 basal medium was prepared in 48 L batches and used to prepare E8 and E6 medium as described below. 48 L of DMEM/F12 with HEPES (Thermo Fisher Scientific, catalog number 11,330,057) was added to a large carboy along with 3.072 g L-Ascorbic acid 2-phosphate sesquimagnesium salt hydrate (Sigma-Aldrich), 931 μL of sodium selenite solution (0.7 mg/mL in PBS; Sigma-Aldrich), and 26.064 g sodium bicarbonate (Sigma-Aldrich). The solution was mixed for 20 min followed by alternating pH and osmolarity tests and adjustments. Osmolarity of the solution was adjusted to 340 ± 5 mOsm/kg using sodium chloride (Fisher Scientific) and tested using a Precision Systems Micro-OSMETTE Model 5004 osmometer. pH of the solution was adjusted to 7.4 ± 0.05 using 5 M sodium hydroxide and measured using a Thermo Scientific Orion Star A211 benchtop pH meter. The solution was mixed for 10 min between each pH and osmolarity adjustment. Final E4 medium was frozen in 500 mL aliquots. Final concentrations in E4 basal medium were 64 mg/L L-Ascorbic acid 2-phosphate sesquimagnesium salt hydrate, 14 μg/L of sodium selenite, and 1743 mg/L sodium bicarbonate (20.75 mM) [27]. Detailed protocols for media preparation are available upon request.

E8 medium

E8 medium was prepared by adding 100 μL of human insulin solution (Sigma-Aldrich), 500 μL of 10 mg/mL of human holo-transferrin (R&D Systems), 500 μL of 100 μg/mL human basic fibroblast growth factor (bFGF; Peprotech), and 500 μL of 2 μg/mL TGFβ1 (Peprotech) to 500 mL of E4. The final concentrations are 2.14 mg/L insulin, 100 μg/L bFGF, 2 μg/L TGFβ1, and 10.7 mg/L holo-transferrin [27]. Media was sterile filtered and stored at 4 °C for a maximum of 2 weeks.

E6 medium

E6 medium was prepared by adding 100 μL of human insulin solution and 500 μL of 10 mg/mL of human holo-transferrin to 500 mL of E4. The final concentrations are 2.14 mg/L insulin and 10.7 mg/L holo-transferrin [28]. The medium was sterile filtered and stored at 4 °C for a maximum of 2 months.

Unconditioned medium (UM)

Unconditioned medium (UM) was prepared as previously described [24]. UM consisted of DMEM/F12 (Thermo Fisher Scientific), 20% Knockout Serum Replacer (Thermo Fisher Scientific), 1× MEM non-essential amino acids (Thermo Fisher Scientific), 1 mM Glutamax (Thermo Fisher Scientific), and 0.1 mM β-mercaptoethanol (Sigma-Aldrich). UM was sterile filtered and stored at 4 °C for a maximum of 2 weeks.

Endothelial cell (EC) medium

Endothelial cell (EC) medium consisted of human Endothelial Serum-Free Medium (Thermo Fisher Scientific) supplemented with 1% platelet-poor plasma-derived bovine serum (Fisher Scientific) [31]. EC medium was supplemented with 20 ng/mL bFGF and 10 μM all-trans retinoic acid (Sigma-Aldrich) during the EC phase prior to subculture and during the first 24 h of subculture, then removed to promote induction of the barrier phenotype [25]. EC medium was sterile filtered and stored at 4 °C for a maximum of 2 weeks.

Maintenance of iPSCs

Cell lines used were IMR90-4 iPSCs [32], CD12 iPSCs [33], CC3 iPSCs [34], and SM14 iPSCs [35, 36]. IMR90-4 and CC3 lines are female. CD12 and SM14 lines are male. All cell lines were thawed directly into E8 medium containing 10 μM Y-27632 (Tocris). 24 h after thaw, cells were changed to E8 medium without Y-27632. E8 medium was changed every day thereafter. All iPSCs were maintained on Matrigel (Corning). Once 70% confluent, iPSCs were passaged by washing cells once with Versene solution (Thermo Fisher Scientific), incubating cells with Versene solution for 5 min at 37 °C, collecting the cells in fresh E8 medium, and distributing the cells at desired ratios to Matrigel-coated plates.

iPSC differentiation to BMECS

Induced pluripotent stem cell were washed once with DPBS (Thermo Fisher Scientific) and incubated with Accutase (Stem Cell Technologies) for 3 min to yield a single cell suspension. Cells were collected via centrifugation, resuspended in E8, and counted using either a hemocytometer or Countess II (Thermo Fisher Scientific). Trypan blue was not used to measure cell viability when using a hemocytometer but was used when measuring cell density using the Countess II. Cells were seeded at densities ranging from 10,000 to 15,600 cells per square centimeter in E8 containing 10 μM Y-27632 (Day −1). Approximately 24 h after seeding, media was changed to UM or E6 medium (Day 0) to induce differentiation. Media was changed every 24 h. Cells were differentiated in UM for 6 days or in E6 medium for 4 days. Next, cells were treated with EC medium containing 20 ng/mL bFGF and 10 μM retinoic acid for 48 h. Following treatment, EC medium was removed, and cells were washed once with DPBS and incubated with Accutase for 20–25 min [37]. Cells were collected via centrifugation and subsequently purified by selective adhesion onto a collagen-fibronectin matrix. In brief, tissue culture polystyrene plates and Transwell filters (polyethylene terephthalate, 0.4 μm pore size, 1.1 cm^2 surface area in 12-well format) were coated with a solution of 400 μg/mL collagen IV (Sigma-Aldrich) and 100 μg/mL fibronectin (Sigma-Aldrich) for a minimum of 1 h for plates and a minimum of 4 h up to overnight for Transwell filters. Cells were subcultured onto plates and filters at a ratio of 1 well of a 6-well plate of differentiated cells to 3 wells of a 12-well plate, 6 wells of a 24-well plate, or 3 Transwell filters. To assess barrier properties, TEER was measured 24 h after subculture using an EVOM2 voltohmmeter with STX3 chopstick electrodes (World Precision Instruments). Following TEER measurement, cells were changed to EC medium containing no bFGF and no RA to induce barrier phenotype. No further media changes occurred after this point. TEER was measured approximately every 24 h thereafter. Experiments were terminated when average TEER fell below 1000 $\Omega \times cm^2$. All reported TEER values are corrected for the resistance due to an empty Transwell filter.

Immunocytochemistry

Cells were washed twice with DPBS and fixed for either 20 min in 4% paraformaldehyde (Sigma-Aldrich) or 10 min in 100% ice-cold methanol. Cells were washed 3 times with DPBS and blocked for a minimum of 1 h in PBS or TBS containing 5% donkey serum and 0.3% Triton X-100 (PBS-DT and TBS-DT, respectively). Cells were incubated with primary antibody diluted in PBS or TBS containing 5% donkey serum (PBSD and TBSD, respectively) or in PBS-DT or TBS-DT overnight at 4 °C. Following primary antibody incubation (see Additional file 1: Table S1), cells were rinsed once with PBS or TBS and washed five times with PBS or TBS for a minimum of 5 min per wash. Cells were incubated in secondary antibody (see Additional file 1: Table S2) diluted in the same buffer as primary antibody for a minimum of 1 h. Following secondary antibody incubation, cells were incubated with 4′,6-Diamidino-2-pheny-lindoldihydrochloride (DAPI; Thermo Fisher Scientific) for 10 min to label nuclei. Cells were rinsed once and washed five times with PBS/TBS and then visualized using a Zeiss AxioObserver Z1 microscope or a Leica DMi8 microscope. An average of three images were taken for each stain and the entire field was visually assessed to ensure that the presented images are representative of the entire dish.

Efflux transporter activity assays

Substrate accumulation

Induced pluripotent stem cell-derived BMECs were purified into 24-well plates and subjected to EC medium lacking bFGF and RA for 24 h prior to efflux assays. For inhibition experiments, BMECs were incubated with 10 μM PSC833 (Sigma-Aldrich) or 10 μM MK-571 (Sigma-Aldrich) for 1 h at 37 °C. Following this incubation, BMECs were incubated with 10 μM rhodamine 123 (Sigma-Aldrich; 488 nm excitation and 540 nm emission) or 10 μM 2′,7′-dichlorodihydrofluorescein diacetate (H_2DCFDA, ThermoFisher, 492 nm excitation and 527 nm emission), with or without their respective inhibitors, for 1 h at 37 °C. Cells were washed three times with DPBS and subsequently lysed using DPBS with 5% Triton X-100 to measure dye accumulation in the cells. Fluorescence was measured on a BioTek Synergy H1 multi-mode microplate reader. For each condition, one well of cells was not lysed. These conserved wells were fixed for 10 min in 100% ice-cold methanol and incubated with DAPI for 10 min. Cells were washed three times with DPBS and imaged. 6 images per condition were taken, and nuclei count per culture area was found using CellProfiler analysis software [38]. Fluorescence is reported on a per-cell basis, normalized to control fluorescence from cells treated with fluorescent substrate but no inhibitor.

Apical-to-basolateral flux

Induced pluripotent stem cell-derived BMECs were purified onto Transwell filters and subjected to EC medium lacking bFGF and RA for 24 h prior to assays. For inhibition experiments, BMECs were incubated with 10 μM PSC833 or 10 μM MK-571 for 1 h at 37 °C. Inhibitor was only included in the apical chamber. Following this incubation, 10 μM rhodamine 123 or 10 μM H_2DCFDA was added to the apical chamber, with or without respective inhibitors, for 1 h at 37 °C. 200 μL of media was then removed from the basolateral chamber and fluorescence was measured on a BioTek Synergy H1 multi-mode microplate reader.

Sodium fluorescein permeability

Induced pluripotent stem cell-derived BMECs were purified onto Transwell filters and subjected to EC medium lacking bFGF and RA for 24 h prior to permeability measurements. Medium was aspirated from the apical and basolateral chambers of each filter and replaced with fresh medium of the same composition to allow for monolayer equilibration. After 1 h, medium from the apical chamber was aspirated and replaced with 0.5 mL of sodium fluorescein (10 μM, Sigma-Aldrich) diluted in fresh medium. Every 30 min, 200 μL of medium was removed from the basolateral chamber and replaced with 200 μL of fresh medium. The same experiment was conducted on an empty filter. After 2 h, fluorescence was measured on a BioTek Synergy H1 multi-mode microplate reader. The rate of accumulation, corrected for media removal and flux across the empty filter, was used to calculate P_e values.

Primary human pericyte culture

Primary human brain vascular pericytes were purchased from ScienCell Research Laboratories. Pericytes were cultured on plates coated with 0.1% gelatin (Sigma-Aldrich) and maintained in DMEM (Corning) supplemented with 10% fetal bovine serum (Thermo Fisher Scientific). Medium was changed every 3 days, and cells were passaged for maintenance when approximately 80% confluent. Pericytes (passage 15) were subcultured onto Matrigel-coated 12-well plates for co-culture experiments when approximately 40% confluent at a ratio of 1 well of a 6-well plate to 3 wells of a 12-well plate. Once co-cultured with iPSC-derived glia, pericytes were maintained in E6 medium with 10 ng/mL CNTF and 10 ng/mL EGF. Pericyte co-culture with BMECs (with or without astrocytes and glial progenitors) was initiated 24 h after BMEC seeding onto Transwell filters. At this time, pericytes were changed to EC medium lacking bFGF and RA. Medium was not changed for the duration of the experiment.

iPSC differentiation to astrocytes

IMR90-4 iPSCs were washed with 2 mL DPBS and incubated with Accutase for 3 min at 37 °C. Cells were collected via centrifugation, resuspended in E8 medium, and counted using a hemocytometer. Cells were seeded at 2×10^5 cells/cm^2 onto Matrigel-coated plates in E8 medium containing 10 μM Y-27632. 24 h after seeding, media was changed to E6 medium containing 10 μM SB431542 (Tocris) and 1 μM dorsomorphin dihydrochloride (Tocris). The medium was changed every 24 h for 6 days. On day 6 of differentiation, strips of cells were mechanically picked from the culture using a P200 pipette and transferred to a Matrigel-coated plate with E6 medium containing 10 ng/mL ciliary neurotrophic factor (CNTF; Peprotech), 10 ng/mL epidermal growth factor (EGF; Peprotech), and 10 μM Y-27632. 72 h after picking, media was changed to E6 medium containing 10 ng/mL CNTF and 10 ng/mL EGF but no Y-27632. The medium was changed every 3 days for 30 days. On day 30, cells were incubated with Accutase for 3 min, collected via centrifugation, and seeded at a ratio of 1 well of a 6-well plate to 1 full 6-well plate. Cells were maintained in E6 medium containing 10 ng/mL CNTF and 10 ng/mL EGF with media changes every 48 h. Cells were passaged when approximately 80% confluent. Cells were cultured through a second passage and frozen in liquid nitrogen in E6 medium containing 10% DMSO (Sigma-Aldrich). Frozen iPSC-derived astrocytes were thawed and cultured for two passages before being seeded for co-culture. Astrocytes were seeded for co-culture at a ratio of 1 well of a 6-well plate to 6 wells of a 12-well plate. Cells were maintained in E6 medium containing 10 ng/mL CNTF and 10 ng/mL EGF when in co-culture with pericytes but were switched to EC medium lacking bFGF and RA upon co-culture with BMECs.

Initiation of co-culture

To initiate co-culture with astrocytes and pericytes, BMECs were subcultured onto Transwell filters as described above. 24 h after subculture, TEER was measured. Transwell filters were then transferred to wells containing astrocytes, pericytes, or astrocytes and pericytes, and medium was changed to EC medium lacking bFGF and RA. BMECs in monoculture served as a control for the experiment. TEER was measured approximately every 24 h. Medium was not changed throughout the duration of the experiment.

Statistical analysis

Data were expressed as mean ± standard deviation. Two-way ANOVA analysis and Student's unpaired t test were used to determine statistical significance for efflux transporter activity assays and TEER values.

Results

Defined medium shortens required differentiation time to BMECs

Previous protocols to differentiate iPSCs to BMECs relied on seeding iPSCs at defined densities, expanding the cells in mTeSR media for 3 days [26], and differentiating the cells for 6 days in UM to immature BMECs [24, 25, 37, 39]. BMECs were expanded in EC medium supplemented with basic fibroblast growth factor (bFGF) and RA and purified onto collagen/fibronectin matrices. Barrier phenotype was then induced by changing to EC medium lacking both bFGF and RA. Peak barrier phenotypes were observed 24 h after this medium change, and it was at this time point that most assays to measure barrier fidelity were conducted. In total, these methods required a minimum of 13 days from time of iPSC seeding to achieving functional, purified BMECs. We sought to improve these established methods in several ways. First, in place of mTeSR, we utilized E8 medium for maintenance [27], as described by others [30]. Next, we removed the 3 day expansion phase prior to differentiation and instead seeded IMR90-4 iPSCs overnight as single cells at densities ranging from 10,000 to 15,600 cells per square centimeter in E8 medium supplemented with Y-27632 before initiating differentiation the following day, a technique that has been utilized in other differentiation protocols [28]. Finally, we explored the use of E6 medium in place of UM during the differentiation process (Fig. 1).

With E6 medium, we were surprised to observe large patches of PECAM-1$^+$ endothelial cells after only 4 days

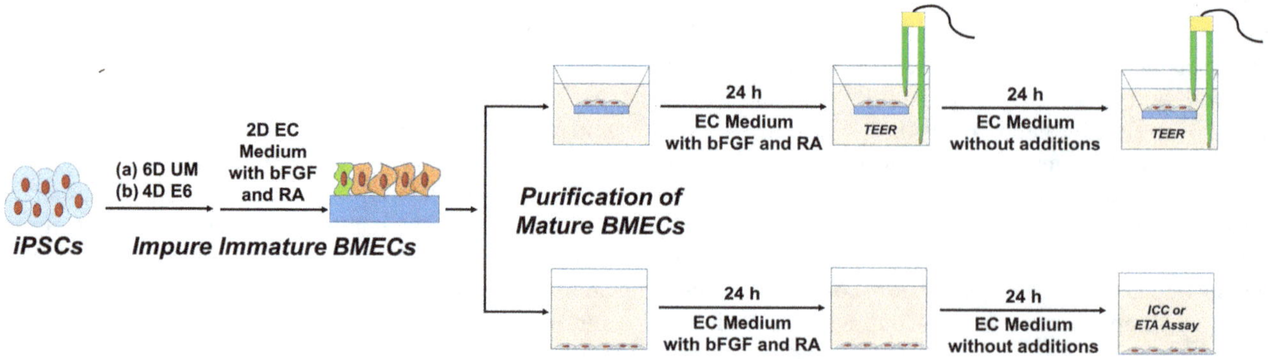

Fig. 1 Differentiation of iPSCs to BMECs. iPSCs were seeded at defined densities and differentiated for either 6 days in unconditioned medium (UM) or for 4 days in defined E6 medium. Impure immature BMECs were subsequently treated for 2 days with endothelial cell (EC) medium supplemented with bFGF and retinoic acid (RA). Mature BMECs were purified onto Transwell filters or plates for 24 h in EC medium supplemented with bFGF and RA. 24 h after purification, barrier was induced by treating cells with EC medium lacking bFGF and RA

of differentiation, which contrasts the time point when endothelium is first observed during UM differentiation (Fig. 2a) [24]. After 48 h in EC medium containing bFGF and RA, expression of PECAM-1, GLUT-1, VE-cadherin, and occludin were observed, indicating acquisition of a BBB phenotype (Fig. 2b). Cells were then purified onto Transwell filters or polystyrene culture plates using updated passaging techniques described by Wilson et al. [37]. Barrier phenotype was evaluated every 24 h by TEER, while immunocytochemistry was used to evaluate expression of endothelial and BBB markers 48 h after barrier induction. Immunocytochemical analysis of E6-derived BMECs showed robust expression of GLUT-1, claudin-5, occludin, VE-cadherin, and PECAM-1 (Fig. 2c), similar to UM-derived BMECs [24, 25]. E6-derived BMECs exhibited a maximum barrier of $4678 \pm 49\ \Omega \times cm^2$, and a minimum barrier stability of $1000\ \Omega \times cm^2$ was observed over 12 days for three independent biological replicates (Fig. 3a). For comparison, UM-derived BMECs exhibited maximum TEER of $3980 \pm 151\ \Omega \times cm^2$ 24 h after barrier induction, a value comparable to previously published results [25], and maintained stability for a similar timeframe as E6-derived BMECs (Fig. 3b).

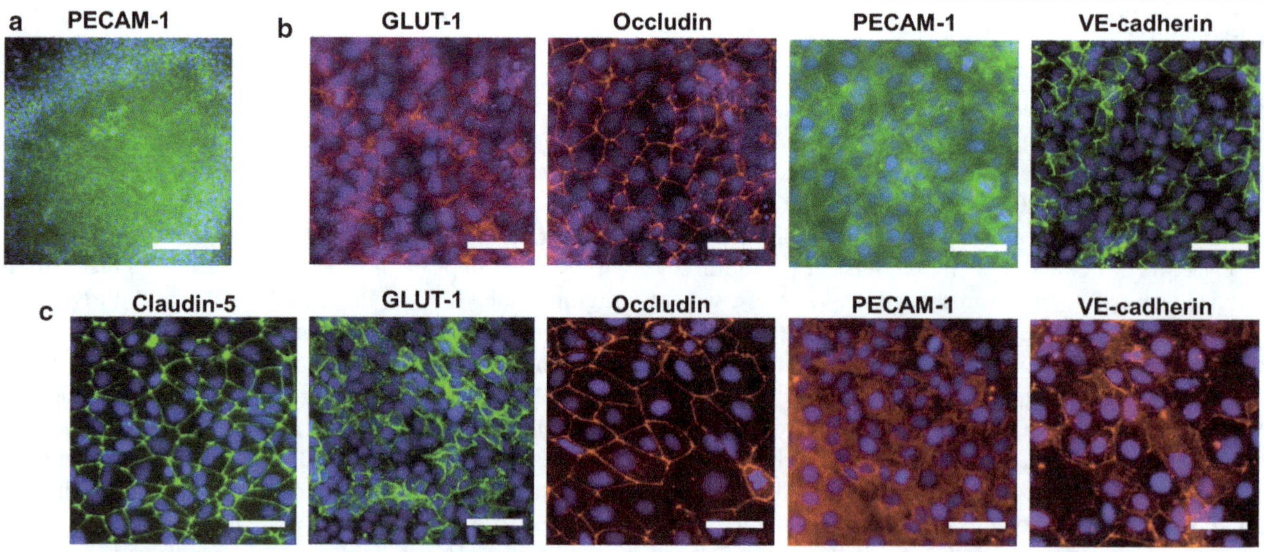

Fig. 2 Immunocytochemical analysis of BBB markers before and after purification. **a** Immunocytochemical detection of PECAM-1 after 4 D E6 medium. *Scale bar* is 200 μm. **b** Immunocytochemical detection of GLUT-1, occludin, PECAM-1, and VE-cadherin after 4 D E6 medium and 2 D EC medium supplemented with bFGF and RA. All *scale bars* are 50 μm. **c** Immunocytochemical detection of claudin-5, GLUT-1, occludin, PECAM-1, and VE-cadherin following purification and induction of barrier phenotype. All *scale bars* are 50 μm

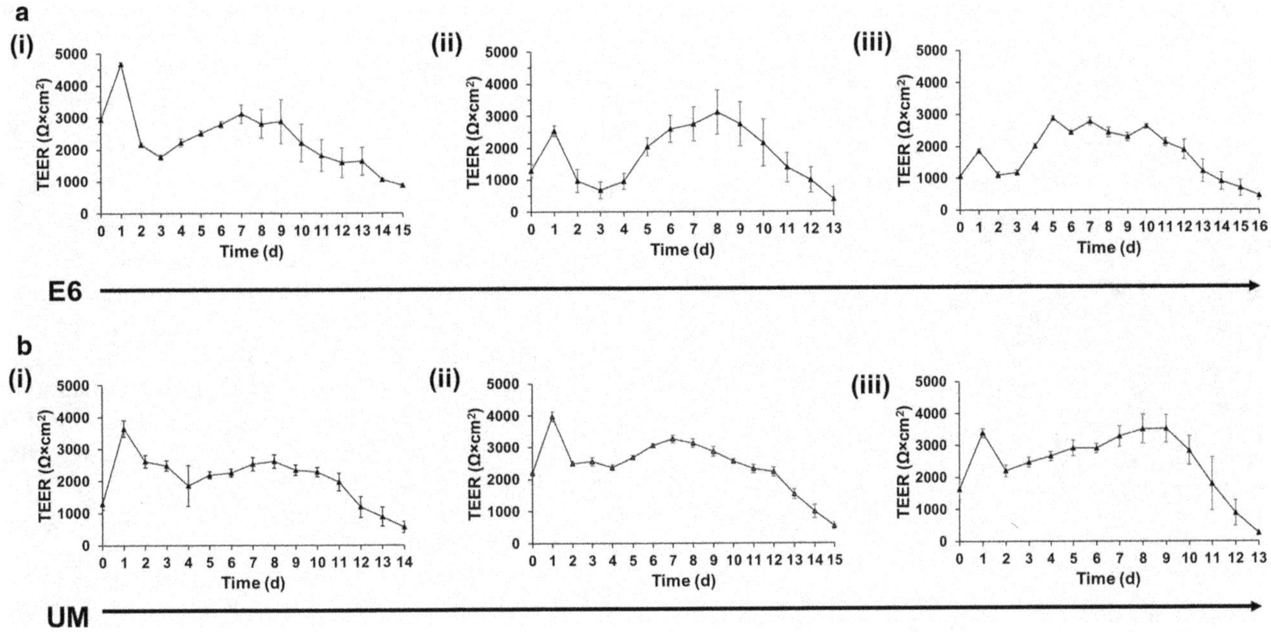

Fig. 3 BMECs differentiated using UM and E6 medium demonstrate equivalent maximum TEER and stability. For each medium, three filters were seeded with BMECs, and TEER was measured in three different positions for each filter. Each plot is the result of one biological replicate (n = 1) with each daily TEER measurement the result of a technical n = 9. Values are reported as mean ± standard deviation of these collective measurements. **a** BMECs differentiated using E6 medium demonstrated maximum TEER values of at least 2500 Ω × cm^2 for a minimum of 11 days in three biological replicates (*i–iii*). TEER was measured approximately every 24 h for the duration of the experiment. **b** BMECs differentiated using UM demonstrated maximum TEER values of at least 2500 Ω × cm^2 for a minimum of 12 days in three biological replicates (*i–iii*). TEER was measured approximately every 24 h for the duration of the experiment

E6-derived BMECs were next evaluated for efflux transporter activity (ETA) and compared to UM-derived BMECs. Purified BMECs were incubated with rhodamine 123, a fluorescent substrate for P-glycoprotein, in the presence and absence of P-glycoprotein inhibitor PSC833. Fluorescence accumulation increased in the presence of PSC833 for both E6-derived BMECs (154 ± 5%) and UM-derived BMECs (151 ± 14%), which indicates inhibition of P-glycoprotein (Fig. 4). Purified BMECs were also incubated with H_2DCFDA, a fluorescent MRP family substrate, in the presence and absence of MK-571, an MRP family inhibitor. Fluorescence accumulation increased in the presence of MK-571 for both E6-derived BMECs (267 ± 19%) and UM-derived BMECs (249 ± 31%), which indicates inhibition of MRP efflux transporters (Fig. 4). Differences in efflux transporter activity for the two sets of BMECs were statistically insignificant for both P-glycoprotein and the MRP family, suggesting that the change in differentiation medium did not have an effect on the efflux transporter activity of BMECs. Overall, these results indicate that using E6 medium to differentiate iPSCs to BMECs, in conjunction with updated seeding methods, reduces differentiation time and yields equivalent functionality as compared to established UM-based differentiation protocols.

Defined medium supports BMEC differentiation in multiple iPSC lines

After demonstrating the successful use of E6 medium to differentiate IMR90-4 iPSCs to BMECs, we sought to confirm the utility of this medium in other iPSC lines. Control iPSC lines CD12 and CC3 as well as iPSC line SM14, from a preclinical PD patient carrying compound heterozygous loss-of-function mutations in *PARK2* associated with familial early-onset PD [34–36], were differentiated to BMECs using E6 medium (Fig. 1). TEER measurements were used to assess barrier fidelity in three independent biological replicates for each line, and TEER exceeding 1000 Ω × cm^2 was measured for a minimum of 8 days, with 5 out of 6 lines exhibiting stability above 1000 Ω × cm^2 for at least 11 days (Fig. 5a-CD12, 5b-CC3, 5c-SM14). This barrier stability was comparable to results achieved in IMR90-4-derived BMECs differentiated in both E6 and UM. Notably, CD12-derived BMECs achieved TEER in excess of 4000 Ω × cm^2 10 days after purification, a maximum value that was also comparable to IMR90-4-derived BMECs.

Next, we sought to validate efflux transporter activity in these lines by conducting directional flux inhibition measurements. When treated with PSC833 and MK-571, CC3- and CD12-derived BMECs exhibited increased

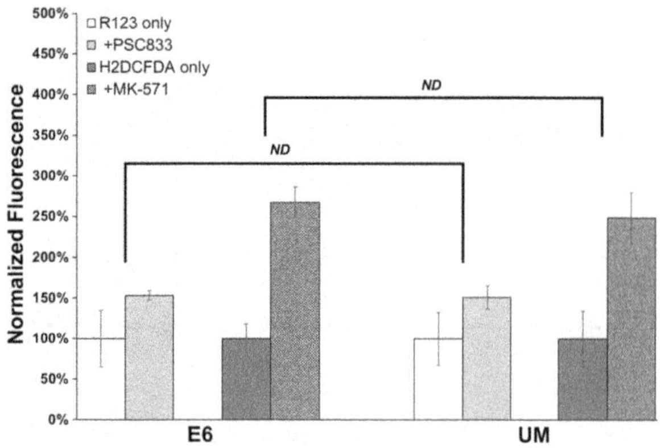

Fig. 4 E6-derived BMECs and UM-derived BMECs demonstrate equivalent efflux transporter activity. E6-derived BMECs and UM-derived BMECs were incubated with rhodamine 123 (R123) or H_2DCFDA in the presence and absence of efflux transporter inhibitors, PSC833 and MK-571, respectively. Fluorescence accumulation within cells incubated with fluorescent substrate in the presence of the desired inhibitor was normalized to fluorescence accumulation in cells incubated with substrate but with no inhibitor. Each condition was performed using triplicate wells, and cell count per condition was calculated as an average from 6 images taken from 1 additional well for each condition. All fluorescence values are normalized on per-cell basis and reported as normalized mean fluorescence ± standard deviation. Two-way ANOVA analysis indicates no statistical difference ($p > 0.05$) in fluorescence accumulation between E6-derived BMECs and UM-derived BMECs. All substrate and inhibitor conditions were repeated in an additional independent differentiation per medium to confirm reported trends

transport of corresponding substrate across the monolayer (Fig. 5d). SM14-derived BMECs, however, showed increased substrate transport across the barrier upon treatment with MK-571 but not PSC833, possibly indicating diminished P-glycoprotein function or polarization. Paracellular permeability of fluorescein (P_e) was less than 1.95×10^{-7} cm/s for all lines, further confirming the passive barrier properties observed by TEER (Fig. 5e). These P_e measurements align with previously published values of BMECs derived using UM [30, 37].

Co-culture with iPSC-derived astrocytes and primary human brain pericytes supports a sustained barrier phenotype

Induced pluripotent stem cell-derived BMECs have previously been shown to gain an elevated barrier phenotype when co-cultured with astrocytes and pericytes [25]. In order to evaluate if BMECs differentiated in E6 medium responded to such cues in a similar manner, iPSCs were differentiated to a mix of astrocytes and glial progenitors [28]. Co-culture of this cell population (49 ± 8% $GFAP^+$, see Additional file 1: Figure S1) with CD12-derived BMECs was initiated 24 h after subculture onto Transwell filters, and co-culture was maintained in EC medium lacking bFGF and RA. Co-cultured cells were seeded in the bottom of the well plates; therefore, no direct contact occurred between BMECs and co-cultured cell types. As such, all observed differences are the result of soluble factors released in the system. Compared to BMECs in monoculture, BMECs in co-culture with glia reached both a higher absolute maximum TEER ($5378 \pm 479\ \Omega \times cm^2$ versus $4227 \pm 370\ \Omega \times cm^2$, $p < 10^{-4}$) and maintained TEER above $1000\ \Omega \times cm^2$ in excess of 22 days (Fig. 6a). BMECs were also co-cultured with primary human brain pericytes (see Additional file 1: Figure S1) and achieved a maximum TEER of $5937 \pm 157\ \Omega \times cm^2$ ($p < 10^{-6}$ versus monoculture) with a stable barrier phenotype above $1000\ \Omega \times cm^2$ for longer than 22 days (Fig. 6a). BMECs co-cultured with both astrocytes and pericytes (35 ± 13% astrocytes, 63 ± 13% pericytes, Figure S1), achieved the highest maximum TEER of $6635 \pm 315\ \Omega \times cm^2$ ($p < 10^{-9}$ versus monoculture, $p < 10^{-4}$ versus astrocyte co-culture, $p < 10^{-3}$ versus pericyte co-culture) and maintained TEER exceeding $1000\ \Omega \times cm^2$ in excess of 22 days. These inductive effects were further verified through co-culture of CC3-derived BMECs with astrocytes and pericytes. A similar statistically significant increase in TEER was observed in co-cultured BMECs versus control BMECs, further validating the responsive nature of E6-derived BMECs to soluble cues from astrocytes and pericytes (Fig. 6b). Co-cultured and control BMECs grown on Transwell filters were stained for claudin-5 and occludin, and no significant phenotypic change was evident between monocultured BMECs on filters, BMECs in co-culture with astrocytes and pericytes, or BMECs grown in well plates (Fig. 2). Thus, the barrier-promoting effects of co-culture with astrocytes and pericytes exceeds effects of the two cell types alone, as expected from previous reports [25]. We note that media was not changed after day 0 to ascertain stability without any external stimulation, and we suspect that partial media exchanges could extend stability further. At present, we are also unsure why the TEER drops precipitously after day 1 and rebounds over the course of a week. We hypothesize this effect may be due to complete removal of bFGF, which is worthy of future exploration.

Discussion

Protocols to differentiate iPSCs to BMECs for in vitro BBB modeling have not necessarily achieved widespread adoption, potentially due in part to the time required to produce purified BMECs and the cost associated with such differentiation and purification. The purpose of this study was to decrease both the time and cost required for such differentiation while still achieving BMECs of comparable performance to established differentiation methods. These advancements will potentially allow

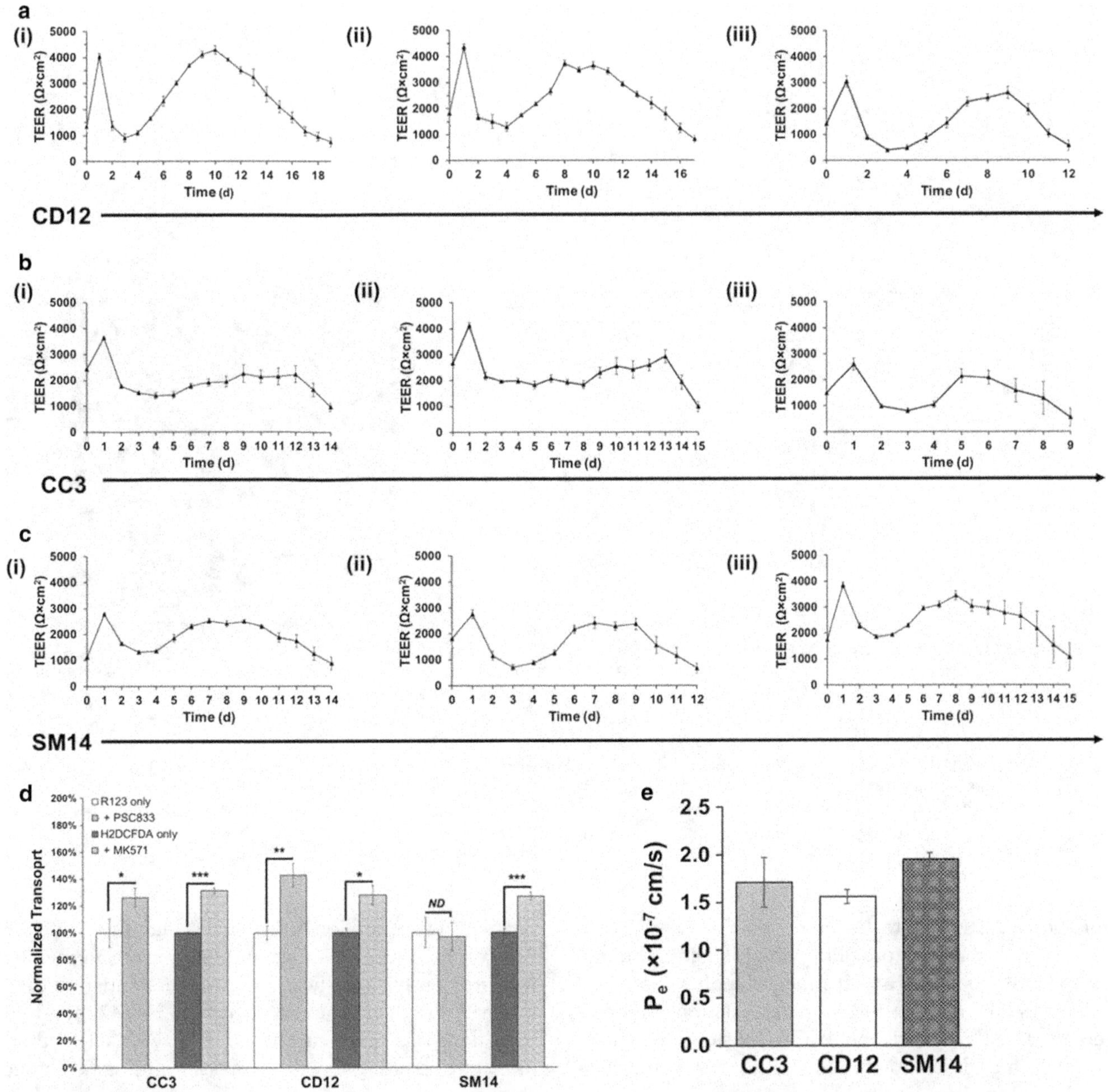

Fig. 5 BMEC differentiation using E6 medium translates to additional iPSC lines. iPSC lines CD12, CC3, and SM14 were differentiated to BMECs with E6 medium as described in Fig. 1, and TEER was measured approximately every 24 h. For each differentiation, three filters were seeded with BMECs, and each filter was measured at three locations on the filter. Each plot is the result of one biological replicate ($n = 1$) with each daily TEER measurement the result of a technical $n = 9$. All values are mean ± standard deviation of these nine total measurements per condition. **a** CD12-derived BMECs achieved maximum TEER values exceeding 4000 $\Omega \times cm^2$ and maintained TEER above 1000 $\Omega \times cm^2$ for a minimum of 11 days in 3 independent biological replicates. **b** CC3-derived BMECs achieved maximum TEER values exceeding 3500 $\Omega \times cm^2$ and maintained TEER above 1000 $\Omega \times cm^2$ for a minimum of 8 days in 3 independent biological replicates. **c** SM14-derived BMECs achieved maximum TEER values exceeding 2500 $\Omega \times cm^2$ and maintained TEER above 1000 $\Omega \times cm^2$ for a minimum of 11 days in 3 independent biological replicates. **d** Apical-to-basolateral flux of rhodamine 123 (R123) and H_2DCFDA was measured across BMECs in the presence or absence of PSC833 and MK-571, respectively. Fluorescence was normalized to cells not treated with inhibitor and reported as normalized mean fluorescence ± standard deviation. Each condition was performed using triplicate filters and statistics were calculated using a technical n of 3. Statistical significance was determined using the Student's unpaired t test (*$p < 0.1$; **$p < 0.05$; ***$p < 0.01$). Data from one biological experiment are shown, and an additional biological replicate was performed for each line to verify the observed trends. **e** The permeability of sodium fluorescein was measured across BMECs. Each experiment was performed using triplicate filters and data are presented as mean ± standard deviation. Biological duplicates were used to verify each measurement. The effective permeability (P_e) was calculated at less than 1.95×10^{-7} cm/s for all lines

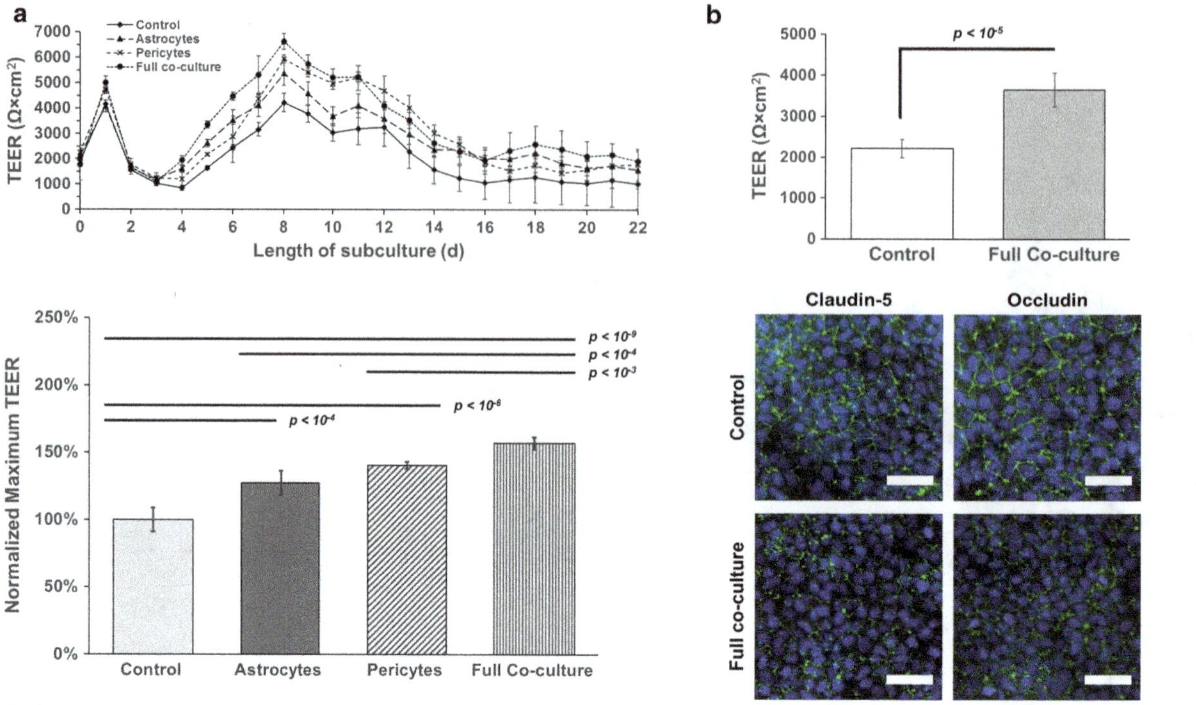

Fig. 6 E6-derived BMECs respond to inductive cues from astrocytes and pericytes. **a** Co-culture of CD12-derived BMECs with astrocytes, pericytes, and a mixture of astrocytes and pericytes achieved maximum TEER values exceeding $4000\ \Omega \times cm^2$ and maintained TEER above $1000\ \Omega \times cm^2$ for a minimum of 22 days under all co-culture conditions. Each condition was conducted on triplicate filters with all BMECs purified from a single differentiation. Each filter was measured at three different locations on the filter each day. Values are mean $\pm$ standard deviation from these collective nine technical replicates per condition per day. Maximum TEER values achieved on day 8 of subculture were normalized to the TEER of the monoculture control. Statistical significance was calculated using Student's unpaired t test. **b** CC3-derived BMECs were co-cultured with a mixture of astrocytes and pericytes, achieving a significant increase in TEER 24 h after barrier induction ($p < 10^{-5}$, Student's unpaired t test). Each condition was conducted on triplicate filters with all BMECs purified from a single differentiation. Each filter was measured at three different locations on the filter each day. Values are mean $\pm$ standard deviation from these collective nine technical replicates per condition per day. BMECs were subsequently stained for occludin and claudin-5 in both control and co-culture conditions. *Scale bars* are 50 μm

iPSC-derived BMECs to be more readily accessible to researchers, thereby providing high-fidelity human in vitro BBB models for a wide range of applications.

In this study, existing BMEC differentiation protocols were modified to exclude the iPSC expansion phase prior to initiation of differentiation [24, 25, 37]. By controlling initial iPSC seeding density [37], maximum TEER values of purified BMECs from such differentiations remained consistently in excess of $2500\ \Omega \times cm^2$, and barrier fidelity, as indicated by TEER above $1000\ \Omega \times cm^2$, was maintained for a minimum of 8 days, as was similarly achieved in a recent microfluidics-based model using UM-derived BMECs [40]. E8 medium was also used for iPSC maintenance in place of mTeSR, as described by others [30]. Given that we routinely use E6 medium (a derivative of E8 medium that lacks growth factors promoting pluripotency) for neural differentiations [28], we further explored its use for differentiating iPSCs to BMECs. Upon differentiation in E6 medium, immunocytochemical analysis unexpectedly showed PECAM-1^+ cells at 4 days of differentiation rather than 6 days. We note that changes in culture methods and differentiation medium have previously been shown to alter differentiation times to lineages such as neuroectoderm [28, 41, 42] and midbrain dopaminergic neurons [41, 43], with all methods ultimately resulting in cells expressing the same characteristic markers. Therefore, it is unsurprising that changes made in differentiation medium resulted in altered differentiation timelines. After establishing this accelerated differentiation timeline from iPSCs to BMECs using E6 medium, BMECs were evaluated for BBB phenotype by TEER measurement and efflux transporter activity. BMECs differentiated in E6 medium maintained a stable barrier above $1000\ \Omega \times cm^2$ for 8 days, longer than previously published reports using similar Transwell-based methods [25, 37], while achieving similar maximum TEER values to UM-derived BMECs. BMECs differentiated using E6 medium and UM also had no statistical difference in efflux transporter activity for P-glycoprotein and MRP family members. BMEC differentiation using

E6 medium was further validated in iPSC lines CD12, CC3, and SM14. CD12- and CC3-derived BMECs demonstrated equivalent maximum TEER and long-term stability as IMR90-4-derived BMECs differentiated in both E6 medium and UM. Notably, CD12-derived BMECs achieved TEER greater than 4000 $\Omega \times cm^2$ on days 9 and 10 of subculture, a value equivalent to the maximum TEER achieved after initial induction of BMEC phenotype. Finally, SM14 iPSCs, which harbor biallelic loss-of-function *PARK2* mutations associated with familial early onset PD, yielded BMECs with maximum TEER and long term stability equivalent to BMECs derived from control lines, similar fluorescein permeability, and equivalent MRP family efflux transporter activity. Interestingly, SM14-derived BMECs did not show active P-glycoprotein in the apical-to-basolateral transport assays. Studies on advanced PD patients have demonstrated increased brain uptake of P-glycoprotein substrates [44]. Our data may indicate that patients with familial PD mutations are predisposed to loss of P-glycoprotein function. However, our results are very preliminary and would need to be rigorously confirmed across multiple iPSC lines from different patients harboring the same mutation. As this manuscript is centered on the utility of E6 medium for in vitro differentiation, we have not pursued these studies herein. Even so, this exciting result indicates researchers can probe mechanisms of BBB regulation in the context of genetic disease or evaluate molecular transport and toxicology over extended experimental time points. Our methods can ostensibly be extended to other iPSC disease lines of interest, provided that the genetic mutation does not impact barrier stability.

To further explore the utility of the model, we investigated the effect of co-culturing BMECs with iPSC-derived astrocytes and primary human brain pericytes. Astrocytes and pericytes are known to aid in induction of BBB phenotype in the developing neurovascular environment [3]. Though co-culture of BMECs with astrocytes and co-culture of BMECs with pericytes individually were both found to increase barrier function as indicated by TEER, co-culture with astrocytes and pericytes concurrently enhanced the TEER above that achieved through co-culture with either cell type alone. This effect has been noted in other in vitro BBB models, though the reported maximum TEER value from co-culture in this study exceeds previously published in vitro TEER values by more than 700 $\Omega \times cm^2$ [25]. Excitingly, this achievement approaches in vivo TEER predictions of 8000 $\Omega \times cm^2$ put forth by Smith and Rapoport [45]. In addition, medium was not changed following barrier induction to minimize external influences on barrier stability. Due to prospective increased metabolic burden in the co-culture system as evidenced by a qualitative decrease in number of co-cultured cells between the start and end of the experiment, we suspect that gradual media changes following barrier induction may further improve the stability of the model by supporting neurovascular health. Owing to the extended barrier phenotype observed, researchers may now conduct long-term experiments without concern that barrier degradation may confound results.

Conclusions

The differentiation of iPSCs to BMECs using defined E6 medium shortened differentiation time and produced BMECs of equivalent performance as BMECs differentiated according to previously published protocols using UM. Stability of the model system has also been greatly improved, with monocultured BMECs exhibiting enhanced stability for greater than 8 days and co-cultured BMECs exhibiting stability of more than 3 weeks. We routinely produce E6 and E8 medium in-house in large batches (see "Methods"), thus substantially reducing the cost of maintenance and differentiation to allow increased throughput of experiments. Thus, the overall improvements described in this manuscript will enable iPSC-derived BMECs to become more accessible to researchers and more broadly enable studies ranging from disease pathogenesis to analyses of repeated drug dosing.

Abbreviations

BBB: blood–brain barrier; BMEC: brain microvascular endothelial cell; iPSC: induced pluripotent stem cell; H_2DCFDA: 2′,7′-dichlorodihydrofluorescein diacetate; R123: rhodamine 123; EC: endothelial cell; UM: unconditioned medium; MRP: multidrug resistance protein; RA: retinoic acid; bFGF: basic fibroblast growth factor; TEER: trans-endothelial electrical resistance; ETA: efflux transporter activity; ICC: immunocytochemistry; CNTF: ciliary neurotrophic factor; EGF: epidermal growth factor; TGFβ1: transforming growth factor beta-1; PD: Parkinson's Disease.

Authors' contributions

EKH, AKB, and AVP performed experiments. EKH and ESL designed the research, analyzed the results, and wrote the paper. MDN and ABB provided CD12, CC3, and SM14 iPSC lines and advised on their culture. All authors read and approved the final manuscript.

Author details

[1] Department of Chemical and Biomolecular Engineering, Vanderbilt University, 2201 West End Ave, Nashville, TN 37235, USA. [2] Department of Biochemistry, Vanderbilt University, 2201 West End Ave, Nashville, TN 37235, USA. [3] Department of Pediatrics, Vanderbilt University Medical Center, 1211 Medical Center Dr, Nashville, TN 37232, USA. [4] Department of Neurology, Vanderbilt University Medical Center, 1211 Medical Center Dr, Nashville, TN 37232, USA.

Acknowledgements

The authors would like to thank Dr. Shannon Faley and Dr. Leon Bellan for assistance with microscopy and use of the Zeiss AxioObserver Z1 microscope. The authors would also like to thank Dr. John Wilson for the use of the BioTek Synergy H1 multi-mode microplate reader and Max Jacobson for his aid in operating the instrument. Helpful comments were provided by Daniel Balikov during manuscript preparation.

Competing interests

The authors declare that they have no competing interests.

Funding

Funding for this work was provided by the School of Engineering at Vanderbilt University (ESL) and NIH Grants ES010563 (ABB) and ES016931 (ABB).

References

1. Zlokovic BV. The blood–brain barrier in health and chronic neurodegenerative disorders. Neuron. 2008;57:178–201.
2. Kniesel U, Wolburg H. Tight junctions of the blood–brain barrier. Cell Mol Neurobiol. 2000;20:57–76.
3. Obermeier B, Daneman R, Ransohoff RM. Development, maintenance and disruption of the blood–brain barrier. Nat Med. 2013;19:1584–96.
4. Butt AM, Jones HC, Abbott NJ. Electrical resistance across the blood–brain barrier in anaesthetized rats: a developmental study. J Physiol. 1990;429:47–62.
5. Olesen SP, Crone C. Electrical resistance of muscle capillary endothelium. Biophys J. 1983;42:31–41.
6. Löscher W, Potschka H. Drug resistance in brain diseases and the role of drug efflux transporters. Nat Rev Neurosci. 2005;6:591–602.
7. Begley DJ. ABC transporters and the blood–brain barrier. Curr Pharm Des. 2004;10:1295–312.
8. Friese MA, Schattling B, Fugger L. Mechanisms of neurodegeneration and axonal dysfunction in multiple sclerosis. Nat Rev Neurol. 2014;10:225–38.
9. Korn A, Golan H, Melamed I, Pascual-Marqui R, Friedman A. Focal cortical dysfunction and blood–brain barrier disruption in patients with Postconcussion syndrome. J Clin Neurophysiol Off Publ Am Electroencephalogr Soc. 2005;22:1–9.
10. Rosell A, Cuadrado E, Ortega-Aznar A, Hernández-Guillamon M, Lo EH, Montaner J. MMP-9–positive neutrophil infiltration is associated to blood–brain barrier breakdown and basal lamina type iv collagen degradation during hemorrhagic transformation after human ischemic stroke. Stroke. 2008;39:1121–6.
11. Sandoval KE, Witt KA. Blood–brain barrier tight junction permeability and ischemic stroke. Neurobiol Dis. 2008;32:200–19.
12. Strbian D, Durukan A, Pitkonen M, Marinkovic I, Tatlisumak E, Pedrono E, et al. The blood–brain barrier is continuously open for several weeks following transient focal cerebral ischemia. Neuroscience. 2008;153:175–81.
13. Barzó P, Marmarou A, Fatouros P, Corwin F, Dunbar J. Magnetic resonance imaging—monitored acute blood–brain barrier changes in experimental traumatic brain injury. J Neurosurg. 1996;85:1113–21.
14. Montagne A, Barnes SR, Sweeney MD, Halliday MR, Sagare AP, Zhao Z, et al. Blood–brain barrier breakdown in the aging human hippocampus. Neuron. 2015;85:296–302.
15. Abbott NJ. Blood–brain barrier structure and function and the challenges for CNS drug delivery. J Inherit Metab Dis. 2013;36:437–49.
16. Helms HC, Abbott NJ, Burek M, Cecchelli R, Couraud P-O, Deli MA, et al. In vitro models of the blood–brain barrier: an overview of commonly used brain endothelial cell culture models and guidelines for their use. J Cereb Blood Flow Metab. 2016;36:862–90.
17. Al Ahmad A, Taboada CB, Gassmann M, Ogunshola OO. Astrocytes and pericytes differentially modulate blood–brain barrier characteristics during development and hypoxic insult. J Cereb Blood Flow Metab. 2011;31:693–705.
18. Al Ahmad A, Gassmann M, Ogunshola OO. Maintaining blood–brain barrier integrity: pericytes perform better than astrocytes during prolonged oxygen deprivation. J Cell Physiol. 2009;218.
19. Abbott NJ. Prediction of blood–brain barrier permeation in drug discovery from in vivo, in vitro and in silico models. Drug Discov Today Technol. 2004;1:407–16.
20. Reichel A. Addressing central nervous system (CNS) penetration in drug discovery: basics and implications of the evolving new concept. Chem Biodivers. 2009;6:2030–49.
21. Syvänen S, Lindhe Ö, Palner M, Kornum BR, Rahman O, Långström B, et al. Species differences in blood–brain barrier transport of three positron emission tomography radioligands with emphasis on P-glycoprotein transport. Drug Metab Dispos. 2009;37:635–43.
22. Bernas MJ, Cardoso FL, Daley SK, Weinand ME, Campos AR, Ferreira AJG, et al. Establishment of primary cultures of human brain microvascular endothelial cells to provide an in vitro cellular model of the blood–brain barrier. Nat Protoc. 2010;5:1265–72.
23. Weksler BB, Subileau EA, Perrière N, Charneau P, Holloway K, Leveque M, et al. Blood–brain barrier-specific properties of a human adult brain endothelial cell line. FASEB J. 2005;19:1872–4.
24. Lippmann ES, Azarin SM, Kay JE, Nessler RA, Wilson HK, Al-Ahmad A, et al. Derivation of blood–brain barrier endothelial cells from human pluripotent stem cells. Nat Biotechnol. 2012;30:783–91.
25. Lippmann ES, Al-Ahmad A, Azarin SM, Palecek SP, Shusta EV. A retinoic acid-enhanced, multicellular human blood–brain barrier model derived from stem cell sources. Sci Rep. 2014;4:4160.
26. Ludwig TE, Levenstein ME, Jones JM, Berggren WT, Mitchen ER, Frane JL, et al. Derivation of human embryonic stem cells in defined conditions. Nat Biotechnol. 2006;24:185–7.
27. Chen G, Gulbranson DR, Hou Z, Bolin JM, Ruotti V, Probasco MD, et al. Chemically defined conditions for human iPSC derivation and culture. Nat Methods. 2011;8:424–9.
28. Lippmann ES, Estevez-Silva MC, Ashton RS. Defined human pluripotent stem cell culture enables highly efficient neuroepithelium derivation without small molecule inhibitors. Stem Cells. 2014;32:1032–42.
29. Lian X, Bao X, Zilberter M, Westman M, Fisahn A, Hsiao C, et al. Chemically defined, albumin-free human cardiomyocyte generation. Nat Methods. 2015;12:595–6.
30. Patel R, Alahmad AJ. Growth-factor reduced Matrigel source influences stem cell derived brain microvascular endothelial cell barrier properties. Fluids Barriers CNS. 2016;13:6.
31. Calabria AR, Weidenfeller C, Jones AR, De Vries HE, Shusta EV. Puromycin-purified rat brain microvascular endothelial cell cultures exhibit improved barrier properties in response to glucocorticoid induction. J Neurochem. 2006;97:922–33.
32. Yu J, Vodyanik MA, Smuga-Otto K, Antosiewicz-Bourget J, Frane JL, Tian S, et al. Induced pluripotent stem cell lines derived from human somatic cells. Science. 2007;318:1917–20.
33. Tidball AM, Neely MD, Chamberlin R, Aboud AA, Kumar KK, Han B, et al. Genomic instability associated with p53 knockdown in the generation of huntington's disease human induced pluripotent stem cells. PLoS ONE. 2016;11:e0150372.
34. Kumar KK, Lowe EW Jr, Aboud AA, Neely MD, Redha R, Bauer JA, et al. Cellular manganese content is developmentally regulated in human dopaminergic neurons. Sci Rep. 2014;4:6801.
35. Aboud AA, Tidball AM, Kumar KK, Neely MD, Ess KC, Erikson KM, et al. Genetic risk for Parkinson's disease correlates with alterations in neuronal manganese sensitivity between two human subjects. Neurotoxicology. 2012;33:1443–9.
36. Aboud AA, Tidball AM, Kumar KK, Neely MD, Han B, Ess KC, et al. PARK2 patient neuroprogenitors show increased mitochondrial sensitivity to copper. Neurobiol Dis. 2015;73:204–12.
37. Wilson HK, Canfield SG, Hjortness MK, Palecek SP, Shusta EV. Exploring the effects of cell seeding density on the differentiation of human pluripotent stem cells to brain microvascular endothelial cells. Fluids Barriers CNS. 2015;12:13.
38. Carpenter AE, Jones TR, Lamprecht MR, Clarke C, Kang IH, Friman O, et al. Cell Profiler: image analysis software for identifying and quantifying cell phenotypes. Genome Biol. 2006;7:R100.
39. Katt ME, Xu ZS, Gerecht S, Searson PC. Human brain microvascular endothelial cells derived from the BC1 iPS cell line exhibit a blood–brain barrier phenotype. PLoS ONE. 2016;11:e0152105.
40. Wang YI, Abaci HE, Shuler ML. Microfluidic blood–brain barrier model provides in vivo-like barrier properties for drug permeability screening. Biotechnol Bioeng. 2017;114:184–94.
41. Chambers SM, Fasano CA, Papapetrou EP, Tomishima M, Sadelain M, Studer L. Highly efficient neural conversion of human ES and iPS cells by dual inhibition of SMAD signaling. Nat Biotechnol. 2009;27:275–80.

42. Pankratz MT, Li X-J, LaVaute TM, Lyons EA, Chen X, Zhang S-C. Directed neural differentiation of human embryonic stem cells via an obligated primitive anterior stage. Stem Cells. 2007;25:1511–20.
43. Kawasaki H, Mizuseki K, Nishikawa S, Kaneko S, Kuwana Y, Nakanishi S, et al. Induction of midbrain dopaminergic neurons from es cells by stromal cell-derived inducing activity. Neuron. 2000;28:31–40.
44. Bartels AL, Willemsen ATM, Kortekaas R, de Jong BM, de Vries R, de Klerk O, et al. Decreased blood–brain barrier P-glycoprotein function in the progression of Parkinson's disease, PSP and MSA. J Neural Transm. 2008;115:1001–9.
45. Smith QR, Rapoport SI. Cerebrovascular permeability coefficients to sodium, potassium, and chloride. J Neurochem. 1986;46:1732–42.

3

Amyloid mis-metabolism in idiopathic normal pressure hydrocephalus

A. Jeppsson[1*], Mikko Höltta[2], H. Zetterberg[2,3,4], K. Blennow[2,3], C. Wikkelsø[1] and Mats Tullberg[1]

Abstract

Background: Patients with idiopathic normal pressure hydrocephalus (iNPH) have reduced cerebrospinal fluid (CSF) concentrations of amyloid-β (Aβ) and α- and β-cleaved soluble forms of amyloid precursor protein (sAPPα and sAPPβ). The aims of this study were to examine if changes could also be seen in the CSF for secreted metabolites of APP-like protein 1 (APLP1) and to explore the prognostic value of amyloid-related CSF biomarkers, as well as markers of neuronal injury and astroglial activation, as regards to clinical outcome after shunt surgery.

Methods: Twenty patients diagnosed with iNPH, 10 improved and 10 unchanged by shunt surgery, and 20 neurologically healthy controls were included. All patients were examined clinically prior to surgery and at 6-month follow-up after surgery using the iNPH scale. Lumbar puncture was performed pre-operatively. CSF samples were analyzed for neurofilament light (NFL), Aβ isoforms Aβ38, Aβ40 and Aβ42, sAPPα, sAPPβ, APLP1 β-derived peptides APL1β25, APL1β 27 and APL1β 28 and YKL40 by immunochemical methods.

Results: The concentrations of all soluble forms of APP, all Aβ isoforms and APL1β28 were lower, whilst APL1β25 and APL1β27 were higher in the CSF of iNPH patients compared to controls. There was no difference in biomarker concentrations between patients who improved after surgery and those who remained unchanged.

Conclusions: The reduced CSF concentrations of Aβ38, Aβ40, Aβ42, sAPPα and sAPPβ suggest that APP expression could be downregulated in iNPH. In contrast, APLP1 concentration in the CSF seems relatively unchanged. The increase of APL1β25 and APL1β27 in combination with a slight decreased APL1β28 could be caused by more available γ-secretase due to reduced availability of its primary substrate, APP. The data did not support the use of these markers as indicators of shunt responsiveness.

Keywords: Neurodegeneration, Normal pressure hydrocephalus, Cerebrospinal fluid, Amyloid, NFL, YKL40, Prediction , APLP1

Background

Idiopathic normal pressure hydrocephalus (iNPH) is a condition with gait and balance disturbances, cognitive decline and urinary incontinence in combination with enlarged cerebral ventricles [1, 2]. Shunt treatment improves more than 80 % of the patients [3]. Without surgery, the clinical course is progressive and a delay in treatment means a loss of function that cannot be restored [4]. Being one of the few treatable neurodegenerative conditions, an accurate diagnosis and identification of patients who will benefit from shunt surgery is essential. The use of CSF biomarkers for such purposes has been identified as one of the priorities for hydrocephalus research [5].

Patients with iNPH exhibit suppressed CSF concentrations of amyloid-β (Aβ) and the precursors soluble amyloid precursor protein α-, and β- (sAPPα, sAPPβ), in combination with elevated neurofilament light protein (NFL) [6–9]. Hypothetically, this is thought to be due to a downregulation of APP in the periventricular tissue possibly caused by changed amyloid metabolism and/or a reduced clearance of extracellular fluid into CSF leading to lowered concentrations of APP-derived proteins in CSF [6].

Amyloid-like protein 1 (APLP1)-derived peptides are processed by similar enzymatic pathways as APP and share

*Correspondence: anna.jeppsson@neuro.gu.se
[1] Hydrocephalus Research Unit, Institute of Neuroscience and Physiology, The Sahlgrenska Academy, University of Gothenburg, 413 45 Gothenburg, Sweden

related structural domains and functions [10–12]. APLP1 is processed into short Aβ-like peptides (APL1β25, 1β27 and 1β28) [13]. APLP1 is a substrate for the enzyme γ-secretase and the ratio of APLP1-derived APL1β28 to total APL1β is a surrogate marker for Aβ42 production in the central nervous system [13, 14]. Recently, it was reported that γ-secretase was higher in brain biopsies from iNPH patients with amyloid plaques than in those without [15].

The aim of this study was to examine CSF concentrations of APLP1-derived peptides in iNPH, especially if the APL1β28 form was increased, and to explore the prognostic value of amyloid-related CSF biomarkers. For this purpose, we analyzed the APP-derived peptides sAPPα, sAPPβ, Aβ38, Aβ40 and Aβ42, the APLP1derived peptides APL1β25, APL1β27 and APL1β28 in CSF in 20 patients with iNPH (10 improved and 10 unchanged by shunt operation) and 20 neurologically healthy controls.

Methods

Study populations

Ten iNPH patients improved after shunt surgery and 10 non-improved were retrospectively selected. All were diagnosed in accordance with the international guidelines [16]. The patients were selected from our local database at the hydrocephalus unit at Sahlgrenska University Hospital on the premises that full medical data pre- and postoperatively were available and that there was sufficient CSF stored to perform the analyses. In all, the database contained 176 patients. From the database, the 10 patients who benefitted the most from surgery (as defined by improvement in the iNPH scale) and fulfilled the inclusion criteria were selected. In the group that did not benefit from surgery, medical records were scanned in order to establish that at time for follow-up all shunts were working, none had complications and that that there be no other known cause for non-improvement. Patients who had complications that could be attributed to shunt surgery were excluded. In all, the groups were selected in order to magnify the difference in responsiveness to shunt surgery within the clinical material and analyze two clearly-distinguishable extreme groups as regards to shunt responsiveness.

The improved 10 patients consisted of five men and five women, aged 70.3 ± 3.20 (mean ± SD) and the 10 unimproved patients (<5 points at the iNPH scale) consisted of seven men and three women aged 71.6 ± 8 (mean ± SD). The groups did not differ significantly in terms of comorbidities, preoperative MMSE scores, extent of white matter lesions (WML), age or sickness duration. The baseline clinical data of the different groups are outlined in Table 1.

All patients were examined clinically prior to surgery and 6 months after by the iNPH scale, composed of items assessing gait, cognition, continence and balance [17]. The extent of WML was rated by the Wahlund scale from MRI or CT scans at the time for diagnosis [18]. Lumbar puncture was performed preoperatively with the patient in recumbent position. In the improved group the median improvement was 26 points and in the non-improved group the median was 1 point (Table 2). All patients received a ventriculo-peritoneal shunt with a programmable valve with an anti-siphon device and a Rickham reservoir. All had working shunts and none had complications at the time for evaluation.

Table 1 Clinical characteristics of iNPH patients at baseline

	Improved n = 10	Non-improved n = 10	
Age (mean ± SD)	70.3 ± 3.2	71.6 ± 8.0	ns
Sex (male/female)	5/5	7/3	ns
Sickness duration (month)	42 ± 21	34 ± 28	ns
Diabetes (y/n)	2/8	2/8	ns
Hypertension (y/n)	5/5	6/4	ns
Cardiovascular disease (y/n)	2/8	1/9	ns
MMSE (median, IQ-range)	23 (22–28)	26 (24–28)	ns
WML (median, IQ-range)	6 (4–10)	11 (5–20)	ns
Evans index (median, IQ-range)	0.43 (0.38–0.46)	0.39 (0.36–0.41)	ns

Twenty control subjects were chosen from a population of volunteers who had given consent to CSF sampling prior to knee surgery. The controls had no history of neurological or psychiatric disease, a normal clinical neurological examination and a normal mini-mental state examination score. They consisted of eight men and 12 women aged 71.2 (±6.4). There was no difference in age between the three subcategories (controls, iNPH improved and iNPH non-improved).

CSF analyses

Amyloid β isoforms (Aβ38, Aβ40, and Aβ42) were analyzed by electrochemiluminescence assays (Meso Scale Discovery, Gaithersburg, MD, USA). The APLP1-derived peptides APL1β25, APL1β27, and APL1β28 were analyzed using a commercial ELISA (IBL International, Hamburg, Germany). The samples were analyzed according to the kit insert with minor modifications. The CSF samples were diluted 1:20 for APL1β25, 1:10 for APL1β27, and 1:5 for APL1β28 by the dilution buffer contained in the kit. All samples were analyzed in duplicate and the CV % for standards and samples was <5 %.

NFL was measured by ELISA technology using a commercial kit (NF-Light, UmanDiagnostics, Umeå, Sweden) with a lower limit of detection of 50 ng/L. For astroglia activation, CSF YKL-40 concentration was measured by

Table 2 iNPH scale score pre op, post op and outcome (median and IQ-range)

	Pre op		Post op		Outcome	
	Improved	Non-improved	Improved	Non improved	Improved	Non-improved
	n = 10	n = 10	n = 10	n = 10	n = 10	n = 10
Gait domain	33 (16–48)	54 (35–69)	84 (57–100)	50 (34–81)	49 (26 to 57)	−1 (−6 to 11)
Cognitive domain	64 (37–73)	60 (46–80)	75 (57–85)	69 (48–80)	10 (6 to 21)	3 (−6 to 11)
Continence domain	60 (20–80)	80 (60–80)	90 (75–100)	70 (55–80)	30 (0 to 45)	0 (−20 to 5)
Balance domain	67 (67–71)	67 (67–83)	75 (67–87)	67 (67–83)	0 (−4 to 20)	0 (−16 to 0)
Total iNPH score	50 (36–64)	63 (56–70)	77.3 (71–87)	64 (52–71)	26 (21 to 30)	1 (−3 to 3)

solid phase sandwich ELISA (R&D Systems, Inc., Minneapolis, Minnesota, USA) according to the manufacturer's instructions. All analyses were performed batch-wise on one occasion by board-certified laboratory technicians at the Clinical Neurochemistry Laboratory at Sahlgrenska University Hospital, Mölndal, Sweden. Intra-assay coefficients of variation were below 10 %.

Statistics

Non-parametric methods were used for analyses. For comparisons between two groups the Mann–Whitney U test was performed and for comparisons between the three subgroups, the Kruskal–Wallis test was performed. For comparison of two proportions, Fisher's exact test was used. For association between two independent variables, the Spearman rank order correlation was chosen. The level of significance chosen was $p = 0.05$, if not otherwise stated. No correction for the mass-significance effect was made in order to avoid type II errors. Statistical analyses were made using IBM® SPSS® Statistics for Windows version 21.

Results

CSF concentrations of sAPPα, sAPPβ, Aβ38, Aβ40, Aβ42 and APL1β28 were significantly lower and APL1β25 and 27 significantly higher in iNPH patients compared to healthy controls. Levels of NFL and YKL 40 did not differ between iNPH patients and healthy controls (Table 3; Fig. 1). The APL1β28/total APL1β ratio and the Aβ42/to total Aβ ratio was lower in patients with iNPH in comparison with healthy controls (Fig. 2).

There were no differences in any of the CSF biomarkers between improved and non-improved iNPH patients (Table 4).

Discussion

Our data showing substantially reduced CSF concentrations of Aβ38, Aβ40, Aβ42, sAPPα and sAPPβ in patients with iNPH, confirm earlier results [6–9, 11, 19–22]. In contrast, APLP1 in CSF was mildly but significantly, changed with an increase in APL1β25 and APL1β27 and a slight decrease of APL1β28, compared with controls. The ratios APL1β28/total APL1β and Aβ42/total Aβ were reduced in patients with iNPH. However, there were no differences in any CSF biomarker between improved and non-improved iNPH patients after treatment with shunt surgery.

This explorative study was in part designed to identify predictive alterations in the amyloid CSF pattern. We included two small groups representing iNPH patients that benefitted the most and those without any response to surgical treatment with shunting, in order to identify possible differences. However, we found no differences in CSF biomarkers between improved and non-improved patients. The low number of cases in each group may have been a limitation in this study. However, if there are subtle variances in CSF amyloid concentrations linked to responsiveness that could be identified in larger sample sets, we believe that these would be of minor clinical importance. Lumbar CSF as opposed to ventricular CSF was analysed to enhance the practical applicability of the generated results. Ventricular CSF might however provide a different pattern as it probably mirrors brain metabolic processes more accurately.

The reduced CSF concentrations of Aβ38, Aβ40, Aβ42, sAPPα and sAPPβ in iNPH is consistent with earlier findings [6, 7, 9, 11, 19–23], and compatible with a reduction in the concentrations of APP-derived proteins in the CSF of iNPH-patients. iNPH is a disorder of disturbed CSF dynamics and/or consequences thereof. Recent insights into the glymphatic system, has provided possibilities for a new route for clearance of excess fluid and interstitial metabolites, including Aβ, from the brain parenchyma [24, 25], together with clearance of Aβ across the blood–brain barrier (BBB) via the LRP-1 receptor [26]. In the glymphatic system, there may be a para arterial influx of CSF from the subarachnoid space into the brain parenchyma where convective flow of interstitial fluid (ISF) helps to clear metabolic waste by para venous clearance towards the cervical lymph system, a system that seems to impair with aging [25, 27]. However, clear evidence

Table 3 Biomarker levels in iNPH and controls (median and IQ range)

	iNPH n = 20	Controls n = 20
NFL (ng/L)	1185 (731–2103)	938 (610–2141)
APL1β25 (ng/L)	2591 (2296–2951) ↑	2180 (1898–2386)***
APL1β27 (ng/L)	1083 (887–1177) ↑	874 (796–964)***
APL1β28 (ng/L)	1423 (1317–1550) ↓	1621 (1422–1797)**
Aβ38 (ng/L)	502 (266–625) ↓	1114 (819–1445)***
Aβ40 (ng/L)	3676 (2190–4748) ↓	7682 (6366–9809)***
Aβ42 (ng/L)	241 (144–405) ↓	754 (493–1058)***
sAPPα (ng/mL)	207 (157–259) ↓	416 (323–665)***
sAPPβ (ng/mL)	119 (92–170) ↓	280 (182–389)***
YKL40 (ng/mL)	122 (90–167)	137 (104–177)

Arrows indicating biomarker levels in iNPH in comparison with controls

ns non-significant

* $p \leq 0.05$; ** $p \leq 0.01$; *** $p \leq 0.001$

for this clearance is still lacking. In iNPH the CSF flow above the convexities is reduced and redirected into the ventricles and iNPH patients often present with a disproportionately enlarged subarachnoid-space [28, 29]. These findings could hypothetically be in accordance with a disturbance of CSF/ISF exchange as the dilated paravascular spaces could impair CSF/ISF exchange. Although speculative, it could be hypothesized that the reduced concentrations of APP-derived proteins in the CSF of INPH patients could be due to stagnation of the flow in the periventricular ISF with reduced clearance of Aβ. This, however, remains to be proven. Regardless, levels of APP-derived proteins in CSF are affected by both production and clearance of APP, and also by the ISF/CSF itself. This could make estimates of tissue levels in relation to CSF concentration problematic in patients with iNPH [30].

CSF APP-derived proteins increase after surgery, more in improved patients than in those that do not improve

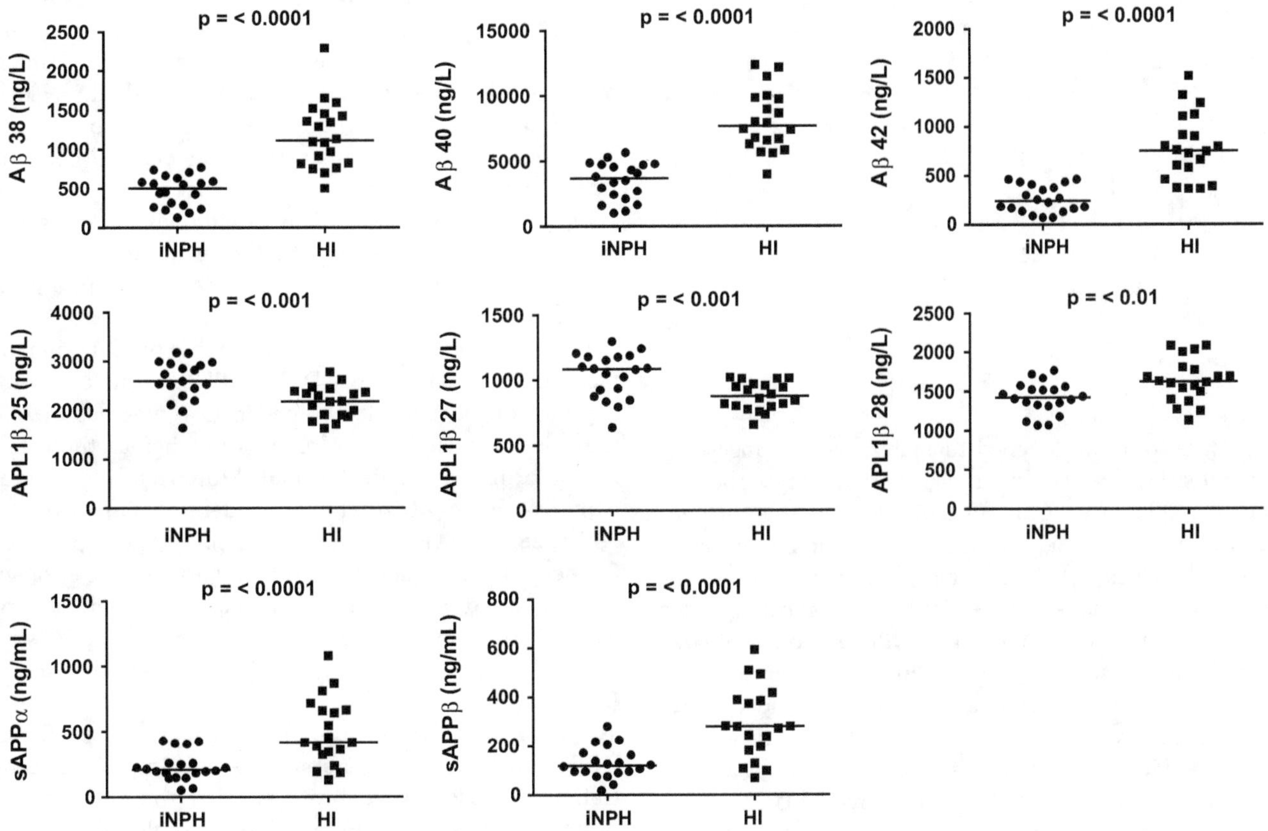

Fig. 1 Scatter plot showing CSF concentrations of Amyloids (Aβ38, 40, 42), APLP1 derivates (APL1β25, 27, 28) and amyloid precursor proteins (sAPPα, β) in 20 patients with iNPH and 20 controls. Medians are indicated by horizontal lines. P values indicate the level of significance. The differences between the difference in concentrations of APLP1-derived proteins are, although statistically significant, more modest

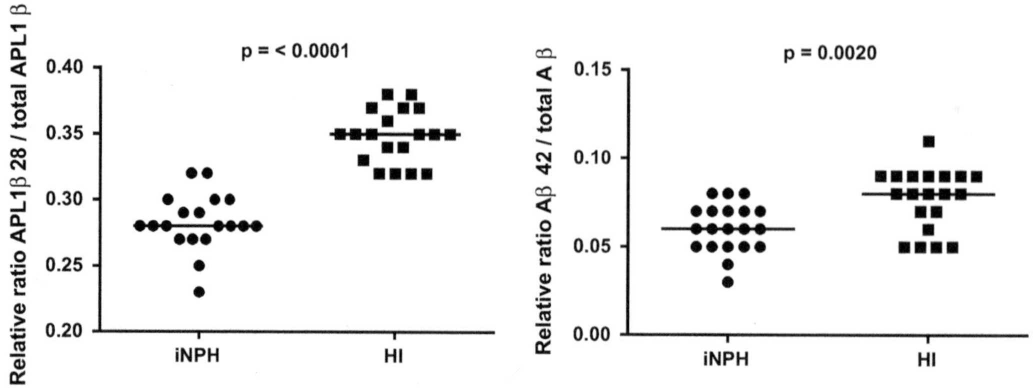

Fig. 2 The relative ratios of APL1β28 to total APL1β and Aβ42 to total Aβ in CSF in 20 patients with iNPH and 20 Controls. P values show the level of significance

Table 4 Levels of biomarkers in improved vs non-improved iNPH patents (median and IQ-range)

	Improved n = 10	Non-improved n = 10	
NFL (ng/L)	1186 (869–1670)	1085 (699–2432)	ns
APL1β25 (ng/L)	2532 (2174–2958)	2820 (2401–2954)	ns
APL1β27 (ng/L)	1067 (900–1157)	1085 (867–1214)	ns
APL1β28 (ng/L)	1423 (1264–1568)	1458 (1291–1562)	ns
Aβ38 (ng/L)	500 (308–605)	503 (224–677)	ns
Aβ40 (ng/L)	3731 (2642–4740)	3677 (1522–4789)	ns
Aβ42 (ng/L)	241 (155–370)	244 (122–438)	ns
sAPPα (ng/mL)	205 (175–279)	212 (144–297)	ns
sAPPβ (ng/mL)	114 (95–155)	127 (75–181)	ns
YKL40 (ng/mL)	122 (99–153)	134 (84–180)	ns

ns non-significant

[6, 11]. Even if not designed to analyze such changes, the present study does not contradict these findings. The presumed reduction in CSF concentrations of the amyloid-derived proteins could reflect a pathophysiological aspect of iNPH that is not directly linked with prediction. The irreversibility in non-improved iNPH patients could be due to either tissue damage related to iNPH or damage related to other factors such as co-morbidities e.g. cerebrovascular lesions, as there was a tendency of more profound WML in the non-improved group even if not reaching statistical significance. However, cerebrovascular disease is not a negative predictor of outcome after shunt surgery [31].

Contrary to the profound alterations in APP metabolites, the APLP1-derived peptides showed only minor changes with a small elevation in APL1β25 and APL1β27 and a slight reduction of APL1β28. APP and APLP1 are processed by the same enzymes, including γ-secretase [10, 12, 13, 32], and the results could indicate that the two substrates compete with each other at the active site of γ-secretase. If APP expression is reduced, as most data suggest it is in iNPH, there would be more γ-secretase available for the processing of APLP1. The processing occurs by γ-secretase cleaving at amino acid 28 of the membrane-spanning β-domain of APLP1 and then working its way towards the N-terminus of the protein. Increased processing of APLP1 by γ-secretase would thus result in decreased concentration of APL1β and increased concentrations of the shorter forms [33, 34]. This is exactly what we observe in iNPH. Over-expression of APP results in a decrease of APL1β, which supports this substrate competition hypothesis [35].

There is a difference in APP-metabolite production pattern between iNPH and AD. In iNPH there is a general suppression of APP-metabolites in CSF whereas in AD, there is an isolated Aβ42 reduction, whereas the other Aβ-isoforms are unaffected [36]. Moreover, the internal composition of Aβ production differs as shown in the APL1β28/total APL1β ratio. In our opinion, this provides further evidence against a common pathological etiology and might aid in the differential diagnosis of iNPH from AD by CSF biomarkers [37].

Conclusions

This data lends further support to a diagnostic profile in iNPH consisting of a general reduction in CSF concentration of APP-derived proteins. That the amyloid-like proteins behave in a different pattern could support the specificity and importance of the APP-down-regulation in iNPH. The study indicates that the biomarker profile in iNPH is consistent between patients who improve by shunt insertion and those who do not; therefore, our results do not lend support to the idea that these markers can be used for predictive purposes, but rather as an aid in the diagnosis of iNPH. Further studies will be needed to replicate the results and to expand the knowledge on the role of a possible altered amyloid metabolism for the pathogenesis of iNPH and the potential use of markers of amyloid metabolism to identify shunt responders needs to be further elucidated.

Abbreviations

iNPH: idiopathic normal pressure hydrocephalus; CSF: cerebrospinal fluid; Aβ: amyloid-β; sAPPα: α-cleaved soluble forms of amyloid precursor protein; sAPPβ: β-cleaved soluble forms of amyloid precursor protein; APLP1: APP-like protein 1; APL1β: APLP1 β-derived Aβ-like peptide; NFL: neurofilament light; WML: white matter lesion; ISF: interstitial fluid; BBB: blood–brain barrier.

Authors' contributions

AJ carried out the statistical analysis, participated in the design of the study and conceived the study, drafted the manuscript and participated in the coordination of the study. MK, HZ and KB carried out the laboratory analysis, participated in the design of the study and conceived the study. CW and MT conceived of the study and participated in the design and coordination and helped to write the manuscript. All authors read and approved the final manuscript.

Author details

[1] Hydrocephalus Research Unit, Institute of Neuroscience and Physiology, The Sahlgrenska Academy, University of Gothenburg, 413 45 Gothenburg, Sweden. [2] Department of Psychiatry and Neurochemistry, Institute of Neuroscience and Physiology, the Sahlgrenska Academy, University of Gothenburg, Gothenburg, Sweden. [3] Clinical Neurochemistry Laboratory, Sahlgrenska University Hospital, Molndal, Sweden. [4] Department of Molecular Neuroscience, UCL Institute of Neurology, Queen Square, London, UK.

Acknowledgements

The authors would like to thank the patients, and the staff at the Hydrocephalus Research Unit and the Clinical Neurochemistry Laboratory, especially Per Hellström who provided highly valuable help on statistical and clinical matters.

Competing interests

K. B. has served as a consultant and at advisory boards for IBL International, Fujirebio Europe and Roche Diagnostics. C. W. receives honoraria for lecturing and consulting by Codman, Johnson and Johnson. The other authors have no competing interests.

Study funding

This study was supported by grants from the Swedish Research Council, the European Research Council, Swedish State Support for Clinical Research (LUA-ALF), the Knut and Alice Wallenberg Foundation, the Torsten Söderberg Foundation, the Swedish Brain Foundation, Frimurarestiftelsen, the Göteborg Foundation for Neurological Research and the Neurological Research Foundation. The sponsors were not involved in the study design, in the collection, analysis and interpretation data; in the writing of the report; or in the decision to submit the paper for publication.

References

1. Hakim S, Adams RD. The special clinical problem of symptomatic hydrocephalus with normal cerebrospinal fluid pressure. Observations on cerebrospinal fluid hydrodynamics. J Neurol Sci. 1965;2:307–27.
2. Fisher CM. The clinical picture in occult hydrocephalus. Clin Neurosurg. 1977;24:270–84.
3. Klinge P, Hellström P, Tans J, Wikkelsø C. One-year outcome in the European multicentre study on iNPH. Acta Neurol Scand. 2012;126:145–53.
4. Andrén K, Wikkelsø C, Tisell M, Hellström P. Natural course of idiopathic normal pressure hydrocephalus. J Neurol Neurosurg Psychiatry. 2014;85:806–10.
5. McAllister JP, Williams MA, Walker ML, Kestle JRW, Relkin NR, Anderson AM, et al. An update on research priorities in hydrocephalus: overview of the third National Institutes of Health-sponsored symposium "opportunities for hydrocephalus research: pathways to better outcomes". J Neurosurg. 2015;123:1427–38.
6. Jeppsson A, Zetterberg H, Blennow K, Wikkelsø C. Idiopathic normal-pressure hydrocephalus Pathophysiology and diagnosis by CSF biomarkers. Neurology. 2013;80:1385–92.
7. Miyajima M, Nakajima M, Ogino I, Miyata H, Motoi Y, Arai H. Soluble amyloid precursor protein α in the cerebrospinal fluid as a diagnostic and prognostic biomarker for idiopathic normal pressure hydrocephalus. Eur J Neurol. 2013;20:236–42.
8. Ågren-Wilsson A, Lekman A, Sjöberg W, Rosengren L, Blennow K, Bergenheim AT, et al. CSF biomarkers in the evaluation of idiopathic normal pressure hydrocephalus. Acta Neurol Scand. 2007;116:333–9.
9. Ray B, Reyes PF, Lahiri DK. Biochemical studies in normal pressure hydrocephalus (NPH) patients: change in CSF levels of amyloid precursor protein (APP), amyloid-beta (Aβ) peptide and phospho-tau. J Psychiatr Res. 2011;45:539–47.
10. Eggert S, Paliga K, Soba P, Evin G, Masters CL, Weidemann A, et al. The proteolytic processing of the amyloid precursor protein gene family members APLP-1 and APLP-2 involves α-, β-, γ-, and ε-Like cleavages: modulation of APLP-1 processing by N-glycosylation. J Biol Chem. 2004;279:18146–56.
11. Moriya M, Miyajima M, Nakajima M, Ogino I, Arai H. Impact of cerebrospinal fluid shunting for idiopathic normal pressure hydrocephalus on the amyloid cascade. PLoS One. 2015;10(3):e0119973.
12. Jacobsen KT, Iverfeldt K. Amyloid precursor protein and its homologues: a family of proteolysis-dependent receptors. Cell Mol Life Sci. 2009;66:2299–318.
13. Yanagida K, Okochi M, Tagami S, Nakayama T, Kodama TS, Nishitomi K, et al. The 28-amino acid form of an APLPl-derived Aβ-like peptide is a surrogate marker for Aβ42 production in the central nervous system. EMBO Mol Med. 2009;1:223–35.
14. Tagami S, Okochi M, Yanagida K, Kodama T, Arai T, Kuwano R, et al. Relative ratio and level of amyloid-β 42 surrogate in cerebrospinal fluid of familial alzheimer disease patients with presenilin 1 mutations. Neurodegener Dis. 2014;13:166–70.
15. Laiterä T, Sarajärvi T, Haapasalo A, Puli L, Kauppinen T, Mäkinen P, et al. Increased γ-secretase activity in idiopathic normal pressure hydrocephalus patients with β-amyloid pathology. PLoS One. 2014;9(4):e93717.
16. Relkin N, Marmarou A, Klinge P, Bergsneider M, Black PM. Diagnosing idiopathic normal-pressure hydrocephalus. Neurosurgery. 2005;57:S4–16 **(discussion ii–v)**.
17. Hellström P, Klinge P, Tans J, Wikkelsø C. A new scale for assessment of severity and outcome in iNPH. Acta Neurol Scand. 2012;126:229–37.
18. Wahlund LO, Barkhof F, Fazekas F, Bronge L, Augustin M, Sjögren M, et al. A new rating scale for age-related white matter changes applicable to MRI and CT. Stroke. 2001;32:1318–22.
19. Tarnaris A, Toma AK, Pullen E, Chapman MD, Petzold A, Cipolotti L, et al. Cognitive, biochemical, and imaging profile of patients suffering from idiopathic normal pressure hydrocephalus. Alzheimers Dement. 2011;7:501–8.
20. Lins H, Wichart I, Bancher C, Wallesch CW, Jellinger KA, Rösier N. Immunoreactivities of amyloid β peptide(1-42) and total τ protein in lumbar cerebrospinal fluid of patients with normal pressure hydrocephalus. J Neural Transm. 2004;111:273–80.
21. Hulstaert F, Blennow K, Ivanoiu A, Schoonderwaldt HC, Riemenschneider M, De Deyn PP, et al. Improved discrimination of AD patients using β-amyloid (1–42) and tau levels in CSF. Neurology. 1999;52:1555–62.
22. Kapaki EN, Paraskevas GP, Tzerakis NG, Sfagos C, Seretis A, Kararizou E, et al. Cerebrospinal fluid tau, phospho-tau181 and β-amyloid 1–42 in idiopathic normal pressure hydrocephalus: a discrimination from Alzheimer's disease. Eur J Neurol. 2007;14:168–73.

23. Leinonen V, Menon LG, Carroll RS, Dello Iacono D, Grevet J, Jääskeläinen JE, et al. Cerebrospinal fluid biomarkers in idiopathic normal pressure hydrocephalus. Int J Alzheimers Dis. 2011;2011:312526. doi:10.4061/2011/312526.
24. Xie L, Kang H, Xu Q, Chen MJ, Liao Y, Thiyagarajan M, et al. Sleep drives metabolite clearance from the adult brain. Science. 2013;342:373–7.
25. Iliff JJ, Wang M, Liao Y, Plogg BA, Peng W, Gundersen GA, et al. A paravascular pathway facilitates CSF flow through the brain parenchyma and the clearance of interstitial solutes, including amyloid beta. Sci Transl Med. 2012;4:147ra11.
26. Shibata M, Yamada S, Ram Kumar S, Calero M, Bading J, Frangione B, et al. Clearance of Alzheimer's amyloid-β1-40 peptide from brain by LDL receptor-related protein-1 at the blood-brain barrier. J Clin Invest. 2000;106:1489–99.
27. Kress BT, Iliff JJ, Xia M, Wang M, Wei HS, Zeppenfeld D, et al. Impairment of paravascular clearance pathways in the aging brain. Ann Neurol. 2014;76:845–61.
28. Hashimoto M, Ishikawa M, Mori E, Kuwana N. Diagnosis of idiopathic normal pressure hydrocephalus is supported by MRI-based scheme: a prospective cohort study. Cerebrospinal Fluid Res. 2010;7:1.
29. Larsson A, Arlig A, Bergh AC, Bilting M, Jacobsson L, Stephensen H, et al. Quantitative SPECT cisternography in normal pressure hydrocephalus. Acta Neurol Scand. 1994;90:190–6.
30. Laiterä T, Kurki MI, Pursiheimo JP, Zetterberg H, Helisalmi S, Rauramaa T, et al. The expression of transthyretin and amyloid-β protein precursor is altered in the brain of idiopathic normal pressure hydrocephalus patients. J Alzheimers Dis. 2015;48:959–68.
31. Tullberg M, Jensen C, Ekholm S, Wikkelsø C. Normal pressure hydrocephalus: vascular white matter changes on MR images must not exclude patients from shunt surgery. AJNR Am J Neuroradiol. 2001;22:1665–73.
32. Sjödin S, Andersson KKA, Mercken M, Zetterberg H, Borghys H, Blennow K, et al. APLP1 as a cerebrospinal fluid biomarker for γ-secretase modulator treatment. Alzheimers Res Ther. 2015;7:1.
33. Portelius E, Price E, Brinkmalm G, Stiteler M, Olsson M, Persson R, et al. A novel pathway for amyloid precursor protein processing. Neurobiol Aging. 2011;32:1090–8.
34. Selkoe DJ, Wolfe MS. Presenilin: running with scissors in the membrane. Cell. 2007;131:215–21.
35. Portelius E, Hölttä M, Soininen H, Bjerke M, Zetterberg H, Westerlund A, et al. Altered cerebrospinal fluid levels of amyloid β and amyloid precursor-like protein 1 peptides in Down's syndrome. Neuromol Med. 2014;16:510–6.
36. Blennow K, Hampel H. CSF markers for incipient Alzheimer's disease. Lancet Neurol. 2003;2:605–13.
37. Graff-Radford NR. Alzheimer CSF biomarkers may be misleading in normal-pressure hydrocephalus. Neurology. 2014;83:1573–5.

4

The MRZ reaction in primary progressive multiple sclerosis

Tilman Hottenrott[1*], Rick Dersch[1], Benjamin Berger[1], Sebastian Rauer[1,3], Daniela Huzly[2] and Oliver Stich[1]

Abstract

Background: The MRZ reaction (MRZR), composed of the three antibody indices (AI) against measles, rubella and varicella zoster virus and found positive in the majority of relapsing-remitting multiple sclerosis (RRMS) patients, is absent in other inflammatory neurological diseases (OIND). So far, it has been uncertain whether its differential diagnostic promise extends to patients with primary-progressive multiple sclerosis (PPMS).

Objective: To investigate the prevalence of MRZR in PPMS compared to RRMS and OIND patients.

Methods: MRZR was assessed in patients with PPMS (n = 103), RRMS (n = 100) and OIND (n = 48). Both stringency levels for MRZR testing, MRZR-1 (≥1 AI positive) and MRZR-2 (≥2 AI positive), were applied.

Results: Prevalence of positive MRZR-1 was 83.5% in PPMS and 67.8% in RRMS ($p < 0.05$). A positive MRZR-2 was found in 54.4% of PPMS and in 43.0% of RRMS patients (not significant). Compared to both MS subgroups, OIND patients exhibit lower frequencies of positive MRZR (MRZR-1: 22.9%, MRZR-2: 8.3%; $p < 0.0001$ each).

Conclusion: Positive MRZR was at least as frequent in PPMS as in RRMS and much less frequent in OIND, confirming its promise as a potentially useful diagnostic tool for distinguishing both MS course types from OIND.

Keywords: Primary progressive multiple sclerosis, PPMS, Intrathecal polyspecific antiviral immune response, MRZ reaction, MRZR, Oligoclonal bands, OCB

Background

Multiple sclerosis (MS) is a chronic inflammatory autoimmune central nervous system (CNS) disorder displaying a variable disease course. At clinical onset, more than 85% of MS patients are classified as having relapsing-remitting MS (RRMS) [1]. These patients are predominately female and typically 20–30 years old at presentation of initial symptoms [1]. The remaining 10–15% of MS patients exhibit primary progressive MS (PPMS), characterised by a continuous worsening of symptoms from the onset, when patients are typically between 30 and 50 years old [1, 2]. PPMS affects men and women with similar frequency [1]. Both types of disease course exhibit inflammatory changes in the cerebrospinal fluid (CSF), e.g. the presence of oligoclonal bands (OCB), and inflammatory lesions in CNS detectable by magnetic resonance imaging (MRI) [1–3]. Diagnosis of PPMS and RRMS across the world today widely follows the 2010 revision of the McDonald criteria [4]. These require for PPMS a continuous disease progression of more than one year and that at least two of three additional criteria are met, one which is the presence of OCB in CSF. CSF analysis is no longer crucial for RRMS diagnosis, as here McDonald criteria primarily rely on clinical and MRI findings [4]. Despite their above mentioned similarities it is still a matter of debate whether PPMS and RRMS share sufficient underlying pathophysiological characteristics to be regarded as phenotypes of the same disorder and accordingly it cannot be taken as given that both will exhibit the MRZ reaction (MRZR) with similar frequency [3].

MRZR, first described in 1992, is a polyspecific, intrathecal humoral immune response to the three most frequent neurotropic viruses found in many RRMS patients: measles (M), rubella (R) and varicella zoster (Z),

*Correspondence: tilman.hottenrott@uniklinik-freiburg.de
[1] Department of Neurology and Neurophysiology, University Medical Center Freiburg, Breisacher Strasse 64, 79106 Freiburg, Germany

assessed using the three respective antibody indices (AI) [5]. A positive AI usually indicates intrathecal synthesis of antibodies against the respective pathogen, which is or recently was present in patient CSF. The absence of virus DNA in the CSF of MS patients with positive MRZ-AI led to the hypothesis of a 'bystander reaction', described as polyspecific B cell activation within the CNS [6]. While the pathophysiological role of MRZR may require further research, the interest in clinical practice is its potential to contribute to alternative diagnosis of MS. Whereas a positive MRZR is found in many RRMS patients, a few studies have shown negative MRZR in most patients with other autoimmune inflammatory neurological diseases (OIND) such as neuromyelitis optica (NMO), paraneoplastic neurological syndromes (PND), neurosarcoidosis (NS), acute disseminated encephalomyelitis (ADEM) and autoimmune encephalitis (AIE) [5, 7–9]. Additionally, MRZR has also been shown to be widely negative in patients with infectious CNS diseases which can mimic MS, such as Lyme neuroborreliosis and HTLV-I associated myelopathy [10, 11].

Studies showing a high prevalence of positive MRZR in MS to date are certainly fully applicable to RRMS; however the proportion of PPMS patients studied has been small, where any were included. Given current uncertainty about the similarity of PPMS and RRMS pathophysiology, and lack of understanding of the mechanisms linking MRZR to MS, our specific aim was to investigate MRZR in patients with PPMS.

Another limitation of previous studies has been the use of different criteria for positive MRZR. Some studies required only a single positive AI to constitute positive MRZR (MRZR-1), concluding that the prevalence of positive MRZR in MS is up to more than 90% [5], whereas others have required at least two AI positives for positive MRZR (MRZR-2), resulting in estimates of prevalence in MS of even below 50% [12].

This study investigated the prevalence of MRZR indicated by both the laxer MRZR-1 and the stricter MRZR-2 in a large cohort of PPMS patients. Results were compared to the prevalence of MRZR among patients with RRMS and some OIND.

Methods

Patients

This is a retrospective study in which all patients were treated at the University Medical Centre Freiburg in Germany between 2003 and 2015. Lumbar puncture (LP) had already been performed for all patients—for clinical purposes only and after written consent. CSF and serum samples were taken on the same day and stored according to consensus protocol for the standardization of CSF collection and biobanking [13]. Haemolytic CSF specimens were excluded. Diagnosis of MS was established according to the 2010 revised McDonald criteria, with particularly careful exclusion of relevant differential diagnoses [4]. All PPMS patients in the MS cohort were included for whom an MRZR measurement had been recorded or could be performed with existing CSF and serum samples. The MS cohort was screened for those with a recorded MRZR result, and from this set of MS patients, 100 RRMS patients were randomly drawn. The OIND group consisted of 48 patients for whom MRZR results were available from previous research, and unlike MS groups the OIND group did not include patients treated in 2015 [9]. Data concerning the ethnicity and immunization status of study patients was not available. The ethics committee of University Medical Centre Freiburg approved the study.

MRZR and CSF analysis

All MRZR assessments were performed at the Department of Virology of the University of Freiburg between 2003 and 2015. All other CSF measurements relevant to this study were carried out in the CSF laboratory at the Department of Neurology. The CSF laboratory at the Department of Neurology regularly takes part in the External Quality Control of Diagnostic Assays and Tests (EQAS) for CSF diagnostics, including protein analytics, and the laboratory at the Department of Virology regularly takes part in the EQAS for virus diagnostics, including virus serology. Both EQAS procedures are performed by Instand e.V. (Gesellschaft zur Förderung der Qualitätssicherung in medizinischen Laboratorien e.V.; Düsseldorf; Germany).

Total immunoglobulin (Ig) concentrations in serum and CSF were detected nephelometrically (ProSpect System, Siemens, Germany), whereas measles-, rubella- and varicella-IgG (IgGspec) levels in CSF and serum were measured by enzyme linked immunosorbent assay (Serion *classic* ELISA, Germany), both according to the manufacturer's instructions. MRZR was determined from the three respective virus-specific AI which were calculated as follows: $AI = Q_{IgG[spec]}/Q_{IgG[total]}$, if $Q_{IgG[total]} < Q_{lim}$, and $AI = Q_{IgG[spec]}/Q_{lim}$, if $Q_{IgG[total]} > Q_{lim}$ according to Reiber's formula [14]. For a positive AI finding the threshold of $AI \geq 1.5$ was applied [9, 10, 12, 15]. Previous studies have varied as to how many positive AIs are required for positive MRZR. In this study, MRZR-2 is used to refer to the MRZR definition requiring two or more positive AI, and MRZR-1 to refer to the MRZR definition requiring only one or more positive AI. Where an AI could not be calculated because no antibodies were detected in the CSF, AI was considered to be 1.0 (negative). CSF laboratory records were used which routinely include total CSF cell count, significant quantitative intrathecal antibody synthesis (defined as ≥10%), IgG index, QIgG, IgG concentration in CSF and presence or absence of oligoclonal bands (OCB) according to the Reibergrams and the CSF consensus report [16]. Detection of OCB for patients was performed using a highly sensitive isoelectric focusing technique on agarose gel followed by immunofixation (Hydragel Isofocusing, sebia, France) [17]. A positive OCB finding is defined as two or more OCB [16].

Statistical analysis

Statistical testing of differences between groups on gender, prevalence of positive AI, MRZR, intrathecal Ig synthesis and OCB was performed using Fisher's exact test (two-tailed). Differences of mean values of AI, total CSF cell count, intrathecal Ig synthesis, QIgG, IgG concentrations in CSF and age between groups were tested using Student's *t* test (two-tailed). A p value <0.05 was regarded as statistically significant. The correlation between MRZR and OCB status was measured using the Phi correlation coefficient (ϕ). A correlation coefficient between 0.2 and 0.4 was considered as weak, between 0.4 and 0.6 as intermediate and >0.6 as strong.

Results

Study population

The complete 2003–2015 cohort consisting of 1668 patients with a recorded MS diagnosis was retrospectively screened for MS subtype, RRMS or PPMS, following the 2010 McDonald criteria [4]. 236 PPMS patients (14.1%) were found of whom 96 had to be excluded due to missing CSF/serum samples and 37 due to insufficient clinical data, resulting in a PPMS group of 103 well-characterized patients. A random sample of 100 RRMS patients already tested for MRZR for clinical reasons was drawn from the same MS cohort. Additionally, an existing group of 48 patients with OIND was drawn on for comparison. Twenty-two of this OIND group had been diagnosed with neurosarcoidosis (NS), 19 with autoimmune encephalitis (AIE) and 7 with acute disseminated encephalomyelitis (ADEM). Table 1 shows key demographic features of the three study groups.

Virus-specific antibody indices (AI)

Results of AI tests of the three study groups are shown in Table 2. No statistically significant differences were found between the two MS groups in respect of frequency of one, two or three positive AIs and mean values of any of the three AI (M, R and Z). However, a positive AI for M and R was statistically significantly more frequent in PPMS compared to RRMS. Compared to both MS subgroups, the OIND group showed lower mean AI values and less frequent positive AI for all three viruses.

MRZR

In accordance with AI findings, positive MRZR was found in a minority of OIND patients (MRZR-2: 8.3%, MRZR-1: 22.9%), statistically significantly less than in either of the MS subtypes (PPMS MRZR-2: 54.4%, PPMS MRZR-1: 83.5%; RRMS MRZR-2: 43.0%, RRMS MRZR-1: 69.0%—see Fig. 1).

Merging the two MS subtypes (PPMS and RRMS, n = 203) confirms that frequencies of both positive MRZR-2 (48.8%) and MRZR-1 (76.4%) among MS patients are statistically significantly different to those found in the OIND group ($p < 0.0001$ each).

Comparison of MRZR results with previous studies

Table 3 presents MRZR results from the present study alongside those from previous studies. For these studies, findings from both MRZR definitions (MRZR-2 and MRZR-1) are listed where these could be reconstructed from the data provided in the relevant publication.

OCB

As can be seen from Fig. 2, the prevalence of positive OCB in CSF was similar in the two MS groups (93.2% for PPMS and 87.0% for RRMS) and significantly higher than in the OIND group (31.2%).

OCB and MRZR

As presented in Tables 4 and 5, there was a weakly positive correlation between OCB and MRZR status (applying to both MRZR-2 and MRZR-1) in the combined MS group. Among the few OCB negative MS patients,

Table 1 Demographic data of all study patients

Study group	PPMS (n = 103)	RRMS (n = 100)	OIND (n = 48)	Comparison statistics
Gender, females in %	60.2	73.0	41.7	p < 0.05 for both MS groups vs. OIND; between MS groups: n.s.
Mean age in years at LP (range; SD)	51.3 (25–78; 10.0)	40.0 (19–74; 11.3)	51.8 (4–84; 18.4)	p < 0.0001 for PPMS and OIND vs. RRMS; between PPMS and OIND: n.s.

PPMS primary progressive multiple sclerosis, *RRMS* relapsing-remitting multiple sclerosis, *OIND* other autoimmune inflammatory neurological diseases comprising 22 patients with neurosarcoidosis (NS), 19 with autoimmune encephalitis (AIE) and 7 with acute disseminated encephalomyelitis (ADEM), *n* number of patients, *LP* lumbar puncture, *SD* standard deviation, *n.s.* not significant

Table 2 Antibody indexes for all study patients

	PPMS (n = 103)	RRMS (n = 100)	OIND (n = 48)	Comparison statistics
Patients with 0 positive AI	16.5%	31.0%	77.1%	p < 0.0001 for both MS groups vs. OIND; p < 0.05 between MS groups
Patients with 1 positive AI	29.1%	26.0%	14.6%	all comparisons: n.s.
Patients with 2 positive AI	25.2%	25.0%	6.3%	p < 0.01 for both MS groups vs. OIND; between MS groups: n.s.
Patients with 3 positive AI	29.1%	18.0%	2.1%	p < 0.01 for both MS groups vs. OIND; between MS groups: n.s.
Positive AI for M	62.1%	48.0%	6.3%	p < 0.001 for both MS groups vs. OIND; p < 0.05 between MS groups
Positive AI for R	57.3%	43.0%	12.5%	p < 0.001 for both MS groups vs. OIND; p < 0.05 between MS groups
Positive AI for Z	48.5%	39.0%	14.6%	p < 0.05 for both MS groups vs. OIND; between MS groups: n.s.
Mean AI for M (range; SD)	3.3 (0.8–20.3; 3.2)	3.2 (0.6–52.2; 6.3)	1.0 (0.6–2.6; 0.3)	p < 0.01 for both MS groups vs. OIND; between MS groups: n.s.
Mean AI for R (range; SD)	3.1 (0.5–24.0; 4.0)	3.0 (0.5–19.8; 4.0)	1.2 (0.6-8.3; 1.2)	p < 0.01 for both MS groups vs. OIND; between MS groups: n.s.
Mean AI for Z (range; SD)	3.0 (0.6–19.8; 3.7)	2.5 (0.6–25.4; 3.5)	1.2 (0.4–3.8; 0.6)	p < 0.05 for both MS groups vs. OIND; between MS groups: n.s.

PPMS primary progressive multiple sclerosis, *RRMS* relapsing-remitting multiple sclerosis, *OIND* other autoimmune inflammatory neurological diseases, *positive AI* antibody index for measles (M), rubella (R) or varicella zoster (Z) ≥1.5, *n.s.* not significant

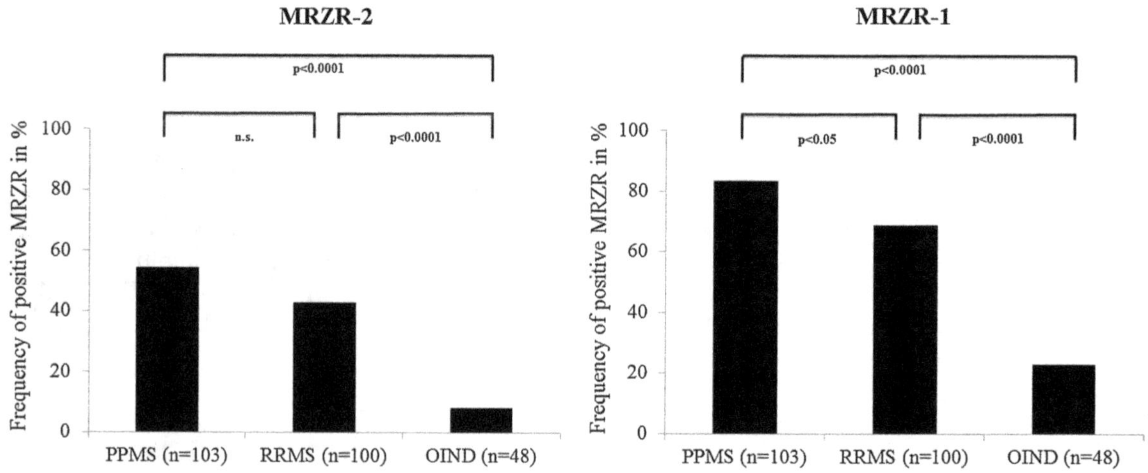

Fig. 1 Frequency of positive MRZR-2 and MRZR-1 in patients with PPMS, RRMS and OIND. Frequency of positive MRZR-2 and MRZR-1 in patients with primary progressive multiple sclerosis (PPMS), relapsing-remitting multiple sclerosis (RRMS) and other autoimmune inflammatory neurological diseases (OIND). *MRZR-2* one or more positive AI, *MRZR-1* two or more positive AI, *n.s.* not significant

15.0 and 30.0% showed positive MRZR-2 and MRZR-1 respectively.

CSF routine findings in MS patients

Inflammatory CSF changes were found in 93.2% of PPMS patients and in 87% of RRMS patients (n.s.). The most frequent pathological CSF finding was positive OCB (see above) followed by quantitative intrathecal IgG synthesis (51.5% in PPMS patients and 50.0% in RRMS; n.s.), elevated total CSF cell count (PPMS: 22.3%, RRMS: 43.0%; p < 0.01), quantitative intrathecal IgM synthesis (PPMS: 8.7%, RRMS: 14.8%; n.s.) and quantitative intrathecal IgA synthesis (PPMS: 7.8%, RRMS: 8.0%; n.s.). The data from the routine CSF analyses are presented in Table 6.

Discussion

To our knowledge, this is the first systematic investigation of the MRZR in a distinct PPMS cohort of reasonable size, and comparison with RRMS and OIND. The two main results are that positive MRZR is at least as frequent in PPMS as in RRMS patients and significantly more frequent than among OIND patients.

Study population

PPMS patients showed typical demographic features: a more balanced gender distribution and a higher average age than RRMS patients [3, 18]. It has to be mentioned that diagnosis of RRMS can usually now be made earlier than at the mean age of this cohort (39 years). The high

Table 3 A comparison of MRZR studies in multiple sclerosis patients

Study	Number of MS patients (MS subtypes)	Positive MRZR-2	Positive MRZR-1
Present study	n = 203 (PPMS: n = 103, RRMS: n = 100)	49%	76%
Reiber et al. [15]	n = 177 (no data concerning subtype)	[67%]	89%
Felgenhauer et al. [5]	n = 100 (no data concerning subtype)	[72%]	94%
Rosche et al. [24]	n = 68 (RRMS: n = 61, CIS: n = 7)	58%	[n.a.]
Brettschneider et al. [12]	n = 49 (CIS patients who converted to MS within 2 years)	47%	[n.a.]
Brecht et al.[a] [19]	n = 46 (RRMS: n = 26, SPMS: n = 12, PPMS: n = 8)	[24%]	46%
Jarius et al. [7]	n = 42 (RRMS: n = 29, SPMS: n = 4, CIS: n = 9)	88%	[n.a.]
Bednarova et al. [10]	n = 42 (no data concerning subtype)	[47%]	88%
Hottenrott et al. [9]	n = 33 (RRMS: n = 14, SPMS: n = 5, PPMS: n = 14)	70%	[82%]
Kulakowska et al.[b] [22]	n = 27 (RRMS: n = 21, PPMS: n = 6)	[56%]	81%
Tumani et al. [23]	n = 26 (no data concerning subtype)	[n.a.]	73%
Robinson-Agramonte et al. [21]	n = 23 (incomplete data concerning subtype)	[48%]	100%

The studies are presented in descending order of number of patients

Numbers in brackets were calculated by the author from data available in the respective article where possible

MRZR-1 one or more positive antibody indices (AI) for measles (M), rubella (R) and varicella zoster (Z), *MRZR-2* two or more positive AI, *CIS* clinical isolated syndrome, *SPMS* secondary progressive multiple sclerosis, *PPMS* primary progressive multiple sclerosis, *RRMS* relapsing-remitting multiple sclerosis, *n.a.* not available

[a] This study investigated only OCB-negative MS patients

[b] This study included AI for HSV

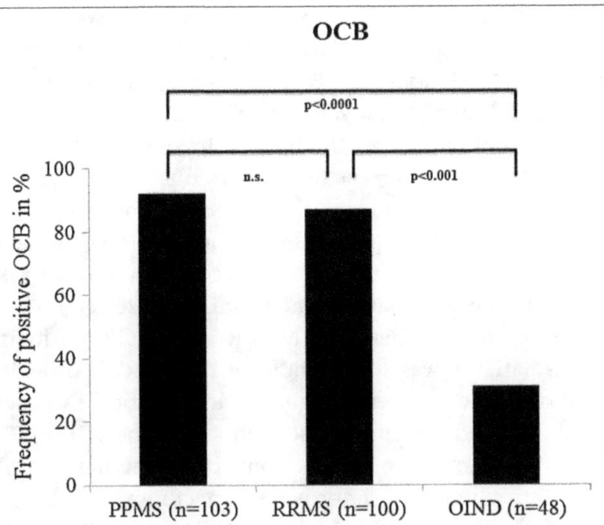

Fig. 2 Prevalence of OCB in CSF of patients with PPMS, RRMS and OIND. Prevalence of oligoclonal bands (OCB) in cerebrospinal fluid (CSF) of patients with primary progressive multiple sclerosis (PPMS), relapsing-remitting multiple sclerosis (RRMS) and other autoimmune inflammatory neurological diseases (OIND), *n.s.* not significant

average age of RRMS patients might be a consequence of selection bias, as discussed below.

AI and MRZR

Frequencies of positive AI and AI mean values in both MS groups (M > R > Z) were similar compared to a previous study but inverse in OIND patients (M < R < Z, Table 2) [15]. The rather low frequency of positive MRZR-2 in the OIND group indicates that MRZR-2 might be particularly helpful in distinguishing both MS subtypes from OIND. The less rigorous MRZR-1 is clearly less specific, showing more false positive results in OIND. This was also found in another recent study in tertiary care, where MRZ-1 was found to be positive in 19% of patients with OIND (well in line with the 23% in our OIND group) and 8% of patients with other non-inflammatory neurological diseases (OND), whereas none of these 53 patients were MRZR-2 positive [19]. Up to now, there is no indication of a pathophysiological role of any of the three MRZ viruses in MS pathogenesis, unlike in the case of the Epstein-Barr-virus (EBV) where it was shown that after EBV infection the risk of developing MS is increased [20].

Table 3 illustrates how inconsistent results of MRZR studies can appear if differences in definition (MRZR-2 vs. MRZR-1) are not considered. After clearly distinguishing between MRZR-2 and MRZR-1, the MRZR results from this study align quite well with most previous research. The study shows positive MRZR-1 in 76% of MS patients, which is less frequent than in some earlier studies [5, 10, 15, 21]. But, the frequency of positive MRZR-1 is closely in line with two other recent studies [22, 23]. Furthermore, several studies established a similar frequency of MRZR-2 positives of around 50% [10, 12, 21, 22, 24]. Exceptionally, Jarius et al. reported a considerably higher proportion of positive MRZR-2 (88%) in their MS cohort, which was used in two MRZR studies

Table 4 Correlation between the presence of oligoclonal bands and MRZR-2 in patients with multiple sclerosis

Combined MS group (n = 203)	OCB positive	OCB negative		Association metrics
MRZR-2 positive	96	3	99	
MRZR-2 negative	87	17	104	
	183	20	203	$\phi = 0.22$

OCB positive ≥2 oligoclonal bands in CSF, *MRZR-1* one or more positive antibody indices (AI) for measles (M), rubella (R) and varicella zoster (Z), *MRZR-2* two or more positive AI, *positive AI* AI ≥ 1.5, combined MS group: all primary progressive multiple sclerosis patients (n = 103) and relapsing-remitting multiple sclerosis patients (n = 100), ϕ Phi correlation coefficient

Table 5 Correlation between the presence of oligoclonal bands and MRZR-1 in patients with multiple sclerosis

Combined MS group (n = 203)	OCB positive	OCB negative		Association metrics
MRZR-1 positive	149	6	155	
MRZR-1 negative	34	14	48	
	183	20	203	$\phi = 0.36$

OCB positive ≥2 oligoclonal bands in CSF, *MRZR-1* one or more positive antibody indices (AI) for measles (M), rubella (R) and varicella zoster (Z), *MRZR-2* two or more positive AI, *positive AI* AI ≥ 1.5, combined MS group: all primary progressive multiple sclerosis patients (n = 103) and relapsing-remitting multiple sclerosis patients (n = 100), ϕ Phi correlation coefficient

[7, 8]. Reasons for this divergence remain elusive, but selection bias is a conceivable explanation. Unfortunately, study reports did not include a detailed description of patient selection. In the present study, there may have been selection bias in the RRMS group, due to including patients with MRZR already previously performed for clinical reasons. Though such a bias might have contributed to their unexpectedly high mean age, this was actually similar to the mean age of MS patients in an even larger retrospective CSF study (not addressing MRZR) [25]. There is a lower risk of selection bias in the PPMS group because all available PPMS patients were included in the analysis, where possible. This is supported by the fact that our PPMS group matches demographic characteristics of PPMS patients studied elsewhere very well [1, 3, 18]. Limitations of this study include the monocenter cohort, the retrospective design and the lack of data concerning ethnicity and vaccination status of enrolled patients. Infection rates and vaccination status in respect of the three MRZ viruses can influence MRZR results, as has been demonstrated for the rubella virus in Cuba [21]. Therefore, verification of the MRZR results for PPMS patients with known vaccination status, and expansion to a multicenter prospective study, including populations from different parts of the world, would be a valuable next step.

OCB and other CSF routine parameters

As expected, a high and very similar prevalence of OCB of around 90% was found in PPMS and RRMS patients-confirming the high sensitivity of this CSF parameter for both MS subgroups. The prevalence of OCB in PPMS and RRMS patients found here matches the findings of a previous monocenter Canadian study investigating 451 MS patients with CSF analyses performed between 1993 and 2007 [25]. In that study positive OCB was reported in 91% of RRMS and in 85% of PPMS patients.

Though the high prevalence of OCB in MS patients can be useful, a diagnostic disadvantage of OCB is their high prevalence in related conditions of diagnostic importance, in particular OIND. For example, OCB can be found in 40% of patients with neurosarcoidosis and in 50% of patients with neurologic complications of systemic lupus erythematosus (neuro-SLE) [9, 26].

The correlation between MRZR and OCB positivity in MS patients was weak, showing that MRZR provides additional, independent diagnostic information as previously reported for clinical isolated syndrome (CIS) [12]. One important issue in this context is whether MRZR tests can potentially improve the accuracy of diagnosis based on the 2010 revised McDonald criteria [4].

Table 6 Results of routine CSF analysis for MS patients

	PPMS (n = 103)	RRMS (n = 100)	Comparison statistics
Total CSF cell count in/µl (range; SD)	4.1 (1–43; 5.9)	8.9 (1–47; 10.3)	$p < 0.001$
Intrathecal IgG synthesis in % (range; SD)	19.8 (0–75.4; 21.8)	21.6 (0–84.3; 25.0)	n.s.
Intrathecal IgA synthesis in % (range; SD)	3.8 (0–54.9; 12.6)	2.1 (0–47.4; 7.5)	n.s.
Intrathecal IgM synthesis in % (range; SD)	5.0 (0–92.4; 17.0)	6.1 (0–88.3; 16.8)	n.s.
IgG index (range; SD)	0.93 (0.45–2.83; 0.42)	1.02 (0.23–4.0; 0.65)	n.s.
QIgG × 10^{-3} (range; SD)	5.3 (2.0–16.9; 3.1)	5.2 (1.0–15.8; 3.3)	n.s.
IgG concentration in CSF in mg/l (range; SD)	60.7 (19.4–217.0; 42.4)	55.9 (9.1–206.0; 39.8)	n.s.

PPMS primary progressive multiple sclerosis, *RRMS* relapsing-remitting multiple sclerosis, *IgG* immunoglobuline G, *IgA* immunoglobuline A, *IgM* immunoglobuline M, *QIgG* quotient of IgG, *SD* standard deviation, *n.s* not significant. All group values are expressed as means

Referring to Tables 4 and 5, it appears that a combination of MRZR and OCB criteria could extend diagnostic sensitivity for the small proportion of OCB negative MS patients with 15% MRZR-2 positive and 30% MRZR-1 positive results. This seemingly contradicts findings in a group of 177 MS patients in which no patient was found MRZR positive and OCB negative [15]. This led the authors to recommend testing for MRZR only in OCB positive patients. However, the very high OCB prevalence in that study group (98%) meant that there were only three or four OCB negative patients, so that it could easily be a result of chance that none of these patients were found MRZR positive. MRZR/OCB findings of the present study are in line with a recent study in which MRZR-2 positives made up even 24% of 46 OCB negative MS patients [19]. Apart from that, MRZ-specific OCB were found in nearly 50% of MS patients without routine OCB [17]. Taking these results together, testing for MRZR in OCB negative patients with suspected MS appears well justified.

Considering the other CSF routine parameters, only the total cell count differed between the two MS subgroups: RRMS patients more often showed an elevated total cell count and a higher mean total cell count compared to PPMS patients. All Ig parameters (total IgG concentration in CSF, QIgG and intrathecal IgG/M/A synthesis) were similar between PPMS and RRMS patients paralleling the MRZR-2 results and indicating that these two MS subgroups seemingly display similar humoral immune responses in CSF.

Conclusions

Positive MRZR has now been shown to be at least as frequent in PPMS patients as in RRMS, suggesting MRZR could be used in the diagnostic workup for both subtypes of MS in a similar way. MRZR has also been found to be less prevalent in OIND patients compared to OCB indicating that particularly the stricter MRZR-2 measure may well be helpful in the critical task of distinguishing OIND from MS. Altogether, these study results further support the significance of CSF analysis as an important tool to ensure alternative diagnoses of MS are promptly detected and properly treated [27].

Authors' contributions

TH initiated this study and drafted the manuscript. RD performed the statistical analysis and helped to draft the manuscript. BB helped to draft the manuscript. DH supervised performance of the immunoassays in the Institute of Virology. OS and SR participated in study design and helped to draft the manuscript. All authors read and approved the final manuscript.

Author details

[1] Department of Neurology and Neurophysiology, University Medical Center Freiburg, Breisacher Strasse 64, 79106 Freiburg, Germany. [2] University Medical Center Freiburg, Institute of Virology, Hermann-Herder-Strasse 11, 79104 Freiburg, Germany. [3] Ravo Diagnostika GmbH, Oltmannsstrasse 5, 79100 Freiburg, Germany.

Acknowledgements

Special thanks are due to the staff of the Institute of Virology who performed the immunoassays, to the staff of the CSF laboratory at the Department of Neurology who analysed the CSF/serum samples and especially to Simon Robinson who helped to improve linguistic clarity. This research received no specific grant from any funding agency in the public, commercial or not-for-profit sectors.

Competing interests

TH received travel grants from Bayer Vital GmbH and Novartis. RD reports no competing interests with this study. BB received travel grants from Bayer Vital GmbH, Ipsen and Genzyme. DH received lecture fees from Serion. OS and SR report receiving consulting and lecture fees, grant and research support from Baxter, Bayer Vital GmbH, Biogen Idec, Genzyme, Merck Serono, Novartis, RG, Sanofi-Aventis and Teva. Furthermore, SR indicates that he is a founding executive board member of ravo Diagnostika GmbH (Oltmannsstrasse 5, D-79100 Freiburg, Germany), which is selling in vitro diagnostic medical devices for the detection of infectious diseases and paraneoplastic autoantibodies.

Funding

This research received no specific grant from any funding agency in the public, commercial or not-for-profit sectors. The cost of the article-processing charge was covered by the Albert Ludwig University of Freiburg.

References

1. Lublin FD, Reingold SC. Defining the clinical course of multiple sclerosis: results of an international survey. National Multiple Sclerosis Society (USA) Advisory Committee on Clinical Trials of New Agents in Multiple Sclerosis. Neurology. 1996;46:907–11.
2. Runmarker B, Andersen O. Prognostic factors in a multiple sclerosis incidence cohort with twenty-five years of follow-up. Brain. 1993;116:117–34.
3. Antel J, Antel S, Caramanos Z, et al. Primary progressive multiple sclerosis: part of the MS disease spectrum or separate disease entity? Acta Neuropathol. 2012;123:627–38.
4. Polman CH, Reingold SC, Banwell B, et al. Diagnostic criteria for multiple sclerosis: 2010 revisions to the McDonald criteria. Ann Neurol. 2011;69:292–302.
5. Felgenhauer K, Reiber H. The diagnostic significance of antibody specificity indices in multiple sclerosis and herpes virus induced diseases of the nervous system. Clin Investig. 1992;70:28–37.
6. Godec MS, Asher DM, Murray RS, et al. Absence of measles, mumps, and rubella viral genomic sequences from multiple sclerosis brain tissue by polymerase chain reaction. Ann Neurol. 1992;32:401–4.
7. Jarius S, Franciotta D, Bergamaschi R, et al. Polyspecific, antiviral immune response distinguishes multiple sclerosis and neuromyelitis optica. J Neurol Neurosurg Psychiatry. 2008;79:1134–6.
8. Jarius S, Eichhorn P, Jacobi C, et al. The intrathecal, polyspecific antiviral immune response: specific for MS or a general marker of CNS autoimmunity? J Neurol Sci. 2009;280:98–100.
9. Hottenrott T, Dersch R, Berger B, et al. The intrathecal, polyspecific antiviral immune response in neurosarcoidosis, acute disseminated encephalomyelitis and autoimmune encephalitis compared to multiple sclerosis in a tertiary hospital cohort. Fluids Barriers CNS. 2015;12:27.
10. Bednarova J, Stourac P, Adam P. Relevance of immunological variables in neuroborreliosis and multiple sclerosis. Acta Neurol Scand. 2005;112:97–102.
11. Puccioni-Sohler M, Kitze B, Felgenhauer K, et al. The value of CSF analysis for the differential diagnosis of HTLV-I associated myelopathy and multiple sclerosis. Arq Neuropsiquiatr. 1995;53:760–5.
12. Brettschneider J, Tumani H, Kiechle U, et al. IgG antibodies against measles, rubella, and varicella zoster virus predict conversion to multiple sclerosis in clinically isolated syndrome. PLoS ONE. 2009;4:e7638.
13. Teunissen CE, Petzold A, Bennett JL, et al. A consensus protocol for the standardization of cerebrospinal fluid collection and biobanking. Neurology. 2009;73:1914–22.
14. Reiber H, Lange P. Quantification of virus-specific antibodies in cerebrospinal fluid and serum: sensitive and specific detection of antibody synthesis in brain. Clin Chem. 1991;37:1153–60.

15. Reiber H, Ungefehr S, Jacobi C. The intrathecal, polyspecific and oligoclonal immune response in multiple sclerosis. Mult Scler. 1998;4:111–7.
16. Andersson M, Alvarez-Cermeño J, Bernardi G, et al. Cerebrospinal fluid in the diagnosis of multiple sclerosis: a consensus report. J Neurol Neurosurg Psychiatry. 1994;57:897–902.
17. Stich O, Kluge J, Speck J, et al. Oligoclonal restriction of antiviral immunoreaction in oligoclonal band-negative MS patients. Acta Neurol Scand. 2014;. doi:10.1111/ane.12350.
18. Cottrell DA, Kremenchutzky M, Rice GP, et al. The natural history of multiple sclerosis: a geographically based study. 5. The clinical features and natural history of primary progressive multiple sclerosis. Brain. 1999;122:625–39.
19. Brecht I, Weissbrich B, Braun J, et al. Intrathecal, polyspecific antiviral immune response in oligoclonal band negative multiple sclerosis. PLoS ONE. 2012;7:e40431.
20. Levin LI, Munger KL, O'Reilly EJ, et al. Primary infection with the Epstein-Barr virus and risk of multiple sclerosis. Ann Neurol. 2010;67:824–30.
21. Robinson-Agramonte M, Reiber H, Cabrera-Gomez JA, et al. Intrathecal polyspecific immune response to neurotropic viruses in multiple sclerosis: a comparative report from Cuban patients. Acta Neurol Scand. 2007;115:312–8.
22. Kułakowska A, Mroczko B, Mantur M, et al. Multiplexing analysis of the polyspecific intrathecal immune response in multiple sclerosis. Methods. 2012;56:528–31.
23. Tumani H, Tourtellotte WW, Peter JB, et al. Acute optic neuritis: combined immunological markers and magnetic resonance imaging predict subsequent development of multiple sclerosis. The Optic Neuritis Study Group. J Neurol Sci. 1998;155:44–9.
24. Rosche B, Laurent S, Conradi S, et al. Measles IgG antibody index correlates with T2 lesion load on MRI in patients with early multiple sclerosis. PLoS ONE. 2012;7:e28094.
25. Siritho S, Freedman MS. The prognostic significance of cerebrospinal fluid in multiple sclerosis. J Neurol Sci. 2009;279:21–5.
26. Deisenhammer F, Bartos A, Egg R, et al. Guidelines on routine cerebrospinal fluid analysis. Report from an EFNS task force. Eur J Neurol. 2006;13:913–22.
27. Tumani H, Deisenhammer F, Giovannoni G, et al. Revised McDonald criteria: the persisting importance of cerebrospinal fluid analysis. Ann Neurol. 2011;70:520 **(author reply 521)**.

5

The choroid plexus as a site of damage in hemorrhagic and ischemic stroke and its role in responding to injury

Jianming Xiang[1], Lisa J. Routhe[2], D. Andrew Wilkinson[1], Ya Hua[1], Torben Moos[2], Guohua Xi[1] and Richard F. Keep[1,3*]

Abstract

While the impact of hemorrhagic and ischemic strokes on the blood–brain barrier has been extensively studied, the impact of these types of stroke on the choroid plexus, site of the blood-CSF barrier, has received much less attention. The purpose of this review is to examine evidence of choroid plexus injury in clinical and preclinical studies of intraventricular hemorrhage, subarachnoid hemorrhage, intracerebral hemorrhage and ischemic stroke. It then discusses evidence that the choroid plexuses are important in the response to brain injury, with potential roles in limiting damage. The overall aim of the review is to highlight deficiencies in our knowledge on the impact of hemorrhagic and ischemic strokes on the choroid plexus, particularly with reference to intraventricular hemorrhage, and to suggest that a greater understanding of the response of the choroid plexus to stroke may open new avenues for brain protection.

Keywords: Intraventricular hemorrhage, Subarachnoid hemorrhage, Intracerebral hemorrhage, Cerebral ischemia, Choroid plexus, Cerebrospinal fluid, Blood–brain barrier

Background

The choroid plexuses (CPs) are present in the lateral, third and fourth ventricles of the brain (LVCP, 3rd CP, 4th CP). Each CP is comprised of epithelial cells surrounding a richly vascularized core [1]. Compared to the cerebral capillaries that form the blood–brain barrier (BBB), CP capillaries are leakier with the endothelial cells having fenestrations, reflecting the role of the CPs in CSF secretion [2–6]. The CPs are the site of the blood-CSF barrier, with the CP epithelial cells being linked by tight junctions that limit paracellular diffusion [1, 7].

Many neurological conditions result in BBB dysfunction, including ischemic and hemorrhagic strokes [8–11]. That dysfunction participates in brain injury by, for example, causing vasogenic brain edema, allowing the entry of potentially neurotoxic compounds from blood to brain, and promoting leukocyte infiltration and neuroinflammation. In contrast to the wealth of studies on BBB injury, much less is known about whether CP injury occurs after stroke [12, 13]. One purpose of the present review is to discuss what is currently known about such injury. It addresses hemorrhagic and ischemic stroke, with a particular focus on the former including intraventricular hemorrhage (IVH), subarachnoid hemorrhage (SAH) and intracerebral hemorrhage (ICH).

Another purpose is to review a body of evidence that the CPs respond to injury (that may be distant from the CP) by releasing factors that protect the brain [14–16]. This has led to experimental studies with CP transplantation for a variety of conditions [17–19]. That section also addresses a related topic, namely the role of the CP in leukocyte entry into the brain after injury. Results on the protective effects of the CP in brain injury/disease may help to inform studies on the role of cerebral endothelial cells.

*Correspondence: rkeep@umich.edu
[1] Department of Neurosurgery, University of Michigan, R5018 BSRB, 109 Zina Pitcher Place, Ann Arbor, MI 48109-2200, USA

Choroid plexus as a site of injury

This section discusses evidence of CP injury in different forms of stroke in humans and animals. In human studies, it discusses morphological (post-mortem), imaging and permeability data to assess injury. One advantage of studies on the CP compared to the BBB is that the CSF (unlike the brain) can be sampled in patients, although it should be noted that CSF composition can reflect changes at both the blood-CSF and blood–brain barriers. In animal studies, the CP itself, as well as the CSF, can be sampled. Inflammatory changes will be discussed in the next section (CP as a responder to injury). Additionally, this section examines whether hemorrhage (particularly bleeding within the ventricles) can cause CP injury. It does not discuss the CP being the site of initial bleeding, although some evidence indicates CP hemorrhage is a major cause of IVH in babies born at full term [20] and can occur at other ages [21, 22].

Intraventricular hemorrhage

IVH commonly occurs in premature infants as a result of germinal matrix hemorrhage. It is a major cause of cerebral palsy in such infants and is often associated with later development of hydrocephalus [23]. In adults, intraventricular extension of bleeding occurs in ~50% of patients with ICH and ~45% of patients with SAH [24, 25]. Such ventricular extension is a risk factor for poor outcome after both ICH and SAH [25–27]. ICH is known to cause perihematomal tissue damage [28] and BBB dysfunction [10]. Clot-derived factors, including hemoglobin, iron and thrombin, play a major role in ICH-induced injury [28]. Despite this evidence in ICH and the proximity of intraventricular blood to the CPs, we did not find clinical studies examining the effects of IVH on the CP epithelial morphology in the literature. Clinically, IVH results in changes in CSF protein concentrations (e.g. [29–33]). While changes in blood-CSF barrier function are one parameter that can affect those concentrations, assessing barrier function from such data is very difficult, particularly in the setting of IVH. Thus, for example, total CSF protein is elevated after IVH [29], but this may reflect protein originating from the initial hemorrhage, protein influx at the BBB as well as the blood-CSF barrier and production from brain parenchyma. Examining the CSF/plasma ratio of specific proteins, such as albumin [30, 32], helps address the latter point, but albumin will still enter CSF from the initial IVH as well as any potential BBB disruption.

In animals, Simard et al. [34] examined a rat IVH model at 2 days and found induction of inflammatory signaling (nuclear factor κB activation) within the CP along with a significant intracellular uptake of IgG. Furthermore, Gram et al. [35] found a marked inflammatory response in a rabbit preterm model of IVH at 1 and 3 days. This was accompanied by CP cell death, caspase activation and pronounced ultrastructural changes. Similar inductions in inflammatory mediators and cell death were obtained in vitro when CP epithelial cells were exposed to met-hemoglobin, heme or CSF from preterm babies with IVH [35]. The hemoglobin scavenger, haptoglobin, prevented the adverse effects of IVH in vivo and hemoglobin or IVH CSF in vitro [35].

In contrast, Pang et al. [36] found only subtle changes in CP morphology at 3 months in a dog IVH model. In comparison, the ependymal lining of the lateral ventricles was destroyed or interrupted in many areas. Interestingly, they also examined the effects of urokinase in their model to lyse the IVH and found that this protected the ependyma but also resulted in CP atrophy in some animals for unknown reasons. While it is possible that there may be species differences in the effects of IVH on the CP, a more likely reason for the differences between the studies are the time points examined. As described below, in SAH and ischemia there is evidence of acute injury followed by a recovery in CP structure, although the latter may be accompanied by a reduction in CP size. Acute studies (1–3 days) in larger species and chronic studies in rodents would be informative (Fig. 1).

As opposed to the paucity of data on CP injury in human IVH or animal models, there is considerable data on damage to the ependymal cells that line the cerebral ventricles. Thus, Fukumizu et al. [37, 38] found marked ependymal damage and loss in human neonatal IVH. Mayfrank et al. [39] used a pig IVH model with and without tissue plasminogen activator-induced fibrinolysis and, similar to Pang et al. [36] in dog, they found marked IVH-induced ependymal damage at 1 and 7 weeks and that was reduced by fibrinolysis. In rat, Simard et al. [34] found that ependymal cells took up IgG at 48 h post IVH and Gao et al. [40] found ependymal damage 1 day after intracerebroventricular (ICV) injection of Fe^{3+}, a degradation product of hemoglobin. These results indicate that there can be acute and chronic ependymal damage after IVH. In the CP after ischemic injury, there is evidence of tissue repair with time (see below). Why this does not happen in the ependyma is uncertain but it might relate to the ability of the CP to shrink in size when shedding dead cells. Because of the physical contact between the ependyma and underlying brain, such shrinkage is not possible for the ependyma.

Subarachnoid hemorrhage

SAH is often associated with extension of blood into the ventricular system (30–50%; [25, 27]). IVH is a risk factor for poor prognosis in SAH and for the development of hydrocephalus and vasospasm [25, 27, 41]. Rosen

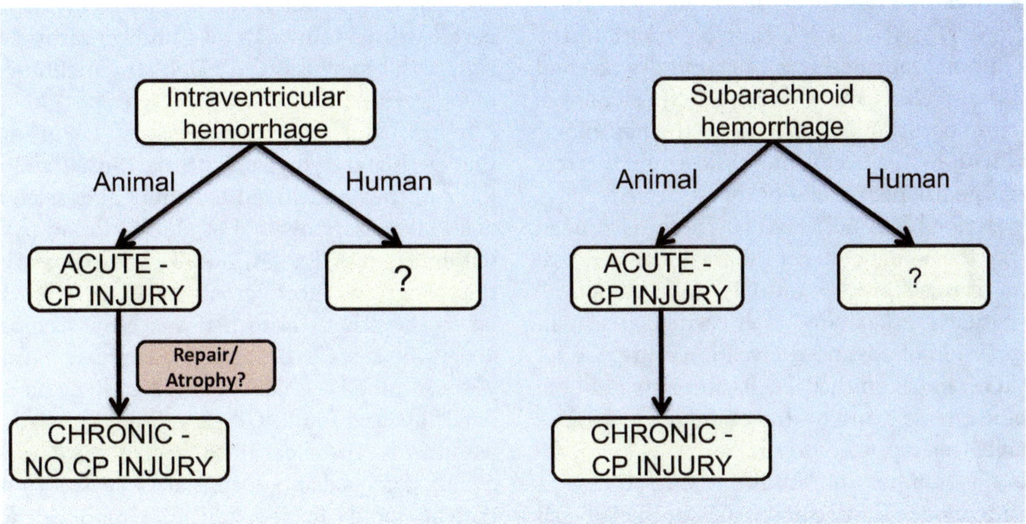

Fig. 1 In general, there is a surprising lack of data on the effects of intraventricular and subarachnoid hemorrhage on choroid plexus (CP) injury, particularly in humans. In intraventricular hemorrhage, there are studies indicating acute CP damage but this may be absent in the long-term. This could reflect repair mechanisms (see Fig. 2 for cerebral ischemia) and there is a need for longitudinal studies in the same model. For subarachnoid hemorrhage, there is evidence for both acute and chronic CP injury

et al. [25] found that hydrocephalus developed in 62% of SAH patients with IVH compared to 26% of patients without IVH. Post-hemorrhagic hydrocephalus is generally assumed to result from a block in the CSF flow pathways or fibrosis at CSF outflow sites [42, 43]. Whether SAH (with or without associated IVH) causes CP injury has not to our knowledge been examined in patients. Given the preclinical data indicating that SAH causes CP damage in animals, this gap in knowledge needs to be corrected.

Several studies using cisterna magna blood injection in rabbits have reported effects on the CP (Fig. 1). Liszczak et al. [44] reported CP changes including electron-dense cytoplasmic inclusions and expansion of the lateral and subcellular spaces. Yilmaz et al. [45] examined both choroidal artery vasospasm and CP injury (using an injury scoring system) at 20 days and found evidence of a correlation between choroidal artery constriction and CP damage after SAH. In another study, the presence of water filled spaces within the CP was examined at 2 and 14 days after SAH [46]. There was a marked increase in the numbers of such spaces, particularly at 2 days and the authors hypothesized that these changes may be related to altered CSF secretion. Furthermore, changes in CP morphology, with reduced epithelial cell and microvillus height, and many TUNEL-positive cells have been reported 10 days after SAH (24% of cells in animals surviving SAH and 42% in animals that died) [47].

As in humans, animal models of SAH can also cause hydrocephalus. Thus, using a endovascular perforation model of SAH (perforation at the internal carotid artery bifurcation), Okobu et al. [48] found evidence of acute hydrocephalus in about 40% in rats. A question that has not been totally resolved is whether there has to be blood in the ventricles to induce CP injury and hydrocephalus, although Okobu et al. [48] found that hydrocephalus was always associated with blood in the ventricular system.

Intracerebral hemorrhage

Intraventricular extension of bleeding is a common finding in ICH and a risk factor for poor outcome [24, 26]. Whether ICH without such IVH can impact CP function has not been examined. Even though there is no extension of blood into the ventricular system, products from clot degradation may move into the CSF [49].

Ischemic stroke

In humans, the blood supply to the LVCP comes from the anterior, lateral posterior and medial posterior choroidal arteries [50]. The blood supply to the third ventricle CP comes from the bilateral medial posterior choroidal arteries [51], while that to the fourth ventricle CP is from the anterior and posterior inferior cerebellar arteries and the superior cerebellar artery [52]. The rich collateral circulation for each of the CPs may help protect them from focal ischemic events. Thus, using magnetic resonance imaging (MRI), only three CP infarcts have been described in the literature. Two related to choroidal artery occlusion [53, 54] and one due to a basilar artery occlusion [55]. Brain infarcts from anterior choroid artery (AChA) occlusion have been described by multiple groups (e.g. [56–59]). The AChA supplies multiple tissues (e.g. the internal capsule, optic tract and the cerebral peduncle; [58]) as well as the LVCPs. Whether changes in LVCP function occur and contribute to the neurological symptoms with AChA occlusion is uncertain. Infarcts related to the medial posterior choroidal arteries have rarely been described [54, 60] (Fig. 2). There have been few studies on the impact of transient global cerebral ischemia (e.g. cardiac arrest) on CP injury/function. However, in patients resuscitated after cardiac arrest, an increased expression of advanced glycation end-product receptors (RAGE) in CP epithelial cells and amyloid beta in both CP blood vessels and on the epithelial basement membrane have been reported [61, 62].

In animals, a number of studies using transient global ischemia models have shown CP epithelial cell death (Fig. 2). Thus, Pulsinelli et al. [63], using permanent bilateral basilar artery occlusion with 30 min transient common carotid artery occlusion (4VO model) in rats, found ischemic necrosis in the CP at 6 h and this is earlier than found in hippocampus suggesting selective vulnerability. Also, using the rat 4VO model, LVCP atrophy (~35%) [64] and histological damage [65] have been reported. Other studies have reported widespread epithelial cell death and CP edema early during reperfusion (0–12 h) after bilateral common carotid artery occlusion (10 min) with hypotension (2VO + hypotension) [66, 67]. Furthermore, CP DNA fragmentation occurred after 2VO + hypotension in rats at 18–24 h [68, 69]. In gerbils with 5 min bilateral common carotid artery occlusion with reperfusion, CP DNA fragmentation was found at ~1 week [70, 71].

In neonatal rats, Rothstein and Levinson [72] found that perinatal hypoxia/ischemia caused cell death in the CP and they concluded that the CP is selectively vulnerable. Likewise, Towfighi et al. [73] found pyknotic nuclei within the rat CP a few hours after hypoxia/ischemia and this progressed to necrosis by 24 h. Interestingly, similar to the adult, those necrotic cells disappeared within 4 days of the CP becoming atrophied. Sivakumar et al. [74] examined the effects of 2 h of hypoxia alone in neonatal rats and found CP morphological signs of injury at 3 and 24 h. These began to resolve at 3 days with the CPs having a normal appearance at 14 days. It should be noted that one study in neonatal mice reported no damage to the CP after hypoxia/ischemia injury [75]. It is interesting, however, that many of these studies report a recovery in CP structure and loss of damaged cells with time [63, 64, 66–69, 73]. This recovery may reflect the loss of damaged cells, the recruitment of new cells or both. The CP atrophy reported by Dienel [64] and Towfighi et al. [73] suggests the former, but there is some evidence for cell recruitment (see below). In terms of blood-CSF barrier function, barrier disruption was reported by Ikeda et al. [70] after bilateral common carotid occlusion in the gerbil. Similarly, Ennis and Keep [76] reported blood-CSF barrier disruption at 6 h after 2VO + hypotension in the rat.

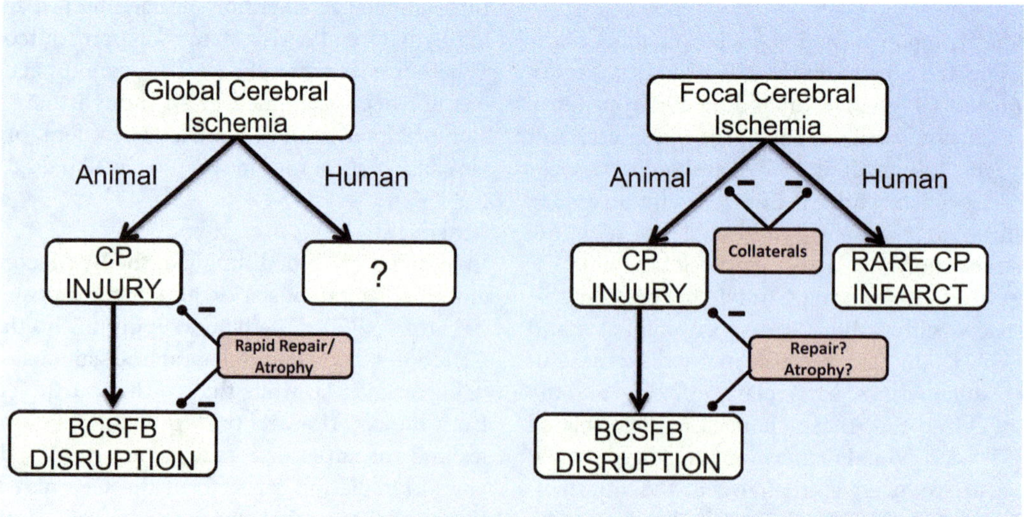

Fig. 2 In animal studies, there is evidence that both transient global cerebral ischemia and focal cerebral ischemia cause choroid plexus (CP) injury and blood-CSF barrier (BSCFB) disruption. There is evidence that the damage after global ischemia is quickly repaired and this probably involves shedding of damaged cells resulting in CP atrophy. This has not been examined in focal cerebral ischemia. In humans, the effects of transient global cerebral ischemia (e.g. cardiac arrest) on the CP have not been examined. There are very rare reports of CP infarcts after focal cerebral ischemia in patients, but the occurrence of CP damage after focal cerebral ischemia is almost certainly limited by the rich collateral circulation to the CP

There have been few studies on CP injury after focal ischemia [76–79] (Fig. 2). It should be noted that the commonly used suture model of middle cerebral artery (MCA) occlusion can result in reduced blood supply to the LVCP [76] as the branch point for the AChA from the internal carotid artery is close to the bifurcation of the MCA [80]. In the rat, Ennis and Keep [76] found a 38% decrease in LVCP blood flow after MCA occlusion and there was a 53% reduction if the animals underwent a tandem common carotid artery occlusion. Nagahiro et al. [79] examined the effects of different durations of tandem MCA and internal carotid occlusion in rats. They found evidence of blood-CSF barrier disruption with MRI using gadolinium-diethylene triamine pentaacetic acid (Gd-DTPA) in animals with 15 and 30 min of ischemia with 6 h of reperfusion, whereas BBB disruption was only found with longer (60 min) periods of ischemia. They did not find evidence of CP morphological changes after 6 h of reperfusion by H&E staining. Li et al. [78], studying 2 h transient MCA occlusion and reperfusion in rats, reported that CP cells became swollen (1–4 days) and that there was bromodeoxyuridine (BrdU) staining indicating cell proliferation, perhaps in compensation for CP cell death. No BrdU staining was observed in the CP in non-ischemic rats. Interestingly, the BrdU staining after MCA occlusion was not limited to the LVCP, but also occurred in the 3rd and 4th CPs indicating effects on proliferation distant to the ischemic parenchyma. Gillardon et al. [77] found evidence of LVCP epithelial cell death (TUNEL staining) after 6 h but not 1.5 h of permanent MCA occlusion in the rat and Ennis and Keep [76] found evidence of LVCP edema after MCA occlusion in rats with and without tandem common artery occlusion.

A number of co-morbidities increase the risk of ischemic stroke and result in more severe brain injury after stroke. These include aging, hypertension, hyperlipidemia and hyperglycemia and they are known to enhance BBB dysfunction after stroke [81]. The effects of such co-morbidities on CP injury after ischemic stroke are unknown. However, even in the absence of stroke, it is known that aging and Alzheimer's disease result in CP dysfunction [5, 82–84].

Choroid plexus as a responder to injury

As well as being a site of injury, the CP may be involved in a neuroprotective response after brain injury. This includes CP secretion of protective factors, the CP as a site of neurogenesis/progenitor cell migration, the CP as a site of leukocyte infiltration (although this may have beneficial and detrimental effects) and potential changes in CSF production (Fig. 3). The evidence on such roles is limited and, therefore, this section discusses brain injury/disease in general and not just stroke. It should be noted that responses can be to brain injuries that are distant to the CP raising the question of how those injuries are 'sensed'.

Growth factor/neuropeptide release

The CPs produce a wide range of peptides/proteins: e.g. adrenomedullin, basic fibroblast growth factor (bFGF)-2, insulin-like growth factor (IGF)-2, transthyretin, transforming growth factor (TGF) β and vasopressin, many of which are secreted into the CSF [14–16]. There they can impact periventricular cells but they may also have an autocrine function since the CPs also possess an array of receptors: e.g. the FGFR1 and FGFR2 for fibroblast growth factor, IGF-1R and IGF-2R for insulin-like growth factor, TβRII for TGFβ, and the vasopressin receptors V_{1a}, V_{1b} and, during development, V_2 [14]. There is evidence of CP-induced neuroprotection via growth factor release in a number of injury and disease states including stroke (see below) and traumatic brain injury [15, 85]. It should be noted, however, that some peptide release by the CP can have adverse effects. Thus, for example, there is evidence that vasopressin exacerbates brain injury after stroke [14].

With respect to animal models of stroke, studies have focused on cerebral ischemia and not the CP response to cerebral hemorrhage. Knuckey et al. [86] found that TGFβ-1, -2 and -3 mRNA expression in the CP increased at day 1 and 2 after transient global ischemia (2VO + hypotension), returning to normal at day 3. Those changes in mRNA expression were not mirrored in altered CP protein expression and it was suggested that increased mRNA levels might reflect secretion into CSF. Increases in CSF TGFβ-1 have been reported in ischemic stroke and SAH [87, 88]. In cerebral ischemia, TGFβ-1 appears to be neuroprotective [89, 90] but it may have an adverse effect in IVH-induced and other forms of hydrocephalus [42, 91].

Hayamizu et al. [92] used immunohistochemistry to examine the effects of transient global cerebral ischemia (2VO + hypotension) on bFGF-2 expression in the CP and found that ischemia caused a marked decrease in cytoplasmic (but not apical or lateral membrane associated) expression from 6 h to 14 days post-ischemia. The loss of cytoplasmic staining was interpreted as reflecting CP to CSF secretion. Since ICV injection of bFGF-2 is protective in animal models of global ischemia [93, 94], this suggests that CP secretion has a protective role. Beilharz et al. [95] examined the response of IGF-1 and -2 and different IGF binding proteins (IGFBP) to hypoxia/ischemia in 3 weeks-old rats. They found that IGFBP-6 mRNA and protein was induced in the CP (as well as the ependymal and reactive glial cells) and hypothesized that IGFBP-6 binds particularly to IGF-2 limiting adverse

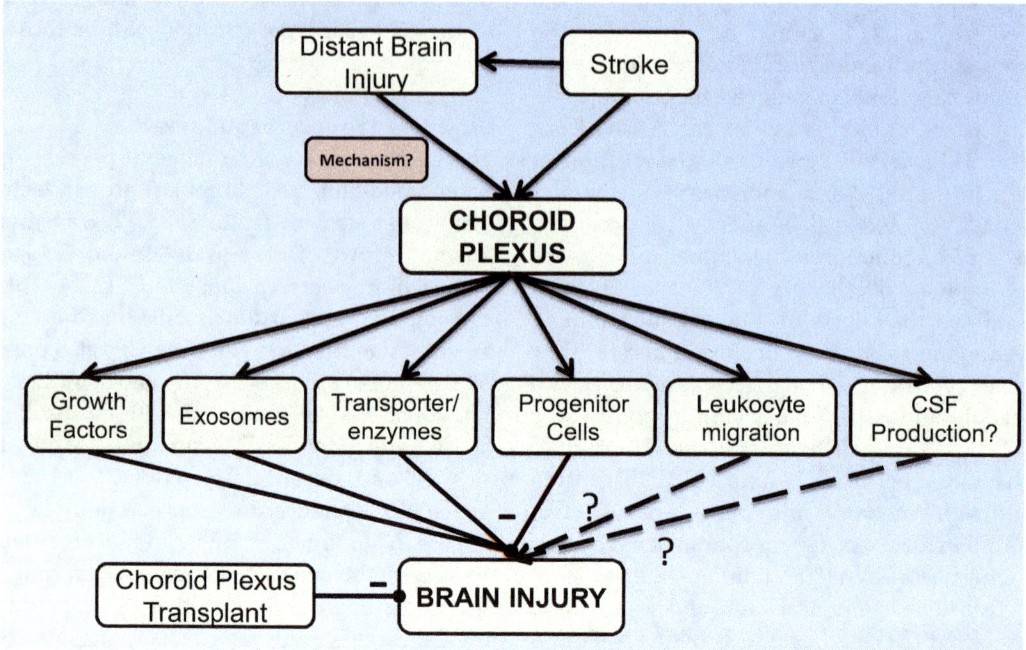

Fig. 3 As well as being a potential site of injury after stroke, the choroid plexus (CP) also responds to stroke in multiple ways that may modify brain injury. It should be noted that the potential protective CP responses may be elicited by injury distant from the CP, indicating an unknown signaling mechanism. While most of the CP responses are thought to be protective, the effects of leukocyte diapedesis and changes in CSF production (if any) are uncertain. Elucidation of protective mechanisms involving the CP led to studies where CPs or CP epithelial cell transplants were used in animals with ischemic stroke with evidence of neuroprotection

effects of IGF-2 after hypoxia/ischemia. Sivakumar et al. [74] found increased VEGF mRNA and protein levels in the CP at different times after 2 h of hypoxia in neonatal rats. VEGF expression is regulated by hypoxia-inducible factor α and VEGF concentrations in CSF are increased by conditions causing brain hypoxia [96]. Additionally, there are multiple papers indicating a protective effect of ICV administered VEGF in ischemic stroke [97–100] suggesting that CP production of VEGF could have protective effects in stroke. However, it should be noted that Liu et al. [101] recently found that ICV administration of an anti-VEGF receptor-2 antibody reduced early brain injury in a mouse SAH model.

A concern with such growth factor studies is that using data on CP mRNA or protein expression to imply secretion into CSF could be misleading. It should be noted, however, that there is also in vitro data indicating such secretion. For example, Borlongan et al. [18] found that CP explants secrete glial-derived neurotrophic factor, brain-derived neurotrophic factor and nerve growth factor. Another concern is the relative importance of the CPs in secreting such factors into CSF after stroke compared to other brain areas. Data using selective inhibition of CP growth factor production during stroke would be very informative (e.g. CP specific inducible KO mice; [102]).

With respect to human stroke, Flood et al. [87] examined CSF TGFβ1 in patients who had hydrocephalus after SAH and found markedly increased CSF levels early and late after SAH. While the initial rise was probably related to platelet-derived TGFβ1, the authors found that late increase in CSF levels correlated with increased CP expression. Adrenomedullin is a vasoactive peptide that is secreted by the CP and other non-BBB areas of the brain. After SAH, there is an early (day 3) and particularly a late (day 8) increase in CSF adrenomedullin that does not correlate with plasma levels. Higher CSF levels were correlated with an increased risk of delayed ischemic neurological deficits, occurrence of hyponatremia and reduced appetite [103, 104]. Whether the elevated CSF adrenomedullin levels are due to increased CP secretion has not been directly examined.

Apart from secreting proteins directly into CSF, recent evidence indicates that CP epithelial cells also secrete exosomes into the CSF [105–107]. These contain proteins, microRNAs and other components and form another type of communications between CP and the brain parenchyma [105–107]. The role of exosomes in the protective effects of the CP in brain injury is still unclear.

Choroid plexus enzymes and transporters

As well as secreting factors that may influence brain damage, the CPs also express many enzymes and transporters that may be important in the response to injury. Thus, unlike the CSF, the CP has high fibrinolytic activity [108, 109] and this may play a role in intraventricular hematoma resolution. In addition, considering the role that iron, as a degradation product of hemoglobin, has in brain injury after cerebral hemorrhage [28, 110, 111], it is noteworthy that the CP expresses a very wide array of iron-handling proteins including transporters: e.g. divalent metal transporter-1, ferroportin, transferrin and transferrin receptor-1 and -2, the iron storage protein ferritin, the heme metabolizing enzyme heme oxygenase-1, and proteins that change the oxidative sate of iron (ceruloplasmin and hephaestin) [112, 113]. The role of the CP in handling hemoglobin and iron after IVH merits further investigation. In relation to Alzheimer's disease, the CP plays a role in regulating amyloid-β degradation and the levels of amyloid-β in the brain were reduced in a mouse model of Alzheimer's disease by CP implants [17].

Choroid plexus transplantation

Because of the evidence that the CP can protect the brain from injury, there have been a number of studies examining the effects of CP transplants on different types of brain injury. Borlongan et al. found that transplanting rat [114] or pig [18] choroid plexus into the CNS protected against cerebral ischemia in rats. Matsumoto et al. [115] also showed similar protection with cultured choroid plexus epithelial cells in rat MCA occlusion. Outside cerebral ischemia, Bolos et al. [17] found that CP epithelial cell transplants reduced amyloid-β deposits, tau hyperphosphorylation and astrocytic reactivity in a mouse model of Alzheimer's disease. They also improved behavioral outcomes including memory tests. Similarly, transplants of CP epithelial cells have enhanced axonal regeneration and locomotor improvement in rat spinal cord injury [19, 116]. Compared to approaches that focus on a single factor (e.g. a growth factor) to promote brain protection/recovery, CP epithelial cells transplants may have an advantage in producing multiple factors. It is also possible that the CP epithelial cells may have a modified response dependent upon the type of injury. Thus, for example, will CP epithelial cells exposed to an ischemic brain produce the same growth factor and express the same enzymes as those exposed to a brain with Alzheimer's disease?

Choroid plexus proliferation and progenitor cells

In the adult CP, there is only a slow turnover of epithelial cells in rodents and primates [117, 118]. However, there is in vitro evidence that injury and growth factors (IGF and epidermal growth factor) can cause CP epithelial cell proliferation [119]. In vivo, Li et al. [78] found increased CP cell proliferation (BrdU positive cells) after MCA occlusion in the rat. The overall impact of such proliferation on CP injury in vivo is as yet uncertain (i.e. can it replace the cell loss caused by stroke?) and some of the BrdU cells were neuronal nuclear antigen (NeuN) and glial fibrillary acidic protein positive leading Li et al. to suggest they were neural precursor cells [78].

There has been considerable interest in the use of exogenous stem cells, either administered systemically or into the brain, to treat different neurological conditions. Endothelial progenitor cells administered intravenously can integrate into the cerebral endothelium after stroke and may be a source of growth factors [120]. Whether that is the case for the CP is unclear. Zhang et al. [121] found that bone marrow-derived endothelial progenitor cells migrated to the CP endothelium after intravenous injection in non-ischemic mice and Beck et al. [122] also found that bone marrow-derived cells given intravenously migrated to the CP in ischemic (MCA occlusion) and non-ischemic mice. They were uncertain whether those cells were integrating into the CP endothelium or migrating through the CP. However, mesenchymal stem cells given ICV can integrate into the CP epithelium [123, 124].

Leukocyte migration at the choroid plexus

In stroke, neuroinflammation may have both detrimental and beneficial effects. Thus, an early influx of leukocytes (particularly neutrophils) into the brain from the blood may exacerbate ischemic and hemorrhagic brain injury [125, 126], but a later inflammation may be beneficial in brain repair [127–129]. In the case of cerebral hemorrhage, infiltrating macrophages/resident microglia have an important role in hematoma resolution via phagocytosis [130, 131]. Infiltrating leukocytes may enter the brain across the BBB or the blood-CSF barrier after a stroke. While there is a wealth of knowledge about leukocyte entry at the BBB in stroke, studies on the role of the CP are very limited. Kowarik et al. [132] compared CSF levels of leukocytes in patients across multiple neurological conditions. For stroke (a mixture of ischemic and hemorrhagic), they examined CSF within 4 weeks of onset. Unlike some conditions (e.g. bacterial or viral meningitis), stroke was not associated with high CSF leukocyte counts nor did it alter the distribution of leukocyte subsets. The majority of CSF leukocytes after stroke were CD4+ T cells (71%) and CD8+ T cells (17%). A fuller time course of such changes in CSF, particularly soon after stroke, would be informative.

The CP is thought to be involved in immune surveillance by trafficking T-lymphocytes [133, 134]. In a model of hypoxia/ischemia with systemic inflammation (lipopolysaccharide; to mimic intrauterine infection) in rats, Yang et al. [135] found an early (4 h) infiltration of T-lymphocytes (CD43+) into the CP. This was blocked by fingolimod (FTY720; a sphingosine-1-phosphate receptor modulator) treatment which also markedly reduced the brain injury in lipopolysaccharide-enhanced hypoxia/ischemia injury. In other neurological conditions, such as multiple sclerosis, traumatic brain injury, spinal cord injury and meningitis, as well as peripheral inflammation, there has been interest in the role of the CP in leukocyte entry into CSF and brain [3, 136, 137]. For example, Szmydynger-Chodobska et al. [138, 139] found that the CP is a site of neutrophil and monocyte entry into the brain after traumatic brain injury (controlled cortical impact). It is interesting that in those studies the CPs are distant from the site of initial injury raising the question as to what signaling mechanisms trigger the diapedesis of leukocytes at the CP.

CSF production

Alterations in CSF production could impact brain injury. Increases could aid in the clearance of neurotoxic factors from the brain (CSF sink effect) but might also exacerbate hydrocephalus. With regards to the latter, choroid plexus hyperplasia and choroid plexus papillomas are associated with CSF hypersecretion and hydrocephalus [140]. Decreases in CSF production might serve to decrease the incidence of hydrocephalus and reduce intracranial pressure, and CP cauterization has been used as a treatment for hydrocephalus [141, 142]. After stroke, there is a lack of data on whether CSF production is changed. However, Holloway and Cassin [143] did report a 33% decline in CSF production with hypoxia in neonatal dogs.

The water channel, aquaporin 1 (Aqp1) is highly expressed in the CP epithelium and Aqp1 knockout mice have reduced CSF secretion [144]. There has, therefore, been an interest in examining the effects of stroke on Aqp1 expression. In the 4VO model of transient global cerebral ischemia, Akdemir et al. [65] reported an increase AQP1 protein expression in the CP epithelium between 24 and 48 h of reperfusion. Similarly, Sveinsdottir et al. [145] found an increase in CP Aqp1 protein expression in a preterm rabbit IVH model. However, at the mRNA level, there was a decrease in expression, an effect replicated in vitro by exposing cultured CP epithelial cells to the CSF of preterm infants with IVH or hemin. The reason for the different protein and mRNA responses are uncertain. Interestingly, Sveinsdottir et al. [145] also examined the expression of another aquaporin, Aqp5. They found a marked increase in both protein and mRNA expression in the preterm rabbit IVH model for that aquaporin and they also found increased Aqp5 mRNA after exposure of CP epithelial cells to hemin in vitro. This merits further investigation.

Injury sensing by the choroid plexus

In the earlier descriptions of stroke-induced CP injury, this review has focused on types of injury that directly impact the CP, including reductions in CP blood flow or blood in the ventricular system adjacent to the CPs. However, there is evidence that events distant from the CPs may trigger protective responses in the CP. For example, traumatic brain injury that does not directly impact the CP results in growth factor production [15, 85], alters CP protein expression (e.g. [146]), and infiltration of leukocytes across the CP [138], and Li et al. [78] found increased cell proliferation in CPs distant to the parenchymal damage induced by a MCA occlusion. How does the CP sense that distant injury and what pathways in the CP are triggered to elicit the protective response? As noted above, the CP expresses a wide range of peptide/protein receptors [14] and these may be involved, but these are as yet largely unaddressed questions.

Choroid plexus and cerebral endothelial responses to stroke

Our knowledge of the effects of stroke on cerebral endothelial cells, the site of the BBB, is much greater than at the CP epithelium. There are also differences in the types of experiment that can be performed in relation to each tissue. For example, with the cerebral endothelium, two-photon microscopy using fluorescently-tagged permeability markers and endothelial proteins (e.g. cells expressing GFP-tagged claudin-5) can be used to study stroke-induced BBB disruption in real time [147]. Such techniques can not currently be used to study the deeply-situated CPs. However, CP studies have an advantage in that CSF can be sampled (in animals and humans) in contrast to the cerebral endothelium studies where adjacent brain interstitial fluid is inaccessible. Thus, for example, the sampling of exosomes released from cerebral endothelial cells is currently limited to cultured cells [148]. While acknowledging that other sites (e.g. ependyma), as well as the CP, may contribute to CSF exosomes, analysis of such exosomes has given insight into exosome cargo in animals and humans in vivo (e.g. proteins, mRNAs and microRNAs [149–151]) as well as the impact of disease on exosomes [152].

Access to CSF has aided examination of the potential roles of the CP in protecting the brain from injury/disease. The results of such CP studies may aid in formulating brain endothelial studies. For example, to what extent will brain endothelial cells fulfil similar protective roles to the CP? While there has been considerable interest in the production of growth factors by neural and endothelial progenitor cells (endogenous and exogenous) after injury [153, 154], the role of the normal cerebral endothelium has received less attention.

Conclusions

There have been surprisingly few studies examining the degree to which hemorrhagic stroke causes CP injury. This is particularly noticeable in the setting of IVH, where the CP is in close proximity to the hemorrhage. In ICH, there is considerable evidence that clot derived factors (e.g. hemoglobin and iron) cause perihematomal injury [28] and are a therapeutic target (intracerebral hemorrhage deferoxamine trial; iDEF—NCT02175225). Further clinical and preclinical studies on the extent to which IVH and SAH cause CP injury are needed as they may identify a therapeutic target.

Because of its rich collateral circulation, focal cerebral ischemia probably rarely causes CP infarction. However, there is evidence suggesting that the CP is selectively vulnerable to ischemia. Further studies on the impact of transient global ischemia (e.g. cardiac arrest) on CP injury in patients are warranted. The finding that the CPs can produce factors that can protect the brain from injury and disease raises many opportunities. The factors involved are probably numerous, making the effects difficult to reproduce pharmacologically (especially within the brain). Hence, there has been an interest in using CP transplants. However, there is a question as to what can trigger the release of protective factors from the CP? Determining the signaling pathway(s) may be a promising therapeutic avenue. It should also be noted that a role of the CP in neuroprotection after IVH or SAH has not really been examined and this may be an important area of research.

Authors' contributions

All the authors contributed to the writing and editing of this manuscript. All authors read and approved the final manuscript.

Author details

[1] Department of Neurosurgery, University of Michigan, R5018 BSRB, 109 Zina Pitcher Place, Ann Arbor, MI 48109-2200, USA. [2] Department of Health Science and Technology, Aalborg University, Aalborg, Denmark. [3] Department of Molecular & Integrative Physiology, University of Michigan, Ann Arbor, USA.

Competing interests

The authors declare that they have no competing interests.

Funding

This work was supported by the National Institutes of Health Grants NS073595, NS079157, NS090925, NS091545, NS093399, NS096917 and NS007222. The content is solely the responsibility of the authors and does not necessarily represent the official views of the NIH. Lisa Juul Routhe is recipient of a Ph.D-stipend obtained from the Lundbeck foundation (Grant No: R191-2015-1360).

References

1. Redzic ZB, Segal MB. The structure of the choroid plexus and the physiology of the choroid plexus epithelium. Adv Drug Deliv Rev. 2004;56(12):1695–716.
2. Damkier HH, Brown PD, Praetorius J. Cerebrospinal fluid secretion by the choroid plexus. Physiol Rev. 2013;93(4):1847–92.
3. Demeestere D, Libert C, Vandenbroucke RE. Clinical implications of leukocyte infiltration at the choroid plexus in (neuro)inflammatory disorders. Drug Discov Today. 2015;20(8):928–41.
4. Hladky SB, Barrand MA. Mechanisms of fluid movement into, through and out of the brain: evaluation of the evidence. Fluids Barriers CNS. 2014;11(1):26.
5. Marques F, Sousa JC, Brito MA, Pahnke J, Santos C, Correia-Neves M, Palha JA. The choroid plexus in health and in disease: dialogues into and out of the brain. Neurobiol Dis. 2016. doi:10.1016/j.nbd.2016.08.011.
6. Spector R, Johanson CE. Sustained choroid plexus function in human elderly and Alzheimer's disease patients. Fluids Barriers CNS. 2013;10(1):28.
7. Tietz S, Engelhardt B. Brain barriers: crosstalk between complex tight junctions and adherens junctions. J Cell Biol. 2015;209(4):493–506.
8. Jickling GC, Liu D, Stamova B, Ander BP, Zhan X, Lu A, Sharp FR. Hemorrhagic transformation after ischemic stroke in animals and humans. J Cereb Blood Flow Metab. 2014;34(2):185–99.
9. Jin R, Yang G, Li G. Molecular insights and therapeutic targets for blood-brain barrier disruption in ischemic stroke: critical role of matrix metalloproteinases and tissue-type plasminogen activator. Neurobiol Dis. 2010;38(3):376–85.
10. Keep RF, Zhou N, Xiang J, Andjelkovic AV, Hua Y, Xi G. Vascular disruption and blood-brain barrier dysfunction in intracerebral hemorrhage. Fluids Barriers CNS. 2014;11:18.
11. Yang Y, Rosenberg GA. Blood-brain barrier breakdown in acute and chronic cerebrovascular disease. Stroke. 2011;42(11):3323–8.
12. Ennis SR, Keep RF. Forebrain ischemia and the blood-cerebrospinal fluid barrier. Acta Neurochir Suppl. 2006;96:276–8.
13. Keep RF, Ennis SR, Xiang J. The blood-CSF barrier and cerebral ischemia. In: Zheng W, Chodobski A, editors. The blood-cerebrospinal fluid barrier. Boca Raton: Taylor & Francis; 2005. p. 345–60.
14. Chodobski A, Szmydynger-Chodobska J. Choroid plexus: target for polypeptides and site of their synthesis. Microsc Res Tech. 2001;52(1):65–82.
15. Johanson C, Stopa E, Baird A, Sharma H. Traumatic brain injury and recovery mechanisms: peptide modulation of periventricular neurogenic regions by the choroid plexus-CSF nexus. J Neural Transm. 2011;118(1):115–33.
16. Redzic ZB, Preston JE, Duncan JA, Chodobski A, Szmydynger-Chodobska J. The choroid plexus-cerebrospinal fluid system: from development to aging. Curr Top Dev Biol. 2005;71:1–52.
17. Bolos M, Antequera D, Aldudo J, Kristen H, Bullido MJ, Carro E. Choroid plexus implants rescue Alzheimer's disease-like pathologies by modulating amyloid-beta degradation. Cell Mol Life Sci. 2014;71(15):2947–55.
18. Borlongan CV, Skinner SJ, Geaney M, Vasconcellos AV, Elliott RB, Emerich DF. Intracerebral transplantation of porcine choroid plexus provides structural and functional neuroprotection in a rodent model of stroke. Stroke. 2004;35(9):2206–10.
19. Ide C, Nakano N, Kanekiyo K. Cell transplantation for the treatment of spinal cord injury—bone marrow stromal cells and choroid plexus epithelial cells. Neural Regen Res. 2016;11(9):1385–8.
20. Lacey DJ, Terplan K. Intraventricular hemorrhage in full-term neonates. Dev Med Child Neurol. 1982;24(3):332–7.
21. Miyasaka Y, Yada K, Ohwada T, Morii S, Kitahara T, Kurata A, Tanaka R. Choroid plexus arteriovenous malformations. Neurol Med Chir. 1992;32(4):201–6.

22. Reeder JD, Kaude JV, Setzer ES. Choroid plexus hemorrhage in premature neonates: recognition by sonography. AJNR Am J Neuroradiol. 1982;3(6):619–22.
23. Ballabh P. Intraventricular hemorrhage in premature infants: mechanism of disease. Pediatr Res. 2010;67(1):1–8.
24. Bhattathiri PS, Gregson B, Prasad KS, Mendelow AD, Investigators S. Intraventricular hemorrhage and hydrocephalus after spontaneous intracerebral hemorrhage: results from the STICH trial. Acta Neurochir Suppl. 2006;96:65–8.
25. Rosen DS, Macdonald RL, Huo D, Goldenberg FD, Novakovic RL, Frank JI, Rosengart AJ. Intraventricular hemorrhage from ruptured aneurysm: clinical characteristics, complications, and outcomes in a large, prospective, multicenter study population. J Neurosurg. 2007;107(2):261–5.
26. Hanley DF. Intraventricular hemorrhage: severity factor and treatment target in spontaneous intracerebral hemorrhage. Stroke. 2009;40(4):1533–8.
27. Jabbarli R, Reinhard M, Roelz R, Shah M, Niesen WD, Kaier K, Taschner C, Weyerbrock A, Velthoven VV. The predictors and clinical impact of intraventricular hemorrhage in patients with aneurysmal subarachnoid hemorrhage. Int J Stroke. 2016;11(1):68–76.
28. Keep RF, Hua Y, Xi G. Intracerebral haemorrhage: mechanisms of injury and therapeutic targets. Lancet Neurol. 2012;11(8):720–31.
29. Hallevi H, Walker KC, Kasam M, Bornstein N, Grotta JC, Savitz SI. Inflammatory response to intraventricular hemorrhage: time course, magnitude and effect of t-PA. J Neurol Sci. 2012;315(1–2):93–5.
30. Kaestner S, Dimitriou I. TGF beta1 and TGF beta2 and their role in post-hemorrhagic hydrocephalus following SAH and IVH. J Neurol Surg Part A Cent Eur Neurosurg. 2013;74(5):279–84.
31. Kramer AH, Jenne CN, Zygun DA, Roberts DJ, Hill MD, Holodinsky JK, Todd S, Kubes P, Wong JH. Intraventricular fibrinolysis with tissue plasminogen activator is associated with transient cerebrospinal fluid inflammation: a randomized controlled trial. J Cereb Blood Flow Metab. 2015;35(8):1241–8.
32. Milman N, Graudal NA, Olsen TS, Wandall JH, Pedersen NS. Cerebrospinal fluid ferritin in patients with meningitis and cerebral infarction or bleeding. Dan Med Bull. 1993;40(4):490–2.
33. Morales DM, Silver SA, Morgan CD, Mercer D, Inder TE, Holtzman DM, Wallendorf MJ, Rao R, McAllister JP, Limbrick DD Jr. Lumbar cerebrospinal fluid biomarkers of posthemorrhagic hydrocephalus of prematurity: amyloid precursor protein, soluble amyloid precursor protein alpha, and L1 cell adhesion molecule. Neurosurgery. 2017;80(1):82–90.
34. Simard PF, Tosun C, Melnichenko L, Ivanova S, Gerzanich V, Simard JM. Inflammation of the choroid plexus and ependymal layer of the ventricle following intraventricular hemorrhage. Transl Stroke Res. 2011;2(2):227–31.
35. Gram M, Sveinsdottir S, Cinthio M, Sveinsdottir K, Hansson SR, Morgelin M, Akerstrom B, Ley D. Extracellular hemoglobin—mediator of inflammation and cell death in the choroid plexus following preterm intraventricular hemorrhage. J Neuroinflammation. 2014;11:200.
36. Pang D, Sclabassi RJ, Horton JA. Lysis of intraventricular blood clot with urokinase in a canine model: Part 3. Effects of intraventricular urokinase on clot lysis and posthemorrhagic hydrocephalus. Neurosurgery. 1986;19(4):553–72.
37. Fukumizu M, Takashima S, Becker LE. Neonatal posthemorrhagic hydrocephalus: neuropathologic and immunohistochemical studies. Pediatr Neurol. 1995;13(3):230–4.
38. Fukumizu M, Takashima S, Becker LE. Glial reaction in periventricular areas of the brainstem in fetal and neonatal posthemorrhagic hydrocephalus and congenital hydrocephalus. Brain Develop. 1996;18(1):40–5.
39. Mayfrank L, Kim Y, Kissler J, Delsing P, Gilsbach JM, Schroder JM, Weis J. Morphological changes following experimental intraventricular haemorrhage and intraventricular fibrinolytic treatment with recombinant tissue plasminogen activator. Acta Neuropathol. 2000;100(5):561–7.
40. Gao F, Liu F, Chen Z, Hua Y, Keep RF, Xi G. Hydrocephalus after intraventricular hemorrhage: the role of thrombin. J Cereb Blood Flow Metab. 2014;34(3):489–94.
41. Wilson TJ, Stetler WR Jr, Davis MC, Giles DA, Khan A, Chaudhary N, Gemmete JJ, Xi G, Thompson BG, Pandey AS. Intraventricular hemorrhage is associated with early hydrocephalus, symptomatic vasospasm, and poor outcome in aneurysmal subarachnoid hemorrhage. J Neurol Surg. 2015;76(2):126–32.
42. Cherian S, Whitelaw A, Thoresen M, Love S. The pathogenesis of neonatal post-hemorrhagic hydrocephalus. Brain Pathol. 2004;14(3):305–11.
43. Whitelaw A, Thoresen M, Pople I. Posthaemorrhagic ventricular dilatation. Arch Dis Child Fetal Neonatal Ed. 2002;86(2):F72–4.
44. Liszczak TM, Black PM, Tzouras A, Foley L, Zervas NT. Morphological changes of the basilar artery, ventricles, and choroid plexus after experimental SAH. J Neurosurg. 1984;61(3):486–93.
45. Yilmaz A, Aydin MD, Kanat A, Musluman AM, Altas S, Aydin Y, Calik M, Gursan N. The effect of choroidal artery vasospasm on choroid plexus injury in subarachnoid hemorrhage: experimental study. Turk Neurosurg. 2011;21(4):477–82.
46. Kanat A, Turkmenoglu O, Aydin MD, Yolas C, Aydin N, Gursan N, Tumkaya L, Demir R. Toward changing of the pathophysiologic basis of acute hydrocephalus after subarachnoid hemorrhage: a preliminary experimental study. World Neurosurg. 2013;80(3–4):390–5.
47. Kotan D, Aydin MD, Gundogdu C, Aygul R, Aydin N, Ulvi H. Parallel development of choroid plexus degeneration and meningeal inflammation in subarachnoid hemorrhage—experimental study. Adv Clin Exp Med. 2014;23(5):699–704.
48. Okubo S, Strahle J, Keep RF, Hua Y, Xi G. Subarachnoid hemorrhage-induced hydrocephalus in rats. Stroke. 2013;44(2):547–50.
49. Norrving B, Olsson JE. The diagnostic value of spectrophotometric analysis of the cerebrospinal fluid in cerebral hematomas. J Neurol Sci. 1979;44(1):105–14.
50. Marinkovic S, Gibo H, Milisavljevic M, Djulejic V, Jovanovic VT. Microanatomy of the intrachoroidal vasculature of the lateral ventricle. Neurosurgery. 2005;57(1 Suppl):22–36 **(discussion 22–36)**.
51. Wolfram-Gabel R, Maillot C, Koritke JG, Laude M. Vascularization of the tela choroidea of the 3rd ventricle in man. Archives d'Anatomie, d'Histologie, et d'Embryologie Normales et Experimentales. 1984;67:3–42.
52. Sharifi M, Ciolkowski M, Krajewski P, Ciszek B. The choroid plexus of the fourth ventricle and its arteries. Folia Morphol. 2005;64(3):194–8.
53. Koral K, Dowling MM, Rollins NK. Choroid plexus infarction in a child. Pediatr Neurol. 2007;37(6):452–3.
54. Liebeskind DS, Hurst RW. Infarction of the choroid plexus. AJNR Am J Neuroradiol. 2004;25(2):289–90.
55. Nabavizadeh SA, Tangestanipoor A, Mowla A, Hurst R, Mamourian AC. Infarction of the choroid plexus in basilar artery occlusion. J Neurol Sci. 2015;358(1–2):467–8.
56. Helgason CM. A new view of anterior choroidal artery territory infarction. J Neurol. 1988;235(7):387–91.
57. Hupperts RM, Lodder J, Heuts-van Raak EP, Kessels F. Infarcts in the anterior choroidal artery territory. Anatomical distribution, clinical syndromes, presumed pathogenesis and early outcome. Brain. 1994;117(Pt 4):825–34.
58. Pezzella FR, Vadala R. Anterior choroidal artery territory infarction. Front Neurol Neurosci. 2012;30:123–7.
59. Takahashi S, Ishii K, Matsumoto K, Higano S, Ishibashi T, Suzuki M, Sakamoto K. The anterior choroidal artery syndrome. II. CT and/or MR in angiographically verified cases. Neuroradiology. 1994;36(5):340–5.
60. Neau JP, Bogousslavsky J. The syndrome of posterior choroidal artery territory infarction. Ann Neurol. 1996;39(6):779–88.
61. Maslinska D, Laure-Kamionowska M, Taraszewska A, Deregowski K, Maslinski S. Immunodistribution of amyloid beta protein (Abeta) and advanced glycation end-product receptors (RAGE) in choroid plexus and ependyma of resuscitated patients. Folia Neuropathol. 2011;49(4):295–300.
62. Wisniewski HM, Maslinska D. Beta-protein immunoreactivity in the human brain after cardiac arrest. Folia Neuropathol. 1996;34(2):65–71.
63. Pulsinelli WA, Brierley JB, Plum F. Temporal profile of neuronal damage in a model of transient forebrain ischemia. Ann Neurol. 1982;11(5):491–8.
64. Dienel GA. Regional accumulation of calcium in postischemic rat brain. J Neurochem. 1984;43(4):913–25.
65. Akdemir G, Kaymaz F, Gursoy-Ozdemir Y, Akalan N, Akdemir ES. The time course changes in expression of aquaporin 4 and aquaporin 1 following global cerebral ischemic edema in rat. Surg Neurol Int. 2016;7:4.

66. Johanson CE, Palm DE, Primiano MJ, McMillan PN, Chan P, Knuckey NW, Stopa EG. Choroid plexus recovery after transient forebrain ischemia: role of growth factors and other repair mechanisms. Cell Mol Neurobiol. 2000;20(2):197–216.
67. Palm D, Knuckey N, Guglielmo M, Watson P, Primiano M, Johanson C. Choroid plexus electrolytes and ultrastructure following transient forebrain ischemia. Am J Physiol. 1995;269(1 Pt 2):R73–9.
68. Ferrand-Drake M. Cell death in the choroid plexus following transient forebrain global ischemia in the rat. Microsc Res Tech. 2001;52(1):130–6.
69. Ferrand-Drake M, Wieloch T. The time-course of DNA fragmentation in the choroid plexus and the CA1 region following transient global ischemia in the rat brain. The effect of intra-ischemic hypothermia. Neuroscience. 1999;93(2):537–49.
70. Ikeda J, Mies G, Nowak TS Jr, Joo F, Klatzo I. Evidence for increased calcium influx across the choroid plexus following brief ischemia of gerbil brain. Neurosci Lett. 1992;142(2):257–9.
71. Kitagawa H, Setoguchi Y, Fukuchi Y, Mitsumoto Y, Koga N, Mori T, Abe K. DNA fragmentation and HSP72 gene expression by adenovirus-mediated gene transfer in postischemic gerbil hippocampus and ventricle. Metab Brain Dis. 1998;13(3):211–23.
72. Rothstein RP, Levison SW. Damage to the choroid plexus, ependyma and subependyma as a consequence of perinatal hypoxia/ischemia. Dev Neurosci. 2002;24(5):426–36.
73. Towfighi J, Zec N, Yager J, Housman C, Vannucci RC. Temporal evolution of neuropathologic changes in an immature rat model of cerebral hypoxia: a light microscopic study. Acta Neuropathol. 1995;90(4):375–86.
74. Sivakumar V, Lu J, Ling EA, Kaur C. Vascular endothelial growth factor and nitric oxide production in response to hypoxia in the choroid plexus in neonatal brain. Brain Pathol. 2008;18(1):71–85.
75. D'Angelo B, Ek CJ, Sandberg M, Mallard C. Expression of the Nrf2-system at the blood-CSF barrier is modulated by neonatal inflammation and hypoxia-ischemia. J Inherit Metab Dis. 2013;36(3):479–90.
76. Ennis SR, Keep RF. The effects of cerebral ischemia on the rat choroid plexus. J Cereb Blood Flow Metab. 2006;26(5):675–83.
77. Gillardon F, Lenz C, Kuschinsky W, Zimmermann M. Evidence for apoptotic cell death in the choroid plexus following focal cerebral ischemia. Neurosci Lett. 1996;207(2):113–6.
78. Li Y, Chen J, Chopp M. Cell proliferation and differentiation from ependymal, subependymal and choroid plexus cells in response to stroke in rats. J Neurol Sci. 2002;193(2):137–46.
79. Nagahiro S, Goto S, Korematsu K, Sumi M, Takahashi M, Ushio Y. Disruption of the blood-cerebrospinal fluid barrier by transient cerebral ischemia. Brain Res. 1994;633(1–2):305–11.
80. He Z, Yang SH, Naritomi H, Yamawaki T, Liu Q, King MA, Day AL, Simpkins JW. Definition of the anterior choroidal artery territory in rats using intraluminal occluding technique. J Neurol Sci. 2000;182(1):16–28.
81. Lucke-Wold BP, Logsdon AF, Turner RC, Rosen CL, Huber JD. Aging, the metabolic syndrome, and ischemic stroke: redefining the approach for studying the blood–brain barrier in a complex neurological disease. Adv Pharmacol. 2014;71:411–49.
82. Serot JM, Bene MC, Faure GC. Comparative immunohistochemical characteristics of human choroid plexus in vascular and Alzheimer's dementia. Hum Pathol. 1994;25(11):1185–90.
83. Serot JM, Zmudka J, Jouanny P. A possible role for CSF turnover and choroid plexus in the pathogenesis of late onset Alzheimer's disease. J Alzheimer's Dis. 2012;30(1):17–26.
84. Vandenbroucke RE. A hidden epithelial barrier in the brain with a central role in regulating brain homeostasis. Implications for aging. Ann Am Thorac Soc. 2016;13(Supplement_5):S407–10.
85. Walter HJ, Berry M, Hill DJ, Cwyfan-Hughes S, Holly JM, Logan A. Distinct sites of insulin-like growth factor (IGF)-II expression and localization in lesioned rat brain: possible roles of IGF binding proteins (IGFBPs) in the mediation of IGF-II activity. Endocrinology. 1999;140(1):520–32.
86. Knuckey NW, Finch P, Palm DE, Primiano MJ, Johanson CE, Flanders KC, Thompson NL. Differential neuronal and astrocytic expression of transforming growth factor beta isoforms in rat hippocampus following transient forebrain ischemia. Brain Res Mol Brain Res. 1996;40(1):1–14.
87. Flood C, Akinwunmi J, Lagord C, Daniel M, Berry M, Jackowski A, Logan A. Transforming growth factor-beta1 in the cerebrospinal fluid of patients with subarachnoid hemorrhage: titers derived from exogenous and endogenous sources. J Cereb Blood Flow Metab. 2001;21(2):157–62.
88. Krupinski J, Vodovotz Y, Li C, Slowik A, Beevers D, Flanders KC, Lip G, Kumar P, Szczudlik A. Inducible nitric oxide production and expression of transforming growth factor-beta1 in serum and CSF after cerebral ischaemic stroke in man. Nitric Oxide. 1998;2(6):442–53.
89. Buisson A, Lesne S, Docagne F, Ali C, Nicole O, MacKenzie ET, Vivien D. Transforming growth factor-beta and ischemic brain injury. Cell Mol Neurobiol. 2003;23(4–5):539–50.
90. Dobolyi A, Vincze C, Pal G, Lovas G. The neuroprotective functions of transforming growth factor beta proteins. Int J Mol Sci. 2012;13(7):8219–58.
91. Aojula A, Botfield H, McAllister JP 2nd, Gonzalez AM, Abdullah O, Logan A, Sinclair A. Diffusion tensor imaging with direct cytopathological validation: characterisation of decorin treatment in experimental juvenile communicating hydrocephalus. Fluids Barriers CNS. 2016;13(1):9.
92. Hayamizu TF, Chan PT, Johanson CE. FGF-2 immunoreactivity in adult rat ependyma and choroid plexus: responses to global forebrain ischemia and intraventricular FGF-2. Neurol Res. 2001;23(4):353–8.
93. Koketsu N, Berlove DJ, Moskowitz MA, Kowall NW, Caday CG, Finklestein SP. Pretreatment with intraventricular basic fibroblast growth factor decreases infarct size following focal cerebral ischemia in rats. Ann Neurol. 1994;35(4):451–7.
94. Nakata N, Kato H, Kogure K. Protective effects of basic fibroblast growth factor against hippocampal neuronal damage following cerebral ischemia in the gerbil. Brain Res. 1993;605(2):354–6.
95. Beilharz EJ, Russo VC, Butler G, Baker NL, Connor B, Sirimanne ES, Dragunow M, Werther GA, Gluckman PD, Williams CE, et al. Co-ordinated and cellular specific induction of the components of the IGF/IGFBP axis in the rat brain following hypoxic-ischemic injury. Brain Res Mol Brain Res. 1998;59(2):119–34.
96. Scheufler KM, Drevs J, van Velthoven V, Reusch P, Klisch J, Augustin HG, Zentner J, Marme D. Implications of vascular endothelial growth factor, sFlt-1, and sTie-2 in plasma, serum and cerebrospinal fluid during cerebral ischemia in man. J Cereb Blood Flow Metab. 2003;23(1):99–110.
97. Harrigan MR, Ennis SR, Sullivan SE, Keep RF. Effects of intraventricular infusion of vascular endothelial growth factor on cerebral blood flow, edema, and infarct volume. Acta Neurochir (Wien). 2003;145(1):49–53.
98. Jin K, Zhu Y, Sun Y, Mao XO, Xie L, Greenberg DA. Vascular endothelial growth factor (VEGF) stimulates neurogenesis in vitro and in vivo. Proc Natl Acad Sci USA. 2002;99(18):11946–50.
99. Kaya D, Gursoy-Ozdemir Y, Yemisci M, Tuncer N, Aktan S, Dalkara T. VEGF protects brain against focal ischemia without increasing blood–brain permeability when administered intracerebroventricularly. J Cereb Blood Flow Metab. 2005;25(9):1111–8.
100. Sun Y, Jin K, Xie L, Childs J, Mao XO, Logvinova A, Greenberg DA. VEGF-induced neuroprotection, neurogenesis, and angiogenesis after focal cerebral ischemia. J Clin Investig. 2003;111(12):1843–51.
101. Liu L, Fujimoto M, Kawakita F, Nakano F, Imanaka-Yoshida K, Yoshida T, Suzuki H. Anti-vascular endothelial growth factor treatment suppresses early brain injury after subarachnoid hemorrhage in mice. Mol Neurobiol. 2016;53(7):4529–38.
102. Crouthamel MH, Kelly EJ, Ho RJ. Development and characterization of transgenic mouse models for conditional gene knockout in the blood-brain and blood-CSF barriers. Transgenic Res. 2012;21(1):113–30.
103. Kubo Y, Koji T, Kashimura H, Otawara Y, Ogawa A, Ogasawara K. Adrenomedullin concentration in the cerebrospinal fluid is related to appetite loss and delayed ischemic neurological deficits after subarachnoid hemorrhage. Neurol Res. 2013;35(7):713–8.
104. Kubo Y, Ogasawara K, Kakino S, Kashimura H, Yoshida K, Ogawa A. Cerebrospinal fluid adrenomedullin concentration correlates with hyponatremia and delayed ischemic neurological deficits after subarachnoid hemorrhage. Cerebrovasc Dis. 2008;25(1–2):164–9.
105. Balusu S, Van Wonterghem E, De Rycke R, Raemdonck K, Stremersch S, Gevaert K, Brkic M, Demeestere D, Vanhooren V, Hendrix A, et al. Identification of a novel mechanism of blood-brain communication during peripheral inflammation via choroid plexus-derived extracellular vesicles. EMBO Mol Med. 2016;8(10):1162–83.
106. Grapp M, Wrede A, Schweizer M, Huwel S, Galla HJ, Snaidero N, Simons M, Buckers J, Low PS, Urlaub H, et al. Choroid plexus transcytosis and

exosome shuttling deliver folate into brain parenchyma. Nat Commun. 2013;4:2123.
107. Tietje A, Maron KN, Wei Y, Feliciano DM. Cerebrospinal fluid extracellular vesicles undergo age dependent declines and contain known and novel non-coding RNAs. PLoS ONE. 2014;9(11):e113116.
108. Fodstad H, Kok P, Algers G. Fibrinolytic activity of cerebral tissue after experimental subarachnoid haemorrhage: inhibitory effect of tranexamic acid (AMCA). Acta Neurol Scand. 1981;64(1):29–46.
109. Masuda T, Dohrmann GJ, Kwaan HC, Erickson RK, Wollman RL. Fibrinolytic activity in experimental intracerebral hematoma. J Neurosurg. 1988;68(2):274–8.
110. Gao C, Du H, Hua Y, Keep RF, Strahle J, Xi G. Role of red blood cell lysis and iron in hydrocephalus after intraventricular hemorrhage. J Cereb Blood Flow Metab. 2014;34(6):1070–5.
111. Strahle JM, Garton T, Bazzi AA, Kilaru H, Garton HJ, Maher CO, Muraszko KM, Keep RF, Xi G. Role of hemoglobin and iron in hydrocephalus after neonatal intraventricular hemorrhage. Neurosurgery. 2014;75(6):696–705 **(discussion 706)**.
112. Mesquita SD, Ferreira AC, Sousa JC, Santos NC, Correia-Neves M, Sousa N, Palha JA, Marques F. Modulation of iron metabolism in aging and in Alzheimer's disease: relevance of the choroid plexus. Front Cell Neurosci. 2012;6:25.
113. Rouault TA, Zhang DL, Jeong SY. Brain iron homeostasis, the choroid plexus, and localization of iron transport proteins. Metab Brain Dis. 2009;24(4):673–84.
114. Borlongan CV, Skinner SJ, Geaney M, Vasconcellos AV, Elliott RB, Emerich DF. CNS grafts of rat choroid plexus protect against cerebral ischemia in adult rats. NeuroReport. 2004;15(10):1543–7.
115. Matsumoto N, Taguchi A, Kitayama H, Watanabe Y, Ohta M, Yoshihara T, Itokazu Y, Dezawa M, Suzuki Y, Sugimoto H, et al. Transplantation of cultured choroid plexus epithelial cells via cerebrospinal fluid shows prominent neuroprotective effects against acute ischemic brain injury in the rat. Neurosci Lett. 2010;469(3):283–8.
116. Kanekiyo K, Nakano N, Noda T, Yamada Y, Suzuki Y, Ohta M, Yokota A, Fukushima M, Ide C. Transplantation of choroid plexus epithelial cells into contusion-injured spinal cord of rats. Restor Neurol Neurosci. 2016;34(3):347–66.
117. Chauhan AN, Lewis PD. A quantitative study of cell proliferation in ependyma and choroid plexus in the postnatal rat brain. Neuropathol Appl Neurobiol. 1979;5(4):303–9.
118. Kaplan MS. Proliferation of epithelial cells in the adult primate choroid plexus. Anat Rec. 1980;197(4):495–502.
119. Barkho BZ, Monuki ES. Proliferation of cultured mouse choroid plexus epithelial cells. PLoS ONE. 2015;10(3):e0121738.
120. Malinovskaya NA, Komleva YK, Salmin VV, Morgun AV, Shuvaev AN, Panina YA, Boitsova EB, Salmina AB. Endothelial progenitor cells physiology and metabolic plasticity in brain angiogenesis and blood–brain barrier modeling. Front Physiols. 2016;7:599.
121. Zhang ZG, Zhang L, Jiang Q, Chopp M. Bone marrow-derived endothelial progenitor cells participate in cerebral neovascularization after focal cerebral ischemia in the adult mouse. Circ Res. 2002;90(3):284–8.
122. Beck H, Voswinckel R, Wagner S, Ziegelhoeffer T, Heil M, Helisch A, Schaper W, Acker T, Hatzopoulos AK, Plate KH. Participation of bone marrow-derived cells in long-term repair processes after experimental stroke. J Cereb Blood Flow Metab. 2003;23(6):709–17.
123. Hamisha KN, Tfilin M, Yanai J, Turgeman G. Mesenchymal stem cells can prevent alterations in behavior and neurogenesis induced by Ass25-35 administration. J Mol Neurosci. 2015;55(4):1006–13.
124. Violatto MB, Santangelo C, Capelli C, Frapolli R, Ferrari R, Sitia L, Tortarolo M, Talamini L, Previdi S, Moscatelli D, et al. Longitudinal tracking of triple labeled umbilical cord derived mesenchymal stromal cells in a mouse model of amyotrophic lateral sclerosis. Stem Cell Res. 2015;15(1):243–53.
125. Petrovic-Djergovic D, Goonewardena SN, Pinsky DJ. Inflammatory Disequilibrium in Stroke. Circ Res. 2016;119(1):142–58.
126. Wang J. Preclinical and clinical research on inflammation after intracerebral hemorrhage. Prog Neurobiol. 2010;92(4):463–77.
127. Iadecola C, Anrather J. The immunology of stroke: from mechanisms to translation. Nat Med. 2011;17(7):796–808.
128. Kim JY, Park J, Chang JY, Kim SH, Lee JE. Inflammation after ischemic stroke: the role of leukocytes and glial cells. Exp Neurobiol. 2016;25(5):241–51.
129. Vexler ZS, Yenari MA. Does inflammation after stroke affect the developing brain differently than adult brain? Dev Neurosci. 2009;31(5):378–93.
130. Schallner N, Pandit R, LeBlanc R 3rd, Thomas AJ, Ogilvy CS, Zuckerbraun BS, Gallo D, Otterbein LE, Hanafy KA. Microglia regulate blood clearance in subarachnoid hemorrhage by heme oxygenase-1. J Clin Investig. 2015;125(7):2609–25.
131. Zhao X, Sun G, Ting SM, Song S, Zhang J, Edwards NJ, Aronowski J. Cleaning up after ICH: the role of Nrf2 in modulating microglia function and hematoma clearance. J Neurochem. 2015;133(1):144–52.
132. Kowarik MC, Grummel V, Wemlinger S, Buck D, Weber MS, Berthele A, Hemmer B. Immune cell subtyping in the cerebrospinal fluid of patients with neurological diseases. J Neurol. 2014;261(1):130–43.
133. Baruch K, Ron-Harel N, Gal H, Deczkowska A, Shifrut E, Ndifon W, Mirlas-Neisberg N, Cardon M, Vaknin I, Cahalon L, et al. CNS-specific immunity at the choroid plexus shifts toward destructive Th2 inflammation in brain aging. Proc Natl Acad Sci USA. 2013;110(6):2264–9.
134. Ritzel RM, Crapser J, Patel AR, Verma R, Grenier JM, Chauhan A, Jellison ER, McCullough LD. Age-associated resident memory CD8 T cells in the central nervous system are primed to potentiate inflammation after ischemic brain injury. J Immunol. 2016;196(8):3318–30.
135. Yang D, Sun YY, Bhaumik SK, Li Y, Baumann JM, Lin X, Zhang Y, Lin SH, Dunn RS, Liu CY, et al. Blocking lymphocyte trafficking with FTY720 prevents inflammation-sensitized hypoxic-ischemic brain injury in newborns. J Neurosci. 2014;34(49):16467–81.
136. Coisne C, Engelhardt B. Tight junctions in brain barriers during central nervous system inflammation. Antioxid Redox Signal. 2011;15(5):1285–303.
137. Shrestha B, Paul D, Pachter JS. Alterations in tight junction protein and IgG permeability accompany leukocyte extravasation across the choroid plexus during neuroinflammation. J Neuropathol Exp Neurol. 2014;73(11):1047–61.
138. Szmydynger-Chodobska J, Strazielle N, Gandy JR, Keefe TH, Zink BJ, Ghersi-Egea JF, Chodobski A. Posttraumatic invasion of monocytes across the blood-cerebrospinal fluid barrier. J Cereb Blood Flow Metab. 2012;32(1):93–104.
139. Szmydynger-Chodobska J, Strazielle N, Zink BJ, Ghersi-Egea JF, Chodobski A. The role of the choroid plexus in neutrophil invasion after traumatic brain injury. J Cereb Blood Flow Metab. 2009;29(9):1503–16.
140. Karimy JK, Duran D, Hu JK, Gavankar C, Gaillard JR, Bayri Y, Rice H, DiLuna ML, Gerzanich V, Marc Simard J, et al. Cerebrospinal fluid hypersecretion in pediatric hydrocephalus. Neurosurg Focus. 2016;41(5):E10.
141. Scarff JE. The treatment of nonobstructive (communicating) hydrocephalus by endoscopic cauterization of the choroid plexuses. J Neurosurg. 1970;33(1):1–18.
142. Weil AG, Westwick H, Wang S, Alotaibi NM, Elkaim L, Ibrahim GM, Wang AC, Ariani RT, Crevier L, Myers B, et al. Efficacy and safety of endoscopic third ventriculostomy and choroid plexus cauterization for infantile hydrocephalus: a systematic review and meta-analysis. Child's Nerv Syst. 2016;32(11):2119–31.
143. Holloway LS Jr, Cassin S. Cerebrospinal fluid dynamics in the newborn dog during normoxia and hypoxia. Am J Physiol. 1972;223(3):499–502.
144. Oshio K, Watanabe H, Song Y, Verkman AS, Manley GT. Reduced cerebrospinal fluid production and intracranial pressure in mice lacking choroid plexus water channel Aquaporin-1. FASEB J. 2005;19(1):76–8.
145. Sveinsdottir S, Gram M, Cinthio M, Sveinsdottir K, Morgelin M, Ley D. Altered expression of aquaporin 1 and 5 in the choroid plexus following preterm intraventricular hemorrhage. Dev Neurosci. 2014;36(6):542–51.
146. Podvin S, Gonzalez AM, Miller MC, Dang X, Botfield H, Donahue JE, Kurabi A, Boissaud-Cooke M, Rossi R, Leadbeater WE, et al. Esophageal cancer related gene-4 is a choroid plexus-derived injury response gene: evidence for a biphasic response in early and late brain injury. PLoS ONE. 2011;6(9):e24609.
147. Knowland D, Arac A, Sekiguchi KJ, Hsu M, Lutz SE, Perrino J, Steinberg GK, Barres BA, Nimmerjahn A, Agalliu D. Stepwise recruitment of transcellular and paracellular pathways underlies blood-brain barrier breakdown in stroke. Neuron. 2014;82(3):603–17.

148. Andras IE, Toborek M. Extracellular vesicles of the blood-brain barrier. Tissue Barriers. 2016;4(1):e1131804.
149. Chiasserini D, van Weering JR, Piersma SR, Pham TV, Malekzadeh A, Teunissen CE, de Wit H, Jimenez CR. Proteomic analysis of cerebrospinal fluid extracellular vesicles: a comprehensive dataset. J Proteom. 2014;106:191–204.
150. Street JM, Barran PE, Mackay CL, Weidt S, Balmforth C, Walsh TS, Chalmers RT, Webb DJ, Dear JW. Identification and proteomic profiling of exosomes in human cerebrospinal fluid. J Transl Med. 2012;10:5.
151. Yagi Y, Ohkubo T, Kawaji H, Machida A, Miyata H, Goda S, Roy S, Hayashizaki Y, Suzuki H, Yokota T. Next-generation sequencing-based small RNA profiling of cerebrospinal fluid exosomes. Neurosci Lett. 2017;636:48–57.
152. Yang Y, Keene CD, Peskind ER, Galasko DR, Hu SC, Cudaback E, Wilson AM, Li G, Yu CE, Montine KS, et al. Cerebrospinal fluid particles in Alzheimer disease and Parkinson disease. J Neuropathol Exp Neurol. 2015;74(7):672–87.
153. Chen J, Venkat P, Zacharek A, Chopp M. Neurorestorative therapy for stroke. Front Hum Neurosci. 2014;8:382.
154. Zhang ZG, Chopp M. Neurorestorative therapies for stroke: underlying mechanisms and translation to the clinic. Lancet Neurol. 2009;8(5):491–500.

6

Evolutionary development of embryonic cerebrospinal fluid composition and regulation: an open research field with implications for brain development and function

David Bueno* and Jordi Garcia-Fernàndez

Abstract

Within the consolidated field of evolutionary development, there is emerging research on evolutionary aspects of central nervous system development and its implications for adult brain structure and function, including behaviour. The central nervous system is one of the most intriguing systems in complex metazoans, as it controls all body and mind functions. Its failure is responsible for a number of severe and largely incurable diseases, including neurological and neurodegenerative ones. Moreover, the evolution of the nervous system is thought to be a critical step in the adaptive radiation of vertebrates. Brain formation is initiated early during development. Most embryological, genetic and evolutionary studies have focused on brain neurogenesis and regionalisation, including the formation and function of organising centres, and the comparison of homolog gene expression and function among model organisms from different taxa. The architecture of the vertebrate brain primordium also reveals the existence of connected internal cavities, the cephalic vesicles, which in fetuses and adults become the ventricular system of the brain. During embryonic and fetal development, brain cavities and ventricles are filled with a complex, protein-rich fluid called cerebrospinal fluid (CSF). However, CSF has not been widely analysed from either an embryological or evolutionary perspective. Recently, it has been demonstrated in higher vertebrates that embryonic cerebrospinal fluid has key functions in delivering diffusible signals and nutrients to the developing brain, thus contributing to the proliferation, differentiation and survival of neural progenitor cells, and to the expansion and patterning of the brain. Moreover, it has been shown that the composition and homeostasis of CSF are tightly controlled in a time-dependent manner from the closure of the anterior neuropore, just before the initiation of primary neurogenesis, up to the formation of functional choroid plexuses. In this review, we draw together existing literature about the formation, function and homeostatic regulation of embryonic cerebrospinal fluid, from the closure of the anterior neuropore to the formation of functional fetal choroid plexuses, from an evolutionary perspective. The relevance of these processes to the normal functions and diseases of adult brain will also be discussed.

Keywords: Neuro-evo-devo, Embryonic cerebrospinal fluid (eCSF), Blood-eCSF interface, Primary neurogenesis, Neural progenitor cells, Brain development, Cephalic vesicles

Background

From its embryonic beginnings and throughout adult life, the vertebrate brain is organised around an extraordinarily dynamic and complex fluid called cerebrospinal fluid (CSF). The study of CSF attracts growing interest in brain development research, as it is an active signalling medium containing growth factors and signalling molecules involved in the regulation of multiple cell functions in the central nervous system (CNS), including brain development, homeostasis and disease (for general reviews, see [1–7]). Today, several research findings have generated sufficient evidence to support

*Correspondence: dbueno@ub.edu
Department of Genetics, Microbiology and Statistics, Unit of Biomedical, Evolutionary and Developmental Genetics, Faculty of Biological Sciences, University of Barcelona, Av. Diagonal 643, 08028 Barcelona, Catalonia, Spain

the hypothesis that embryonic CSF (eCSF) is involved in nearly all aspects of embryonic brain development.

Evo-devo (evolutionary development) has flourished in the last 20 years, since initial studies were published in the 1980s by Nobel Laureates Edward B. Lewis, Christiane Nüsslein-Volhard and Eric Wieschaus. In these studies, some of the genes important in *Drosophila* fruit fly development, for example the *Hox* genes, were found to be broadly conserved among metazoans [8–10]. Even functions of these genes appeared to be conserved, as *Hox* vertebrate genes could substitute, at least partially, for missing homolog *Drosophila hox* genes. More recently, variation in the nervous system of metazoans has also begun to be examined from an evo-devo perspective. This has led to the emergence of the term evo-devo-neuro [11] or neuro-evo-devo [12]. A nearly ubiquitous theme in evo-devo studies on CNS is the search for cellular and/or molecular causes of evolutionary change in development trajectories. Just as the field of evo-devo has shed light on how diversity in animal body plans are variations on a few developmental themes [13, 14], so the study of neuro-evo-devo is beginning to illuminate how morphological and functional diversity in the brain are variations on developmental and neurochemical themes [15, 16].

Most of molecular evo-devo research has focused on the functional comparison of homologous genes. In this respect, the genes that specify brain patterning early in development are highly conserved in bilaterians [17–20]. A comparative analysis of these genes in different taxa has provided insights into the early origin of the central nervous system and regional brain homologies in vertebrates and invertebrates. For example, all known bilaterian nervous systems are established via transforming growth factor β (TGF-β) family signalling, which arranges dorsoventral polarity, except in nematodes [17, 21, 22]. However, the chordate nervous system is dorsoventrally inverted compared with protostomes, and it has been suggested that hemichordates represent an intermediate body plan [23] (see Fig. 1 for a general cladistics phylogenetic tree). Similarly, anterior–posterior patterning is in part defined by *Otd/Otx* (anterior) and *Unpg/Gbx* (posterior) expression, with *Pax2/5/8* expressed at the intersection [24–26]. Likewise, comparisons of patterning genes after the establishment of the anterior–posterior axis have identified evolutionary relationships among brain regions in bilaterians from very distant taxa. For example, expression of *Pax6* and *Emx1* specify the pallial telencephalon, whereas *Dlx* and *Nkx2.1* specify subpallial regions [27, 28] (for a review, see [12]). Interestingly, invertebrate mushroom bodies have similar evolutionary origins to the pallium of vertebrates, as annelid mushroom bodies are also specified by *Pax6* and *Emx1* expression [29].

We will not continue with this line of argument as it is beyond the scope of this paper, except to cite another example of classic evo-devo research related to brain evolutionary development that has been analysed by the authors of this review and their collaborators to which we will return later. A comparison of the structure and expression of *Evx* genes in the cephalochordate amphioxus (which belongs to the sister group of vertebrates) and its vertebrate homologs linked invertebrate and vertebrate *Evx* functions across different taxa, and pointed to crucial evolutionary vertebrate innovations for brain development at the level of molecular and morphological regionalisation [30]. Amphioxus has been reported to have two *Evx* genes that are genomically linked. *AmphiEvxA* is prototypical to the vertebrate *Evx1* and *Evx2* genes with respect to its sequence and expression, whilst *AmphiEvxB* is very divergent. Mapping the expression of *AmphiEvxA* onto a phylogeny showed a role in gastrulation, dorsal–ventral patterning, tailbud formation and neurogenesis. This suggests that basic *Evx* function has been retained throughout bilaterian evolution. Interestingly for brain evolutionary development, *AmphiEvxA* is not expressed in amphioxus in the region homologous to the vertebrate midbrain–hindbrain boundary, a well-known organising centre for brain development that is also called the isthmic organiser (IsO). This observation is consistent with the elaboration of the full organiser properties of this region being a vertebrate innovation. Later in this paper, we will go back to this organising centre, as its maintenance during early embryonic brain development also depends on the actions exerted by the eCSF [31].

To cite a final example, in this case also related to some aspects of animal behaviour, it has been reported that gonadotropin-releasing hormone, which is produced by the pituitary gland located at the base of the brain in vertebrates, is also produced in the most anterior part of the amphioxus body. This hormone is a key player in the control of vertebrate reproduction, and it has been shown to display seasonal variations in the Cephalochordate amphioxus with respect to their reproductive cycle. This suggests that it plays an ancient role in the control of reproduction in all chordates, even before the evolution of a defined pituitary gland [32]. However, despite the explosion of evo-devo studies on some morphological traits, the impact of behavioural factors upon speciation has scarcely been analysed [11], although it has been said that the elaborate and complex nervous system of amniotes is correlated with their behavioural repertoire [33].

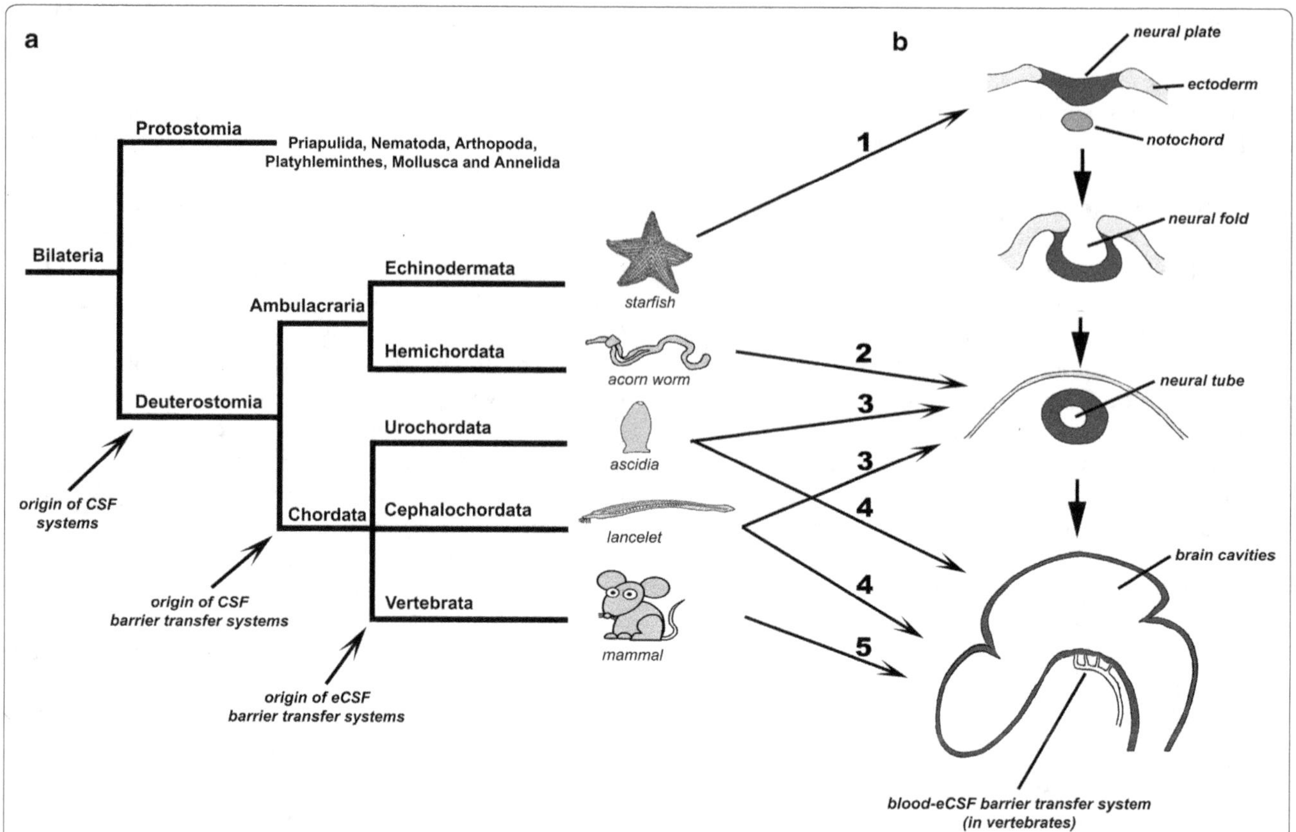

Fig. 1 Phylogeny and ontogeny of the CNS. **a** Phylogenetic relationships among main deuterostome clades, as cited in the text. **b** Ontogeny of the CNS, including the brain, in vertebrates. The origin of the different elements of the CSF system has been indicated. Similarities between deuterostome clades and CNS development in vertebrates have also been indicated. *1* Adult starfish possess a neural plate-like nervous system similar to one from early vertebrate embryos, before the formation of the neural tube; *2* Adult Hemichordata possess a hollow dorsal nerve chord similar to one from vertebrate embryos before the closure of the anterior neuropore; *3* Urochordata and cephalochordata larvae possess a hollow dorsal nerve chord anteriorly open similar to one from vertebrate embryos before the closure of the anterior neuropore; *4* Urochordata and cephalochordata adults possess a closed dorsal nerve chord similar to one from vertebrate embryos after the closure of the anterior neuropore; *5* In vertebrates, the neural tube becomes a physiologically sealed system from a very early developmental stage and the site of the embryonic transfer system is depicted

Similarly, very little work has been done on brain cephalic vesicles from the evo-devo perspective, and the same is true for both CSF in general and eCSF in particular. In this regard, from fetal stages through adult life, it has long been known that CSF is primarily produced by choroid plexuses. It has been shown that choroid plexus is derived from the same embryonic primordium as the hindbrain roof plate, and that it develops in a patterned, segmental manner, from lineage-restricted compartments expressing Wnt1 [34]. Moreover, it has also been shown that molecular heterogeneity between telencephalic and hindbrain choroid plexi contributes to region-specific, age-dependent protein secretion in vitro, which may contribute to dynamic signalling gradients across the mammalian cerebroventricular system [35]. However, eCSF has a role in vertebrate brain development at a much earlier stage, at least just after the closure of the anterior neuropore and before the initiation of brain primary neurogenesis, prior to the existence of a functional choroid plexus (for general reviews, see [1, 2, 4]).

The main objective of this review is to demonstrate that the evolutionary development of the embryonic brain cavity system, including the eCSF it contains and the mechanisms controlling its formation and homeostasis, must also be taken into account to get a better overall understanding of brain development, CNS evolution, and neurological diseases. To present our thesis in an ordered way, we will first review data on evolutionary changes of the brain cavities in metazoans, primarily in the deuterostome lineage. We will then review research on eCSF function and composition, and on its formation and homeostasis regulation, much of which has been developed by the authors and their collaborators over the last 10 years. Finally, we will integrate all these data in a comprehensive thesis about the actual importance of the developmental evolution of the brain cavities and eCSF, in the light of mammalian brain development and human diseases, with some comments on behavioural aspects.

Embryonic CSF evolutionary aspects: from the origin of deuterostomes to vertebrates

In vertebrates, brain formation begins early during development. Generally speaking, its development involves several distinct phases (Fig. 1; for a general description of central CNS development, see [36–38]). First, a portion of the dorsal ectoderm develops into neural ectoderm and forms the neural plate, which is in contact with the amniotic fluid in amniotes (reptiles, birds and mammals) or with the surrounding water in the anamniotes (fish and amphibians). Second, the neural plate folds longitudinally to form the neural tube, which becomes the rudiment of the CNS, trapping some of the surrounding fluid within its lumen. The tube still remains in contact with the environmental fluids through the open neuropores. Then, the neural tube polarises into a posterior spinal cord and an anterior expanded brain. Initially, the embryonic brain is a hollow fluid-filled vesicle surrounded by a pseudo-monostratified neuroepithelium. The subsequent closure of the anterior neuropore enables the organism to exert some control over CSF formation and composition for the first time. Thus, the CSF composition can become independent of environmental fluids. Finally, histogenesis of the neuroepithelium occurs. Interestingly, from the evo-devo perspective, this developmental process parallels evolutionary aspects of brain cavities and CSF formation and regulation in the deuterostome metazoan lineage (Fig. 1).

Metazoan phylogeny classifies the vertebrata as a subphylum of the phylum Chordata, which also includes two other subphyla, the Urochordata and the Cephalochordata. Within this scheme, the phylum Chordata is included in a major group, the Deuterostomia, which also includes the phyla Echinodermata and Hemichordata. These last two phyla are in turn grouped in the clade Ambulacraria. Chordates invariably possess a notochord and a dorsal neural tube, and share tadpole-type larvae containing the notochord and a hollow nerve cord. However, Ambulacrarians have dipleurula-type larvae containing a hydrocoel. It has been proposed that the evolutionary occurrence of tadpole-type larvae with a hollow nerve chord was fundamental to the origin of chordates [39]. The sister group of Deuterostomia are the Protostomia, including the clades Priapulida, Nematoda, Arthopoda, Platyhelminthes, Mollusca and Annelida, none of which exhibit a hollow nerve tube with an internal lumen or brain cavities.

It is thought that the CSF system evolved in the deuterostome lineage from the ancestor of Ambulacraria and Chordata, as a way to maintain the chemical environment required for the functioning of CNS cells, including the neuroendocrine pathways [40]. In this context, it has been said that the system of CSF-contacting neurons has a special role in taking up, transforming and emitting nonsynaptic signals mediated by this brain fluid. Most CSF-contacting neurons send dendritic processes into the CSF of the brain ventricles or central canal, where they form terminals bearing stereocilia. The axons of these CSF-contacting neurons transmit information taken up by dendrites and perikarya to synaptic zones of various brain areas. The importance of nonsynaptic signal transmission in the function of nervous tissue has been confirmed, and it has been considered that its evolutionary origin could be the deuterostome ancestors, before the split between Ambulacraria and Chordata clades (reviewed by [41]).

Echinoderms, such as starfish, have a neural plate-like nervous system. The neurons of the radial nerves and "brain" are always in contact with seawater, which allows them to directly detect its chemical composition and other physical parameters such as water temperature, and modulate the activity of the nervous system and overall animal behaviour accordingly (Fig. 1) [40, 42–44]. However, the open nature of this neural plate-like nervous system means that it cannot respond to neuroendocrine or other molecular signalling pathways. In contrast, Hemichordata, such as the acorn worm *Saccoglossus kowalevskii*, which may represent an intermediate body plan [23], exhibit both dorsal and ventral nerve cords. While the ventral cord runs only as far as the collar, the dorsal cord reaches into the proboscis, and is often hollow.

Regarding the phylum Chordata, the development of the cephalochordate amphioxus *Branchiostoma lanceolatum*, includes a larval stage in which the neural plate is folded longitudinally to form a neural tube, but the anterior neuropore remains open throughout this stage. This allows seawater to enter the ventricular lumen of the lancelet larval "brain". Thus seawater represents the first "internal" fluid environment of lancelet brain which consequently depends directly—but not necessarily exclusively—on the external environment [40, 41]. In these organisms, nearly all neurons are found to be in direct contact with the internal fluid of the neural tube-like central nervous system. However, when lancelets reach adulthood, the anterior neuropore closes and the ventricular lumen of the "brain" becomes a closed system (Fig. 1). Thus, the composition of this fluid no longer depends directly on the surrounding water environment, but largely on the activity and metabolism of the organism. This modified sea water constitutes the primary CSF.

At this stage, the regulatory function of CSF-contacting neurons likely become important through their interaction with the metabolic state of the brain tissue [44–46].

Similarly, the development of the Urochordate ascidia *Ciona intestinalis,* includes a larval stage in which the neural plate is folded longitudinally to form a neural tube, but the anterior neuropore also remains open (Fig. 1). Unlike lancelet larval development, ascidians follow an invariant pattern of embryonic cleavage, and their larval CNS possess fewer than 400 cells, most of which are in direct contact with the internal fluid of the neural tube-like central nervous system, as revealed by cell lineage studies [47–49]. Nevertheless, as in Cephalochordates, when ascidians reach adulthood the anterior neuropore closes and the ventricular lumen of the "brain" becomes a closed system, which includes a sensory vesicle (Fig. 1).

In lancelets and ascidians, nearly all neurons contact the lumen of the central nervous system. Consequently, it has been suggested that the CSF-contacting neurons of vertebrates are derived from an ancient epithelial neuron-type of the ectoderm, and thereby represent a phylogenetically old cell type, the "protoneuron" [50]. In mammals, only the CSF-contacting neurons of the spinal cord retain their ancient structure; the rest of the neurons no longer contact CSF [41].

Finally, in vertebrates, the anterior neuropore closes very early in neural tube development, just before primary neurogenesis starts, and thus the composition of the CSF contained within the cephalic cavities depends exclusively on the surrounding tissue and on the rest of the embryo from this stage. Environmental conditions are no longer directly detected by CNS neurons, and this function is passed to specific sensory organs. This opens up the possibility of precisely regulating CSF composition and homeostasis. The gain in CSF regulation implies, or has been paralleled by, a gain in morphological and physiological neural complexity. Thus, it has been reported that, at least in mammals, CSF is essential for the formation of the layers of neurons [51, 52] in the evolutionary progressively enlarged cerebral cortex, including the highly developed neocortex [53], a brain region that is absent in fish and amphibians (anamniotes).

CSF composition and homeostasis in vertebrate fetal and adult brains are tightly regulated by the choroid plexus, whose epithelial cells establish a blood-CSF barrier [54, 55] (reviewed by [56]). The choroid plexus is a vascular structure in the brain ventricles that secretes CSF by promoting the transport of certain molecules and electrolytes from blood plasma and producing others that are delivered directly to the ventricles [57–61]. All vertebrates analysed, from fish to mammals, possess a set of choroid plexuses [40, 56] and it has been described that the choroid plexus increases in complexity among the various vertebrate classes. However, no choroid plexus has been detected in non-vertebrate chordates, such as Cephalochordates. Acting in parallel, CNS homeostasis in adult vertebrates is also controlled by the blood–brain barrier (BBB) vessels in the brain, which significantly impede entry from the blood to the brain of virtually all molecules, except those that are small and lipophilic. However, BBB vessels also allow sets of small and large hydrophilic molecules, e.g., gene products, to enter the brain via various transport processes (reviewed by [62]). Control of eCSF production and homeostasis in vertebrate embryos from the closure of the anterior neuropore to the formation of functional choroid plexuses during fetal stages has not been analysed until recently. This developmental stage is particularly interesting for brain formation, since it is mainly characterised by rapid brain anlagen growth and initiation of primary neurogenesis in the neural progenitor cells lining the cavities.

Embryonic CSF function: from neural progenitor cell functions to the establishment of organising centres

CSF has intrigued philosophers, physicians and scientists for a long time. The earliest mention of a fluid within the brain dates back to ancient Egypt [5], and the first studies of barriers in the brain are attributed to Herophilus (335-280 BCE), who described the choroid plexus. The first reports on CSF functions are attributed to Galen of Pergamon (129-200/216). Studies on eCSF are much more recent, dating back to the mid-twentieth century. Due to its specific molecules and mechanical properties, it has been determined that eCSF plays several crucial roles during the early stages of brain development and may influence adult brain function.

Using several experimental approaches, mainly in zebrafish, chick and mouse embryos, it has been reported that the progressive increase in eCSF volume exerts positive pressure against the neuroepithelial walls and generates an expansive force, which contributes to brain expansion [63–65]. Moreover, as proteoglycans are the major components of the extracellular matrix found in embryo brain cavities, it has been suggested that the special osmotic properties of chondroitin sulfate proteoglycan and other proteoglycans in eCSF may cause water retention in the cavities [66, 67]. This would contribute to the generation and regulation of inner cephalic hydrostatic pressure.

Studies on in vitro cultures of neuroectodermal explants from chick and rat embryos at E4 and E12.5 (E stands for embryonic development day) respectively, which correspond to the stage at which the anterior neuropore has just closed and brain primary neurogenesis is initiated, have shown that diffusible molecules contained within eCSF, including growth factors and cytokines, contribute to the regulation of some basic neural progenitor cell functions, i.e., their survival, proliferation, and differentiation [68–70]. Furthermore, it has been reported that neuroectodermal tissue explants cultured with only a chemically defined medium show lower numbers of proliferating cells, an increased number of apoptotic cells, and a severe decrease in the number of cells engaged in the process of neural differentiation compared to control embryos. However, when the medium is supplemented with eCSF, these basic cellular parameters remain close to those of embryos developed in ovo (for chicks) or in utero (for rats). It has also been reported that repeatedly draining eCSF from embryonic zebrafish brain vesicles not only prevents brain enlargement due to the lack of hydrostatic pressure (see paragraph above), but also decreases the rate of cell survival [63], paralleling the effects reported in amniotes (at least in birds and mammals). Moreover, the particular effect of the eCSF on neural progenitor cells depends on the developmental stages from which both the fluid and the cells have been obtained. This suggests that the composition of the eCSF varies with time, as does the receptiveness of the cells, most probably through developmentally regulated specific receptors [52, 71, 72].

Most of the proteins identified in the eCSF (see the section below on *eCSF protein content*) have known physiological functions during embryonic development in systems other than CSF that nevertheless are consistent with the overall roles reported for eCSF during CNS development [73, 74]. Thus, functional in vivo and in vitro analysis of some of these molecules at the beginning of primary neurogenesis, before the formation of functional choroid plexuses, has revealed specific roles in the function of eCSF in neuroepithelial progenitor cell behaviour. For example, it has been reported that immunoblocking of active FGF2 in eCSF in chick embryos severely disrupts neuroepithelial stem cell proliferation and differentiation [75]. Similarly, it has been reported that the LDL lipid fraction, transported by apolipoprotein B in eCSF, is also involved in regulating neuroepithelial progenitor cell proliferation and differentiation in the same system [76].

Other reports in chick embryos have shown that retinol-binding protein (RBP) is responsible for transporting all-trans-retinol from the embryonic plasma to the eCSF (as detected by high-performance liquid chromatography), from where it reaches the neuroepithelium to be transformed into retinoic acid by the retinoic acid-synthesising enzymes expressed in this embryonic tissue; and that the presence of these molecules is necessary both in vivo and in vitro to maintain basic neuroepithelial cell parameters (i.e., proliferation and differentiation [77, 78]). Interestingly, a parallel situation has been described recently in zebrafish embryos [79]. This suggests that at least some of the basic mechanisms in which eCSF is involved during early brain development are conserved among vertebrates. It has also been shown that large glycoprotein SCO-spondin contributes to the control of neuroepithelial cell proliferation via eCSF in chick embryos [80], and that eCSF contained in nanovesicles carrying evolutionarily-conserved molecules promotes neural stem cell proliferation [81]. Other findings include the capacity of eCSF to activate neurogenesis of neural precursors within the subventricular zone of the adult mouse brain [82].

Therefore, eCSF contains specific molecules that affect neural progenitor cell behaviour. In addition, eCSF has been reported to be involved in regulating the expression of genes that are known to be implicated in brain patterning [31]. Thus, when dorsal mesencephalic neuroepithelial explants lacking IsO (a known organising centre for mesencephalon and brain development) or explants including IsO are cultured in a chemically defined medium but in the absence of eCSF, the typical expression of dorsal mesencephalic and IsO genes, i.e., *Otx2* and *Fgf8* respectively, is disrupted. Conversely, when dorsal mesencephalic explants including IsO are cultured in an eCSF-supplemented medium, they do express these genes. Interestingly, when dorsal mesencephalic explants lacking IsO are cultured with an eCSF-supplemented medium, they also show ectopic expression domains of *Shh* in the mesencephalic neuroectoderm, even though this gene is typically expressed in the ventral, but not the dorsal, neuroectoderm. Only the concurrence of eCSF and IsO allow this tissue to mimic its typical pattern of gene expression, which suggests that IsO and some molecules in eCSF act synergistically in brain development, as is the case for the retinoic acid system [77, 78]. It is worth noting that the elaboration of the full organiser properties of this region [30] and embryonic control over eCSF composition are both vertebrate innovations that act synergistically in brain development [31].

Moreover, the presence of folate and some of its derivatives within fetal CSF has been reported [83], as well as the presence of reduced-folate carriers within the neuroepithelium from E9.0 in mouse embryos [84, 85]. Folate is known to prevent neural tube defects when supplemented prior to conception, and it has also been reported to contribute to the establishment of epigenetic modifications [86–88], which in turn are crucial for CNS development [89], including adult behaviour [90–93]. Taken together, the results of all the studies mentioned in this section point to the crucial role of this embryonic fluid in the regulation of basic neural progenitor cell function and CNS development, before the formation of a functional choroid plexus. This may have implications for adult brain function.

Embryonic CSF protein content: from extracellular matrix components to growth factors

Classic studies performed on several species (chick embryos at developmental stages E2.5 to E6.5; sheep fetuses at E35 and E60; and rats from E12 to E22 and neonatal) showed that eCSF has a higher concentration of total proteins than adult CSF [94–100]; reviewed by [101]. Initially, individual proteins were identified based on crossed immunoelectrophoresis or by SDS-PAGE protein separation and molecular mass inference. More recent and accurate proteomic analyses of avian and mammalian eCSF have confirmed and greatly expanded most of the initial findings. The first reports to use conventional proteomic techniques (2D-electrophoresis, in-gel digestion, and ESI–MS/MS mass spectrometry analysis) were carried out on chick and rat eCSF at E4 and E12.5, respectively, which corresponds to the developmental stages when there is maximum neuroepithelial progenitor cell proliferation, and coincides with the beginning of brain neural differentiation. These studies showed the presence of dozens of specific proteins within this fluid, most of which may be involved in brain development, by inference from their roles in systems other than CSF [73, 74]. They include gene products involved in extracellular matrix, osmotic pressure and ion carriers, cell death and quiescence, apolipoproteins, retinol and vitamin D carriers, and antioxidant and antimicrobial products, among others (for a comparative review, see [101]).

From the evolutionary point of view, the most remarkable dissimilarity between chick and rat eCSF proteomes is the presence of enzymes and enzyme regulators in rat eCSF, as well as an increased number of members of the apolipoprotein family. Only two different apolipoproteins have been identified in chicks, AI and AIV, whereas at least five have been found in rats, including AI and AIV, as well as B, E, and M. These differences may be related to the higher complexity of the CNS in mammals, although apolipoprotein B was later identified in chick eCSF by Western-blot analysis using specific antibodies [76]. These dissimilarities may also be due to differences in the timing of choroid plexus formation between the two species. In this regard, E4.5 chick embryos correspond to a developmental stage that is 2.5 days before the first appearance of the choroid plexus. However, in E12.5 rat embryos, transthyretin-positive choroid plexus primordium starts to be detected, although it is probably not fully functional, as suggested by the coexistence of a specific, temporary embryonic blood-eCSF barrier [102] (see the section below on *eCSF composition and regulation*).

An extensive and thorough proteome analysis of rat and human eCSF from several different stages and locations of brain vesicles [i.e., E12.5, E14.5 from both the lateral and fourth ventricles, and E17.5 during cortical development in rats; and Carnegie Stage 20 (CG20) in humans] has also been reported [103]. They identified 423, 318, 249, and 382 proteins, respectively, in rats, and 188 proteins in humans, 130 of which are shared with rats. Although differences in protein number between rat and human eCSF has not been fully explained, it has been suggested it may be due to the difficulty in experimentally matching stages of embryonic cortical development between humans and rats [103], as the composition of this fluid has been proved to be highly dynamic. The categorisation of these proteins based on their molecular function and action on biological processes are almost identical, which suggest that they represent essential eCSF functions. They include several growth factors and cytokines. Similar results were obtained more recently by Bueno, Miyan and Parvas on eCSF from chick and rat embryos at E4 and E13 respectively, using a high-performance liquid chromatography ion-trap column coupled to an ESI MS/MS mass spectrometer, which is a more sensitive technique (unpublished results).

Other studies have examined the presence of growth factors and cytokines within eCSF by immunohistochemical procedures, since these molecules, crucial for controlling developmental processes, exert their actions at very low concentrations, and thus are not usually detected by conventional proteomic techniques. For example, Western-blot analyses of both avian and mammalian eCSF using specific antibodies have revealed the presence of fibroblast growth factor 2 (*Fgf2*) [75], epidermal growth factor (*Egf*) [104], and leukemia inhibitory factor [105], which are known to be involved in the regulation of a number of developmental processes. Taken together, these studies, whose overall results are relatively similar, have proved to be complementary. They reinforce the putative capacity of eCSF to influence the behaviour of neuroepithelial cells and CNS development through its constituent molecules, including behavioural aspects of adult brain function.

It has been reported that a number of neurological and neurodegenerative diseases, including dementia and schizophrenia, involve alterations in CSF protein content, which in some cases is also being used in diagnostics (see, for example, [101, 106–110]). It is tempting to speculate that abnormal eCSF composition early during CNS development may favour the appearance of these diseases during adulthood, due to interference with developmental mechanisms.

Regulation of embryonic CSF composition: the importance of the blood-eCSF barrier for controlling eCSF homeostasis in early brain development

As discussed in previous sections, the evolutionary development of brain cavities in vertebrates has provided the opportunity to tightly control eCSF composition and homeostasis from very early brain development stages. This in turn may allow this fluid to act as a mechanism for establishing neuroendocrine pathways and enabling a progressive increase in brain complexity. As described above, this hypothesis is supported by the particular effect of the specific molecules on neuroepithelial progenitor cell behaviour and on the establishment of organising centres, which are crucial for CNS development and functionality. The hypothesis is also supported by the molecular content of eCSF, as revealed by proteomic analyses and other technical approaches. However, to achieve this, barrier systems are required to control eCSF formation, composition and homeostasis from early brain developmental stages.

In fetuses and adults, there are several barrier systems that control the internal environment of the brain, such as the blood–brain barrier between the lumen of cerebral blood vessels and the brain parenchyma, the blood-CSF barrier between choroid plexus blood vessels and adult and fetal CSF, and the outer CSF-brain barrier between the subarachnoid space and overlying structures. The integrity of these barriers is crucial, as both the stability and specificity of this fluid environment are essential for normal brain development and function [111]. The barriers significantly impede the passage of virtually all molecules from the blood to the CSF, except for small, lipophilic ones, and some sets of both small and large hydrophilic molecules, such as proteins, that can enter the CSF by specific transport processes.

In avian and mammalian embryos, an inner CSF-brain barrier between the eCSF and the brain parenchyma has been reported that impedes the passage of virtually all molecules [102, 112]. However, the fact that eCSF content has proven crucial for these stages of CNS development implies the need for a physiological blood-eCSF transfer system that controls the initial composition and homeostasis of eCSF, before the formation of functional fetal choroid plexuses. This need is reinforced by the fact that most of the abundant protein fractions contained within the eCSF are produced outside of the brain anlagen, and thus they have to be transferred from the embryonic serum to the eCSF by crossing an inner eCSF-brain barrier [112]. In this context, the existence of an inner eCSF-brain barrier has been demonstrated by the microinjection of a small-sized 3 kDa tracer, biotin dextran amine(BDA3000), into the cephalic cavity, or conversely into the outflow of the heart of embryos at different embryonic days during chick development [102]. It has been shown that this inert tracer cannot cross the inner and temporary eCSF-brain barrier transfer area from day E4 on, i.e., after the closure of the anterior neuropore coinciding with the initiation of brain primary neurogenesis. However there exists a small subset of endothelial cells and adjacent neuroepithelial cells that remove the tracer from the brain cavities into the circulation. This subset of cells, which is located in the ventral mesencephalon and in the most anterior part of the ventral prosencephalon, lateral to the floor plate, may act as a temporary functional barrier transfer system, to control eCSF composition and homeostasis [102]. A number of studies published during the last 6 years, conducted primarily on chick embryos from E3 to E5 and on rat embryos at an equivalent developmental stage from E12.7 to E13.7, have demonstrated the existence of this functional, dynamic barrier transfer system. It is formed by endothelial cells of specific blood vessels and by columnar cells of the differentiating neuroepithelium. The system is active from closure of the anterior neuropore, at the beginning of brain primary neurogenesis and before the choroid plexus becomes functionally active. It contributes to the brain's internal milieu at this crucial stage of development (see [1, 2] for a review; see Table 1 for a chronology including main aspects of embryonic blood–brain barrier transfer system in chick and rat).

It has been reported that from chick E3, eCSF has a complex protein composition that differs from that of blood plasma, and that the relative concentration of these proteins varies during development and with respect to adult CSF [95–97, 99, 100]. Initially, eCSF is derived from trapped amniotic fluid. However, after the closure of the anterior neuropore, the brain cavities become physiologically sealed enabling the tight regulation of eCSF composition. Furthermore, it has been demonstrated in mice that amniotic fluid and eCSF proteomes begin to diverge during development after the closure of the anterior neuropore, and that these changes in protein composition allow neural progenitor cell self-renewal [113]. This suggests that the composition of eCSF is somehow regulated from this initial stage of brain development to fulfil specific functions on neuroepithelial progenitor cells. Various experiments have demonstrated that the transport

Table 1 Chronology of the embryonic blood–brain barrier transport system formation

Morphological or physiological aspect	Embryonic day (E)	
	Chick	Rat
Closure of anterior neuropore/initial differentiation of eCSF protein content	E1.7–E2	E10.5–E11
Brain cavity becomes physiologically sealed	E3.5–E4	E12.4–E12.7
Transient embryonic blood–brain barrier starts to be physiologically functional	A bit before E4	A bit before E12.7

of proteins from the blood plasma to the eCSF and vice versa in chick embryos at E4 and E5 is tightly regulated, as is the homeostatic control, which is crucial for eCSF function in brain development [102, 114]. These experiments included the quantification of endogenous chick proteins present in both the blood plasma and the eCSF (ovalbumin, retinol-binding protein, fibroblast growth factor No. 2, and immunoglobulin IgY), as well as the microinjection of several proteins of different molecular size into the brain cavities or alternatively into the outflow of the heart of chick embryos at E4 to examine the properties of this blood-eCSF barrier transfer system. The proteins used in the microinjection experiments included both endogenous chick proteins that are normally present in the eCSF or conversely not normally detected within this fluid, and proteins from sources other than chicks (bovine serum albumin, myosin heavy chain from rabbit, fibroblast growth factor No. 2, plasma retinol-binding protein, a recombinant protein from glutathione-S transferase from *Schistosoma japonicum*, alcohol dehydrogenase from *Drosophila lebanonensis*, and ovalbumin). These experiments demonstrated that the physiological ratio of chick endogenous proteins between the eCSF and the blood plasma is regulated developmentally, as the transfer rates varied from E3 to E5 according to their activity in brain development. It was also shown that the transfer of both chick endogenous proteins and microinjected proteins across the blood-eCSF interface was highly protein-specific. In other words, proteins that are not normally present within eCSF are never transferred from the blood serum to the brain cavity when microinjected into the outflow of the heart, and they are also rapidly removed from the eCSF when microinjected into the brain cavities. Interestingly, the ratio of transfer for these proteins was tightly regulated and never exceeded the physiological ratios for any developmental stage, even when the proteins were injected at levels 10- to 100-fold higher than normal physiological conditions [102].

A histological analysis of protein transfer across the blood-eCSF barrier transfer system demonstrated that it occurs only in a specific embryonic region, located in the brain stem lateral to the floor plate, in the ventral mesencephalon and the most anterior part of the ventral prosencephalon [102] (Fig. 1). This location does not coincide with the area where the fetal choroid plexus will start to develop, i.e., from an invagination of the dorsal roof plate along the midline of the neural tube. Therefore, this transient embryonic blood-eCSF barrier function appears to be independent of the choroid plexus, and probably fulfils a function that is temporarily lacking after the formation of a physiologically-sealed brain. Immunohistological analysis has also revealed that protein transport across this transient blood-eCSF barrier uses transcellular routes by means of caveolae [115]. It has also revealed the existence, in the same neuroepithelial and endothelial cells, of water and ion channels (i.e., *Aqp1*, *Aqp4*, and *Kir4.1* [116]) and glucose transporter (*Glut 1*) in both chick and rat embryos at an equivalent developmental stage [115].

Concluding remarks

Many of the world's first human civilisations developed along riverbanks and seashores, as they used the nearby fluid medium as a food resource. As civilisations developed over time and gained social and technological complexity, they also used the fluid pathways provided by rivers, lakes, seas and oceans to promote transport and cohesion between near and far territories. These activities included the trading of goods and news by postal services, to which people responded by adapting both their individual and collective behaviour to the changing environment. Over time, civilisations modified these fluid pathways to better serve their needs, for example by constructing harbours, dams and canals to regulate water influx, and docking for transport and irrigation. These cultural and technological human modifications of the fluid environment in some ways parallel and serve as an analogy of the evolutionary developmental changes that occur in CNS with regard to the existence of internal brain cavities filled with CSF, and with respect to CSF and eCSF composition and homeostasis regulation, as reviewed in this paper.

Thus, as human civilisations gain social complexity through the progressive use and control of fluid mediums, so does the CNS of deuterostomes with respect to the variety and complexity of neural cells and brain regionalisation. The vertebrate brain is organised, from its embryonic origins and throughout adult life, around this extraordinarily dynamic and complex fluid. CSF composition and homeostasis is tightly regulated from the closure of the anterior neuropore, just before brain primary neurogenesis starts. In contrast, in other deuterostomes, such as cephalochordates and Urochordates, CSF regulation starts during adulthood or is never present (as in Ambulacrarians). Hence, the evolutionary development of brain cavity systems, CSF, and CSF composition and regulation are milestones in vertebrate (and human) brain evolutionary development. They need to be further analysed to fully understand brain function, and may have implications for the increase in behavioural repertoire.

It will be interesting to investigate, in the light of evolution, whether the blood-eCSF embryonic barrier transfer system initially developed when brain cavities become sealed in early brain developmental stages, and thus is specific to the vertebrate lineage. Alternatively, it may represent the initial chordate evolutionary condition and may also be present in adult cephalochordates and urochordates, which have a closed cephalic cavity, but no choroid plexuses. If the latter is the case, the blood-eCSF embryonic barrier transfer system has been heterochronically reused in vertebrate embryos before the newly developed and far more complex choroid plexus is fully active.

Conclusions

Controlling CSF composition and homeostasis is a milestone in the development and evolution of the CNS in deuterostome metazoans, especially in chordates and vertebrates. In higher vertebrates, eCSF formation is tightly regulated by a transient blood–brain barrier transfer system located ventrally in the cephalic cavities from very early stages of brain development, just after the closure of the anterior neuropore, before choroid plexus becomes physiologically functional. It is known that gene products and other molecules contained within this fluid exert crucial functions on neuroepithelial progenitor cell survival, proliferation, differentiation and patterning. The evolutionary development of these barriers and transfer systems has contributed to the increase in brain complexity. Thus, further and deeper examination of the mechanisms regulating CSF composition and homeostasis as well as the functions it exerts on neuroepithelial progenitor cells in model organisms from different deuterostome taxa may provide new and important data for the evolutionary and developmental comprehension of the vertebrate brain.

Abbreviations

CSF: cerebrospinal fluid; CNS: central nervous system; E: embryonic day after conception; eCSF: embryonic cerebrospinal fluid.

Authors' contributions

The authors have contributed equally to this review. Both authors read and approved the final manuscript.

Acknowledgements

This review was supported by grant BFU2014-58908-P (from Ministerio de Economía y Competitividad) to JGF.

Competing interests

The authors declare that they have no competing interests.

References

1. Bueno D, Parvas M, Garcia-Fernàndez J. The embryonic blood-cerebrospinal fluid barrier function before the formation of the fetal choroid plexus: role in cerebrospinal fluid formation and homeostasis. Croat Med J. 2014;55:306–16.
2. Bueno D, Parvas M, Hermelo I, Garcia-Fernàndez J. Embryonic blood-cerebrospinal fluid barrier formation and function. Front Neurosci. 2014;8:343.
3. Ek CJ, Dziegielewska KM, Habgood MD, Saunders NR. Barriers in the developing brain and neurotoxicology. Neurotoxicology. 2012;33:586–604.
4. Gato A, Desmond ME. Why the embryo still matters: CSF and the neuroepithelium as interdependent regulators of embryonic brain growth, morphogenesis and histiogenesis. Dev Biol. 2009;327:263–72.
5. Liddelow SA. Fluids and barriers of the CNS: a historical viewpoint. Fluids Barriers CNS. 2011;8:2.
6. Liddelow SA. Development of the choroid plexus and blood-CSF barrier. Front Neurosci. 2015;9:32.
7. Stolp HB, Liddelow SA, Sá-Pereira I, Dziegielewska KM, Saunders NR. Immune responses at brain barriers and implications for brain development and neurological function in later life. Front Integr Neurosci. 2013;7:61.
8. Cohen B. Nobel committee rewards pioneers of development studies in fruitflies. Nature. 1995;377:465.
9. Raju TN. The Nobel chronicles. Edward B Lewis(b 1918), Christiane Nüsslein-Volhard (b 1942), and Eric Francis Wieschaus (b 1947). Lancet. 1995;2000(356):81.
10. Roush W. Nobel prizes: fly development work bears prize-winning fruit. Science. 1995;270:380–1.
11. Yamamoto D. Evo-Devo-Neuro approach to behavior. J Neurogenet. 2013;27:68.
12. O'Connell LA. Evolutionary development of neural systems in vertebrates and beyond. J Neurogenet. 2013;27:69–85.
13. Carroll SB. Evo-devo and an expanding evolutionary synthesis: a genetic theory of morphological evolution. Cell. 2008;134:25–36.
14. Goodman CS, Coughlin BC. The evolution of evo-devo biology. Proc Natl Acad Sci USA. 2000;97:4424–5.
15. Arendt D, Denes AS, Jekely G, Tessmar-Raible K. The evolution of nervous system centralisation. Philos Trans R Soc Lond B Biol Sci. 2008;363:1523–8.
16. Reiner A, Wullimann MF. The gain in the brain is plain when evo meets devo. BioEssays. 2004;26:1026–30.
17. Denes AS, Jekely G, Steinmetz PR, Raible F, Snyman H, Prud'homme B, Ferrier DE, Balavoine G, Arendt D. Molecular architecture of annelid nerve cord supports common origin of nervous system centralisation in bilateria. Cell. 2007;129:277–88.
18. Puelles L, Rubenstein JLR. Forebrain gene expression domains and the evolving prosomeric model. Trends Neurosci. 2003;26:469–76.
19. Rubenstein JLR, Puelles L. Homeobox gene expression during development of the vertebrate brain. Curr Top Dev Biol. 1994;29:1–63.
20. Striedter GF. Principles of brain evolution. 1st ed. Sunderland: Sinauer; 2005.
21. Lowe CJ, Terasaki M, Wu M, Freeman RM, Runft L, Kwan K, et al. Dorsoventral patterning in hemichordates: insights into early chordate evolution. PLoS Biol. 2006;4:e291.
22. Mizutani CM, Nie Q, Wan FY, Zhang YT, Vilmos P, Sousa-Neves R, et al. Formation of the BMP activity gradient in the Drosophila embryo. Dev Cell. 2005;8:915–24.
23. Lacalli TC. The emergence of the chordate body plan: some puzzles and problems. Acta Zoologica. 2010;1:4–10.
24. Farris SM. Evolutionary convergence of higher brain centers spanning the protostome-deuterostome boundary. Brain Behav Evol. 2008;72:106–22.
25. Lichtneckert R, Reichert H. Insights into the urbilaterian brain: conserved genetic patterning mechanisms in insect and vertebrate brain development. Heredity. 2005;94:465–77.
26. Schilling TF, Knight RD. Origins of anteroposterior patterning and Hox gene regulation during chordate evolution. Philos Trans R Soc B Biol Sci. 2001;356:1599–613.
27. Medina L, Abellan A. Development and evolution of the pallium. Semin Cell Dev Biol. 2009;20:698–711.
28. Moreno N, Gonzalez A, Retaux S. Development and evolution of the subpallium. Semin Cell Dev Biol. 2009;20:735–43.

29. Tomer R, Denes AS, Tessmar-Raible K, Arendt D. Profiling by image registration reveals common origin of annelid mushroom bodies and vertebrate pallium. Cell. 2010;142:800–9.
30. Ferrier DE, Minguillón C, Cebrián C, Garcia-Fernàndez J. Amphioxus Evx genes: implications for the evolution of the midbrain–hindbrain boundary and the chordate tailbud. Dev Biol. 2001;237:270–81.
31. Parada C, Martín C, Alonso MI, Moro JA, Bueno D, Gato A. Embryonic cerebrospinal fluid collaborates with the isthmic organiser to regulate mesencephalic gene expression. J Neurosci Res. 2005;82:333–45.
32. Chambery A, Parente A, Topo E, Garcia-Fernàndez J, D'Aniello S. Characterisation and putative role of a type I gonadotropin-releasing hormone in the cephalochordate amphioxus. Endocrinology. 2009;150:812–20.
33. Nomura T, Kawaguchi M, Ono K, Murakami Y. Reptiles: a new model for brain evo-devo research. J Exp Zool B Mol Dev Evol. 2013;320:57–73.
34. Awatramani R, Soriano P, Rodriguez C, Mai JJ, Dymecki SM. Cryptic boundaries in roof plate and choroid plexus identified by intersectional gene activation. Nat Genet. 2003;35:70–5.
35. Lun MP, Johnson MB, Broadbelt KG, Watanabe M, Kang YJ, Chau KF, et al. Spatially heterogeneous choroid plexus transcriptomes encode positional identity and contribute to regional CSF production. J Neurosci. 2015;35:4903–16.
36. Smith JL, Schoenwolf GC. Neurulation: coming to closure. Trends Neurosci. 1997;20:510–7.
37. Copp AJ, Greene ND, Murdoch JN. The genetic basis of mammalian neurulation. Nat Rev Genet. 2003;4:784–93.
38. Copp AJ. Neurulation in the cranial region–normal and abnormal. J Anat. 2005;207:623–35.
39. Satoh N, Rokhsar D, Nishikawa T. Chordate evolution and the three-phylum system. Proc Biol Sci. 2014;281:20141729.
40. Brocklehurst G. The significance of the evolution of the cerebrospinal fluid system. Ann Rev Coll Surg Engl. 1979;61:349–56.
41. Vígh B, Manzano e Silva MJ, Frank CL, Vincze C, Czirok SJ, Szabó A, et al. The system of cerebrospinal fluid-contacting neurons. Its supposed role in the nonsynaptic signal transmission of the brain. Histol Histopathol. 2004;19:607–28.
42. Vígh B, Vígh-Teichmann I, Manzano e Silva MJ, van den Pol AN. Cerebrospinal fluid-contacting neurons of the central canal and terminal ventricle in various vertebrates. Cell Tissue Res. 1983;231:615–21.
43. Vígh-Teichmann I, Vígh B. Cerebrospinal fluid (CSF) contacting dendrite terminals (Landolt's clubs) in the pineal organ of Chimera monstrosa. In: Functional morphology of neuroendocrine systems. Evolutionary and environmental aspects. 1st ed. Berlin: Springer-Verlag; 1986.
44. Vígh-Teichmann I, Vígh B. The cerebrospinal fluid-contacting neuron: a peculiar cell type of the central nervous system. Immunocytochemical aspects. Arch Histol Cytol. 1989;52(Suppl):195–207.
45. Vígh B, Vígh-Teichmann I. Comparison between CSF contacting neurons and cells of the radial nerve of some echinoderms. Anat Anz. 1982;76:461–3.
46. Vígh-Teichmann I, Vígh B. The system of cerebrospinal fluid contacting neurons. Arch Histol Jpn. 1983;46:427–68.
47. Cole AG, Meinertzhagen IA. The central nervous system of the ascidian larva: mitotic history of cells forming the neural tube in late embryonic *Ciona intestinalis*. Dev Biol. 2004;271:239–62.
48. Meinertzhagen IA, Okamura Y. The larval ascidian nervous system: the chordate brain from its small beginnings. Trends Neurosci. 2001;24:401–10.
49. Taniguchi K, Nishida H. Tracing cell fate in brain formation during embryogenesis of the ascidian *Halocynthia roretzi*. Dev Growth Differ. 2004;46:163–80.
50. Vígh B, Vígh-Teichmann I. The cerebrospinal fluid contacting neurosecretory cell: A protoneuron. In: Farner DS, Lederis K editors. Molecules cells systems. New York:Plenum Press; 1982. p. 458–60.
51. Miyan JA, Nabiyouni M, Zendah M. Development of the brain: a vital role for cerebrospinal fluid. Can J Physiol Pharmacol. 2003;81:317–28.
52. Miyan JA, Zendah M, Mashayekhi F, Owen-Lynch PJ. Cerebrospinal fluid supports viability and proliferation of cortical cells in vitro, mirroring in vivo development. Cerebrospinal Fluid Res. 2006;3:2.
53. Taverna E, Götz M, Huttner WB. The cell biology of neurogenesis: toward an understanding of the development and evolution of the neocortex. Annu Rev Cell Dev Biol. 2014;30:465–502.
54. Møllgård K, Lauritzen B, Saunders NR. Double replica technique applied to choroid plexus from early foetal sheep: completeness and complexity of tight junctions. J Neurocytol. 1979;8:139–49.
55. Tauc M, Vignon X, Bouchaud C. Evidence for the effectiveness of the blood–CSF barrier in the fetal rat choroid plexus. A freeze-fracture and peroxidase diffusion study. Tissue Cell. 1984;16:65–74.
56. Bill BR, Korzh V. Choroid plexus in developmental and evolutionary perspective. Front Neurosci. 2014;14(8):363.
57. Dziegielewska KM, Ek J, Habgood MD, Saunders NR. Development of the choroid plexus. Microsc Res Tech. 2001;52:5–20.
58. Johansson PA, Dziegielewska KM, Liddelow SA, Saunders NR. The blood-CSF barrier explained: when development is not immaturity. BioEssays. 2008;30:237–48.
59. Johansson PA, Irmler M, Acampora D, Beckers J, Simeone A, Gotz M. The transcription factor Otx2 regulates choroid plexus development and function. Development. 2013;140:1055–66.
60. Lehtinen MK, Walsh CA. Neurogenesis at the brain-cerebrospinal fluid interface. Annu Rev Cell Dev Biol. 2011;27:653–79.
61. Lehtinen MK, Bjornsson CS, Dymecki SM, Gilbertson RJ, Holtzman DM, Monuki ES. The choroid plexus and cerebrospinal fluid: emerging roles in development, disease, and therapy. J Neurosci. 2013;33:17553–9.
62. Rubin LL, Staddon JM. The cell biology of the blood-brain barrier. Annu Rev Neurosci. 1999;22:11–28.
63. Chang JT, Sive H. Manual drainage of the zebrafish embryonic brain ventricles. J Vis Exp. 2012;70:e4243.
64. Desmond ME, Jacobson AG. Embryonic brain enlargement requires cerebrospinal fluid pressure. Dev Biol. 1977;57:188–98.
65. Desmond ME, Levitan ML. Brain expansion in the chick embryo initiated by experimentally produced occlusion of the spinal neurocoel. Anat Rec. 2002;268:147–59.
66. Alonso MI, Gato A, Moro JA, Barbosa E. Disruption of proteoglycans in neural tube fluid by beta-D-xyloside alters brain enlargement in chick embryos. Anat Rec. 1998;252:499–508.
67. Alonso MI, Gato A, Moro JA, Martin P, Barbosa E. Involvement of sulfated proteoglycans in embryonic brain expansion at earliest stages of development in rat embryos. Cells Tissues Organs. 1999;165:1–9.
68. Gato A, Moro JA, Alonso MI, Bueno D, De La Mano A, Martín C. Embryonic cerebrospinal fluid regulates neuroepithelial survival, proliferation, and neurogenesis in chick embryos. Anat Rec A Discov Mol Cell Evol Biol. 2005;284:475–84.
69. Martin C, Alonso MI, Santiago C, Moro JA, De la Mano A, Carretero R, et al. Early embryonic brain development in rats requires the trophic influence of cerebrospinal fluid. Int J Dev Neurosci. 2009;27:733–40.
70. Gato A, Alonso MI, Martín C, Carnicero E, Moro JA, De la Mano A, et al. Embryonic cerebrospinal fluid in brain development: neural progenitor control. Croat Med J. 2014;55:299–305.
71. Nabiuni M, Rasouli J, Parivar K, Kochesfehani HM, Irian S, Miyan JA. In vitro effects of fetal rat cerebrospinal fluid on viability and neuronal differentiation of PC12 cells. Fluids Barriers CNS. 2012;9:8.
72. Yari S, Parivar K, Nabiuni M, Keramatipour M. Effect of embryonic cerebrospinal fluid on proliferation and differentiation of neuroprogenitor cells. Cell J. 2013;15:29–36.
73. Parada C, Gato A, Bueno D. Mammalian embryonic cerebrospinal fluid proteome has greater apolipoprotein and enzyme pattern complexity than the avian proteome. J Proteome Res. 2005;4:2420–8.
74. Parada C, Gato A, Aparicio M, Bueno D. Proteome analysis of chick embryonic cerebrospinal fluid. Proteomics. 2006;6:312–20.
75. Martin C, Bueno D, Alonso MI, Moro JA, Callejo S, Parada C, et al. FGF2 plays a key role in embryonic cerebrospinal fluid trophic properties over chick embryo neuroepithelial stem cells. Dev Biol. 2006;297:402–16.
76. Parada C, Escolà-Gil JC, Bueno D. Low-density lipoproteins from embryonic cerebrospinal fluid are required for neural differentiation. J Neurosci Res. 2008;86:2674–84.
77. Parada C, Gato A, Bueno D. All-trans retinol and retinol-binding protein from embryonic cerebrospinal fluid exhibit dynamic behaviour during early central nervous system development. NeuroReport. 2008;19:945–50.
78. Alonso MI, Martín C, Carnicero E, Bueno D, Gato A. Cerebrospinal fluid control of neurogenesis induced by retinoic acid during early brain development. Dev Dyn. 2011;240:1650–9.

79. Chang JT, Lehtinen MK, Sive H. Zebrafish cerebrospinal fluid mediates cell survival through a retinoid signaling pathway. Dev Neurobiol. 2016;76:75–92.
80. Vera A, Stanic K, Montecinos H, Torrejón M, Marcellini S, Caprile T. SCO-spondin from embryonic cerebrospinal fluid is required for neurogenesis during early brain development. Front Cell Neurosci. 2013;7:80.
81. Feliciano DM, Zhang S, Nasrallah CM, Lisgo SN, Bordey A. Embryonic cerebrospinal fluid nanovesicles carry evolutionarily conserved molecules and promote neural stem cell amplification. PLoS One. 2014;9:e88810.
82. Carnicero E, Alonso MI, Carretero R, Lamus F, Moro JA, de la Mano A, et al. Embryonic cerebrospinal fluid activates neurogenesis of neural precursors within the subventricular zone of the adult mouse brain. Cells Tissues Organs. 2013;198:398–404.
83. Cains S, Shepherd A, Nabiuni M, Owen-Lynch PJ, Miyan J. Addressing a folate imbalance in fetal cerebrospinal fluid can decrease the incidence of congenital hydrocephalus. J Neuropathol Exp Neurol. 2009;68:404–16.
84. Maddox DM, Manlapat A, Roon P, Prasad P, Ganapathy V, Smith SB. Reduced-folate carrier (RFC) is expressed in placenta and yolk sac, as well as in cells of the developing forebrain, hindbrain, neural tube, craniofacial region, eye, limb buds and heart. BMC Dev Biol. 2003;3:6.
85. Saitsu H, Ishibashi M, Nakano H, Shiota K. Spatial and temporal expression of folate-binding protein 1 (Fbp1) is closely associated with anterior neural tube closure in mice. Dev Dyn. 2003;226:112–7.
86. Choi SW, Mason JB. Folate and carcinogenesis: an integrated scheme. J Nutr. 2000;130:129–32.
87. Lucock M. Folic acid: nutritional biochemistry, molecular biology, and role in disease processes. Mol Genet Metab. 2000;71:121–38.
88. Meethal SV, Hogan KJ, Mayanil CS, Iskandar BJ. Folate and epigenetic mechanisms in neural tube development and defects. Childs Nerv Syst. 2013;29:1427–33.
89. Juliandi B, Abematsu M, Nakashima K. Epigenetic regulation in neural stem cell differentiation. Dev Growth Differ. 2010;52:493–504.
90. Butler AA, Webb WM, Lubin FD. Regulatory RNAs and control of epigenetic mechanisms: expectations for cognition and cognitive dysfunction. Epigenomics. 2016;8:135–51.
91. Roth TL. Epigenetics of neurobiology and behavior during development and adulthood. Dev Psychobiol. 2012;54:590–7.
92. Senut MC, Cingolani P, Sen A, Kruger A, Shaik A, Hirsch H, et al. Epigenetic of early-life lead exposure and effects on brain development. Epigenomics. 2012;4:665–74.
93. Lv J, Xin Y, Zhou W, Qiu Z. The epigenetic switches for neural development and psychiatric disorders. J Genet Genomics. 2013;40:339–46.
94. Birge WJ, Rose AD, Haywood JR, Doolin PF. Development of the blood-cerebrospinal fluid barrier to proteins and differentiation of cerebrospinal fluid in the chick embryo. Dev Biol. 1974;41:245–54.
95. Checiu I, Prelipceanu O, Popescu O. The role of cerebrospinal fluid during embryonic development. A biochemical study. Morphol Embryol. 1984;30:243–50.
96. Dziegielewska KM, Evans CA, Fossan G. Proteins in cerebrospinal fluid and plasma of fetal sheep during development. J Physiol. 1980;300:441–55.
97. Dziegielewska KM, Evans CA, Fossan G, Lorscheider FL, Malinowska DH, Mřllgĺrd K, et al. Proteins in cerebrospinal fluid and plasma of fetal sheep during development. J Physiol. 1980;300:441–55.
98. Dziegielewska KM, Evans CA, Lai PC. Proteins in cerebrospinal fluid and plasma of fetal rats during development. Dev Biol. 1981;83:193–200.
99. Fielitz W, Esteves A, Moro R. Protein composition of cerebrospinal fluid in the developing chick embryo. Brain Res. 1984;315:111–5.
100. Gato A, Martín P, Alonso MI, Martín C, Pulgar MA, Moro JA. Analysis of cerebro-spinal fluid protein composition in early developmental stages in chick embryos. J Exp Zool A Comp Exp Biol. 2004;301:280–9.
101. Parada C, Parvas M, Bueno D. Cerebrospinal fluid proteomes: from neural development to neurodegenerative diseases. Curr Proteomics. 2007;4:89–106.
102. Parvas M, Parada C, Bueno D. A blood-CSF barrier function controls embryonic CSF protein composition and homeostasis during early CNS development. Dev Biol. 2008;321:51–63.
103. Zappaterra MD, Lisgo SN, Lindsay S, Gygi SP, Walsh CA, Ballif BA. A comparative proteomic analysis of human and rat embryonic cerebrospinal fluid. J Proteome Res. 2007;6:3537–48.
104. Birecree E, King LEJ, Nanney LB. Epidermal growth factor and its receptor in the developing human nervous system. Brain Res Dev Brain Res. 1991;60:145–54.
105. Hatta T, Matsumoto A, Ono A, Udagawa J, Nimura M, Hashimoto R, et al. Quantitative analyses of leukemia inhibitory factor in the cerebrospinal fluid in mouse embryos. NeuroReport. 2006;17:1863–6.
106. Abdelhak A, Junker A, Brettschneider J, Kassubek J, Ludolph AC, Otto M, et al. Brain-specific cytoskeletal damage markers in cerebrospinal fluid: is there a common pattern between amyotrophic lateral sclerosis and primary progressive multiple sclerosis? Int J Mol Sci. 2015;16:17565–88.
107. Del Campo M, Jongbloed W, Twaalfhoven HA, Veerhuis R, Blankenstein MA, Teunissen CE. Facilitating the validation of novel protein biomarkers for dementia: an optimal workflow for the development of sandwich immunoassays. Front Neurol. 2015;6:202.
108. Oertel-Knöchel V, Bittner RA, Knöchel C, Prvulovic D, Hampel H. Discovery and development of integrative biological markers for schizophrenia. Prog Neurobiol. 2011;95:686–702.
109. Simon MJ, Iliff JJ. Regulation of cerebrospinal fluid (CSF) flow in neurodegenerative, neurovascular and neuroinflammatory disease. Biochim Biophys Acta. 2016;1862:442–51.
110. Sui X, Liu J, Yang X. Cerebrospinal fluid biomarkers of Alzheimer's disease. Neurosci Bull. 2014;30(2):233–42.
111. Davson H, Segal MB. Physiology of the CSF and blood-brain barriers. Florida: CRC Press; 1996.
112. Parvas M, Rius M, Bueno D. Most of the abundant protein fractions of embryonic cerebrospinal fluid are produced out of the brain anlagen. Open Proteomics J. 2008;1:1–4.
113. Chau KF, Springel MW, Broadbelt KG, Park HY, Topal S, Lun MP, et al. Progressive differentiation and instructive capacities of amniotic fluid and cerebrospinal fluid proteomes following neural tube closure. Dev Cell. 2015;35:789–802.
114. Castells A, Parvas M, Bueno D. Homeostasis of cerebrospinal fluid has a role in early brain development. NeuroReport. 2012;23:917–21.
115. Parvas M, Bueno D. The embryonic blood-CSF barrier has molecular elements for specific glucose transport and for the general transport of molecules via transcellular routes. Adv Biosci Biotechnol. 2010;1:315–21.
116. Parvas M, Bueno D. The embryonic blood-CSF barrier has molecular elements to control E-CSF osmolarity during early CNS development. J Neurosci Res. 2010;88:1205–12.

7

NIH workshop report on the trans-agency blood–brain interface workshop 2016: exploring key challenges and opportunities associated with the blood, brain and their interface

Margaret J. Ochocinska[1*], Berislav V. Zlokovic[2], Peter C. Searson[3], A. Tamara Crowder[4], Richard P. Kraig[5], Julia Y. Ljubimova[6], Todd G. Mainprize[7], William A. Banks[8], Ronald Q. Warren[9], Andrei Kindzelski[9], William Timmer[10] and Christina H. Liu[10]

Abstract

A trans-agency workshop on the blood–brain interface (BBI), sponsored by the National Heart, Lung and Blood Institute, the National Cancer Institute and the Combat Casualty Care Research Program at the Department of Defense, was conducted in Bethesda MD on June 7–8, 2016. The workshop was structured into four sessions: (1) blood sciences; (2) exosome therapeutics; (3) next generation in vitro blood–brain barrier (BBB) models; and (4) BBB delivery and targeting. The first day of the workshop focused on the physiology of the blood and neuro-vascular unit, blood or biofluid-based molecular markers, extracellular vesicles associated with brain injury, and how these entities can be employed to better evaluate injury states and/or deliver therapeutics. The second day of the workshop focused on technical advances in in vitro models, BBB manipulations and nanoparticle-based drug carrier designs, with the goal of improving drug delivery to the central nervous system. The presentations and discussions underscored the role of the BBI in brain injury, as well as the role of the BBB as both a limiting factor and a potential conduit for drug delivery to the brain. At the conclusion of the meeting, the participants discussed challenges and opportunities confronting BBI translational researchers. In particular, the participants recommended using BBI translational research to stimulate advances in diagnostics, as well as targeted delivery approaches for detection and therapy of both brain injury and disease.

Keywords: Blood–brain barrier, Extracellular vesicles, Exosomes, Cancer, Neurodegeneration, Traumatic brain injury, Therapeutics, Delivery

Background

The goal of the trans-agency blood–brain interface (BBI) workshop was to bring together experts to examine key challenges and develop recommendations for further studies of the interface between the circulatory system and the brain. The interagency workshop was designed to include sessions on the interface itself as well as sessions on blood biomarkers, targeted drug delivery, and brain disorders that release biomarkers into the circulation (Additional file 1).

A common scientific theme that has recently emerged is the role of the immune system and the inflammasome (e.g., innate immune system sensors for immediate response to molecular signals from the injured site or invading microbes). Another emerging area is the role of extracellular vesicles (EV), including exosomes and

*Correspondence: Margaret.Ochocinska@nih.gov
[1] National Heart, Lung, and Blood Institute, National Institutes of Health, 6701 Rockledge Dr., Room 9149, Bethesda, MD 20892-7950, USA

microparticles, and how they can be harnessed for both diagnostic and targeted drug delivery applications. It should be noted that the nomenclature and classification of these cell-derived vesicles is still in progress [1].

Experts in the blood sciences, BBB biology, BBB modeling and technology development—including exosome therapeutics, platform technologies, and nanotechnology—were invited to the workshop to present their latest ideas and research. The workshop presentations and ensuing interdisciplinary discussions highlighted the potential of technologies for diagnostics and therapy development and the need for collaborations across the various groups represented at the meeting. The workshop concluded by generating a set of recommendations to facilitate future development in this promising yet under-represented field.

Keynote presentation I: MRI-guided focused ultrasound surgery to open the blood–brain barrier in the treatment of brain tumors

Dr. Todd Mainprize discussed the potential of MRI-guided focused ultrasound surgery to create openings in the BBB. Dr. Mainprize noted that glioblastoma is the most malignant brain tumor, characterized by a very poor prognosis. Many therapeutic approaches have been developed to treat glioblastoma but do not improve patient survival, in part due to the lack of effective drug delivery through the BBB. Several methods have been employed to circumvent the BBB and more effectively deliver therapeutics to the brain, including direct intratumoral injection, osmotic disruption following intra-arterial carotid delivery, and convection-enhanced delivery.

Ultrasound has been used in medical applications since the early 1900s and has been used for therapeutic purposes in the CNS since the 1950s. Dr. Mainprize pointed out that more recently, magnetic resonance-guided focused ultrasound (MRgFUS), which is a non-invasive procedure that reversibly opens the BBB without damage to the surrounding neurons, has been employed for targeted drug delivery to the brain [2]. Recent studies involving non-human primates [3] investigated the effectiveness and characteristics of BBB opening by MRgFUS. A clinical trial, designed to establish the feasibility, safety and preliminary efficacy of MRgFUS to open the BBB for the delivery of chemotherapeutic agents in brain tumors, has been approved by Health Canada. This single-site Phase I study (NCT02343991), is currently recruiting patients ($n = 6$ max) at the University of Toronto, ON, Canada. Preliminary results have shown an increase in gadolinium uptake (indicative of BBB opening) in the sonicated area of the brain. Treatment with intravenous (IV) doxorubicin, which has very poor oral bioavailability, showed a two to threefold increase in concentration via targeted delivery to the brain tumor. Dr. Mainprize cautioned that the results of this limited interventional trial are preliminary, but suggest that MRgFUS may provide a new method to deliver therapeutic agents into the brain.

Blood science session: Part I (Fig. 1)

The blood–brain barrier and neurodegeneration

Blood vessels in the brain are organized in parallel with the major neurologic circuits tasked with sensation, memory and motion. Tight interrelationships between these circuits may reflect key functional roles the vasculature plays in normal neuronal function, disease and aging [4]. Dr. Berislav Zlokovic discussed the role of the BBB in neurologic disorders, with an emphasis on targets and treatments. He discussed: (1) how defects in blood vessels and the neurovascular unit can lead to BBB breakdown and neurodegeneration (Fig. 1a) [4], (2) the effects of genetic risk factors for Alzheimer's disease (AD) on blood vessels and BBB [5], and (3) the importance of new neurovascular imaging techniques and biomarkers in predicting cognitive impairment [6]. Potential therapeutic targets and treatments directed at the neurovascular unit in AD and stroke were described, including inhibition of the receptor for advanced glycation end-products in AD [7] and protection of the BBB and the neurovascular unit by protease activated protein C in stroke.

Microfluidics for blood research: from disease simulation to patient-specific phenotyping to diagnostics

Dr. Scott Diamond discussed how the quantitation of blood function during thrombosis and hemostasis can be achieved through a combination of systems biology, patient-specific high throughput phenotyping, as well as microfluidics, which is a multidisciplinary field that focuses on the science and technology of fluid flow on a submillimeter scale (Fig. 1b) [8, 9]. Advances in anticoagulation techniques allow the study of platelet function alone, platelet and thrombin function, and thrombosis via both the contact and extrinsic pathways [10]. In addition to blood function, Dr. Diamond's laboratory also includes studies on the interaction of patient blood with cultured endothelium in microfluidic environments. This is part of a larger effort to recreate the neurovascular unit while maintaining flow and measuring the resistivity of the system. However, the phenotypic variability and lack of standardization of cultured human brain endothelium remains a challenge. Dr. Diamond explained that the development of endothelial permeability assays in vitro will help facilitate the evaluation of trans-endothelial transport mechanisms under flow conditions. Compared to animal models, microfluidics offers a highly reproducible and translatable model with improved control

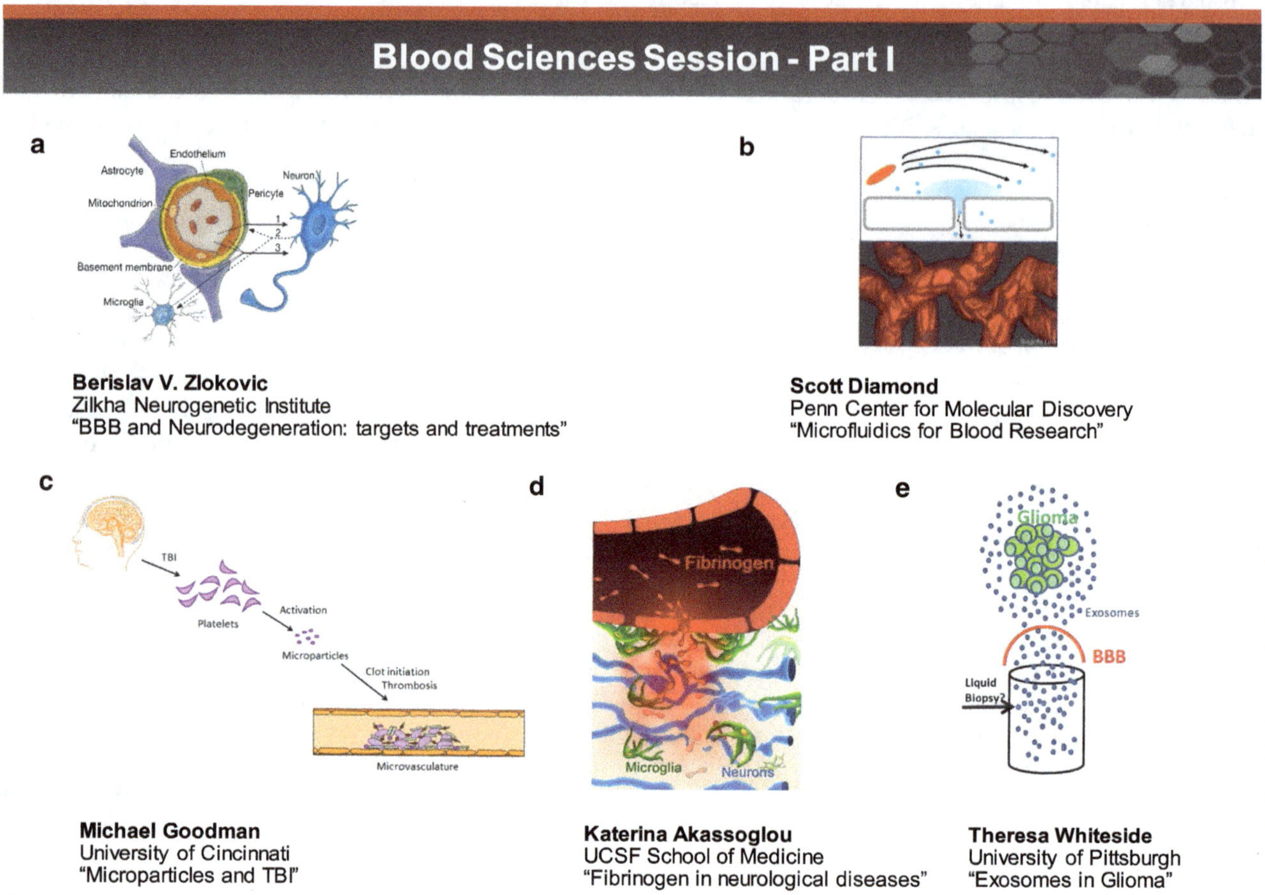

Fig. 1 Blood sciences session—Part I. Part I of the blood sciences session focused on the physiology of the blood and neurovascular unit, biofluid-based molecular markers, and extracellular vesicles associated with brain injury and disease progression. The presentations explored how these entities are transported between brain and blood and can be employed to evaluate injury states or deliver therapeutics. **a** Endothelial cells, pericytes, neurons and glia constitute an interconnected functional cellular network, collectively referred to as the neurovascular unit. Dr. Berislav Zlokovic discussed how defects in blood vessels and the neurovascular unit can lead to BBB breakdown and neurodegeneration (image reprinted with permission from [107]). **b** The Diamond laboratory uses a combination of microfluidics, patient-specific high throughput phenotyping, and systems biology to quantify blood function in the hemodynamic and pharmacological context of thrombosis and hemostasis. Image courtesy of Dr. Diamond. **c** Dr. Michael Goodman discussed how traumatic brain injury (TBI) induces systemic alterations in the aggregation of platelets aggregation and as well as the generation and function of microparticles (MP). Image courtesy of Dr. Goodman. **d** Dr. Katerina Akassoglou identified fibrinogen as a novel molecular link between blood–brain barrier disruption, activation of CNS innate immunity, and neurodegeneration. Image courtesy of Dr. Akassoglou. **e** Dr. Theresa Whiteside noted that genetic and molecular cargo of exosomes found in plasma of glioma patients resembles that of tumor cells and suggested that tumor derived exosomes hold promise as biomarkers of prognosis, as a source of liquid biopsy. Image courtesy of Dr. Whiteside

and visualization capabilities. Dr. Diamond concluded that microfluidic systems can also aid in optimization of nanoparticle formulations, measuring changes in blood chemistry and platelet function during trauma [11] or stroke, and the determination of novel cellular signaling pathways that regulate the BBB.

Microparticles impact coagulation after traumatic brain injury

Dr. Michael Goodman discussed how traumatic brain injury (TBI) induces systemic alterations in the aggregation of platelets as well as the generation and function of microparticles (MP), which are cell-derived extracellular vesicles (EVs) in the 0.1–1 μm range (Fig. 1c) [12]. Dr. Goodman began by noting that the pathophysiology that drives the subacute, persistent hypercoagulable state commonly seen after TBI is not well understood. Alterations in platelet and MP numbers and function caused by TBI, have been suggested as possible causes; however, the contributions of platelets and MPs are currently unknown. Dr. Goodman emphasized that further opportunities remain to determine the direct effect of injury-derived MPs on platelet function and endothelial activation. Studies examining the ability of MPs to traverse the BBB have yet to be performed. Future research will need to focus on the multitude of physiologic and pathologic functions of specific cell-derived MPs in response to injury [13–16].

Fibrinogen in neurological diseases: mechanisms, imaging, therapeutics

A key challenge for the BBB field is the limited understanding of the consequences of blood proteins in the CNS and their contribution to neuronal dysfunction. Protection of the CNS from leakage of plasma proteins by the BBB is compromised in a wide range of neuroimmune and neurodegenerative diseases, as well as after TBI. Dr. Katerina Akassoglou identified fibrinogen as a novel molecular link between blood and brain barrier disruption (BBBD), activation of CNS innate immunity, and neurodegeneration (Fig. 1d) [17]. Following fibrinogen conversion to pro-inflammatory fibrin, the CD11b/CD18 integrin receptor (also known as Mac-1 and complement receptor 3) is activated on microglial cells [18, 19]. Genetic disruption of the fibrin/CD11b interaction suppresses this microglial activation process and results in a reduction of neurologic symptoms, inflammation, demyelination, and axonal damage in experimental autoimmune encephalomyelitis (EAE) [17, 20, 21]. Dr. Akassoglou concluded that targeting the functions of fibrin in the CNS without affecting its beneficial effects in hemostasis holds promise for therapeutic intervention, and suggested that studies of fibrin-induced neuroinflammation in neurological diseases associated with fibrin deposition and microglial activation, such as TBI and AD, are also warranted.

Exosomes in glioma: their potential as carriers of information between the tumor and immune cells

Exosomes, the smallest (30–150 nm) of cell-derived extracellular vesicles (EVs) are present in all body fluids and serve as carriers of information between tumors, immune cells and normal tissue cells. Dr. Theresa Whiteside presented her research involving exosomes in glioma. Dr. Whiteside noted that genetic and molecular cargo of exosomes found in plasma of glioma patients resembles that of tumor cells and suggested that tumor derived exosomes hold promise as biomarkers of prognosis, as a source of liquid biopsy (Fig. 1e). Studies determined that changes in total exosomal protein and mRNA levels could serve as surrogate markers of immunological and clinical responses in glioma patients receiving anti-tumor vaccines [22]. Results from a Phase I/II clinical trial (NCT00766753) indicated that protein and mRNA expression levels for immune-related genes in exosomes (isolated from glioma patients' plasma) were useful in predicting glioma patients' response to dendritic cell (DC)-based vaccination therapy, and could potentially serve as surrogate markers of anti-tumor immune activity and survival.

Blood science session: Part II (Fig. 2)

BBB integrity is critical for preserving brain function following injury (e.g., TBI). Dr. Tamara Crowder emphasized the unique set of challenges for managing BBB integrity in combat-related TBI. Treatment of combat casualties is often complicated by polytrauma and medics must balance lifesaving measures for TBI in combination with hemorrhage, burn, and/or amputation to give the casualty the best chance of survival. The primary goal of the Defense Health Agency's Neurotrauma program is to decrease TBI-related morbidity and mortality, mitigate secondary brain injury, and to facilitate interventions and capabilities for improved patient care. Tools and technologies are currently being developed to improve capabilities for assessment and monitoring of CNS trauma to: (1) explore the relationship among the post-traumatic cerebral blood, autoregulation and the neurovascular unit; and (2) leverage different transporters at the BBIs to regulate the brain metabolomics and pharmacologic microenvironment. According to Dr. Crowder, these tools and technologies offer opportunities to improve clinical practice following brain injury.

Monitoring the central nervous system through peripheral biofluids

The ability to monitor the CNS would advance our knowledge of disease pathogenicity, facilitate clinical care, and support the development of new therapies. Dr. Kendall Van Keuren-Jensen discussed the need for accessible biomarkers in order to allow more frequent monitoring of the CNS and the potential to improve patient care. The presence of RNA in body fluids and its relative stability when transported via EVs or carrier proteins has captured significant attention as a source for biomarker discovery (Fig. 2a). Dr. Van Keuren-Jensen's laboratory identified CNS-enriched RNA transcripts in saliva, plasma/serum, urine, and cerebrospinal fluid (CSF). The potential of extracellular RNAs (exRNAs) for monitoring CNS diseases was demonstrated by the finding that microRNA-34c is upregulated in the hippocampus of AD patients and in mouse models of cognitive impairment [23, 24]. MicroRNA-34c was also found to be upregulated in serum and plasma from patients with dementia in two independent studies [25, 26]. The promise of exRNAs as biomarkers for the CNS is considerable; however, the field is still at an early stage in understanding their specificity and reproducibility.

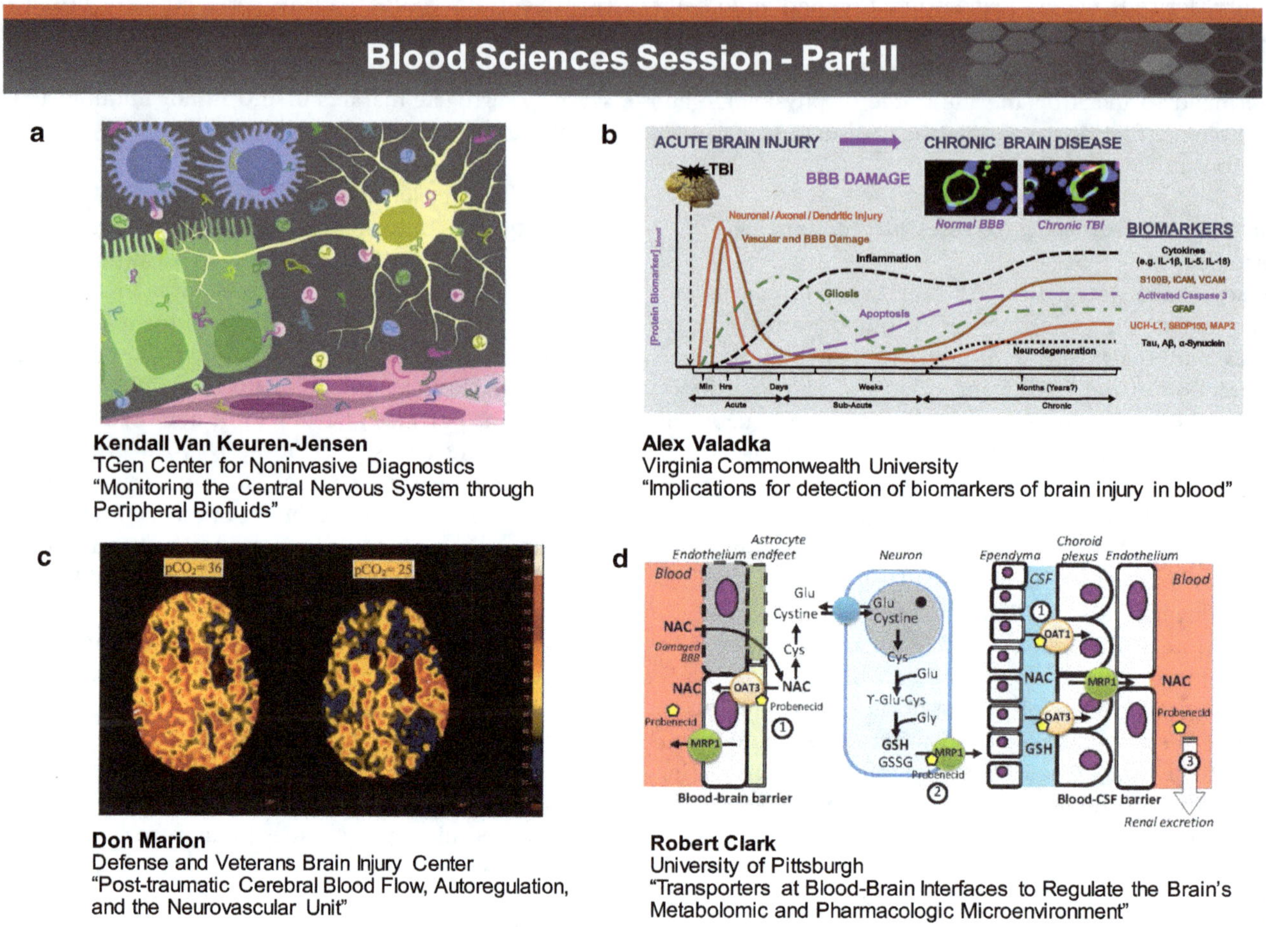

Fig. 2 Blood sciences session—Part II. Tools and technologies are currently being developed to improve capabilities for assessment and monitoring of CNS trauma to: (1) explore the relationship among the post-traumatic cerebral blood, autoregulation and the neurovascular unit; and (2) leverage different transporters at the BBIs to regulate the brain metabolomics and pharmacologic microenvironment. **a** Dr. Kendall Van Keuren-Jensen discussed the need for accessible biomarkers to allow more frequent monitoring of the CNS and the potential to improve patient care. The presence of RNA in body fluids and its relative stability when transported via EVs or carrier proteins has captured significant attention as a source for biomarker discovery. Image courtesy of the NIH exRNA Communication Program. **b** Dr. Alex Valadka noted that differences in markers released by neuronal and glial cells may make possible the diagnosis of specific subtypes of TBI based on distinct patterns and ratios of glial and neuronal markers. Image courtesy of Dr. Valadka. **c** Brain trauma can result in an immediate decrease in the cerebral blood flow, resulting in loss, or fluctuations in multiple physiological control systems including blood pressure and chemical autoregulation. Image courtesy of Dr. Marion. **d** Dr. Robert Clark reported on the importance of membrane transporters at the BBI. These membrane transporters are responsible for efflux of exogenous substrates (e.g. drugs) at the BBB and CSF-blood barriers; impacting the brain's microenvironment. Image courtesy of Dr. Clark

Studying the blood–brain barrier: perspectives from understanding the biokinetics of biomarkers of brain injury

Numerous studies have documented the potential clinical utility of blood-based biomarkers of TBI. Dr. Alex Valadka noted that differences in markers released by neuronal and glial cells may make possible the diagnosis of specific subtypes of TBI based on distinct patterns and ratios of glial and neuronal markers (Fig. 2b). Most of the published literature fails to distinguish between the movement of substrates across the BBI. One resulting issue is that the presence of biomarkers that are known to appear in the blood after non-CNS trauma, or even after exercise, may be erroneously interpreted as evidence of TBI. Properly designed preclinical and clinical studies of posttraumatic changes in the biokinetics of blood-based biomarkers can significantly advance our understanding of pathological responses to TBI, both acutely and long-term [27–31].

Post-traumatic cerebral blood flow, autoregulation, and the neurovascular unit

Brain trauma can result in an immediate decrease in the cerebral blood flow (CBF), resulting in loss, or fluctuations in multiple physiological control systems including blood pressure and chemical autoregulation (Fig. 2c). Dr. Donald Marion noted that a significant number of severe blast TBI victims develop pseudoaneurysms and vasospasm [32–34] as the result of vascular pathology [35]. With regard to BBB integrity, reduction in CBF during hypoxia in mice closely relates to areas with compromised BBB [36]. Dr. Marion showed that there is a mismatch between cerebral metabolism and blood flow after TBI, and that such a mismatch can induce local ischemia and an increase in the penumbra surrounding the primary contusion after prophylactic hyperventilation (pCO_2 < 35 mmHg) therapy. In addition, within contusions and the surrounding parenchyma, CO_2 vasoreactivity may be nearly three times the normal level, suggesting hypersensitivity to hyperventilation therapy. These findings changed the acute care practice for severe TBI from aggressive hyperventilation in the 1980's to maintaining pCO_2 at 35-40 mmHg in 2016.

Employing transporters at blood–brain interfaces to regulate the brain's metabolomic and pharmacologic microenvironment

Dr. Robert Clark reported on the importance of membrane transporters at the BBI. These membrane transporters are responsible for efflux of exogenous substrates (e.g. drugs) at the BBB and CSF-blood barriers, impacting the brain's microenvironment (Fig. 2d). Dr. Clark stressed that many xenobiotics that cross the BBB are transported out of the brain in a dynamic and surprisingly rapid fashion. Both the impact of brain injury on transporter expression and function [37], and the impact of transporter expression and function on recovery after brain injury were discussed [38]. Importantly, there is potential to capitalize on membrane transporters to optimize brain exposure to potentially neuroprotective compounds [39, 40]. Dr. Clark's group recently showed that co-administration of probenecid (an FDA approved antibiotic adjuvant) increases serum and brain *N*-acetyl cysteine (NAC) exposure [41]. NAC, which is also FDA approved, may be an effective countermeasure for blast-induced TBI [42]. Dr. Clark noted that repurposing combinations of transporter inhibitors/inducers and neuroprotective substrates is a promising strategy for clinical translation.

Exosome therapeutics session (Fig. 3)

In vivo tracking of dendritic cell exosomes delivered to brain

Dr. Richard Kraig reported that interferon gamma (IFN)-stimulated dendritic cells (SDCs) release SDC-derived exosomes (SDC-exos) containing specific miRNAs which promote myelination and reduce oxidative stress when administered to brain slice cultures (Fig. 3a) [43]. These effects emulate those seen after slice exposure to exosomes derived from the serum of animals that experienced environmental enrichment (i.e., increased physical, intellectual and social activity) [44]. According to Dr. Kraig, SDC-exos not only increase myelin levels days after nasal administration to naïve animals but also increase remyelination in vivo after lysolecithin-induced exposure, a chemical model of multiple sclerosis and reduced oxidative stress. Using fluorescently labelled SDC-exos, Dr. Kraig and his coworkers tracked SDC-exos movement into brain after nasal delivery. SDC-exos quickly entered via the olfactory route, passed along the interstitial space to the CSF and entered brain from the pial surface and perivascular space, a path consistent with that seen for soluble agents [45]. These results support the use of SDC-exos as a novel cell-based therapeutic to mitigate the impact of neurodegenerative disorders [46]. Future challenges will be to manufacture SDC-exos via standards and quantities needed for human studies.

High content proteomics/lipidomics analysis: on a path toward understanding the mechanisms of exosome-mediated cellular uptake and blood–brain barrier crossing

Dr. Anastasia Khvorova noted that exosomes or EVs have received much attention as vehicles for oligonucleotide (ONT) delivery, as well as endogenous carriers of disease biomarkers for diagnostic purposes. Currently, efficient non-toxic ONT delivery to the CNS represents a significant barrier to the treatment of neurological disorders, such as Huntington's disease [47]. EVs have the potential to act as "native" ONT delivery vehicles, but robust and scalable methods for loading therapeutic RNA cargo into EVs such as exosomes are lacking. Dr. Khvorova and colleagues showed that hydrophobically modified small interfering RNA (siRNA) can be efficiently loaded into exosomes without altering vesicle size, distribution or integrity, and promote efficient neuronal internalization and *Huntingtin* RNA silencing in vitro and in vivo. Dr. Khvorova and coworkers are now examining the surface lipid and protein composition of EV membranes to better understand how these elements contribute to EV function (Fig. 3b).

Exosome-like nanoparticles delivering therapeutic agents through an intranasal route inhibit brain tumor progression

Dr. Huang Ge Zhang noted that although the efficacy of using mammalian cell derived exosomes and nanovectors as vehicles for intranasal delivery of therapeutic agents has been demonstrated [48, 49], biosafety, cytotoxicity considerations and large scale production have presented obstacles to their clinical use [50–52]. Dr. Zhang described a novel approach for grapefruit derived nanovector (GNV)-mediated intranasal delivery of RNA

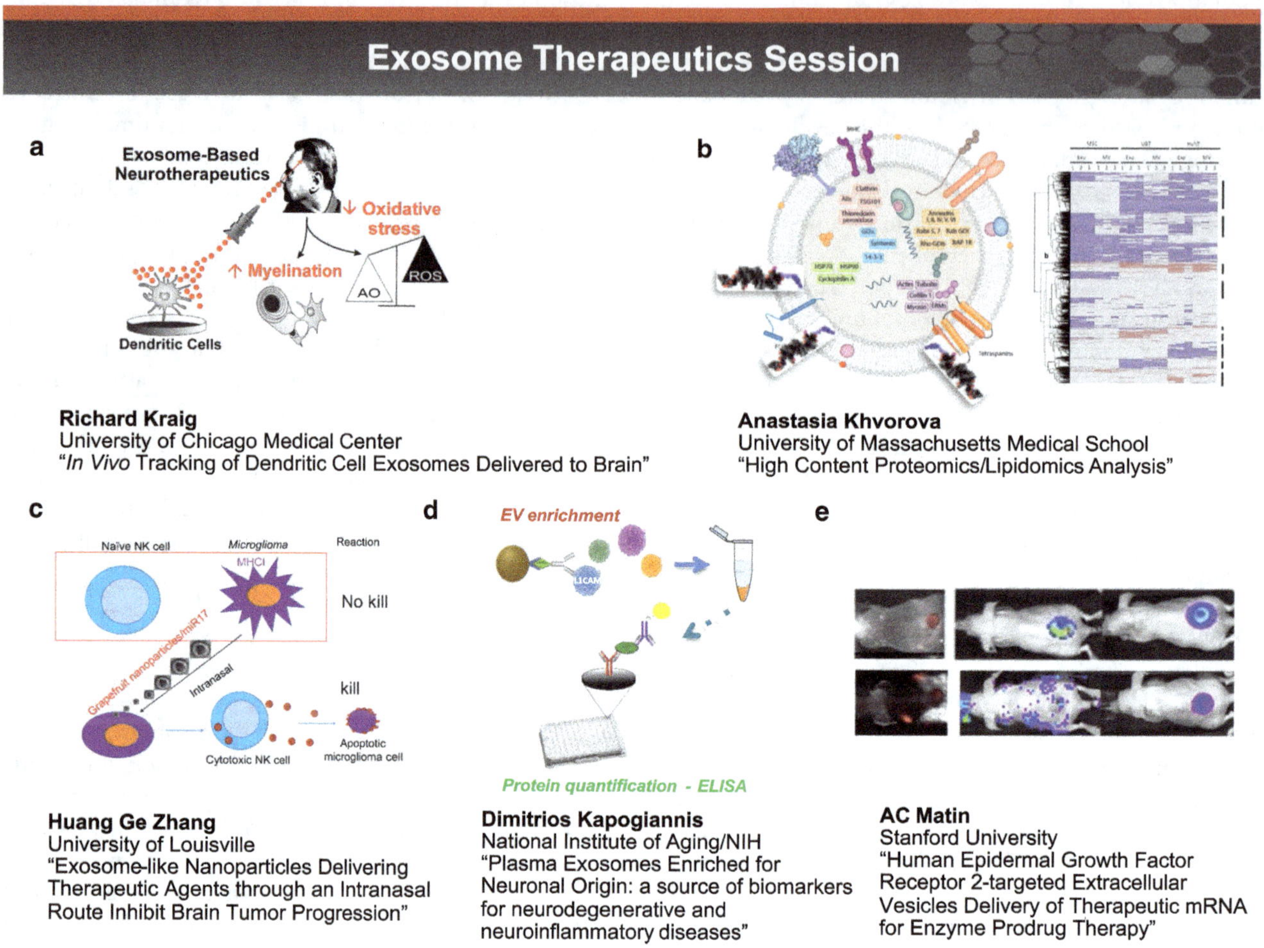

Fig. 3 Exosome therapeutics session. Exosomes, the smallest (30–150 nm) type of cell-derived extracellular vesicles, are present in all body fluids and serve as carriers of information across the body in both health and disease. This session focused on the emerging role of exosomes, in particular how they can be harnessed for both diagnostic and targeted drug delivery applications. **a** Dr. Richard Kraig reported that interferon gamma (IFN)-stimulated dendritic cells (SDCs) release SDC-derived exosomes (SDC-exos) containing specific miRNAs which promote myelination and reduce oxidative stress when administered to brain slice cultures. Image courtesy of Dr. Kraig. **b** Dr. Anastasia Khvorova and coworkers are examining the surface lipid and protein composition of EV membranes (left image modified from [108]) through high content proteomics and lipidomics analysis to better understand how these elements contribute to EV function. Right image courtesy of Dr. Khvorova. **c** Dr. Huang Ge Zhang described a novel approach for grapefruit derived nanovector (GNV)-mediated intranasal delivery of RNA in general and therapeutic miR17 specifically to brain tumor cells as a proof of concept. miR17-mediated downregulation of MHC1 expressed on tumor cells leads to activation of Natural Killer (NK) cells and targeting of tumor cells. Image courtesy of Dr. Zhang. **d** Dr. Dimitrios Kapogiannis and coworkers developed a method for enriching peripheral blood EVs of neuronal origin using L1 cell adhesion molecule (L1CAM) immunoprecipitation. In case-controlled studies, L1CAM + EVs showed diagnostic differences for AD, and perhaps fronto-temporal dementia, multiple sclerosis, and TBI. Image courtesy of Dr. Kapogiannis. **e** By using EVs as the "body's antigen delivery system" for targeting a novel prodrug 6-chloro-9-nitro-5-oxo-5H-benzo(a)phenoxazine (CNOB)/ChrR6 regimen specifically to HER2 positive cancer, the cytotoxic product of this regimen, 9-Amino-6-chloro-5H-benzo(a)phenoxazine-5-one (MCHB), can be visualized noninvasively in living mice. Image reprinted with permission from [58]

in general and therapeutic miR17 specifically to brain tumor cells as a proof of concept (Fig. 3c). The data suggest that RNA, including miR17, is effectively delivered to the brain by GNVs without observable side effects. GNVs coated with folic acid (FA-GNVs) were enhanced for targeting the GNVs to a folate receptor positive GL26 brain tumor. Intranasal administration of miR17 carried by FA-GNVs led to rapid delivery of miR17 to the brain and selective uptake by GL-26 tumor cells. Mice treated intranasally with FA-pGNV/miR17 had delayed brain tumor growth. These results demonstrate that nanovector-mediated intranasal delivery may provide a noninvasive therapeutic approach for treating brain related disease.

Plasma exosomes enriched for neuronal origin: a source of biomarkers for neurodegenerative and neuroinflammatory diseases

EV movement into and out of brain has considerable diagnostic and therapeutic potential for nervous system disorders. Dr. Dimitrios Kapogiannis and coworkers developed a method for enriching peripheral blood EVs of neuronal origin using L1 cell adhesion molecule (L1CAM) immunoprecipitation (Fig. 3d). In case-controlled studies, L1CAM + EVs showed diagnostic differences for AD, and perhaps fronto-temporal dementia, multiple sclerosis, and TBI. Regarding AD, patients have much higher p-T181-tau, p-S396-tau, and Aβ42 (pathogenic proteins for tangle and plaque pathology), as well as Ser-phosphorylated insulin receptor substrate-1 (IRS-1), and lysosomal enzymes [53–55]. Ongoing studies based on samples from large-scale longitudinal studies will determine full diagnostic and predictive potential. According to Dr. Kapogiannis, the key challenges for EV-based diagnostic biomarkers for neurological diseases are (1) elucidating factors (at the levels of EV cargo, endothelial/astrocytic/immune cells) that determine which subset of brain EVs cross the BBB and whether active selection occurs; (2) factors determining rates of transfer and clearance; (3) intra subject variance of EV-derived biomarkers over time; and (4) variability of cargo molecules within an EV population.

Human epidermal growth factor receptor 2-targeted extracellular vesicles delivery of therapeutic mRNA for enzyme Prodrug therapy

Human Epidermal Growth Factor Receptor 2 (HER2) is overexpressed in aggressive breast cancers and metastasis to the brain is a major complication of breast cancer. Dr. A.C. Matin and coworkers have constructed human DC-derived exosomes capable of specifically targeting HER2 positive cancer. By using EVs as the "body's antigen delivery system" for targeting a novel prodrug 6-chloro-9-nitro-5-oxo-5H-benzo(a)phenoxazine (CNOB)/ChrR6 regimen specifically to HER2 positive cancer, the cytotoxic product of this regimen, 9-Amino-6-chloro-5H-benzo(a)phenoxazine-5-one (MCHB), can be visualized noninvasively in living mice (Fig. 3e) [56–59]. These exosomes confer CNOB activating capability specifically on HER2 positive cells [unpublished], and can also deliver genes in vivo [60]. A cranial window model in mice showed that EVs can cross the cancerous BBI. Using a HER2 positive cell line that metastasizes to the brain, Dr. Matin's group is testing the efficacy of the directed exosomes and CNOB to treat brain tumors. These approaches have the potential to treat any cancer overexpressing a marker and by using patient-specific DCs, EV-based therapy holds the promise of personalized medicine.

Keynote presentation II: from blood–brain barrier to blood–brain interface: new opportunities for CNS drug delivery

Dr. William Banks emphasized that the BBB acts as a complex interface regulating the exchange of nutrients, informational molecules, and other substances between the CNS and blood. The properties of this interface are not only due to the physical aspects of the barrier, but also to enzymatic activity and brain-to-blood transporters. Dr. Banks noted that the BBB also serves the nutritional, homeostatic, and communication needs of the CNS. For example, BBB transporters for gastrointestinal peptides are key to the gut-brain axis, and BBB transport and secretion of cytokines/chemokines and regulation of CNS immune cell trafficking are key in the neuroimmune axis. The BBB communicates with pericytes, astrocytes, and other cells forming the neurovascular unit. This communication informs the BBB as the needs of the CNS change with, for example, development, fasting, or sleep. Similarly, the BBB adapts to diseases, but maladaptation or malfunction of the BBB is involved in several diseases, including multiple sclerosis, AD, TBI, and obesity. This complexity of the BBB provides a wealth of special opportunities for drug delivery. For example, (1) BBB transport of phosphorothiolate ONT antisenses which can decrease amyloid protein precursor levels, reversing memory impairments in mouse models of AD, (2) pegylated blockers of leptin transport can induce feeding for potential treatment of anorexia, and (3) exosomes can deliver neurotrophins across the BBB for treating neurodegenerative diseases. Dr. Banks concluded that understanding how the BBIs between the CNS and peripheral tissues interact provides unique approaches for CNS drug development [61–65].

Next generation in vitro BBB models session (Fig. 4)

Recapitulating the neurovascular unit in vitro

The BBB, within the neurovascular unit, comprises approximately 600 km of capillaries formed by highly specialized endothelial cells. The neurovascular unit is supported by pericytes that modulate contractility, and astrocytes that regulate capillary dilation. Together these cells regulate the supply of nutrients and other essential molecules to the brain while maintaining tight control of the microenvironment where neurons and other brain cells function.

The major barriers to achieving a perfusable in vitro model of the human BBB are a source of relevant cells and 3D cell culture methods to build the model [66]. Dr. Peter Searson noted that stem cell technology has the potential to overcome the limitations of animal-derived cells and immortalized cell lines, and provide a source of human brain-specific microvascular endothelial cells,

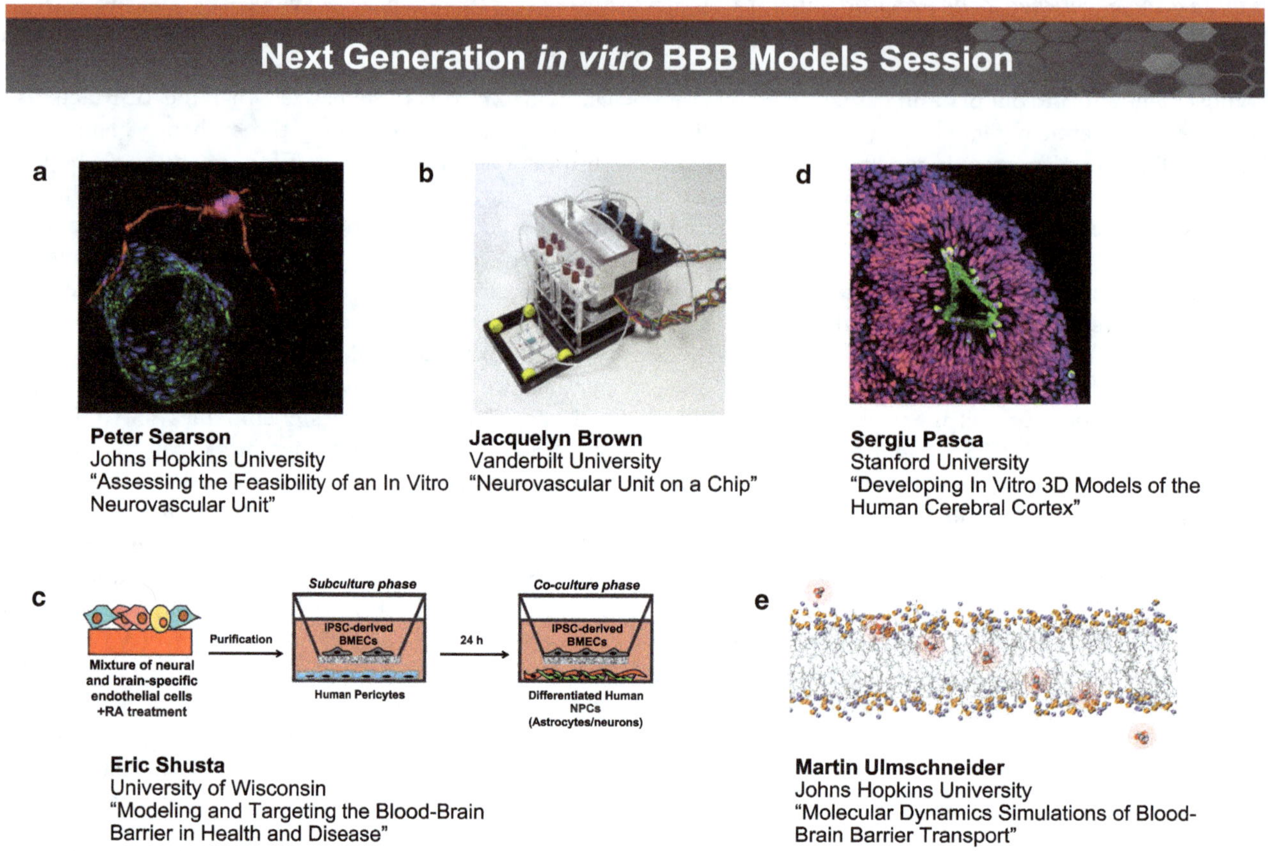

Fig. 4 Next generation in vitro BBB models session. Next generation BBB models span organ-on-a-chip devices and models exploiting organogenesis, microfluidics, 3D printing, and self-organization. These models are enabled by advances in human brain-specific cell lines and tissue engineering, particularly in 3D co-culture and matrix materials. **a** Dr. Peter Searson noted that stem cell technology has the potential to overcome the limitations of animal-derived cells and immortalized cell lines, and provide a source of human brain-specific microvascular endothelial cells, astrocytes, and pericytes. induced pluripotent stem cells (iPSCs) can be used to generate human brain microvascular endothelial cells (hBMECs) for developing perfusable brain capillary networks that capture the important physical and biological characteristics of the BBB in a physiologically relevant geometry. Image courtesy of Dr. Searson. **b** Dr. Jacquelyn Brown and colleagues developed a transwell assay that consists of a monolayer of endothelial cells seeded on a porous membrane that is separated into apical and basolateral chambers on either side of the membrane. These platforms have perfusable vascular and brain chambers on either side of the membrane that can be used to measure solute permeability and asses brain penetration. Image courtesy of Dr. Brown. **c** Dr. Eric Shusta reported how endothelial cells generated from human pluripotent stem cells (hPSCs) can be programmed to possess many BBB attributes, including well-organized tight junctions, polarized efflux transport, and nutrient transporter expression. Image courtesy of Dr. Shusta. **d** Dr. Sergiu Pasca discussed how spheroids of pluripotent stem cells (PSCs) can be programmed to form structures that resemble the human cerebral cortex. Image courtesy of Dr. Pasca. **e** Advances in computational methods have enabled a new generation of tools for modeling BBB transport. Dr. Martin Ulmschneider described how these models can simulate spontaneous transmembrane diffusion of small molecules using unbiased long timescale atomic detail molecular dynamics (MD) techniques. Image courtesy of Dr. Ulmschneider

astrocytes, and pericytes (Fig. 4a). Advances in tissue engineering provide new tools for self-organization of perfusable vascular networks that will provide the foundations for tissue engineered BBB models [67]. For example, the characteristic star-shaped morphology of human astrocytes and the low levels of activation associated with the quiescent state can be recapitulated in novel 3D matrices [68]. Similarly, brain microvascular endothelial cells resist elongation due to shear flow, which may be important in allowing the cells to wrap around and form tight junctions with themselves in brain capillaries [69, 70]. Dr. Searson concluded that these approaches have potential for developing perfusable brain capillary networks that capture the important physical and biological characteristics of the BBB in a physiologically relevant geometry.

Neurovascular unit on a chip: new direction in blood–brain barrier modeling and perfusion

Dr. Jacquelyn Brown described how integrating a monolayer of endothelial cells into a microfluidic platform can form the basis for a new generation of brain-on-a-chip devices (Fig. 4b) [71]. Dr. Brown and colleagues developed a transwell assay that consists of a monolayer of endothelial cells seeded on a porous membrane that is separated into apical and basolateral chambers on either side of the membrane. These platforms have perfusable vascular and brain chambers on either side of the membrane that can be used to measure solute permeability and asses brain penetration. Incorporation of a hydrogel layer on the brain-side of the membrane allows co-culture with astrocytes and pericytes and cell–cell communication with the endothelial cells. This dual-chamber device also provides the high shear forces created by flow for mature tight junction formation in the vascular chamber, while keeping shear stress low in the brain chamber. This next generation brain-on-a-chip device has sufficient cell mass to support a breadth of analytical measurements and is a promising tool for BBB modeling and personalized therapy development.

Modeling and targeting the blood–brain barrier in health and disease

A renewable cell source for human BBB models has the potential to accelerate brain research and pharmaceutical development. Dr. Eric Shusta reported how endothelial cells generated from human pluripotent stem cells (hPSCs) can be programmed to possess many BBB attributes, including well-organized tight junctions, polarized efflux transport, and nutrient transporter expression (Fig. 4c) [72–76]. Importantly, hPSC-derived BBB endothelial cells respond to cues provided by other cells of the neurovascular unit such as human pericytes, astrocytes, and neurons, to generate very tight barrier properties as measured by transendothelial electrical resistance, while exhibiting molecular permeability that correlates well with in vivo brain uptake. Dr. Shusta suggested that using BBB cells derived from patient induced pluripotent stem cell lines is compatible with disease modeling. These cells can be employed for isogenic modeling of the neurovascular unit and evaluation of experimental drug permeability attributes.

Developing tridimensional models of the human cerebral cortex in vitro

Organogenesis involves the self-organization of progenitors and their derivatives into 3D structures of higher cellular complexity. In recent years, 3D culture methods deriving tissue-specific spheroids or organoids from pluripotent stem cells (PSC) have been shown to recapitulate some of these complex cell–cell interactions and tissue cyto-architectures, in contrast to conventional monolayer culture. Dr. Sergiu Pasca discussed how spheroids of PSCs can be programmed to form structures that resemble the human cerebral cortex (Fig. 4d). These floating spheroids grow up to 5 mm in diameter, and include deep and superficial layer pyramidal neurons of the cortex, as well as astrocytes [77, 78]. After developing in culture for ~10 weeks, cortical spheroids display transcriptional characteristics of late mid-fetal human cortex. The emerging neural network activity consists of spontaneous electrical activity, forming functional synapses that can be probed in preparations similar to slice recordings of the animal brain. According to Dr. Pasca, neural spheroid cultures allow detailed examination of human cortical development, function, and disease, and represent a versatile platform for generating other neuronal and glial subtypes in vitro.

Molecular dynamics simulations of blood–brain barrier transport

Advances in computational methods have enabled a new generation of tools for modeling BBB transport. Dr. Martin Ulmschneider described how these models can simulate spontaneous transmembrane diffusion of small molecules using unbiased long timescale atomic detail molecular dynamics (MD) techniques (Fig. 4e) [79–81]. According to Ulmschneider, the key advantage of this approach is that it not only provides the free energy barrier profile for molecular diffusion across both membrane types, but also reveals the molecular transport mechanisms, and allows direct determination of the transport kinetics.

Blood–brain barrier delivery and targeting session (Fig. 5)

Overcoming blood–brain barrier for precise diagnosis, targeting and treatment of primary and metastatic brain tumors

Dr. Julia Ljubimova presented a novel nanotechnology which can overcome the BBB for precise diagnosis, targeting and treatment of primary and metastatic brain tumors. Use of systemically administered novel nanobiopolymers based on a combination of a polymalic acid platform (Polycefin™ family of nano agents), nano drugs and imaging agents, dramatically reduced tumor size by 90% and normalized brain cancer vasculature (Fig. 5a). Such nano drug treatments also significantly protected the brain from edema development [82]. Polycefin nano drug variants were also engineered to treat human Epidermal Growth Factor Receptor (EGFR)-positive lung cancer, triple negative breast cancer, and HER-2/*neu* positive breast tumors in nude mice. The same nano drugs were used to treat brain metastases from lung, triple negative and HER2/*neu* positive breast cancer in a mouse model [83–85]. Further, HER2/*neu* positive breast cancer was treated with a combination nanodrug that blocked HER2/*neu* synthesis and provided an immune system boost by tumor-targeted IL-2 [86]. According to

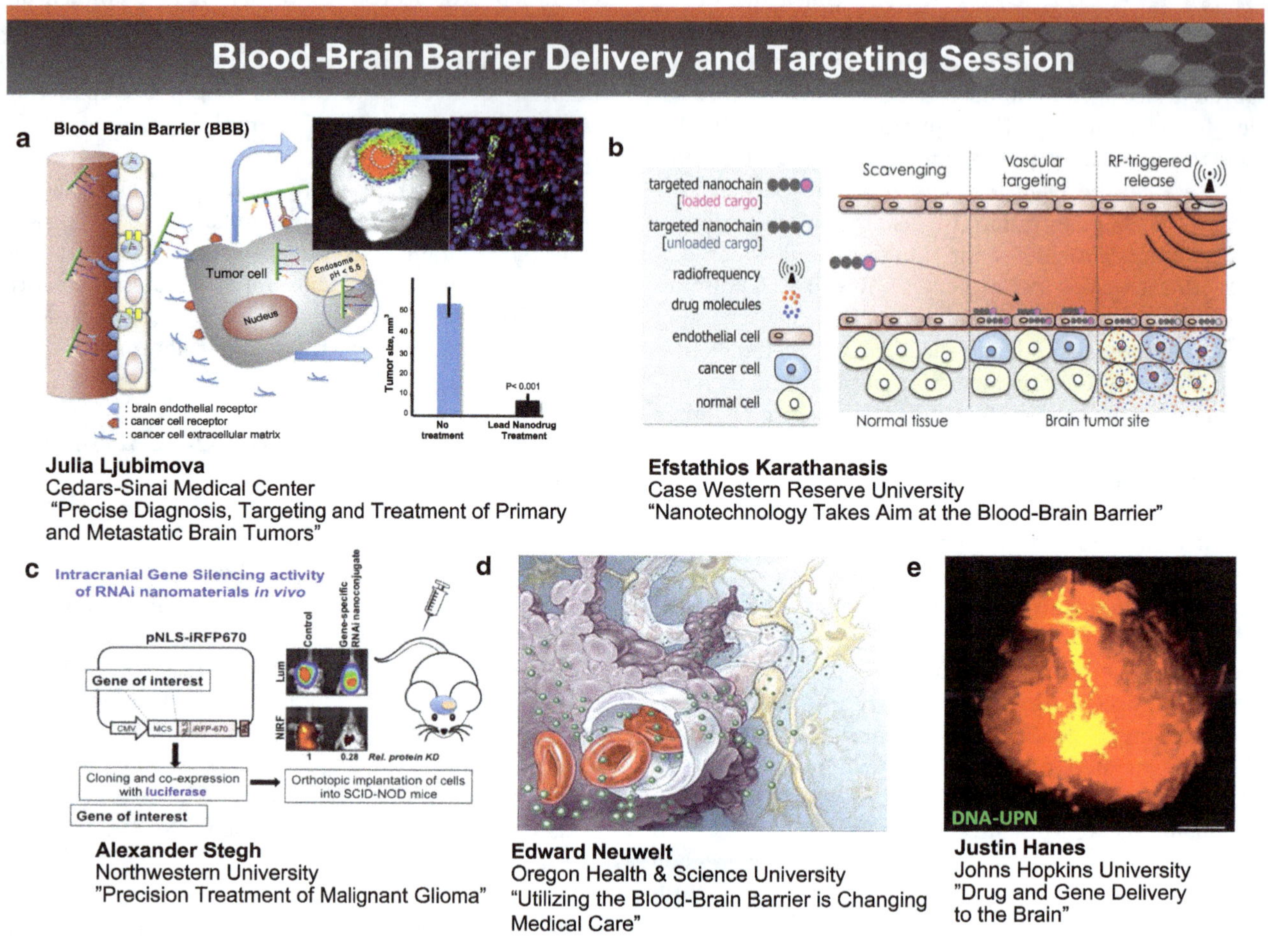

Fig. 5 Blood brain barrier delivery and targeting session. Drug delivery through the BBB to the brain can be enhanced utilizing nanoparticles that are designed to exhibit BBB targeting and/or penetrating capabilities. Evidence of these nanoparticles across the BBB can be accessed via in vivo imaging. **a** Dr. Julia Ljubimova presented a novel nanotechnology which can overcome the BBB for precise diagnosis, targeting and treatment of primary and metastatic brain tumors. Use of systemically administered novel nanobiopolymers based on a combination of a polymalic acid platform (Polycefin™ family of nano agents), nano drugs and imaging agents, dramatically reduced tumor size by 90% and normalized brain cancer vasculature. Image courtesy of Dr. Ljubimova. **b** Dr. Karathanasis' group has developed a new class of multicomponent chain-like nanoparticles, termed nanochains. Due to enhanced site-specific targeting and radiofrequency-triggered drug release, the nanochains facilitate effective delivery of drugs across the BBB into hard-to-reach brain tumors (image reprinted with permission from [91]). **c** Dr. Alexander Stegh and his team developed RNAi-based Spherical Nucleic Acids (SNAs) for the treatment of Glioblastoma multiforme (GBM). Upon IV administration, SNAs cross the BBB and disseminate within intracranial patient-derived xenografts and genetically engineered mouse model tumors. Image courtesy of Dr. Stegh. **d** Dr. Edward Neuwelt emphasized that advances toward penetrating the BBB must consider both normal and abnormal function, as well as the entire neurovascular unit (illustrated here). Image courtesy of Dr. Neuwelt. **e** Dr. Justin Hanes presented a nanoparticle-based platform for drug delivery to the brain. Brain-penetrating DNA nanoparticles (*red color*) spread throughout the entire rat striatum, as compared to standard DNA nanoparticles (*yellow color*) that do not spread as well. Image courtesy of Dr. Panagiotis Mastorakos and the work is a collaboration between Dr. Hanes' research group and that of Prof. Jung Soo Suk

Dr. Ljubimova, these data suggest that nanotechnology can be harnessed for multiple therapeutic interventions.

Nanotechnology takes aim at the blood–brain barrier

In his discussion, Dr. Efstathios Karathanasis noted that aggressive efforts are currently underway to further understand brain tumor's microenvironment and identify brain tumor cell-specific regulators amenable to pharmacologic interventions. While potent, new agents are continuously becoming available, efficient drug delivery to brain tumors remains a limiting factor. This stems from the fact that drug molecules are not specifically designed to overcome the microenvironment of hard-to-treat cancers. To effectively seek and destroy brain tumors, Dr. Karathanasis' group has developed a new class of multicomponent chain-like nanoparticles, termed nanochains [87]. A nanochain particle is comprised of three iron oxide nanospheres and a drug-loaded liposome chemically linked into a 100-nm linear, chain-like assembly. Due to enhanced site-specific targeting and radiofrequency-triggered drug release [88–90], the nanochains facilitate effective delivery of drugs across the BBB into hard-to-reach brain tumors [87], allowing significant expansion of therapies to diseases in the brain where success is currently limited (Fig. 5b) [91].

Spherical nucleic acids for the precision treatment of malignant glioma

Glioblastoma multiforme (GBM) is an incurable cancer, with one of the poorest survival rates of just 14–16 months after diagnosis [92]. Dr. Alexandar Stegh noted that an incomplete understanding of how genetic aberrations influence GBM tumor response to therapy, combined with the lack of effective delivery of drugs to the CNS, have contributed to making GBM one of the most difficult cancers to treat. Dr. Stegh and his team developed RNAi-based Spherical Nucleic Acids (SNAs) for the treatment of GBM. Upon IV administration, SNAs cross the BBB and disseminate within intracranial patient-derived xenografts and genetically engineered mouse model tumors. SNAs potently regulate gene expression via RNA interference, reduce GBM burden, and increase animal survival (Fig. 5c) [93–95]. Dr. Stegh's group has conducted toxicology studies in non-human primates, which will lead to an Investigational New Drug (IND) application and a phase 0 clinical trial in the spring of 2017.

Three areas where studies of the blood–brain barrier change patient care

Current BBB research is focused on improving long term outcomes in patients with primary and metastatic brain tumors. Dr. Edward Neuwelt presented three major research areas: (1) Intra-arterial hyperosmotic mannitol infusion utilizing BBBD transiently increases delivery of chemotherapy, antibodies, and nanoparticles to the brain. Multiple clinical trials have shown its safety and efficacy in methotrexate-based chemotherapy in conjunction with BBBD, particularly in patients with newly diagnosed primary CNS lymphoma [96]. Prospective evaluation of survivors who were treated with BBBD showed stable or improved cognitive status at a median follow-up of 12 years [97]; (2) Neuroimaging with the iron nanoparticle ferumoxytol provides a mechanism to differentiate tumor progression from pseudoprogression, which can resolve the clinical dilemma of continuation of effective therapy or transferring non-responders to novel therapies [98]; and (3) In conjunction with BBBD, thiols, NAC and sodium thiosulfate can protect against cisplatin-induced hearing loss and severe thrombocytopenia [99, 100]. Dr. Neuwelt concluded that advances toward penetrating the BBB must consider both normal and abnormal function, as well as the entire neurovascular unit (Fig. 5d).

Drug and nucleic acid delivery to the brain

Dr. Justin Hanes presented a nanoparticle-based platform for drug delivery to the brain. By analyzing the movements of nanoparticles of various diameters and surface coatings within fresh human and rat brain tissue, his lab discovered that sub-114 nm nanoparticles with a dense surface coverage of polyethylene glycol (PEG) can rapidly penetrate both healthy and tumor brain tissue [101]. Such brain penetrating nanoparticles (BPN) can be used to carry drug or nucleic acid to treat brain tumors following local injection [102]. In addition to local injection, DNA carrying BPN was shown to effectively distribute within the brain following convection enhanced delivery and result in overall level of transgene expression (Fig. 5e). This work was a collaboration between Dr. Hanes' research group and that of Prof. Jung Soo Suk [103–105]. More recently, Dr. Hanes' group collaborated with Dr. Richard Price and colleagues at the University of Virginia to show that systemically-administered BPN can be delivered into desired regions of the brain using image-guided focused ultrasound with microbubbles that temporarily disrupt the BBB [106].

Workshop conclusions

In both health and disease, endothelial cells, neurons, pericytes, and glia constitute a neurovascular unit that regulates the BBB. Bi-directional accessibility and transport of molecules between the blood and brain are dynamically regulated in response to a number of events, such as exercise, stress, and sleep. The integrity of BBB deteriorates with age, and BBB breakdown can lead to entry of neurotoxic blood-derived products to the brain causing inflammation, neuronal injury and neurodegeneration. Sleep-wake disturbances and circadian dysregulation can further affect the neurovascular unit and BBB integrity. Genetic risk factors for AD together with vascular and environmental factors act on blood vessels in the brain resulting in BBB breakdown and dysfunction (e.g., faulty clearance of Amyloid beta). Changes in CBF following TBI, in addition to vascular pathology, can result in BBB dysfunction.

The BBB also poses a tremendous hurdle for systemic delivery of drugs to the brain. Multifunctional imaging and treatment agents utilizing nanoparticles, including EVs, are being designed and tested to cross the BBB through receptor mediated transcytosis and to deliver drugs to brain cells efficiently and safely. Among various delivery routes, intranasal delivery appears to be a promising route to deliver drugs into the brain. Future scientific and clinical developments in treating primary and secondary brain tumors are needed to improve our understanding of targeted brain delivery through the blood and blood-based biomarker development. In vitro models of the neurovascular unit allow us to elucidate the underlying physical and biochemical processes that regulate the BBB, including brain capillaries and microvessels, while simultaneously allowing us to systematically increase the complexity of the model to incorporate the blood component and generate a neuro-vascular-blood unit. Advances in BBB modeling, targeting and therapeutic delivery must also account for both normal and abnormal functions of the neuro-vascular-blood unit.

Research needs and challenges

To date, the role of blood in the BBI (e.g., blood-derived factors, blood-based biomarkers, circulating exosomes) in the pathogenesis of neurological disorders and brain injury states (e.g., brain trauma, stroke, amyotrophic lateral sclerosis, multiple sclerosis, AD) and the underlying neurovascular mechanisms remain largely unknown and under-researched. Speaker presentations and panel discussions highlighted the following overarching research needs and challenges across the interface between the blood and the brain. These can be grouped into three categories:

1. Biophysical/biochemical properties of the BBB
   - Standardize procedures to assess changes in the BBB, employing methods that more accurately reflect changes in physiological analytes and relevant clinical conditions.
   - Develop benchmarks and validate the best practices for models of the neurovascular unit and to incorporate the blood component as an integral part of the neurovascular unit.
   - Determine reproducible protocols for differentiation of iPS cells into brain-specific endothelial cells, astrocytes, and pericytes for cross-laboratory investigations of the neurovascular unit, including the blood component.
   - Develop a consensus "gold standard" approach for BBB-opening for delivery of therapeutics from the blood to the brain.
2. Utilization of EVs in diagnostics and treatments
   - Develop standardized methods to track how exosomes and/or their cargo enter and leave the brain.
   - Develop protocols to stimulate parent cells to produce exosomes of interest with GMP standards.
   - Develop strategies to efficiently load therapeutic cargo into exosomes.
   - Develop methodologies to reduce immunogenicity of exosomes.
   - Optimize methods to deliver exosomes to the brain and target specific cells types.
3. Biomarker discoveries
   - Develop a comprehensive proteomics and RNA sequencing (RNA-Seq) molecular atlas across the BBB in animals and humans for new targets, signaling pathways within the neurovascular unit, drug screens, generation of new transgenic models and new therapies.
   - Determine the origin of extracellular RNA (exRNA) and other biomolecules in peripheral biofluid samples.

Recommendations and opportunities

The following recommendations and opportunities were noted by the speakers:

- Membrane transporters can be capitalized on to optimize brain exposure of potentially neuroprotective compounds in TBI and ischemic brain injury; repurposing transporter inhibitors/inducers should expedite clinical translation of such treatment strategies.
- MPs populations found in peripheral biofluid samples can be a target for assessment of post-TBI or disease progression as well as prophylaxis or amelioration of injury progression.
- Plasma EVs of neural origin can be the source of biomarkers and may provide a unique window for studying organ-specific cellular processes in living humans and to follow responses to experimental treatments. For example, a profile of exosomal peptides may serve as a blood test for AD and other neurological diseases.
- Nanoparticle and EV-based therapies hold the promise of personalized medicine.
- There are opportunities and challenges in developing the building blocks for in vitro models of the neurovascular-blood unit. For example, iPSC-derived brain microvascular endothelial cells can be used as a research tool to explore drug permeability and disease at the human BBB.
- Isogenic patient-derived models of the neurovascular unit can be used for biomarker identification, the study of disease progression, and therapeutic testing.
- Patient-specific neurovascular unit models may complement or replace animal models.
- In silico predictive modeling is advancing rapidly and presenting new exciting opportunities to capture many biological processes.

As our understanding of the complex interactions among the various cellular and molecular components of the BBB and the interdependency of the brain and other organ systems with BBB function grows, more opportunities will reveal themselves to stimulate basic and translational research for developing new diagnostic and treatment modalities related to the neuro-vascular-blood unit.

Abbreviations

AD: Alzheimer's disease; BBB: blood–brain barrier; BBBD: blood–brain barrier disruption; BBI: blood–brain interface; BPN: brain penetrating nanoparticles; CBF: cerebral blood flow; CNS: central nervous system; CSF: cerebrospinal fluid; DC: dendritic cell; EV: extracellular vesicle; exRNA: extracellular RNA; GBM: glioblastoma multiforme; GNV: grapefruit derived nanovector; MP: microparticle; MRgFUS: magnetic resonance-guided focused ultrasound; NAC: *N*-acetyl cysteine; ONT: oligonucleotide; PEG: polyethylene glycol; PSC: pluripotent stem cells; SDC: interferon gamma-stimulated dendritic cell; SDC-exos: interferon gamma-stimulated dendritic cell-derived exosomes; SNAs: spherical nucleic acids; TBI: traumatic brain injury.

Authors' contributions

MJO organized the conference and prepared the workshop report, which all authors reviewed and revised. BVZ, PCS, ATC, RPK, and JYL chaired the workshop sessions and provided session summaries. TGM and WAB provided keynote summaries. WT, RQW, AK, and CHL contributed to the abstract, introduction, and conclusion sections and performed critical revisions of the manuscript. All authors read and approved the final manuscript.

Author details

[1] National Heart, Lung, and Blood Institute, National Institutes of Health, 6701 Rockledge Dr., Room 9149, Bethesda, MD 20892-7950, USA. [2] Zilkha Neurogenetic Institute, Los Angeles, CA, USA. [3] Johns Hopkins School of Medicine, Baltimore, MD, USA. [4] Combat Casualty Care Research Program, Fort Detrick, MD, USA. [5] University of Chicago Medical Center, Chicago, IL, USA. [6] Cedars-Sinai Medical Center, Los Angeles, CA, USA. [7] Sunnybrook Health Science Centre, Toronto, ON, Canada. [8] University of Washington, Seattle, WA, USA. [9] National Heart, Lung, and Blood Institute, National Institutes of Health, Bethesda, MD, USA. [10] National Cancer Institute, National Institutes of Health, Bethesda, MD, USA.

Acknowledgements

The authors would like to thank the workshop speakers for their presentations and contribution to the workshop discussions: Dr. Katerina Akassoglou (UCSF School of Medicine), Dr. Jacquelyn Brown (Vanderbilt University), Dr. Robert Clark (University of Pittsburgh), Dr. Scott Diamond (Penn Center for Molecular Discovery), Dr. Michael Goodman (University of Cincinnati), Dr. Justin Hanes (Johns Hopkins University), Dr. Dimitrios Kapogiannis (National Institute of Aging, NIH), Dr. Efstathios Karathanasis (Case Western Reserve University), Dr. Anastasia Khvorova (University of Massachusetts Medical School), Dr. Donald Marion (Defense and Veterans Brain Injury Center), Dr. A.C. Matin (Stanford University), Dr. Edward Neuwelt (Oregon Health & Science University and the Portland Veterans Affairs Medical Center), Dr. Sergiu Pasca (Stanford University), Dr. Eric Shusta (University of Wisconsin – Madison), Dr. Alexander Stegh (Northwestern University), Dr. Martin Ulmschneider (Johns Hopkins University), Dr. Alex Valadka (Virginia Commonwealth University), Dr. Kendall Van Keuren-Jensen (TGen Center for Noninvasive Diagnostics), Dr. Theresa Whiteside (University of Pittsburgh), Dr. Huang-Ge Zhang (University of Louisville).

Competing interests

The authors declare that they have no competing interests.

References

1. van der Pol E, Boing AN, Harrison P, Sturk A, Nieuwland R. Classification, functions, and clinical relevance of extracellular vesicles. Pharmacol Rev. 2012;64(3):676–705.
2. Hynynen K, McDannold N, Vykhodtseva N, Jolesz FA. Noninvasive MR imaging-guided focal opening of the blood–brain barrier in rabbits. Radiology. 2001;220(3):640–6.
3. McDannold N, Arvanitis CD, Vykhodtseva N, Livingstone MS. Temporary disruption of the blood–brain barrier by use of ultrasound and microbubbles: safety and efficacy evaluation in rhesus macaques. Cancer Res. 2012;72(14):3652–63.
4. Zhao Z, Nelson AR, Betsholtz C, Zlokovic BV. Establishment and dysfunction of the blood–brain barrier. Cell. 2015;163(5):1064–78.
5. Bell RD, Winkler EA, Singh I, Sagare AP, Deane R, Wu Z, Holtzman DM, Betsholtz C, Armulik A, Sallstrom J, et al. Apolipoprotein E controls cerebrovascular integrity via cyclophilin A. Nature. 2012;485(7399):512–6.
6. Montagne A, Barnes SR, Sweeney MD, Halliday MR, Sagare AP, Zhao Z, Toga AW, Jacobs RE, Liu CY, Amezcua L, et al. Blood–brain barrier breakdown in the aging human hippocampus. Neuron. 2015;85(2):296–302.
7. Deane R, Du Yan S, Submamaryan RK, LaRue B, Jovanovic S, Hogg E, Welch D, Manness L, Lin C, Yu J, et al. RAGE mediates amyloid-beta peptide transport across the blood–brain barrier and accumulation in brain. Nat Med. 2003;9(7):907–13.
8. Brass LF, Diamond SL. Transport physics and biorheology in the setting of hemostasis and thrombosis. J Thromb Haemost. 2016;14(5):906–17.
9. Diamond SL. Systems analysis of thrombus formation. Circ Res. 2016;118(9):1348–62.
10. Colace TV, Tormoen GW, McCarty OJ, Diamond SL. Microfluidics and coagulation biology. Annu Rev Biomed Eng. 2013;15:283–303.
11. Li R, Elmongy H, Sims C, Diamond SL. Ex vivo recapitulation of trauma-induced coagulopathy and preliminary assessment of trauma patient platelet function under flow using microfluidic technology. J Trauma Acute Care Surg. 2016;80(3):440–9.
12. Midura EF, Jernigan PL, Kuethe JW, Friend LA, Veile R, Makley AT, Caldwell CC, Goodman MD. Microparticles impact coagulation after traumatic brain injury. J Surg Res. 2015;197(1):25–31.
13. Laroche M, Kutcher ME, Huang MC, Cohen MJ, Manley GT. Coagulopathy after traumatic brain injury. Neurosurgery. 2012;70(6):1334–45.
14. Morel N, Morel O, Petit L, Hugel B, Cochard JF, Freyssinet JM, Sztark F, Dabadie P. Generation of procoagulant microparticles in cerebrospinal fluid and peripheral blood after traumatic brain injury. J Trauma. 2008;64(3):698–704.
15. Nekludov M, Mobarrez F, Gryth D, Bellander BM, Wallen H. Formation of microparticles in the injured brain of patients with severe isolated traumatic brain injury. J Neurotrauma. 2014;31(23):1927–33.
16. Sinauridze EI, Kireev DA, Popenko NY, Pichugin AV, Panteleev MA, Krymskaya OV, Ataullakhanov FI. Platelet microparticle membranes have 50- to 100-fold higher specific procoagulant activity than activated platelets. Thromb Haemost. 2007;97(3):425–34.
17. Davalos D, Akassoglou K. Fibrinogen as a key regulator of inflammation in disease. Semin Immunopathol. 2012;34(1):43–62.
18. Adams RA, Bauer J, Flick MJ, Sikorski SL, Nuriel T, Lassmann H, Degen JL, Akassoglou K. The fibrin-derived gamma377-395 peptide inhibits microglia activation and suppresses relapsing paralysis in central nervous system autoimmune disease. J Exp Med. 2007;204(3):571–82.
19. Ryu JK, Petersen MA, Murray SG, Baeten KM, Meyer-Franke A, Chan JP, Vagena E, Bedard C, Machado MR, Rios Coronado PE, et al. Blood coagulation protein fibrinogen promotes autoimmunity and demyelination via chemokine release and antigen presentation. Nat Commun. 2015;6:8164.
20. Davalos D, Baeten KM, Whitney MA, Mullins ES, Friedman B, Olson ES, Ryu JK, Smirnoff DS, Petersen MA, Bedard C, et al. Early detection of thrombin activity in neuroinflammatory disease. Ann Neurol. 2014;75(2):303–8.
21. Davalos D, Ryu JK, Merlini M, Baeten KM, Le Moan N, Petersen MA, Deerinck TJ, Smirnoff DS, Bedard C, Hakozaki H, et al. Fibrinogen-induced perivascular microglial clustering is required for the development of axonal damage in neuroinflammation. Nat Commun. 2012;3:1227.
22. Muller L, Muller-Haegele S, Mitsuhashi M, Gooding W, Okada H, Whiteside TL. Exosomes isolated from plasma of glioma patients enrolled in

a vaccination trial reflect antitumor immune activity and might predict survival. Oncoimmunology. 2015;4(6):e1008347.
23. Zovoilis A, Agbemenyah HY, Agis-Balboa RC, Stilling RM, Edbauer D, Rao P, Farinelli L, Delalle I, Schmitt A, Falkai P, et al. microRNA-34c is a novel target to treat dementias. EMBO J. 2011;30(20):4299–308.
24. Fiore R, Schratt G. Releasing a tiny molecular brake may improve memory. EMBO J. 2011;30(20):4116–8.
25. Bhatnagar S, Chertkow H, Schipper HM, Yuan Z, Shetty V, Jenkins S, Jones T, Wang E. Increased microRNA-34c abundance in Alzheimer's disease circulating blood plasma. Front Mol Neurosci. 2014;7:2.
26. Burgos K, Malenica I, Metpally R, Courtright A, Rakela B, Beach T, Shill H, Adler C, Sabbagh M, Villa S, et al. Profiles of extracellular miRNA in cerebrospinal fluid and serum from patients with Alzheimer's and Parkinson's diseases correlate with disease status and features of pathology. PLoS ONE. 2014;9(5):e94839.
27. Chodobski A, Zink BJ, Szmydynger-Chodobska J. Blood–brain barrier pathophysiology in traumatic brain injury. Transl Stroke Res. 2011;2(4):492–516.
28. Glushakova OY, Johnson D, Hayes RL. Delayed increases in microvascular pathology after experimental traumatic brain injury are associated with prolonged inflammation, blood–brain barrier disruption, and progressive white matter damage. J Neurotrauma. 2014;31(13):1180–93.
29. Huang XJ, Glushakova O, Mondello S, Van K, Hayes RL, Lyeth BG. Acute temporal profiles of serum levels of UCH-L1 and GFAP and relationships to neuronal and astroglial pathology following traumatic brain injury in rats. J Neurotrauma. 2015;32(16):1179–89.
30. Papa L, Brophy GM, Welch RD, Lewis LM, Braga CF, Tan CN, Ameli NJ, Lopez MA, Haeussler CA, Mendez Giordano DI, et al. Time course and diagnostic accuracy of glial and neuronal blood biomarkers GFAP and UCH-L1 in a large cohort of trauma patients with and without mild traumatic brain injury. JAMA Neurol. 2016;73(5):551–60.
31. Welch RD, Ayaz SI, Lewis LM, Unden J, Chen JY, Mika VH, Saville B, Tyndall JA, Nash M, Buki A, et al. Ability of serum glial fibrillary acidic protein, ubiquitin C-terminal hydrolase-L1, and s100b to differentiate normal and abnormal head computed tomography findings in patients with suspected mild or moderate traumatic brain injury. J Neurotrauma. 2016;33(2):203–14.
32. Armonda RA, Bell RS, Vo AH, Ling G, DeGraba TJ, Crandall B, Ecklund J, Campbell WW. Wartime traumatic cerebral vasospasm: recent review of combat casualties. Neurosurgery. 2006;59(6):1215–25.
33. Ling G, Bandak F, Armonda R, Grant G, Ecklund J. Explosive blast neurotrauma. J Neurotrauma. 2009;26(6):815–25.
34. Razumovsky A, Tigno T, Hochheimer SM, Stephens FL, Bell R, Vo AH, Severson MA, Marshall SA, Oppenheimer SM, Ecker R, et al. Cerebral hemodynamic changes after wartime traumatic brain injury. Acta Neurochir Suppl. 2013;115:87–90.
35. Elder GA, Gama Sosa MA, De Gasperi R, Stone JR, Dickstein DL, Haghighi F, Hof PR, Ahlers ST. Vascular and inflammatory factors in the pathophysiology of blast-induced brain injury. Front Neurol. 2015;6:48.
36. Ek CJ, D'Angelo B, Baburamani AA, Lehner C, Leverin AL, Smith PL, Nilsson H, Svedin P, Hagberg H, Mallard C. Brain barrier properties and cerebral blood flow in neonatal mice exposed to cerebral hypoxia-ischemia. J Cereb Blood Flow Metab. 2015;35(5):818–27.
37. Willyerd FA, Empey PE, Philbrick A, Ikonomovic MD, Puccio AM, Kochanek PM, Okonkwo DO, Clark RS. Expression of ATP-binding cassette transporters B1 and C1 after severe traumatic brain injury in humans. J Neurotrauma. 2016;33(2):226–31.
38. Cousar JL, Conley YP, Willyerd FA, Sarnaik AA, Puccio AM, Empey PE, Kochanek PM, Bell MJ, Okonkwo DO, Clark RS. Influence of ATP-binding cassette polymorphisms on neurological outcome after traumatic brain injury. Neurocrit Care. 2013;19(2):192–8.
39. Chaves C, Shawahna R, Jacob A, Scherrmann JM, Decleves X. Human ABC transporters at blood-CNS interfaces as determinants of CNS drug penetration. Curr Pharm Des. 2014;20(10):1450–62.
40. Sanchez-Covarrubias L, Slosky LM, Thompson BJ, Davis TP, Ronaldson PT. Transporters at CNS barrier sites: obstacles or opportunities for drug delivery? Curr Pharm Des. 2014;20(10):1422–49.
41. Hagos FT, Daood MJ, Ocque JA, Nolin TD, Bayir H, Poloyac SM, Kochanek PM, Clark RS, Empey PE. Probenecid, an organic anion transporter 1 and 3 inhibitor, increases plasma and brain exposure of *N*-acetylcysteine. *Xenobiotica* 2017;47(4):346-53.
42. Hoffer ME, Balaban C, Slade MD, Tsao JW, Hoffer B. Amelioration of acute sequelae of blast induced mild traumatic brain injury by *N*-acetyl cysteine: a double-blind, placebo controlled study. PLoS ONE. 2013;8(1):e54163.
43. Pusic AD, Pusic KM, Clayton BL, Kraig RP. IFN-gamma-stimulated dendritic cell exosomes as a potential therapeutic for remyelination. J Neuroimmunol. 2014;266(1–2):12–23.
44. Pusic AD, Kraig RP. Youth and environmental enrichment generate serum exosomes containing miR-219 that promote CNS myelination. Glia. 2014;62(2):284–99.
45. Lochhead JJ, Wolak DJ, Pizzo ME, Thorne RG. Rapid transport within cerebral perivascular spaces underlies widespread tracer distribution in the brain after intranasal administration. J Cereb Blood Flow Metab. 2015;35(3):371–81.
46. Pusic AD, Pusic KM, Kraig RP. What are exosomes and how can they be used in multiple sclerosis therapy? Expert Rev Neurother. 2014;14(4):353–5.
47. Alterman JF, Hall LM, Coles AH, Hassler MR, Didiot MC, Chase K, Abraham J, Sottosanti E, Johnson E, Sapp E, et al. Hydrophobically modified siRNAs silence huntingtin mRNA in primary neurons and mouse brain. Mol Ther Nucleic Acids. 2015;4:e266.
48. Pathak K, Akhtar N. Nose to brain delivery of nanoformulations for neurotherapeutics in Parkinson's disease: defining the preclinical, clinical and toxicity issues. Curr Drug Deliv. 2016;13(8):1205–21.
49. Bernocchi B, Carpentier R, Lantier I, Ducournau C, Dimier-Poisson I, Betbeder D. Mechanisms allowing protein delivery in nasal mucosa using NPL nanoparticles. J Control Release. 2016;232:42–50.
50. Ali A, Suhail M, Mathew S, Shah MA, Harakeh SM, Ahmad S, Kazmi Z, Alhamdan MA, Chaudhary A, Damanhouri GA, et al. Nanomaterial induced immune responses and cytotoxicity. J Nanosci Nanotechnol. 2016;16(1):40–57.
51. Khalili Fard J, Jafari S, Eghbal MA. A review of molecular mechanisms involved in toxicity of nanoparticles. Adv Pharm Bull. 2015;5(4):447–54.
52. Zhuang X, Xiang X, Grizzle W, Sun D, Zhang S, Axtell RC, Ju S, Mu J, Zhang L, Steinman L, et al. Treatment of brain inflammatory diseases by delivering exosome encapsulated anti-inflammatory drugs from the nasal region to the brain. Mol Ther. 2011;19(10):1769–79.
53. Fiandaca MS, Kapogiannis D, Mapstone M, Boxer A, Eitan E, Schwartz JB, Abner EL, Petersen RC, Federoff HJ, Miller BL, et al. Identification of preclinical Alzheimer's disease by a profile of pathogenic proteins in neurally derived blood exosomes: A case-control study. Alzheimers Dement. 2015;11(6):600–607e601.
54. Goetzl EJ, Boxer A, Schwartz JB, Abner EL, Petersen RC, Miller BL, Kapogiannis D. Altered lysosomal proteins in neural-derived plasma exosomes in preclinical Alzheimer disease. Neurology. 2015;85(1):40–7.
55. Kapogiannis D, Boxer A, Schwartz JB, Abner EL, Biragyn A, Masharani U, Frassetto L, Petersen RC, Miller BL, Goetzl EJ. Dysfunctionally phosphorylated type 1 insulin receptor substrate in neural-derived blood exosomes of preclinical Alzheimer's disease. FASEB J. 2015;29(2):589–96.
56. Barak Y, Nov Y, Ackerley DF, Matin A. Enzyme improvement in the absence of structural knowledge: a novel statistical approach. ISME J. 2008;2(2):171–9.
57. Barak Y, Thorne SH, Ackerley DF, Lynch SV, Contag CH, Matin A. New enzyme for reductive cancer chemotherapy, YieF, and its improvement by directed evolution. Mol Cancer Ther. 2006;5(1):97–103.
58. Thorne SH, Barak Y, Liang W, Bachmann MH, Rao J, Contag CH, Matin A. CNOB/ChrR6, a new prodrug enzyme cancer chemotherapy. Mol Cancer Ther. 2009;8(2):333–41.
59. Wang JH, Endsley AN, Green CE, Matin AC. Utilizing native fluorescence imaging, modeling and simulation to examine pharmacokinetics and therapeutic regimen of a novel anticancer prodrug. BMC Cancer. 2016;16(1):524.
60. Kanada M, Bachmann MH, Hardy JW, Frimannson DO, Bronsart L, Wang A, Sylvester MD, Schmidt TL, Kaspar RL, Butte MJ, et al. Differential fates of biomolecules delivered to target cells via extracellular vesicles. Proc Natl Acad Sci USA. 2015;112(12):E1433–42.
61. Banks WA. The blood–brain barrier in neuroimmunology: tales of separation and assimilation. Brain Behav Immun. 2015;44:1–8.

62. Banks WA. From blood–brain barrier to blood–brain interface: new opportunities for CNS drug delivery. Nat Rev Drug Discov. 2016;15(4):275–92.
63. Banks WA, Kastin AJ. Passage of peptides across the blood–brain barrier: pathophysiological perspectives. Life Sci. 1996;59(23):1923–43.
64. Banks WA, Owen JB, Erickson MA. Insulin in the brain: there and back again. Pharmacol Ther. 2012;136(1):82–93.
65. Erickson MA, Banks WA. Blood–brain barrier dysfunction as a cause and consequence of Alzheimer's disease. J Cereb Blood Flow Metab. 2013;33(10):1500–13.
66. Wong AD, Ye M, Levy AF, Rothstein JD, Bergles DE, Searson PC. The blood–brain barrier: an engineering perspective. Front Neuroeng. 2013;6:7.
67. Bogorad MI, DeStefano J, Karlsson J, Wong AD, Gerecht S, Searson PC. Review: in vitro microvessel models. Lab Chip. 2015;15(22):4242–55.
68. Placone AL, McGuiggan PM, Bergles DE, Guerrero-Cazares H, Quinones-Hinojosa A, Searson PC. Human astrocytes develop physiological morphology and remain quiescent in a novel 3D matrix. Biomaterials. 2015;42:134–43.
69. Katt ME, Xu ZS, Gerecht S, Searson PC. Human brain microvascular endothelial cells derived from the BC1 iPS cell line exhibit a blood–brain Barrier phenotype. PLoS ONE. 2016;11(4):e0152105.
70. Reinitz A, DeStefano J, Ye M, Wong AD, Searson PC. Human brain microvascular endothelial cells resist elongation due to shear stress. Microvasc Res. 2015;99:8–18.
71. Brown JA, Pensabene V, Markov DA, Allwardt V, Neely MD, Shi M, Britt CM, Hoilett OS, Yang Q, Brewer BM, et al. Recreating blood–brain barrier physiology and structure on chip: a novel neurovascular microfluidic bioreactor. Biomicrofluidics. 2015;9(5):054124.
72. Clark PA, Al-Ahmad AJ, Qian T, Zhang RR, Wilson HK, Weichert JP, Palecek SP, Kuo JS, Shusta EV. Analysis of cancer-targeting alkylphosphocholine analogue permeability characteristics using a human induced pluripotent stem cell blood–brain barrier model. Mol Pharm. 2016;13:3341–9.
73. Lippmann ES, Àl-Ahmad A, Azarin SM, Palecek SP, Shusta EV. A retinoic acid-enhanced, multicellular human blood–brain barrier model derived from stem cell sources. Sci Rep. 2014;4:4160.
74. Lippmann ES, Azarin SM, Kay JE, Nessler RA, Wilson HK, Al-Ahmad A, Palecek SP, Shusta EV. Derivation of blood–brain barrier endothelial cells from human pluripotent stem cells. Nat Biotechnol. 2012;30(8):783–91.
75. Stebbins MJ, Wilson HK, Canfield SG, Qian T, Palecek SP, Shusta EV. Differentiation and characterization of human pluripotent stem cell-derived brain microvascular endothelial cells. Methods. 2016;101:93–102.
76. Wilson HK, Canfield SG, Hjortness MK, Palecek SP, Shusta EV. Exploring the effects of cell seeding density on the differentiation of human pluripotent stem cells to brain microvascular endothelial cells. Fluids Barriers CNS. 2015;12:13.
77. Pasca AM, Sloan SA, Clarke LE, Tian Y, Makinson CD, Huber N, Kim CH, Park JY, O'Rourke NA, Nguyen KD, et al. Functional cortical neurons and astrocytes from human pluripotent stem cells in 3D culture. Nat Methods. 2015;12(7):671–8.
78. Pasca SP. Personalized human cortical spheroids. Am J Psychiatry. 2016;173(4):332–3.
79. Ulmschneider JP, Ulmschneider MB, Di Nola A. Monte Carlo vs molecular dynamics for all-atom polypeptide folding simulations. J Phys Chem B. 2006;110(33):16733–42.
80. Ulmschneider JP, Ulmschneider MB. United atom lipid parameters for combination with the optimized potentials for liquid simulations all-atom force field. J Chem Theory Comput. 2009;5(7):1803–13.
81. Ulmschneider JP, Doux JP, Killian JA, Smith JC, Ulmschneider MB. Peptide partitioning and folding into lipid bilayers. J Chem Theory Comput. 2009;5(9):2202–5.
82. Ding H, Inoue S, Ljubimov AV, Patil R, Portilla-Arias J, Hu J, Konda B, Wawrowsky KA, Fujita M, Karabalin N, et al. Inhibition of brain tumor growth by intravenous poly (beta-L-malic acid) nanobioconjugate with pH-dependent drug release [corrected]. Proc Natl Acad Sci USA. 2010;107(42):18143–8.
83. Inoue S, Ding H, Portilla-Arias J, Hu J, Konda B, Fujita M, Espinoza A, Suhane S, Riley M, Gates M, et al. Polymalic acid-based nanobiopolymer provides efficient systemic breast cancer treatment by inhibiting both HER2/neu receptor synthesis and activity. Cancer Res. 2011;71(4):1454–64.
84. Patil R, Ljubimov AV, Gangalum PR, Ding H, Portilla-Arias J, Wagner S, Inoue S, Konda B, Rekechenetskiy A, Chesnokova A, et al. MRI virtual biopsy and treatment of brain metastatic tumors with targeted nanobioconjugates: nanoclinic in the brain. ACS Nano. 2015;9(5):5594–608.
85. Ding H, Gangalum PR, Galstyan A, Fox I, Patil R, Hubbard P, Murali R, Ljubimova JY, Holler E. HER2-positive breast cancer targeting and treatment by a peptide-conjugated mini nanodrug. Nanomedicine. 2017;13:631–9.
86. Ding J, Xu W, Zhang Y, Sun D, Xiao C, Liu D, Zhu X, Chen X. Self-reinforced endocytoses of smart polypeptide nanogels for "on-demand" drug delivery. J Control Release. 2013;172(2):444–55.
87. Peiris PM, Abramowski A, Mcginnity J, Doolittle E, Toy R, Gopalakrishnan R, Shah S, Bauer L, Ghaghada KB, Hoimes C, et al. Treatment of invasive brain tumors using a chain-like nanoparticle. Can Res. 2015;75(7):1356–65.
88. Peiris PM, Bauer L, Toy R, Tran E, Pansky J, Doolittle E, Schmidt E, Hayden E, Mayer A, Keri RA, et al. Enhanced delivery of chemotherapy to tumors using a multicomponent nanochain with radio-frequency-tunable drug release. ACS Nano. 2012;6(5):4157–68.
89. Peiris PM, Toy R, Abramowski A, Vicente P, Tucci S, Bauer L, Mayer A, Tam M, Doolittle E, Pansky J, et al. Treatment of cancer micrometastasis using a multicomponent chain-like nanoparticle. J Control Release. 2014;173:51–8.
90. Peiris PM, Tam M, Vicente P, Abramowski A, Toy R, Bauer L, Mayer A, Pansky J, Doolittle E, Tucci S, et al. On-command drug release from nanochains inhibits growth of breast tumors. Pharm Res. 2014;31(6):1460–8.
91. Karathanasis E, Ghaghada KB. Crossing the barrier: treatment of brain tumors using nanochain particles. Wiley Interdiscip Rev Nanomed Nanobiotechnol. 2016;8(5):678–95.
92. Furnari FB, Fenton T, Bachoo RM, Mukasa A, Stommel JM, Stegh A, Hahn WC, Ligon KL, Louis DN, Brennan C, et al. Malignant astrocytic glioma: genetics, biology, and paths to treatment. Genes Dev. 2007;21(21):2683–710.
93. Kouri FM, Hurley LA, Daniel WL, Day ES, Hua Y, Hao L, Peng CY, Merkel TJ, Queisser MA, Ritner C, et al. miR-182 integrates apoptosis, growth, and differentiation programs in glioblastoma. Genes Dev. 2015;29(7):732–45.
94. Jensen SA, Day ES, Ko CH, Hurley LA, Luciano JP, Kouri FM, Merkel TJ, Luthi AJ, Patel PC, Cutler JI, et al. Spherical nucleic acid nanoparticle conjugates as an RNAi-based therapy for glioblastoma. Sci Transl Med. 2013;5(209):209ra152.
95. Mirkin CA, Stegh AH. Spherical nucleic acids for precision medicine. Oncotarget. 2014;5(1):9–10.
96. Angelov L, Doolittle ND, Kraemer DF, Siegal T, Barnett GH, Peereboom DM, Stevens G, McGregor J, Jahnke K, Lacy CA, et al. Blood–brain barrier disruption and intra-arterial methotrexate-based therapy for newly diagnosed primary CNS lymphoma: a multi-institutional experience. J Clin Oncol. 2009;27(21):3503–9.
97. Doolittle ND, Dosa E, Fu R, Muldoon LL, Maron LM, Lubow MA, Tyson RM, Lacy CA, Kraemer DF, Butler RW, et al. Preservation of cognitive function in primary CNS lymphoma survivors a median of 12 years after enhanced chemotherapy delivery. J Clin Oncol. 2013;31(31):4026–7.
98. Gahramanov S, Varallyay C, Tyson RM, Lacy C, Fu R, Netto JP, Nasseri M, White T, Woltjer RL, Gultekin SH, et al. Diagnosis of pseudoprogression using MRI perfusion in patients with glioblastoma multiforme may predict improved survival. CNS Oncol. 2014;3(6):389–400.
99. Dickey DT, Muldoon LL, Doolittle ND, Peterson DR, Kraemer DF, Neuwelt EA. Effect of *N*-acetylcysteine route of administration on chemoprotection against cisplatin-induced toxicity in rat models. Cancer Chemother Pharmacol. 2008;62(2):235–41.
100. Doolittle ND, Muldoon LL, Culp AY, Neuwelt EA. Delivery of chemotherapeutics across the blood–brain barrier: challenges and advances. Adv Pharmacol. 2014;71:203–43.
101. Nance EA, Woodworth GF, Sailor KA, Shih TY, Xu Q, Swaminathan G, Xiang D, Eberhart C, Hanes J. A dense poly(ethylene glycol) coating improves penetration of large polymeric nanoparticles within brain tissue. Sci Transl Med. 2012;4(149):149ra119.

102. Nance E, Zhang C, Shih TY, Xu Q, Schuster BS, Hanes J. Brain-penetrating nanoparticles improve paclitaxel efficacy in malignant glioma following local administration. ACS Nano. 2014;8(10):10655–64.
103. Kim AJ, Woodworth GF, Boylan NJ, Suk JS, Hanes J. Highly compacted pH-responsive DNA nanoparticles mediate transgene silencing in experimental glioma. J Mater Chem B Mater Biol Med. 2014;2(46):8165–73.
104. Mastorakos P, Song E, Zhang C, Berry S, Park HW, Kim YE, Park JS, Lee S, Suk JS, Hanes J. Biodegradable DNA nanoparticles that provide widespread gene delivery in the brain. Small. 2016;12(5):678–85.
105. Mastorakos P, Zhang C, Berry S, Oh Y, Lee S, Eberhart CG, Woodworth GF, Suk JS, Hanes J. Highly PEGylated DNA nanoparticles provide uniform and widespread gene transfer in the brain. Adv Healthc Mater. 2015;4(7):1023–33.
106. Nance E, Timbie K, Miller GW, Song J, Louttit C, Klibanov AL, Shih TY, Swaminathan G, Tamargo RJ, Woodworth GF, et al. Non-invasive delivery of stealth, brain-penetrating nanoparticles across the blood–brain barrier using MRI-guided focused ultrasound. J Control Release. 2014;189:123–32.
107. Zlokovic BV. The blood-brain barrier in health and chronic neurodegenerative disorders. Neuron. 2008;57(2):178–201.
108. Kourembanas S. Exosomes: vehicles of intercellular signaling, biomarkers, and vectors of cell therapy. Annu Rev Physiol. 2015;77:13–27.

8

Is posture-related craniospinal compliance shift caused by jugular vein collapse?

Manuel Gehlen[1,2*], Vartan Kurtcuoglu[2,3] and Marianne Schmid Daners[4]

Abstract

Background: Postural changes are related to changes in cerebrospinal fluid (CSF) dynamics. While sitting up leads to a decrease in cranial CSF pressure, it also causes shifts in the craniospinal CSF volume and compliance distribution. We hypothesized that jugular vein collapse in upright posture is a major contributor to these shifts in CSF volume and compliance.

Methods: To test this hypothesis, we implemented a mathematical lumped-parameter model of the CSF system and the relevant parts of the cardiovascular system. In this model, the CSF and the venous system are each divided into a cranial and a spinal part. The pressures in these cranial and spinal portions differ by the posture-dependent hydrostatic pressure columns in the connecting vessels. Jugular collapse is represented by a reduction of the hydrostatic pressure difference between cranial and spinal veins. The CSF pressure–volume relationship is implemented as a function of the local CSF to venous pressure gradient. This implies that an increase in CSF volume leads to a simultaneous displacement of blood from adjacent veins. CSF pulsations driven by the cardiovascular system are introduced through a pulsating cranial arterial volume.

Results: In upright posture, the implemented CSF pressure–volume relationship shifts to lower cranial CSF pressures compared to the horizontal position, leading to a decrease in cranial CSF pressure when sitting up. Concurrently, the compliance of the spinal compartment decreases while the one of the cranial compartment increases. With this, in upright posture only 10% of the CSF system's compliance is provided by the spinal compartment compared to 35% in horizontal posture. This reduction in spinal compliance is accompanied by a caudal shift of CSF volume. Also, the ability of the spinal CSF compartment to compensate for cerebral arterial volume pulsations reduces in upright posture, which in turn reduces the calculated craniospinal CSF flow pulsations.

Conclusion: The mathematical model enabled us to isolate the effect of jugular collapse and quantify the induced shifts of compliance and CSF volume. The good concordance of the modelled changes with clinically observed values indicates that jugular collapse can be considered a major contributor to CSF dynamics in upright posture.

Keywords: Craniospinal, Compliance, Cerebrospinal fluid dynamics, Posture

Background

Several pathologies of the central nervous system, like hydrocephalus and syringomyelia, are caused or characterized by altered cerebrospinal fluid (CSF) dynamics. Therefore, the treatment of these conditions typically aims at restoring physiological circulation of CSF and requires profound knowledge of the underlying pathophysiology. However, CSF dynamics are mostly studied in horizontal posture, even though we spend most of our time upright and CSF dynamics fundamentally change with posture. For example, sitting up not only leads to changes in intracranial pressure (ICP), but also to a caudal shift of CSF volume and an inversion of the compliance distribution between the cranial and the

*Correspondence: mgehlen@ethz.ch
[1] Institute for Dynamic Systems and Control, Department of Mechanical and Process Engineering, ETH Zurich, Zurich, Switzerland

spinal part of the CSF system. This inversion of the craniospinal compliance was first observed by Magnaes in a small number of subjects [1]. In a recent study by Alperin et al. [2], the pulse amplitude of craniospinal CSF flow recorded with magnetic resonance imaging (MRI), decreased in sitting posture, which supports the findings of Magnaes. In CSF shunts, anti-siphon devices are used to counteract posture-related changes in pressures. However, the diversity of functional principles on which these devices are based, indicates that the mechanisms of the posture-related changes in CSF dynamics and their link to hemodynamics are largely unknown [2]. Knowing the causalities of these interactions would contribute to the understanding of individual pathologies and to the choice of the most appropriate treatment option, especially in the context of various comorbidities typically seen in these patients.

What we do know is that CSF pressure in equilibrium conditions is a function of venous pressure through Davson's equation [3], and that at least cranial venous pressure changes with posture due to hydrostatic gradients along the blood vessels. Also, cranial venous pressure changes with the state of the jugular veins: when they collapse in upright posture venous resistance increases, reducing both the posture-related decrease in cranial venous pressure and in CSF pressure [4–6].

We hypothesized that the collapse of the jugular veins when upright not only affects mean ICP, but that it also causes the aforementioned caudal shift of CSF volume: interruption of the venous hydrostatic pressure column decreases the cranial CSF to venous pressure gradient by diminishing the reduction in cranial venous pressure when sitting up. Due to the exponential nature of the CSF system's pressure–volume relationship [7], this in turn, increases cranial compliance in upright posture. At the same time, the non-interrupted hydrostatic pressure column leads to an increased CSF to venous pressure gradient below the level of the jugular veins, causing the observed caudal shift of CSF volume. Consequently, the spinal dural sac volume increases, reducing the compliance of the spinal CSF space [1].

We aimed at testing this hypothesis by implementing a mathematical model of the CSF system and the relevant parts of the cardiovascular system. This has enabled us to isolate the effect of jugular vein collapse and quantify the induced shifts of compliance and CSF volume. These estimated changes in CSF dynamics were then compared to the measurements of Magnaes [1]. Testing the hypothesis without a mathematical model would be difficult, as jugular collapse can hardly be avoided in vivo. To allow for further model validation, we computed changes in craniospinal CSF flow secondary to changes in craniospinal compliance distribution. Unlike the distribution of compliance itself, changes in CSF flow can be easily measured with MRI and used as surrogate for changes in compliance distribution. With this, we were able to validate the model by comparing the craniospinal flow rates estimated by the model to reported flow rates recorded in supine and sitting posture [2, 8, 9].

Methods

We used a lumped parameter description of the interaction between the CSF and cardiovascular systems as shown in Fig. 1. As most of the CSF system's compensatory reserve is provided by concurrent venous volume adaptation, the CSF pressure–volume relationship was implemented as a function of the local CSF to venous pressure gradient [10, 11]. This implies that an increase in CSF volume leads to a simultaneous displacement of

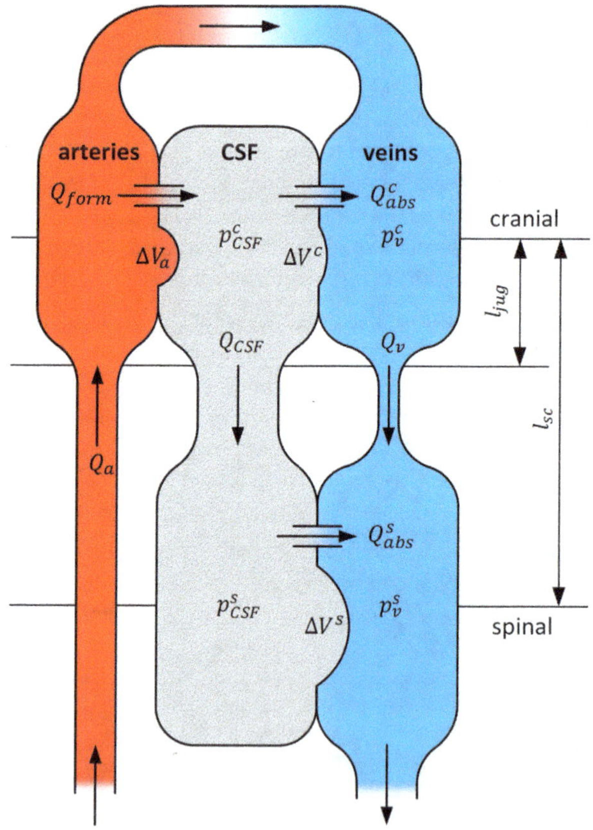

Fig. 1 Model schematic: interaction between CSF and cardiovascular systems in upright posture. In the mathematical model, CSF and venous blood are divided into cranial and spinal compartments. The corresponding pressures at the cranial (p^c_{CSF} and p^c_V) and spinal (p^c_{CSF} and p^c_V) level differ by hydrostatic pressure columns that are characterized by the distances l_{sc} and l_{jug}. The interaction of CSF and venous blood is determined by the local pressure–volume relationships (ΔV^c and ΔV^s). The pulsating arterial blood flow Q_a leads to a pulsating change in the cranial arterial blood volume ΔV_a, which is compensated by craniospinal flows of CSF and venous blood (Q_{CSF} and Q_V). CSF formation (Q_{form}) and absorption (Q_{abs}) are also indicated

venous blood from adjacent veins. In upright posture, hydrostatic pressure gradients between different locations in the CSF space and in the venous system become relevant. In our model, the CSF space and the venous compartment were divided into a cranial and a spinal portion, and CSF and venous pressures were evaluated at these two locations. While in horizontal posture these cranial and spinal pressures are approximately equal, they differ in upright posture due to the hydrostatic gradients in the connecting vessels. If the jugular veins did not collapse in upright posture, spinal and cranial venous pressures would differ by the same hydrostatic pressure column as spinal and cranial CSF pressure, respectively. However, in upright posture and for reasonably low central venous pressures, this hydrostatic pressure gradient is interrupted by the collapsing jugular veins [4, 5]. The collapsed segment of the jugular veins acts as a differential pressure valve with opening pressure equal to ambient pressure. Therefore, in upright posture, cerebral venous outflow is partly redirected through the high-resistance pathway presented by the vertebral veins, and venous pressure at the site of the collapse, is regulated to ambient pressure by the jugular veins [4]. Thus, cerebral venous pressure is only determined by the hydrostatic pressure gradient above the site of the collapse [4, 5]. The reference level of the spinal portion was chosen such that the spinal venous pressure is independent of posture. In contrast to the venous blood vessels, the hydrostatic column in the CSF system was assumed to be uninterrupted.

Cerebrospinal fluid pulsations driven by the cardiovascular system were accounted for through a pulsating cranial arterial volume. The pulsations of this arterial volume were based on recorded flow rates in the internal carotid and vertebral arteries. As CSF competes with the arterial pulsations for the available compliance, the arterial volume was added to the cranial CSF volume. Instantaneous flow rates for CSF and venous blood between cranial and spinal compartments were calculated based on a volume balance, assuming constant cranial volume (Monroe–Kelly doctrine).

Model derivation

Local pressure–volume relationships

The pressure gradient Δp between the CSF pressure p_{CSF} and the venous pressure p_v required for the displacement of venous blood was described by an exponential function:

$$\Delta p = p_{CSF} - p_v = p_1 \cdot e^{E \cdot \Delta V} + p_0, \tag{1}$$

where ΔV is the CSF volume increase from baseline (supine equilibrium), and E, p_1, and p_0 are constants (Table 1). This exponential function was derived from the exponential pressure–volume relation originally described by Marmarou [7, 12, 13]:

$$p_{CSF} = p_1 \cdot e^{E \cdot \Delta V} + p_0^M, \tag{2}$$

where the reference pressure p_0^M is the sum of the postural pressure component p_0 and the venous pressure p_v^s [11, 14]. Describing the pressure–volume relation as a function of the CSF to venous pressure gradient, Δp, allows changes in venous pressure to be accounted for [10, 11]. In the model, the CSF space and the venous compartment were divided into a cranial and a spinal part. Thus, an increase in CSF volume can be compensated by a displacement of venous blood from the cranium (ΔV^c)

Table 1 Parameters, distinctive for normal pressure hydrocephalus

Parameter	Symbol	Value	Unit	Reference
Elastance	E	0.23	mL^{-1}	[9, 16]*
Exponential parameter	p_1	4	mmHg	[16]*
Offset pressure	p_0	3.2	mmHg	[16]*
Rate of CSF formation	Q_{form}	0.35	mL/min	[13]
Total CSF outflow resistance	R_{abs}^{tot}	20.6	mmHg/(mL/min)	[13, 16]*
Relative spinal compliance	k_V	0.35	–	[17]
Spinal venous pressure	p_v^s	5.3	mmHg	[4]
Distance between spinal and cranial reference points	l_{sc}	33.8	cm	[4]
Distance between jugular veins and cranial reference point	l_{jug}	11.0	cm	[4]
Density of CSF	ρ_{CSF}	1000	kg/m^3	
Density of blood	ρ_{blood}	1060	kg/m^3	
Gravitational acceleration	g	9.81	m/s^2	
Relative spinal outflow conduction	k_R	n/a#	–	

* Computed from data given in the referenced work: $E = \ln(RPPC + 1)/\Delta V_a$ [18], $p_1 = ICP_r - p_0 - p_v^s$, $p_0 = p_0^M - p_v^s$, $R_{abs}^{tot} = (ICP_r - p_v^s)/Q_{form}$ [3]

\# The value of this parameter is unknown. It is estimated in this study or from venous vessels adjacent to the spinal canal and the spinal thecal sac (ΔV^s):

$$\Delta V^{tot} = \Delta V^c + \Delta V^s. \quad (3)$$

In horizontal posture, where cranial and spinal CSF as well as venous pressures can be assumed equal ($p^c_{CSF} = p^s_{CSF}$ and $p^c_v = p^s_v$), the combined pressure–volume relationship ΔV^{tot} must be equal to the established relation (Eq. 2). Thus, the local pressure–volume relationships in the spinal and the cranial compartment were implemented as in Eq. 1, but as functions of the respective local CSF to venous pressure gradients:

$$\Delta V^c(p^c_{CSF}) = (1-k_V)\cdot\frac{1}{E}\cdot\ln\left(\frac{p^c_{CSF}-p^c_v-p_0}{p_1}\right) \quad (4)$$

$$\Delta V^s(p^s_{CSF}) = k_V\cdot\frac{1}{E}\cdot\ln\left(\frac{p^s_{CSF}-p^s_v-p_0}{p_1}\right). \quad (5)$$

Here, k_V is a constant that describes the portion of the total compensatory reserve of the CSF system attributed to the spinal compartment. In horizontal posture, k_v is the spinal compliance contribution as measured by Magnaes [1].

Hydrostatic pressure gradients

In upright posture, spinal CSF pressure p^s_{CSF} is higher than the cranial CSF pressure p^c_{CSF} due to the hydrostatic pressure column of length l_{sc}:

$$p^s_{CSF} = p^c_{CSF} + \rho_{CSF}\cdot g\cdot l_{sc}, \quad (6)$$

where l_{sc} is the vertical distance between the reference points of the spinal and the cranial compartments (Fig. 1), ρ_{CSF} is CSF density, and g is gravitational acceleration. p^c_{CSF} is often referred to as ICP. If lumbar CSF pressure is measured, Eq. 6 is accounted for by sensor calibration [4].

For the spinal part of the model, the hydrostatic indifference point of the venous system was chosen as the reference location. Thus, the spinal venous pressure p^s_v was assumed to be independent of posture.

Without collapse of the jugular veins, cranial and spinal venous pressures would also differ by a hydrostatic column of length l_{sc}:

$$p^c_v = p^s_v - \rho_{blood}\cdot g\cdot l_{sc}. \quad (7)$$

However, since venous pressure is equal to ambient pressure at the location where the jugular veins collapse, cerebral venous pressure is determined by the hydrostatic pressure gradient of length l_{jug} instead [4, 5]:

$$p^c_v = -\rho_{blood}\cdot g\cdot l_{jug} \quad (8)$$

l_{jug} is the distance between the upper end of the jugular collapse and the reference point of the cranial compartment.

Using Eqs. 6 and 8, the CSF pressure–volume relationships (Eqs. 4, 5) can also be written, for the upright posture, as a function of only the cranial CSF pressure (p^c_{CSF}):

$$\Delta V^c(p^c_{CSF})\big|_{up} = (1-k_V)\cdot\frac{1}{E}\cdot\ln\left(\frac{p^c_{CSF}+\rho_{blood}\cdot g\cdot l_{jug}-p_0}{p_1}\right) \quad (9)$$

$$\Delta V^s(p^c_{CSF})\big|_{up} = k_V\cdot\frac{1}{E}\cdot\ln\left(\frac{p^c_{CSF}+\rho_{CSF}\cdot g\cdot l_{sc}-p^s_v-p_0}{p_1}\right). \quad (10)$$

Compliance

Compliance C is defined as change of volume relative to the corresponding change in pressure [7]. It was calculated analytically as the slope of the pressure–volume curves (Eqs. 4, 5, 9, 10):

$$C^c(p^c_{CSF})\big|_{hor} = \left.\frac{d\Delta V^c}{dp^c_{CSF}}\right|_{hor} = \frac{1-k_V}{E}\cdot\frac{1}{p^c_{CSF}-p^s_v-p_0} \quad (11)$$

$$C^s(p^c_{CSF})\big|_{hor} = \left.\frac{d\Delta V^s}{dp^c_{CSF}}\right|_{hor} = \frac{k_V}{E}\cdot\frac{1}{p^c_{CSF}-p^s_v-p_0} \quad (12)$$

$$C^c(p^c_{CSF})\big|_{up} = \left.\frac{d\Delta V^c}{dp^c_{CSF}}\right|_{up} = \frac{1-k_V}{E}\cdot\frac{1}{p^c_{CSF}+\rho_{blood}\cdot g\cdot l_{jug}-p_0} \quad (13)$$

$$C^s(p^c_{CSF})\big|_{up} = \left.\frac{d\Delta V^s}{dp^c_{CSF}}\right|_{up} = \frac{k_V}{E}\cdot\frac{1}{p^c_{CSF}+\rho_{CSF}\cdot g\cdot l_{sc}-p^s_v-p_0}. \quad (14)$$

CSF formation and absorption

The rate of CSF formation Q_{form} was implemented as posture independent and constant [13] (Table 1). The cranial and the spinal CSF absorption rates were assumed to be proportional to the local CSF to venous pressure gradient, Δp^i:

$$Q^i_{abs}(\Delta p^i) = \left(p^i_{CSF}-p^i_v\right)/R^i_{abs} \quad (15)$$

where R^i_{abs} is the local CSF outflow resistance. While the overall outflow resistance R^{tot}_{abs} can be determined clinically [15], its craniospinal distribution characterized by the coefficient, k_R, is generally unknown.

$$\frac{1}{R^{tot}_{abs}} = \underbrace{k_R/R^{tot}_{abs}}_{1/R^s_{abs}} + \underbrace{(1-k_R)/R^{tot}_{abs}}_{1/R^c_{abs}} \quad (16)$$

Model parameters

The parameters used for the calculations in this study (Table 1) are characteristic for patients with normal pressure hydrocephalus (NPH). They describe a patient with 12.5 mmHg resting intracranial pressure (ICP_r).

Sensitivity analysis

To analyze the sensitivity of the investigations with respect to the employed parameter values, a three step sensitivity analysis was performed. First, all calculations were repeated with a second parameter set ($E = 0.1$/mL, $p_1 = 10$ mmHg, $p_0 = -5.3$ mmHg, $R_{abs}^{tot} = 13.4$ mmHg/(mL/min)) that describes physiological CSF dynamics [19]. Second, the parameters determining the hydrostatic gradients within the CSF and the venous system (l_{sc}, l_{jug}, and p_v^s) were varied within reported standard deviations ($l_{sc} = 33.8 \pm 2.5$ cm, $p_v^s = 5.3 \pm 2.5$ mmHg) [4] one at a time. Third, the compliance distribution assumed in horizontal position was varied by ±50% ($k_V = 0.35 \pm 0.175$).

Cranial arterial volume

Given that arterial pressure is substantially higher than CSF pressure in all but the most extreme pathologic conditions, arterial blood flow rate to the cranium Q_a was assumed unaffected by CSF dynamics. Therefore, the change in cranial arterial volume can be derived from in vivo measurements of Q_a. We used flow rates recorded by phase-contrast MRI in the internal carotid and vertebral arteries as arterial blood flow, Q_a. These flow rates were obtained from the average of 16 NPH patients [9]. Additionally, the flow rates of a healthy volunteer in supine and sitting position [2] were applied to validate the predicted changes in craniospinal CSF flow.

The flows leaving the cranial arterial compartment are the capillary blood flow and the rate of CSF formation, both of which were assumed non-pulsatile. Therefore, the volume balance in the cranial arterial compartment reduces to

$$\Delta V_a(t) = \int_0^t Q_a(t) - \bar{Q}_a dt, \tag{17}$$

where $\bar{Q}_a$ is the mean arterial flow rate over one cardiac cycle.

Evaluation

Sitting up

Immediately upon sitting up, total CSF volume is identical to the equilibrium volume in horizontal position. In other words, the change in total CSF volume is initially zero. The corresponding CSF pressure in upright posture was determined by numerically solving

$$\Delta V^{tot}\left(p_{CSF}^c\right)\big|_{up} \overset{!}{=} \Delta V^{tot}\left(p_{CSF}^c\right)\big|_{hor} = 0 \tag{18}$$

for the cranial CSF pressure p_{CSF}^c. While total CSF volume will not change immediately after changing posture, a rapid caudal shift of CSF volume through the unrestricted CSF pathways can be expected. This shifted volume corresponds to the change in spinal CSF volume ΔV^s (Eq. 10) evaluated at the above calculated CSF pressure.

Upright equilibrium

The upright equilibrium is reached when CSF absorption and formation rates are equal. However, the pressure-dependent CSF absorption rate can only be calculated for a known craniospinal absorption distribution (k_R). Thus, Magnaes' observation [1] of unchanged total compliance in upright posture was used to determine CSF pressure in upright equilibrium:

$$C^{tot}\left(p_{CSF}^c\right)\big|_{up} \overset{!}{=} C^{tot}\left(p_{CSF}^c\right)\big|_{hor} \tag{19}$$

Then, the ratio k_R that leads to equal CSF formation and absorption at this CSF pressures was calculated:

$$Q_{form} \overset{!}{=} \frac{p_{CSF}^c - p_v^c}{R_{abs}^c} + \frac{p_{CSF}^s - p_v^s}{R_{abs}^s} = \frac{k_R}{R_{abs}^{tot}}\left(p_{CSF}^c - p_v^c\right) + \frac{1-k_R}{R_{abs}^{tot}}\left(p_{CSF}^s - p_v^s\right). \tag{20}$$

Simulation of craniospinal flow rates

Any increase or decrease in volume of one entity (fluids and tissue) within the cranium has to be compensated, respectively, by an equivalent volume decrease or increase of the other entities (Monroe–Kelly doctrine) [20]. Therefore, the pulsating volume increase of arterial blood in the cranium ΔV_a (Eq. 17) has to be compensated by a reduction in CSF or venous blood volume. Similar to changes in cranial CSF volume, a change in the cranial arterial volume can be compensated by either a shift of CSF from or to the spinal compartment or a reduction or increase of cranial venous blood volume. With this, cranial arterial blood directly competes with CSF for the available compliance, and the total amount of displaced venous blood ΔV^{tot} is equal to the sum of changes in CSF volume ΔV_{CSF} and arterial volume $\Delta V_a(t)$:

$$\Delta V_{CSF}(t) + \Delta V_a(t) \overset{!}{=} \Delta V^{tot}\left(p_{CSF}^c\right) \tag{21}$$

Solving this equation for the cranial CSF pressure p_{CSF}^c allows for determining the current pressure-dependent CSF absorption rates and calculating the CSF volume ΔV_{CSF}, which may fluctuate throughout a cardiac cycle:

$$\frac{d}{dt}\Delta V_{CSF}(t) = Q_{form} - Q^c_{abs}(p^c_{CSF}) - Q^s_{abs}(p^c_{CSF}). \quad (22)$$

The CSF volume and the cranial CSF pressure during a cardiac cycle were computed by solving this system of differential–algebraic equations (Eqs. 21, 22) using the Matlab (The MathWorks, Inc., Natick, MA, USA) variable-order solver 'ode15s'.

Based on these computations, the CSF flow rate into the spinal compartment was calculated as the change in spinal CSF volume:

$$Q_{CSF}(t) = \frac{d}{dt}\Delta V^s(p^c_{CSF}(t)), \quad (23)$$

and the craniospinal venous flow rate was calculated based on a volume balance in the cranium:

$$Q_v(t) = Q_a(t) - Q_{CSF}(t). \quad (24)$$

Results

After calculating the local and total pressure–volume relationships of the CSF space in horizontal and upright posture, these correlations were used to derive the local and total compliances. Based on this, CSF volume and pressure in upright posture were determined under the assumption of unchanged CSF volume (Eq. 18) or under the assumption of unchanged total compliance (Eq. 19). The posture-related volume and compliance shifts were then evaluated under these two conditions. Finally, the model output was calculated (Eqs. 21, 22) for one cardiac cycle and the craniospinal flow rates of blood and CSF were derived (Eqs. 23, 24) as a basis for discussion of model validity.

Pressure–volume relationships

In horizontal position, cranial and spinal CSF and venous pressures are equal. The overall pressure–volume relationship was thus described by Eq. 1. In upright posture, the local pressure–volume relationships shifted to lower cranial CSF pressures (Eqs. 9, 10) compared to the horizontal position (Fig. 2a). Hereby, the shift of the spinal pressure–volume relationship $\Delta V^s(p^c_{CSF})$ was determined by the distance between the spinal and the cranial reference point, l_{sc}. With the assumption that the jugular veins collapse in upright posture, the shift of the cranial pressure–volume relationship ($\Delta V^c(p^c_{CSF})$) is reduced to a hydrostatic pressure column of length l_{jug}. The overall pressure–volume relationship $\Delta V^{tot}(p^c_{CSF})$ was found by summation of these two local pressure–volume relationships (Eq. 3).

Compliance

In Fig. 2b, the local compliances derived analytically from the corresponding pressure–volume relationships (Eqs. 11–14) were plotted along with the combined total compliance for horizontal and upright posture. Similar to the total pressure–volume relationship, the total compliance shifted towards lower cranial CSF pressures in upright posture. Due to a steep increase of the cranial compliance at low CSF pressures, the cranial compartment became the dominant source of compliance at cranial CSF pressures below approximately 0 mmHg.

Posture change

The resulting cranial CSF pressure in upright posture without any change in CSF volume, which corresponds

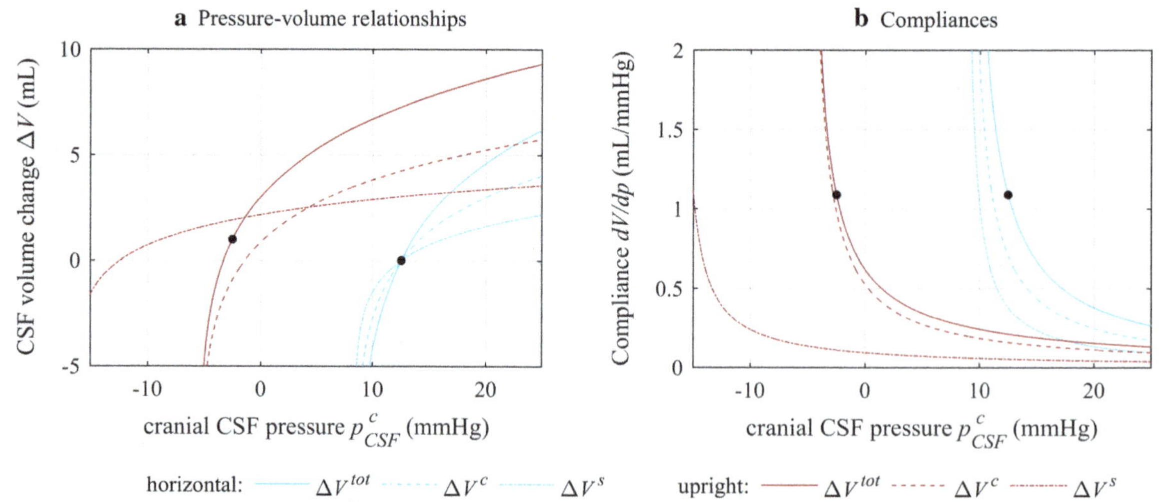

Fig. 2 CSF pressure–volume relationships and compliances in horizontal and upright posture. **a** The cranial and spinal pressure–volume relationships $\Delta V^c(p^c_{CSF})$ and $\Delta V^s(p^c_{CSF})$ are plotted along with the combined overall pressure–volume relationship, $\Delta V^{tot}(p^c_{CSF})$. **b** Visualizes the derivatives of these correlations (Eqs. 11–14), which represent the respective local and total compliances of the CSF system. Equilibrium conditions in both postures are indicated by *black dots*

to the conditions directly after sitting up from horizontal position, was −3.3 mmHg. This decrease in cranial CSF pressure was accompanied by a shift of CSF from the cranial to the spinal compartment (ΔV^s in Table 2). The condition of equal compliance in horizontal and upright posture was satisfied for a cranial CSF pressure of −2.5 mmHg as depicted in Fig. 2b. It required a slight increase in total CSF volume (Table 2). Despite this increase in total CSF volume, the amount of cranial CSF was smaller than in horizontal equilibrium. Furthermore, in equilibrium, the rate of CSF absorption has to match the rate of formation. In upright posture, this was achieved for $k_R = 0.10$. In other words, the spinal resistance to CSF outflow was around nine times the cranial resistance to CSF outflow (Eq. 16). While this meant that in horizontal position 10% of the CSF absorption occurred within the spinal compartment, it equated to 24% spinal absorption in upright posture due to the increased CSF to venous pressure gradient in the spinal compartment.

Compliance shift

As mentioned before, in upright posture the importance of cranial compliance increased for low CSF pressures. In upright equilibrium, only 10% of the total compliance were provided by the spinal compartment. This corresponded to a 71% reduction relative to the spinal compartment's contribution in upright posture (Table 2). Under the condition of no change in total CSF volume after sitting up, the total compliance in upright posture strongly increased due to the steep increase in cranial compliance at low CSF pressure. Consequently, the contribution of the spinal compartment towards overall compliance became even lower.

Cerebral CSF pressure (p^c_{CSF}), total, cranial, and spinal change in CSF volume (ΔV^{tot}, ΔV^c, and ΔV^s), total compliance (C^{tot}), and spinal compliance (C^s) in upright posture are shown in comparison to their reference values in horizontal position. The values were calculated under the two alternative assumed conditions of unchanged volume (Eq. 18) and unchanged total compliance (Eq. 19) relative to the horizontal position.

Table 2 Comparison of CSF pressure, volume and compliance in horizontal and upright posture

Posture condition	Horizontal	Upright	
	–	Eq. 18	Eq. 19
p^c_{CSF} (mmHg)	12.5	−3.3	−2.5
ΔV^{tot} (mL)	0.0	0	1.0
ΔV^c (mL)	0.0	−1.8	−0.9
ΔV^s (mL)	0.0	1.8	1.9
C^{tot} (mL/mmHg)	1.1	1.5	1.1
C^s/C^{tot} (%)	35	8	10
$1-(C^s/C^{tot})/k_V$ (%)	0	77	71

Sensitivity

We analyzed the sensitivity of the reported results to changes in the nominal parameter values (Table 1). This nominal parameter set describes an NPH patient. The physiologic parameter set used to analyze the sensitivity of the model towards changes in the parameters E, p_1, p_0, and R^{tot}_{abs} describes a subject with slightly lower CSF pressure in horizontal position. Also, the calculated cranial CSF pressure in upright posture was lower in the physiologic case (−6.6 mmHg after sitting up and −5.9 mmHg in upright equilibrium) compared to the NPH parameter set. The caudal shift of CSF volume caused by sitting up (ΔV^s in Table 2) was slightly higher (2.1 mL with the physiologic parameter set compared to 1.8 mL in the NPH case). The shift in compliance was not as pronounced as for the NPH parameter set, but the contribution of the spinal compartment to the total compliance still reduced to 18% in upright posture.

For a longer hydrostatic pressure column in the CSF system (l_{sc} = 36.3 cm), the effect of posture increased as the initial volume shift increased to 2.0 mL (not presented in Table 2), and the contribution of the spinal compliance in upright equilibrium decreased to 7%. Conversely, increased spinal venous pressure p^s_v reduced the effect of the jugular vein collapse. Consequently, spinal compliance in upright equilibrium was still 12% and the initial CSF volume shift was reduced to 1.5 mL for 7.7 mmHg spinal venous pressure.

When using different values for the compliance contribution of the spinal compartment in horizontal position (k_V), the caudal shift in CSF volume changed almost proportionally. For example, ΔV^s reduced to 1.0 mL when k_V was reduced by 50% ($k_V = 0.175$) and increased to 4.2 mL when k_V was increased by 50% ($k_V = 0.525$). However, even for such large variations in the compliance distribution (±50%), the reduction of the relative spinal compliance remained between 70 and 82% of its value in horizontal position $(1(C^s/C^{tot})/k_V)$.

Patent jugular veins

Without the collapse of the jugular veins (Eq. 7 instead of Eq. 8) only the difference in density can lead to shifts in CSF volume and compliance distribution when changing posture. In this modified model with patent jugular veins in upright posture, 0.4 mL of CSF flowed from the spinal into the cranial compartment when sitting up from horizontal. Cranial CSF pressure in upright posture decreased further (to −13.3 mmHg) with patent jugular veins compared to the case with collapsed jugular veins (−3.3 mmHg).

Cardiac pulsations

The pulsatile arterial inflow Q_a measured in NPH patients [9] caused a cranial arterial volume pulsation with 1.8 mL stroke volume (difference between maximum and minimum arterial volume, ΔV_a). This change in cranial arterial volume was compensated by craniospinal flows of CSF and venous blood with 0.6 mL and 1.2 mL stroke volume, respectively (Fig. 3, left column). This stroke volume of the craniospinal CSF flow was 35% of the arterial stroke volume, which corresponds to the analytical value of k_V. The total CSF volume hardly changed during one cardiac cycle (less than 1 μL) due to negligible variations in CSF absorption during that short time frame. Nevertheless, the cardiac pulsations caused substantial CSF pressure amplitudes (1.6 mmHg). The pulsation of the spinal CSF volume was directly proportional to the arterial waveform. By definition (Eq. 21), the remaining portion of the pulsatile arterial blood flow was compensated by fluctuations of craniospinal venous blood flow rate Q_v.

In upright posture, this picture changed (Fig. 3, right column). While no change in arterial blood flow was prescribed, craniospinal CSF stroke volume was nevertheless reduced to 10% of the arterial stroke volume (0.2 mL). However, despite these changes in fluid dynamics and changes in absolute pressures, CSF pulse pressure amplitudes remained constant at 1.6 mmHg.

The simulated craniospinal CSF flow pulsations of a healthy subject in horizontal and upright position (Fig. 4) differed from the corresponding measurements in supine and sitting posture [2] by a mean absolute error of 22 and 21 mL/min, respectively. The physiological parameter set ($E = 0.1/\text{mL}$, $p_1 = 10$ mmHg, $p_0 = -5.3$ mmHg, $R^{tot}_{abs} = 13.4\,\text{mmHg}/(\text{mL/min})$) was used for these simulations.

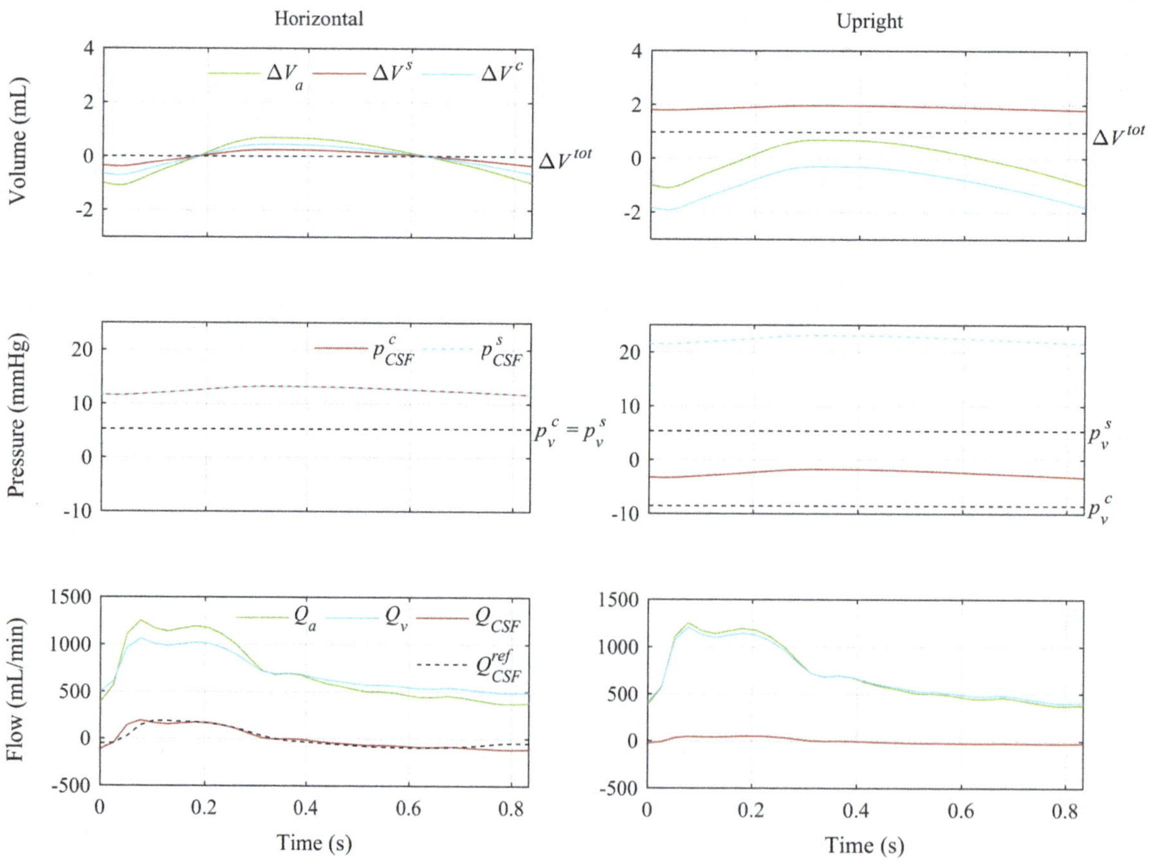

Fig. 3 Effect of arterial pulsation in horizontal and upright posture. During the cardiac cycle, the cranial arterial inflow Q_a (source [9]) leads to fluctuations in cranial arterial volume, ΔV_a. Compensating craniospinal flows of CSF (Q_{CSF}) and venous blood (Q_v), craniospinal CSF distribution (ΔV^c versus ΔV^s), and the corresponding cranial and spinal CSF pressures (p^c_{CSF} and p^s_{CSF}, respectively) are shown for horizontal and upright posture. The corresponding measured CSF flow in supine position [9] is shown as *dashed line*. The flow rates are positive in the directions indicated in (Fig. 1)

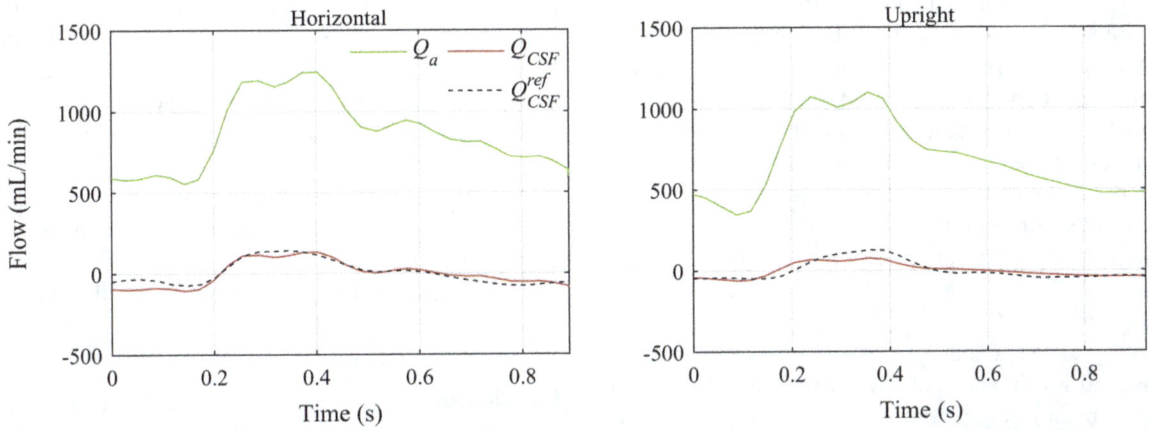

Fig. 4 Comparison of simulated to measured CSF flow pulsation in horizontal and upright posture. Craniospinal CSF flow rates (Q_{CSF}) were simulated in supine and upright posture, based on arterial inflow measured by Alperin et al. [2] in supine and sitting posture. The corresponding measured CSF pulsations are plotted as *dashed lines*

Discussion

Volume and compliance shifts

Our model predicts a posture-dependent shift of the craniospinal compliance distribution caused by a caudal displacement of CSF volume. As previously observed by Magnaes [1], this CSF volume displacement in upright posture reduces the compliance provided by the spinal compartment including the spinal thecal sac. It is induced by the hydrostatic pressure column, which is greater in the CSF system compared to the veins, where it is interrupted by the collapsing jugular veins. The estimated shifts of CSF volume and compliance are in range of the observations of Magnaes [1], although he assumed a much higher contribution of the spinal compartment to compliance than in this study [17]. Furthermore, the posture-dependent shift of the craniospinal compliance distribution was also observed for large variations of the employed parameter values, indicating that our analysis is robust.

Jugular collapse

Without collapsing jugular veins, the model showed neither a caudal shift of CSF volume nor a cranial shift of the compliance distribution. Furthermore, the fall in cranial CSF pressure was greater than that observed clinically [4, 5]. As jugular collapse reduces this fall in pressure in upright posture, the jugular veins may be seen as serving a protective function for the brain. In hydrocephalus patients with ventriculoperitoneal or ventriculoatrial shunts, this protective mechanism is partially bypassed so that, without appropriate siphon prevention, ICP can decrease to levels as low as those predicted by our model without jugular collapse.

Pressure–volume relationship

The exponential pressure–volume relationship of the CSF system is well proven, at least for normal and reasonably increased CSF pressures (relative to the sagittal sinus pressure). However, for sufficiently decreased CSF volume, it implies infinite compliance. This attribute of the exponential pressure–volume relationship becomes especially problematic when applied to the cranial compliance in upright posture, because negative CSF to venous pressure gradients could easily be reached here. However, as such gradients were not reached in this study this limitation does not affect the results or conclusions reported herein. Nonetheless, extrapolation to low CSF pressures would be invalid (Fig. 2). Therefore, a more accurate description of the pressure–volume relationships would need to be used to study the effect of shunting on CSF dynamics [16, 21].

Only considering the mean venous pressure as counter-pressure for the pressure–volume relationship might seem simplistic, as venous pressure varies over the different generations of venous vessels. However, the implemented pressure–volume relationship captures this venous pressure variation and distribution with its exponential shape [22].

The only mechanism of compliance included in the model is the displacement of venous blood. While this mechanism is accepted as the main contributor to compliance in the cranium [10], this is less clear for the rest of the craniospinal space, especially for the spinal thecal sac. However, due to the high distensibility of venous vessels [23], tissue pressure strongly correlates with venous pressure throughout the body. Therefore, it is reasonable to assume that venous pressure is the relevant counter-pressure to compliance in the entire CSF system. If the surrounding tissue itself could provide elastic recoil, part of the pressure–volume relation would have to be modelled independent of venous pressure. This would only then decrease the modelled compliance shift, if the elastic tissue were located intracranially, since the counter-pressure of the spinal compartment is already assumed to be independent of posture due to its proximity to the venous hydrostatic indifference point [4].

CSF absorption

Before Magnaes [1] determined the craniospinal compliance distribution in some of his patients, similar experiments had been done in adult cats [7]. While in cats the spinal compartment appeared to be less important for compliance, it was still responsible for a significant portion of CSF absorption (16%). Similar proportions of the craniospinal CSF absorption distribution were predicted by our model under the condition of posture-independent total compliance. While this result supports the hypothesis that there is spinal CSF absorption, the exact proportion predicted by the model is sensitive to the employed equilibrium pressure in upright posture. Furthermore, the lengths of hydrostatic pressure columns were calculated based on the assumption of 100% cranial absorption [4]. Taking spinal absorption into account, the estimated value of l_{jug} would slightly increase, which would decrease the compliance shift predicted by our model.

Craniospinal flows

Pulsatile arterial inflow into the cranium were compensated by simultaneous craniospinal outflow of CSF and venous blood. Stroke volume and amplitude of the calculated CSF pulsations (Figs. 3, 4) were very close to the respective values measured in vivo [2, 8, 9]. Even the reduction in CSF stroke volume was predicted well (Fig. 4). These are strong indications that the increased resistance of the jugular veins in upright posture is responsible for the shift in compliance observed in vivo. Jugular vein collapse can thus be considered a major contributor to CSF dynamics in upright posture. The calculated overall CSF volume hardly changed within a cardiac cycle. Therefore, the ratio of the estimated CSF and the applied arterial stroke volumes was equal to the contribution of the spinal compartment to the overall compliance. In MRI measurements, CSF and even more so the venous pulses are delayed compared to the arterial input. At least some of this delay can be attributed to wave propagation due to vascular distensibility [23]. In the model, these phase shifts between the calculated craniospinal waves were ignored with the implicit assumption of instantaneous transmission of pressures throughout the craniospinal space. However, when assuming that most of the phase shift originates from a wave propagation delay, it does not influence the compliance distribution estimated from the ratio of CSF and arterial stroke volume. In addition to being delayed, recorded venous pulsations appear damped compared to the modelled pulsations. This damping is probably caused by the Windkessel effect in the larger veins, which is not included in our model. However, the craniospinal venous flow rate is not only difficult to model, it is also difficult to measure with MRI as, especially in upright posture it is distributed over numerous small vessels.

Conclusion

Our results support the hypothesis that the jugular veins play an important role in posture-related changes of CSF dynamics, as their collapse in upright posture induces substantial changes in CSF pressure and compliance.

Abbreviations

CSF: cerebrospinal fluid; ICP: intracranial pressure; MRI: magnet-resonance imaging; NPH: normal pressure hydrocephalus.

Authors' contributions

All authors designed the study and interpreted the data. MG performed the calculations, analyzed the data, and drafted the manuscript. VK and MSD critically revised the manuscript. All authors read and approved the final manuscript.

Author details

[1] Institute for Dynamic Systems and Control, Department of Mechanical and Process Engineering, ETH Zurich, Zurich, Switzerland. [2] The Interface Group, Institute of Physiology, University of Zurich, Zurich, Switzerland. [3] Neuroscience Center Zurich, and the Zurich Center for Integrative Human Physiology, University of Zurich, Zurich, Switzerland. [4] Product Development Group Zurich, Department of Mechanical and Process Engineering, ETH Zurich, Zurich, Switzerland.

Competing interests

The authors declare that they have no competing interests.

Funding

The presented study was supported by grants from the Swiss Academy of Engineering Sciences (2014-080), the 3R Research Foundation (140-14), and the Swiss National Science Foundation through NCCR Kidney.CH.

References

1. Magnæs B. Clinical studies of cranial and spinal compliance and the craniospinal flow of cerebrospinal fluid. Br J Neurosurg. 1989;3(6):659–68.
2. Alperin N, Lee SH, Sivaramakrishnan A, Hushek SG. Quantifying the effect of posture on intracranial physiology in humans by MRI flow studies. J Magn Reson Imaging. 2005;22(5):591–6.
3. Davson H, Hollingsworth G, Segal M. The mechanism of drainage of the cerebrospinal fluid. Brain. 1970;93(4):665–78.
4. Qvarlander S, Sundstrom N, Malm J, Eklund A. Postural effects on intracranial pressure: modelling and clinical evaluation. J Appl Physiol. 2013;115(10):1474–80.

5. Petersen LG, Petersen JCG, Andresen M, Secher NH, Juhler M. Postural influence on intracranial and cerebral perfusion pressure in ambulatory neurosurgical patients. Am J Physiol Regul Integr Comp Physiol. 2016;310(1):R100–4.
6. Gisolf J, Van Lieshout JJ, Van Heusden K, Pott F, Stok WJ, Karemaker JM. Human cerebral venous outflow pathway depends on posture and central venous pressure. J Physiol. 2004;560(1):317–27. doi:10.1113/-jphysiol.2004.070409.
7. Marmarou A, Shulman K, LaMorgese J. Compartmental analysis of compliance and outflow resistance of the cerebrospinal fluid system. J Neurosurg. 1975;43(5):523–34.
8. Yiallourou TI, Schmid Daners M, Kurtcuoglu V, Haba-Rubio J, Heinzer R, Fornani E, et al. Continuous positive airway pressure alters cranial blood flow and cerebrospinal fluid dynamics at the craniovertebral junction. Interdiscip Neurosurg. 2015;2(3):152–9.
9. Qvarlander S, Ambarki K, Wåhlin A, Jacobsson J, Birgander R, Malm J, et al. Cerebrospinal fluid and blood flow patterns in idiopathic normal pressure hydrocephalus. Acta Neurol Scand. 2016. doi:10.1111/ane.12636.
10. Stevens S, Lakin W. Local compliance effects on the global pressure–volume relationship in models of intracranial pressure dynamics. Math Comput Modell Dyn Syst. 2000;6(4):445–65. doi:10.1076/-mcmd.6.4.445.3655.
11. Gehlen M, Kurtcuoglu V, Schmid Daners M. Patient specific hardware-in-the-loop testing of cerebrospinal fluid shunt systems. IEEE Trans Biomed Eng. 2016;63(2):348–58.
12. Avezaat CJJ, van Eijndhoven JHM. Clinical observations on the relationship between cerebrospinal fluid pulse pressure and intracranial pressure. Acta Neurochir (Wien). 1986;79(1):13–29. doi:10.1007/-BF01403461.
13. Czosnyka M, Czosnyka Z, Momjian S, Pickard JD. Cerebrospinal fluid dynamics. Physiol Meas. 2004;25(5):R51–76.
14. Raabe A, Czosnyka M, Piper I, Seifert V. Monitoring of intracranial compliance: correction for a change in body position. Acta Neurochir (Wien). 1999;141(1):31–6.
15. Rigamonti D. Adult hydrocephalus. Cambridge: Cambridge University Press; 2014.
16. Qvarlander S, Lundkvist B, Koskinen LOD, Malm J, Eklund A. Pulsatility in CSF dynamics: pathophysiology of idiopathic normal pressure hydrocephalus. J Neurol Neurosurg Psychiatry. 2013;84(7):735–41.
17. Wåhlin A, Ambarki K, Birgander R, Alperin N, Malm J, Eklund A. Assessment of craniospinal pressure-volume indices. Am J Neuroradiol. 2010;31(9):1645–50.
18. Lenfeldt N, Andersson N, Ågren-Wilsson A, Bergenheim AT, Koskinen LOD, Eklund A, et al. Cerebrospinal fluid pulse pressure method: a possible substitute for the examination of B waves. J Neurosurg. 2004;101(6):944–50.
19. Schmid Daners M, Bottan S, Guzzella L, Poulikakos D, Kurtcuoglu V. Craniospinal pressure–volume dynamics in phantom models. IEEE Trans Biomed Eng. 2012;59(12):3482–90.
20. Greitz D, Wirestam R, Franck A, Nordell B, Thomsen C, Ståhlberg F. Pulsatile brain movement and associated hydrodynamics studied by magnetic resonance phase imaging. Neuroradiology. 1992;34(5):370–80.
21. Drake JM, Tenti G, Sivalsganathan S. Computer modelling of siphoning for CSF shunt design evaluation. Pediatr Neurosurg. 1994;21(1):6–15.
22. Cirovic S, Walsh C, Fraser W. Mathematical study of the role of non-linear venous compliance in the cranial volume-pressure test. Med Biol Eng Comput. 2003;41(5):579–88.
23. Hall JE, Guyton AC. Textbook of medical physiology. Philadelphia: Saunders; 2011.

9

The role of perfusion and diffusion MRI in the assessment of patients affected by probable idiopathic normal pressure hydrocephalus

Francesco Tuniz[1], Maria Caterina Vescovi[1*], Daniele Bagatto[2], Daniela Drigo[3], Maria Cristina De Colle[2], Marta Maieron[4] and Miran Skrap[1]

Abstract

Background: Invasive tests measuring resistance to cerebral spinal fluid (CSF) outflow and the effect of temporary drainage of CSF are used to select candidates affected by idiopathic normal pressure hydrocephalus (iNPH) for shunt surgery. Neither test, however, completely excludes patients from treatment. Perfusion and diffusion magnetic resonance imaging (MRI) are non-invasive techniques that might be of value in selecting patients for surgical treatment and understanding brain changes in iNPH patients. The aim of this study was to understand the role of perfusion and diffusion MRI in selecting candidates for shunt surgery and to investigate the relationship between cerebral perfusion and possible microstructural changes in brain tissue before and after invasive tests, and after ventricular-peritoneal (VP) shunt implantation, to better clarify pathophysiological mechanisms underlying iNPH.

Methods: Twenty-three consecutive patients with probable iNPH were included in this study. Patients underwent a clinical and neuroradiological evaluation before and after invasive tests, and after surgery. Only patients who showed a positive result in at least one of the invasive tests were submitted for VP shunt implantation. Perfusion and diffusion magnetic resonance imaging (MRI) was performed before and after invasive tests and after shunt surgery.

Results: Thirteen patients underwent surgery and all showed clinical improvement after VP shunt implantation and a significant increase in perfusion in both periventricular white matter (PVWM) and basal ganglia (BG) regions. The 10 patients that did not have surgery showed after invasive tests, a significant reduction in perfusion in both PVWM and BG regions. Comparing the changes in perfusion with those of diffusion in positive patients we found a significant positive correlation in BG and a significant inverse correlation in PVWM area.

Conclusions: Perfusion MRI is a non-invasive technique that could be useful together with invasive tests in selecting patients for surgical treatment. Furthermore, the relationship between perfusion and diffusion data could better clarify pathophysiological mechanisms underlying iNPH. In PVWM area we suggest that interstitial edema could reduce microvascular blood flow and interfere with the blood supply to these regions. In BG regions we suggest that a chronic hypoxic insult caused by blood hypo-perfusion produces a chronic cytotoxic edema. Both in PVWM and in BG regions, pathophysiological mechanisms could be modified after VP-shunt implantation.

Keywords: Diffusion, Hydrocephalus, iNPH, MRI, Perfusion, Shunt

*Correspondence: mariacaterina.vescovi@gmail.com
[1] Department of Neurosurgery, AOU-UD "Santa Maria della Misericordia", Piazzale S.M. della Misericordia, 33100 Udine, Italy
Full list of author information is available at the end of the article

Background

Idiopathic normal pressure hydrocephalus (iNPH) is a condition characterized by ventricular enlargement and normal intracranial pressure (ICP) caused by disturbed cerebral spinal fluid (CSF) dynamics [1]. The cause is still unknown. The iNPH signs are typically subcortical, characterized by slow progressive impairment of gait and balance, cognitive deterioration and urinary incontinence [2]. Treatment of iNPH patients with ventricular-peritoneal or ventricular-atrial shunts is successful, with an improvement rate of more than 80% in recent short-term studies, and an acceptable complication rate [3–7]. At present, clinicians have two invasive predictive tests to select patient candidates for surgery: a test measuring compliance of craniospinal space or resistance to CSF outflow (Rout), and a test measuring the effect on symptoms of temporary drainage of CSF (CSF tap test) [8–10]. These tests are, however, not totally specific or sensitive and can be used for selecting patients for shunt surgery but not for excluding patients from treatment [11, 12]. Better methods for the identification of responders and non-responders are required. Cerebral blood flow (CBF) is reduced in iNPH patients, mainly in the frontal cortex and in accordance with the subcortical symptomatology, in the basal ganglia, in the thalami and also in the periventricular white matter (PVWM) [13–19]. As the subcortical and periventricular regions seem to be of special interest in iNPH, magnetic resonance (MR) perfusion imaging with its relatively high resolution and sensitivity for deep structures might be of value as a diagnostic and predictive tool [20]. Some authors have also investigated the role of diffusion MRI in determining brain parenchymal damage in PVWM and basal ganglia (BG) areas and the role of apparent diffusion coefficient (ADC) in predicting surgical outcome [21–26].

The aims of this study were to investigate (a) the relationship between cerebral perfusion and microstructural damage of brain tissue as measured by perfusion and diffusion MRI in PVWM and BG areas before, after invasive tests, and after surgery and (b) the potential role of perfusion and diffusion MRI in selecting patients for VP-shunt implantation.

Methods

Patients selection and clinical evaluation

Twenty-three patients diagnosed with probable iNPH were prospectively included between January 2013 and December 2014. Inclusion criteria for probable iNPH were based on iNPH Guidelines: presence of a gait disturbance in combination with cognitive and/or urinary symptoms and an Evans' Index > 0.30 in the absence of any known cause for secondary hydrocephalus [2]. All patients underwent neuropsychological, physiotherapeutic and neurological examinations, and performance was assessed in the four domains of gait, neuropsychology, balance and continence, yielding separate scores as well as a total score on a recently published iNPH scale [27]. Domain and total scores all range from 0 to 100 with 0 representing the most severe condition and 100 representing normal performance among healthy individuals aged 70–74. This study was approved by our Institutional Review Board and an informed consent was acquired from each patient involved in this study.

Invasive tests

A lumbar infusion test and a tap test were performed on each patient in same procedure. Lumbar puncture was performed in the morning and mean CSF basal pressure was recorded. A lumbar infusion test was then performed using the constant rate infusion method and Rout was calculated. After the infusion test was completed, CSF was drained until the pressure returned to baseline. Then, a tap test was performed, draining 50 ml of CSF. A value of Rout greater than 13 mmHg/min/ml was considered a predictor for good outcome after shunt implantation [28, 29], as well as a good response to the CSF tap test. The response to CSF tap test was expressed as the mean of the percentage change in all motor and psychometric tests compared with the previously achieved results. An increase of 5% was considered significant [11].

Patient groups

Patients were divided into two groups. Those who resulted positive in at least one of the invasive tests underwent ventricular-peritoneal shunt implantation (positive patients, PP); when both invasive tests were negative, patients were denied the surgical procedure (negative patients, NP).

Surgical procedure

All positive patients underwent ventricular-peritoneal shunt implantation. The right ventricular frontal horn was chosen for all patients and a Codman® Hakim® programmable valve with pre-chamber was implanted. The pressure of the valve was set with regards to the level of clinical impairment, the neuroradiological images and response to the invasive tests. Two days after surgical intervention a head CT-scan was performed to rule out surgical complications and to verify the correct placement of the ventricular catheter. All patients were discharged from hospital 5 to 7 days after ventricular-peritoneal shunt implantation with a good clinical recovery. One month after the ventricular peritoneal shunt positioning, positive patients repeated the clinical evaluation.

MRI study

MRI was performed for each patient before and after invasive tests and one month after ventricular peritoneal shunt implantation (timing was chosen to permit good recovery after the surgical procedure). For each patient, perfusion and diffusion sequences were acquired and values for relative cerebral blood flow (rCBF) and apparent diffusion coefficient (ADC) were extrapolated.

Examinations were performed on a 3.0T magnet (Achieva; Philips Medical Systems, Best, The Netherlands).

At the first MRI examination, all patients before diffusion tensor imaging (DTI) and perfusion-weighted imaging (PWI) studies, also underwent a standard brain MRI protocol that included non-enhanced axial inversion recovery (IR) T1-weighted images, sagittal 3D T2-weighted images and axial fluid attenuated inversion recovery (FLAIR) sequences. During the second and third MRI examinations, only DTI and PWI sequences were performed.

Perfusion MRI

Dynamic Susceptibility Contrast-Enhanced (DSC) MR imaging was performed using gradient echo planar T2*—weighted sequence with the following parameters: TR = 1708 ms, TE = 40 ms, inplane resolution = 1.75 × 1.75 mm, slice thickness = 4 mm, number of slices = 25, slice GAP = 0 mm.

Ten seconds after the start of image acquisition, a bolus of a 1.0 mmol/ml gadobutrol formula (Gadovist; Schering Bayer Pharma, Leverkusen, Germany) in a dose of 0.1 mmol/kg of body weight (as indicated by the manufacturer) was injected via a 20-gauge catheter placed in the antecubital vein. Contrast administration was performed using an automatic injector (MEDRAD Spectris Solaris EP MR injection System, Indianola PA, USA) at a rate of 5 ml/s and was followed by a saline bolus (20 ml at 5 ml/s). The dynamic images were post-processed using the vendor specific software on the MRI scanner. For each patient, two different examiners, one neurosurgeon and one neuroradiologist, placed sixteen regions of interest (ROIs) in the same basal ganglia region (i.e. nucleus caudatus, putamen, striatum) and in PVWM area. Six ROIs were also positioned in cortical occipital region. Careful positioning avoided inclusion of other anatomical structures. During image post-processing the two examiners were blinded to patient clinical evaluations and invasive test results, thus ensuring that results were unbiased. As an example, Fig. 1 show ROIs positioned in the periventricular and basal ganglia regions. For each ROI value the relative cerebral blood flow (rCBF), relative cerebral blood volume (rCMV) and mean transit time (MTT) were calculated. In the present study, we used the rCBF as parameter of choice, using the mean cortical occipital rCBF as internal reference.

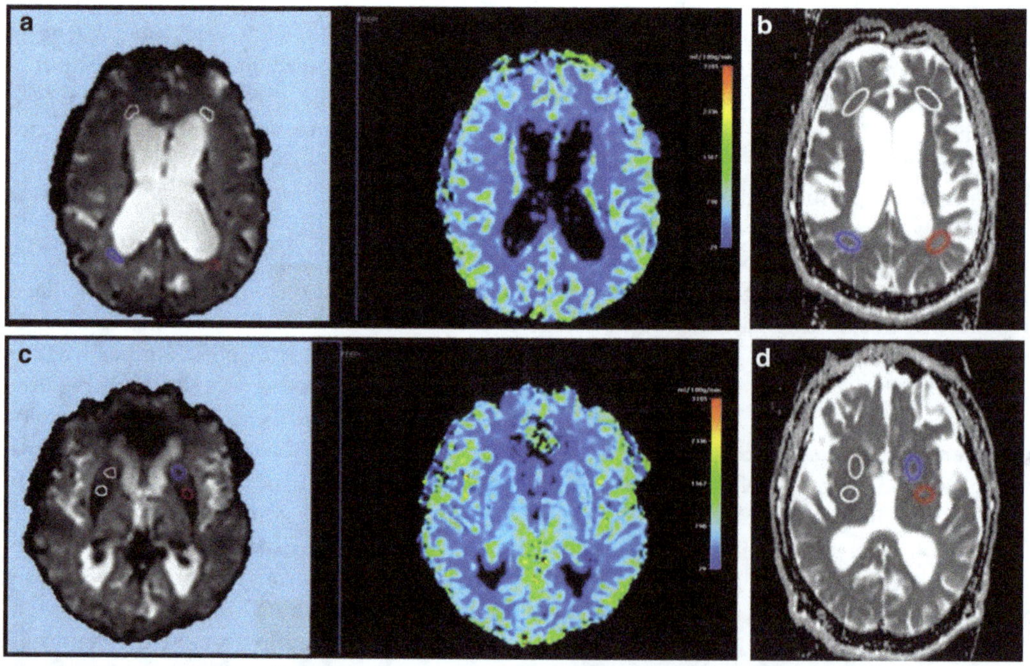

Fig. 1 MR images of patient G. **a, c** Regions of interest (ROIs) positioned on perfusion maps in periventricular and basal ganglia region respectively. **b, d** ROIs positioned on ADC diffusion maps in periventricular and basal ganglia region respectively

Diffusion study

Diffusion-weighted images were acquired before administration of contrast medium using a diffusion-weighted single-shot echo-planar sequence with diffusion gradients along the fifteen directions and effective b-values of 0 and 1000 s/mm^2. ADC and fractional anisotropy (FA) maps were automatically generated by the software employed in the MRI scanner console. Scan parameters of DTI sequence were as follows: TR = 7204 ms, TE = 62 ms, inplane resolution = 1.62 × 1.62 mm, slice thickness = 2 mm, number of slices = 60, slice GAP = 0 mm.

ADC values were calculated in ROIs positioned in basal ganglia and PVWM area and overlapped the perfusion ROIs.

Statistical analysis

Descriptive analysis was performed: median, interquartile range (IQR), mean and standard deviation (SD) were calculated. The parameters of perfusion and diffusion between PP versus NP groups and within subjects were compared by Wilcoxon Mann–Whitney test and Wilcoxon signed rank sum test, respectively. For statistical analysis we applied relative perfusion values, which were calculated using estimates for the occipital cortex as an internal reference [20]. Differences in mean values of perfusion and diffusion from baseline to post-surgery were estimated for each patient. Spearman correlation was calculated. The alpha level was set to 0.05 for all tests. The statistical analysis was performed using Epi Info™ v. 3.5.1 and Microsoft Excel software.

Results

Thirteen patients (56.53%) had at least one positive result in the invasive tests. We referred to this patient group as positive patients (PP). Ten patients (43.47%) conversely had no positive result either in the lumbar infusion test or in the tap test. We referred to this patient group as negative patients (NP).

In the PP group, six patients were male (46.15%) and seven patients were female (53.85%); in the NP group, four patients were male (40%), and six patients were female (60%). For the PP the mean age was 72.5 ± 6.94 years, whereas for NP mean age was 70.7 ± 6.78 years. Regarding invasive tests results in the PP group 10 patients had a Rout greater than 13 mmHg/min/ml (76.92%) and 10 patients had a positive result in the tap test, showing a clinical improvement greater than 5% (Table 1). In the NP group no patient showed clinical improvement after the tap test or a Rout greater than 13 mmHg/min/ml (Table 2).

Considering clinical characteristics, in the PP group, clinical basal score ranged from 44.00 to 84.75 with an average value of 61.54 ± 10.13. In the NP group, baseline clinical score ranged from 22.50 to 78.25 with an average value of 57.97 ± 16.51. No significant differences were demonstrated between the two groups, either in total clinical score or singular domain.

After invasive tests were performed, 10 patients of the PP group showed clinical improvement with a clinical score increase of more than 5%. Average improvement rate was 26.45% ± 19.47% (Table 1). None of the NP showed clinical improvement greater than 5% after the tap test.

Table 1 Positive patients (PP) personal and clinical data

Patient	Sex	Age (years)	Rout (mmHg/min/ml)	Tap test	Total clinical score and its % variation				
					Basal	Post-test	% Variation	Post-surgery	% Variation
A	Male	82	10.40	Positive	60.75	78.25	28.81	84.75	39.51
B	Female	72	13.20	Positive	54.25	69.50	28.11	88.25	62.67
C	Female	68	17.90	Positive	36.50	79.75	25.59	88.25	38.98
D	Female	69	6.10	Positive	55.00	76.50	39.09	95.75	74.09
E	Female	73	22.50	Positive	65.75	81.00	23.19	89.75	36.50
F	Female	74	14.90	Negative	62.75	62.75	0.00	82.25	31.08
G	Male	77	18.20	Positive	53.25	84.75	59.15	88.25	65.73
H	Male	56	15.00	Positive	84.75	98.75	16.52	98.75	16.52
I	Female	75	13.60	Positive	57.75	82.25	42.42	82.25	42.42
L	Male	80	14.00	Positive	44.00	69.50	57.95	69.50	57.95
M	Male	65	11.30	Positive	74.50	88.50	18.79	93.25	25.17
N	Male	79	15.00	Negative	59.25	61.75	4.22	79.75	34.60
O	Female	73	13.60	Negative	64.50	64.50	0.00	84.75	31.40

Table 2 Negative patients (NP) personal and clinical data

Patient	Sex	Age (years)	Rout (mmHg/min/ml)	Tap test	Total basal clinical score
1	Female	75	8.60	Negative	49.00
2	Male	67	5.10	Negative	22.50
3	Female	74	11.10	Negative	73.25
4	Male	59	11.40	Negative	78.25
5	Female	66	10.00	Negative	69.50
6	Female	72	9.50	Negative	51.75
7	Female	69	7.90	Negative	45.75
8	Female	81	12.20	Negative	67.00
9	Male	79	10.40	Negative	66.00
10	Male	65	11.30	Negative	56.75

PP patients were clinically evaluated again 1 month after ventriculo-peritoneal shunt implantation. In the third clinical evaluation all PP patients showed clinical improvement after shunt implantation. Average improvement rate with respect to basal evaluation was 42.82% ± 17.15%. In Table 1 PP personal data, results of invasive tests and clinical score at basal, post-test and post-surgery evaluation are reported. In Table 2 the same data for NP are summarized.

Perfusion and diffusion values of PP group are reported in Table 3 for the periventricular and basal ganglia regions. Values were obtained during the baseline radiological study, after invasive test examination and after shunt implantation. In Table 4 the same values are summarized for the NP group.

Basal values of perfusion and diffusion between the PP and NP groups were compared. No significant differences were demonstrated at basal evaluation either in the periventricular region, or in the basal ganglia region. The post-invasive test values of perfusion and ADC were also compared between the PP and NP groups and a significant difference was found for perfusion values in both the periventricular and the basal ganglia areas between two patient groups. No significant differences were demonstrated in either region for ADC values (Table 5).

Perfusion changes within the PP and NP groups were analysed from basal to post-test and after surgery procedure. A significant improvement of perfusion was found in PP group both in BG region and PVWM area, while NP group shows a significant decrease in the same regions. In Figs. 2 and 3 periventricular and basal ganglia perfusion variation from baseline evaluation to post-surgery assessment in positive patients (PP) are represented. When considering diffusion measurements within each group, results are different. We found a significant decrease of ADC values in PVWM area and a significant increase in BG regions in PP group. In NP group statistical significance was not reached either in PVWM area or in BG. In Table 5 the median and IQR of perfusion and diffusion of PP and NP groups and statistical analysis are reported.

We also investigated the relationship between the clinical score, ADC values, perfusion values and their variation in PP group. Only the correlations that have an impact on clinical and pathophysiological conditions are reported:

- Clinical score and periventricular ADC values in basal and post-test evaluation: a significant inverse correlation was demonstrated ($r_s = -0.51$ and $r_s = -0.56$ respectively). In post-surgery evaluation no significant correlation was detected ($r_s = -0.46$).
- Periventricular perfusion and ADC variation from basal to post-surgery evaluation: a significant inverse correlation was reached ($r_s = -0.52$).
- Spearman correlation of differential values of perfusion and ADC in basal ganglia from basal to post-surgery evaluation: a significant direct correlation was reached ($r_s = 0.57$).

Discussion

Changes in cerebral blood perfusion in iNPH patients compared with aged-matched controls, and changes in brain tissue microstructure, have already been demonstrated by multiple studies [13, 14, 16–20, 24]. In this study we considered only patients with probable iNPH. Patients were recruited over a limited period of 24 months and were prospectively followed; clinical and radiological evaluations were made at the beginning, after invasive tests and after shunt procedure. The patient population was divided into two sub-groups: patients who had at least one positive response to invasive tests and who had undergone surgical treatment (PP group), and patients who did not show any improvement after the tap test or a significantly high Rout (NP group). After

Table 3 Positive patients (PP) perfusion and diffusion values

Patients	Perfusion mean values (rate)[a]						Diffusion mean values (ADC mm^2/sec)[b]					
	Periventricular white matter			Basal ganglia			Periventricular white matter			Basal ganglia		
	Basal evaluation	Post-test evaluation	After surgery evaluation	Basal evaluation	Post-test evaluation	After surgery evaluation	Basal evaluation	Post-test evaluation	After surgery evaluation	Basal evaluation	Post-test evaluation	After surgery evaluation
A	0.85	1.11	1.34	1.46	2.22	2.45	1107.84	1075.96	1122.28	662.71	763.95	811.15
B	0.59	0.71	0.84	1.12	1.33	1.38	917.99	893.31	875.20	753.40	781.38	762.25
C	0.64	1.03	1.08	1.24	1.89	2.02	787.90	814.88	812.00	677.18	683.95	697.66
D	0.64	0.90	1.52	1.35	1.85	2.87	1271.25	1037.63	908.98	729.51	778.29	908.98
E	0.51	1.08	0.98	0.89	2.00	1.90	857.25	819.58	801.34	701.10	725.04	778.50
F	0.58	1.40	1.47	1.07	2.39	2.36	993.28	925.93	941.58	725.03	727.94	734.56
G	0.61	0.91	0.78	1.00	1.54	1.17	947.41	925.24	925.48	752.65	752.26	772.91
H	0.51	0.68	0.76	1.05	1.16	1.51	821.90	840.56	840.85	684.59	667.03	698.10
I	0.58	0.68	0.84	1.01	1.02	1.46	881.43	859.48	834.24	682.03	749.88	742.79
L	0.37	0.57	0.77	1.10	1.01	1.29	1116.04	1071.39	1056.63	675.35	621.00	746.25
M	0.91	1.02	1.24	1.42	1.78	2.12	872.51	832.69	841.56	694.99	672.75	734.56
N	0.59	0.71	0.84	1.12	1.33	1.38	917.99	893.31	875.20	753.40	781.38	762.25
O	0.64	0.90	1.52	1.35	1.85	2.87	1271.25	1037.63	908.98	729.51	778.29	908.98

[a] Perfusion rates are expressed relative to that in the occipital cortex

[b] Diffusion is expressed using apparent diffusion coefficient (ADC) parameter

Table 4 Negative patients (NP) perfusion and diffusion values

Patients	Perfusion mean values (rate)[a]				Diffusion mean values (ADC mm^2/s)[b]			
	Periventricular white matter		Basal ganglia		Periventricular white matter		Basal ganglia	
	Basal evaluation	Post-test evaluation	Basal evaluation	Post-test evaluation	Basal evaluation	Post-test evaluation	Basal evaluation	Post-test evaluation
1	0.36	0.25	0.75	0.48	1638.29	1612.69	745.14	757.73
2	0.57	0.49	1.29	1.10	1351.23	1371.06	734.81	722.08
3	0.53	0.30	1.34	0.83	1067.76	1003.93	736.24	749.36
4	0.76	0.58	1.44	1.15	863.78	822.19	647.24	681.00
5	0.56	0.49	1.10	0.97	864.50	877.64	763.63	754.95
6	0.53	0.33	1.34	0.87	1156.39	1066.43	823.74	835.61
7	0.93	0.78	1.63	1.33	765.13	778.51	676.38	669.20
8	0.62	0.58	1.30	1.14	940.13	952.58	851.38	844.83
9	0.43	0.20	1.24	0.73	666.65	620.79	447.24	482.25
10	0.62	0.49	1.30	1.18	1454.26	1354.30	1000.11	1009.74

[a] Perfusion rates are expressed relative to that in the occipital cortex

[b] Diffusion is expressed using apparent diffusion coefficient (ADC) parameter

Table 5 Median and IQR of perfusion and diffusion of PP and NP groups and statistical analysis

Region	RMN	Patient group	Time			p value**		
			Basal median value (IQR)	Post test median value (IQR)	Post surgery median value (IQR)	Basal vs. post-test	Basal vs. post-surgery	Post test vs. post-surgery
Periventricular region	Perfusion	PP	0.59 (0.58–0.64)	0.90 (0.71–1.03)	0.98 (0.84–1.34)	0.0014	0.0014	0.0156
		NP	0.56 (0.53–0.62)	0.49 (0.31–0.56)	–	0.0051		
		p value*	ns	0.003				
	Diffusion	PP	917.99 (872.51–1107.84)	893.31 (840.56–1037.63)	875.2 (840.85–925.48)	0.0071	0.0071	ns
		NP	1003.94 (863.96–1302.52)	978.25 (836.05–1282.33)	–	ns		
		p value*	ns	ns				
Basal ganglia	Perfusion	PP	1.12 (1.05–1.35)	1.78 (1.33–1.89)	1.9 (1.38–2.36)	0.0024	0.0015	0.0329
		NP	1.30 (1.25–1.25)	1.03 (0.84–1.15)	–	0.0051		
		p value*	ns	0.001				
	Diffusion	PP	701.10 (681.03–729.51)	749.88 (683.95–778.29)	762.25 (734.56–778.5)	ns	0.0015	0.0158
		NP	742.59 (690.98–808.71)	752.16 (691.27–816.14)	–	ns		
		p value*	ns	ns				

* Wilcoxon Mann–Whitney test

** Wilcoxon signed rank sum test

initial clinical data analysis, neither the total clinical score nor the singular domain score showed significant differences between the two groups of patients.

Perfusion MRI

To evaluate cerebral perfusion we used a DSC MRI perfusion sequence, a non-invasive technique. This technique suffers from specific problems related to CBV and CBF quantification in absolute terms. For inter-subject comparison or follow-up evaluation relative perfusion estimates are usually used. We chose occipital cortical perfusion as the internal reference assuming that this region would be less affected by global perfusion reduction [19, 20, 30–32].

The PVWM and BG perfusion data obtained at the beginning of the study (basal values) are consistent with

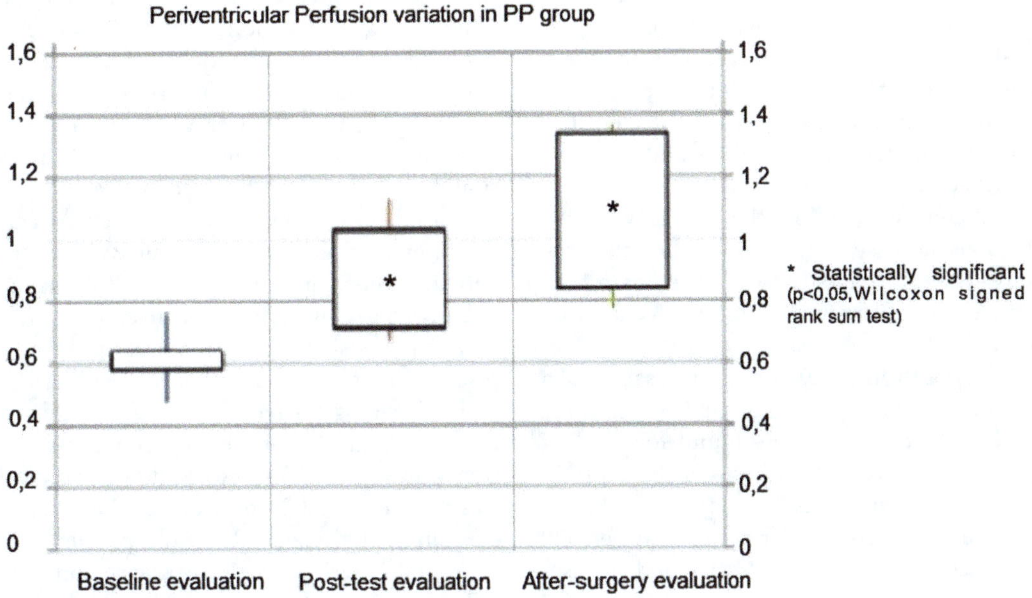

Fig. 2 Periventricular white matter perfusion changes in positive patients (PP). On the vertical axis relative perfusion values are reported [mean rCBF Periventricular/mean rCBF Occipital]. Rectangles represent data inter-quartile range (IQR) and straight lines represent standard deviation (SD). Data are represented for baseline evaluation, after test evaluation and post-surgery assessment. Asterisk indicates when the variation was statistically significant

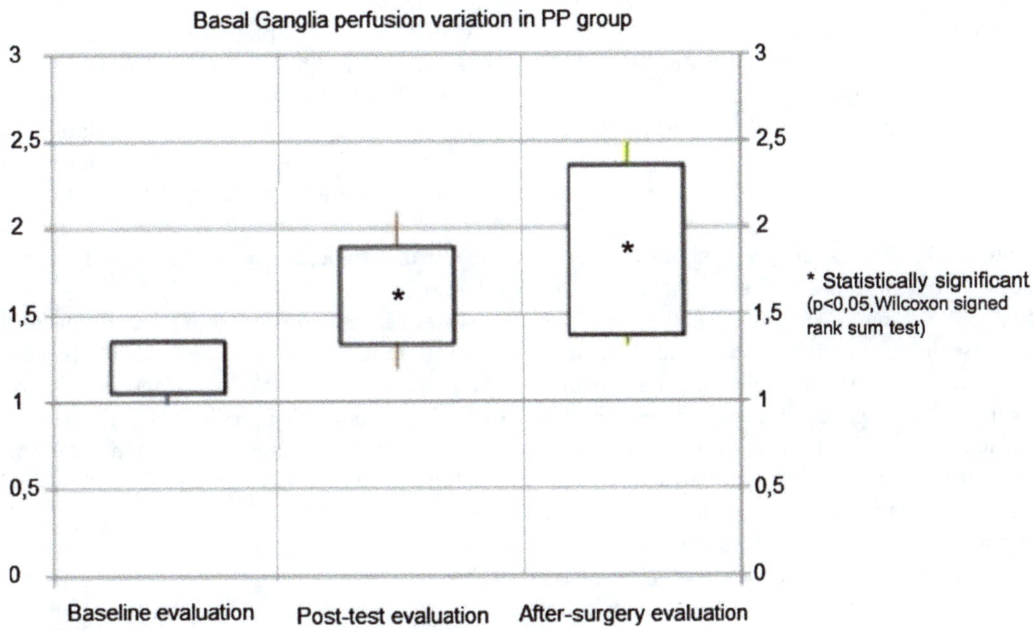

Fig. 3 Basal ganglia perfusion changes in positive patients (PP). On the vertical axis relative perfusion values are reported [mean rCBF Basal Ganglia/mean rCBF Occipital]. Rectangles represent data inter-quartile range (IQR) and straight lines represent standard deviation (SD). Data are represented for baseline evaluation, after test evaluation and post-surgery assessment

values available in the literature for iNPH [20]. In the baseline evaluation no significant differences were demonstrated in perfusion values between PP and NP groups either in PVWM region or in basal ganglia. Likewise no significant difference was obtained in ADC values. Given these results, the authors could not identify a radiological perfusion or diffusion marker for selecting patients to submit to surgery without carrying out invasive tests.

Perfusion values showed a different response between the two groups after performing the invasive tests. In the PP group, perfusion increased significantly both in the periventricular and basal ganglia areas and the same result was achieved after VP shunt. In the PP group we detected clinical improvement in the majority of the cases related to an increase of the CBF values after the invasive tests were performed. These results is are consistent with the ones in literature [32]. NP, on the other hand, showed a significant decrease in perfusion values after invasive tests both in PVWM and in basal ganglia areas and no clinical improvement was achieved in these patients. Significant differences were found for PVWM and basal ganglia perfusion values between PP and NP after performing the invasive tests.

Given the different perfusion patterns between PP and NP, we suggest that perfusion MRI could be useful together with invasive tests in selecting patients for surgical treatment. As an example, three PP patients (F) (N) (O) presented a Rout slightly above the threshold value and no clinical improvement after tap test. All these patients, however, showed a good improvement in perfusion values in PVWM and BG. Patients were subsequently submitted to surgery. A month after VP-shunt implantation these patients showed good clinical improvement and CBF values increased even more. This finding suggests that perfusion MRI (a non-invasive technique) could enhance the selection of candidates for VP shunt implantation.

Diffusion MRI

In the PP group ADC values decrease significantly in PVWM area due, in our opinion, to the interstitial edema reduction after CSF drainage. However, in BG region a significant increase in ADC values was observed. This phenomenon could be related to relief of the chronic hypoxic environment caused by hydrocephalus. In the NP group no significant variation of ADC values was observed. Correlating clinical and radiological data, the authors found a significant inverse correlation between clinical score and periventricular diffusion values in the PP group in basal and post-test evaluations (i.e. patients with higher diffusion values in PVWM area showed a worse clinical score in the baseline exam). The authors speculated that PVWM diffusion values are related to trans-ependymal interstitial edema; this result is consistent with the findings in literature [19, 22, 33].

Pathophysiological considerations

Comparing perfusion and diffusion data from basal to post-surgical evaluation, the authors found a significant inverse correlation in PP group. For higher diffusion values, we found lower CBF values. The authors hypothesized that interstitial edema could reduce microvascular blood flow and interfere with the blood supply of these regions. After VP shunt implantation, more CSF was drained; diffusion values decreased (expression of reduced interstitial edema) and perfusion values increased. Draining CSF acutely or chronically decreased the interstitial edema present in PVWM areas in iNPH patients, improving regional blood perfusion and consequently achieving clinical improvement.

When considering the basal ganglia region, the researchers found data that may describe a different pathophysiological mechanism. A significant direct correlation in the PP group between perfusion and diffusion values from baseline to the postsurgical evaluation was demonstrated. In previous studies, a chronic hypoxic environment caused by hydrocephalus has been demonstrated [17, 18, 20]. Researchers considered that the diffusion values calculated in basal ganglia areas could be conditioned mainly by the chronic hypoxic environment causing cytotoxic damage [25, 26, 33], as opposed to what happens in the periventricular areas where the mechanism underlying the chronic damage of the white matter is mainly induced by the interstitial trans-ependymal edema.

After VP shunt implantation, perfusion improved consistently in the basal ganglia; consequently the chronic hypoxic insult decreased as the cytotoxic edema, and diffusion values increase. We postulate that since correlation is significant only when considering variation from the baseline to postsurgical evaluation, a significant amount of time (several weeks) is required to modify the chronic hypoxic environment and improve cytotoxic edema.

Moreover we argued that this different pathophysiological mechanism between periventricular and basal ganglia areas could be explained by the heterogeneity of brain areas and different tissue structure: white matter (with predominance of axons) in PVWM, grey matter (with predominance of cellular bodies) in BG [26].

Study limitations

There are some underlying limitations of this study. First of all, because of the limited number of patients that influenced the statistical analysis; we were not able to predict some important statistical measures such as positive predictive value of perfusion MRI for selecting patients as candidates for surgery. Another limitation is related to the absence of data that could be derived from negative patients after a hypothetical VP shunt implantation (due to obvious ethical reasons). Those clinical and radiological data could be relevant to confirm the pathophysiological mechanisms we postulate and to point out the role of perfusion and diffusion MRI in the patient selection process.

Conclusions

This study (despite the limited number of patients) allowed us to observe prospectively diffusion and perfusion changes in probable iNPH patient candidates for a VP shunt. Perfusion MRI (a non-invasive technique) was found to be useful, together with invasive tests, for selecting patients for surgery, increasing the specificity in selected cases. Relationships between diffusion and perfusion values estimated with MRI have been studied and a hypothesis has been proposed to better clarify the pathophysiological mechanisms in iNPH. Further studies conducted on a wider patient population will be required to validate the results observed in this prospective cohort investigation.

Abbreviations

ADC: apparent diffusion coefficient; BG: basal ganglia; CSF: cerebral spinal fluid; DTI: diffusion tensor imaging; FA: fractional anisotropy; FLAIR: fluid attenuated inversion recovery; ICP: intracranial pressure; iNPH: idiopathic normal pressure hydrocephalus; IR: inversion recovery; MRI: magnetic resonance imaging; MTT: mean transit time; NP: negative patients; PP: positive patients; PVWM: periventricular white matter; PWI: perfusion weighted imaging; rCBF: relative cerebral blood flow; rCMV: relative cerebral blood volume; ROI: region of interest; VP: ventricular-peritoneal.

Authors' contributions

All authors have contributed equally in the development of this clinical study. All authors read and approved the final manuscript.

Author details

[1] Department of Neurosurgery, AOU-UD "Santa Maria della Misericordia", Piazzale S.M. della Misericordia, 33100 Udine, Italy. [2] Department of Neuroradiology, AOU-UD "Santa Maria della Misericordia", Udine, Italy. [3] Institute of Epidemiology, AOU-UD "Santa Maria della Misericordia", Udine, Italy. [4] Department of Physics, AOU-UD "Santa Maria della Misericordia", Udine, Italy.

Funding

No funding received from any Institution and/or Foundation.

References

1. Hakim S, Adams RD. The special clinical problem of symptomatic hydrocephalus with normal cerebrospinal fluid pressure. Observations on cerebrospinal fluid hydrodynamics. J Neurol Sci. 1965;2:307–27.
2. Relkin N, Marmarou A, Klinge P, Bergsneider M, Black PM. Diagnosing idiopathic normal-pressure hydrocephalus. Neurosurgery. 2005;57(Suppl 3):S4–16.
3. Cage TA, Auguste KI, Wrensch M, Wu YW, Gupta N. Self-reported functional outcome after surgical intervention in patients with idiopathic normal pressure hydrocephalus. J Clin Neurosci. 2011;18:649–54.
4. Eide PK, Sorteberg W. Diagnostic intracranial pressure monitoring and surgical management in idiopathic normal pressure hydrocephalus: a 6-year review of 214 patients. Neurosurgery. 2010;66:80–91.
5. Hashimoto M, Ishikawa M, Mori E, Kuwana N. Diagnosis of idiopathic normal pressure hydrocephalus is supported by MRI-based scheme: a prospective cohort study. Cerebrospinal Fluid Res. 2010;7:18.
6. Klinge P, Hellström P, Tans J, Wikkelsø C, on behalf of the European iNPH Multicentre Study Group. One-year outcome in the European multicenter study on iNPH. Acta Neurol Scand. 2012;126:145–53.
7. Lemcke J, Meier U. Improved outcome in shunted iNPH with a combination of a Codman Hakim programmable valve and an Aesculap-Miethke Shunt Assistant. Cent Eur Neurosurg. 2010;71:113–6.
8. Katzman R, Hussey F. A simple constant-infusion manometric test for measurement of CSF absorption I. rationale and method. Neurology. 1970;20:534–44.
9. Eklund A, Smielewski P, Chambers I, et al. Assessment of cerebrospinal fluid outflow resistance. Med Biol Eng Comput. 2007;45:719–35.
10. Tans JT, Poortvliet DC. CSF outflow resistance and pressure-volume index determined by steady-state and bolus infusions. Clin Neurol Neurosurg. 1985;87:159–65.
11. Wikkelsø C, Hellström P, Klinge P, Tans J, on behalf of the European iNPH Multicentre Study Group. The European iNPH Multicentre Study on the predictive values of resistance to CSF outflow and the CSF Tap Test in patients with idiopathic normal pressure hydrocephalus. J Neurol Neurosurg Psychiatry. 2013;84(5):562–8.
12. Marmarou A, Bergsneider M, Klinge P, Relkin N, Black PM. The value of supplemental prognostic tests for the preoperative assessment of idiopathic normal pressure hydrocephalus. Neurosurgery. 2005;57(3 Suppl):S17–28.
13. Owler BK, Pickard JD. Normal pressure hydrocephalus and cerebral blood flow: a review. Acta Neurol Scand. 2001;104:325–42.
14. Owler BK, Momjian S, Czosnyka Z, et al. Normal pressure hydrocephalus and cerebral blood flow: a PET study of baseline values. J Cereb Blood Flow Metab. 2004;24:17–23.
15. Owler BK, Pena A, Momjian S, et al. Changes in cerebral blood flow during cerebrospinal fluid pressure manipulation in patients with normal pressure hydrocephalus: a methodological study. J Cereb Blood Flow Metab. 2004;24:579–87.
16. Momjian S, Owler BK, Czosnyka Z, Czosnyka M, Pena A, Pickard JD. Pattern of white matter regional cerebral blood flow and autoregulation in normal pressure hydrocephalus. Brain. 2004;127:965–72.
17. Klinge PM, Samii A, Muhlendyck A, et al. Cerebral hypoperfusion and delayed hippocampal response after induction of adult kaolin hydrocephalus. Stroke. 2003;34:193–9.
18. Luciano MG, Skarupa DJ, Booth AM, Wood AS, Brant CL, Gdowski MJ. Cerebrovascular adaptation in chronic hydrocephalus. J Cereb Blood Flow Metab. 2001;21:285–94.
19. Calamante F. Perfusion MRI using dynamic-susceptibility contrast MRI: quantification issues in patient studies. Top Magn Reson Imaging. 2010;21(2):75–85.
20. Ziegelitz D, Starck G, Kristiansen D, et al. Cerebral perfusion measured by dynamic susceptibility contrast MRI is reduced in patients with idiopathic normal pressure hydrocephalus. J Magn Reson Imaging. 2014;39(6):1533–42.
21. Aygok G, Marmarou A, Fatouros P, Young H. Brain tissue water content in patients with idiopathic normal pressure hydrocephalus. Acta Neurochir Suppl. 2006;96:348–51.
22. Demura K, Mase M, Miyati T, et al. Changes of fractional anisotropy and apparent diffusion coefficient in patients with idiopathic normal pressure hydrocephalus. Acta Neurochir Suppl. 2012;113:29–32.
23. Ng SE, Low AM, Tang KK, Lim WE, Kwok RK. Idiopathic normal pressure hydrocephalus: correlating magnetic resonance imaging biomarkers with clinical response. Ann Acad Med Singap. 2009;38(9):803–8.
24. Corkill RG, Garnett MR, Blamire AM, Rajagopalan B, Cadoux-Hudson TA, Styles P. Multi-modal MRI in normal pressure hydrocephalus identifies pre-operative haemodynamic and diffusion coefficient changes in normal appearing white matter correlating with surgical outcome. Clin Neurol Neurosurg. 2003;105(3):193–202.
25. Shevtsov MA, Senkevich KA, Kim AV, et al. Changes of fractional anisotropy (FA) and apparent diffusion coefficient (ADC) in the model of experimental acute hydrocephalus in rabbits. Acta Neurochir (Wien). 2015;157(4):689–98.
26. Chu BC, Miyasaka K. The clinical application of diffusion weighted magnetic resonance imaging to acute cerebrovascular disorders. No To Shinkei. 1998;50(9):787–95.
27. Hellstrom P, Klinge P, Tans J, Wikkelso C. A new scale for assessment of severity and outcome in iNPH. Acta Neurol Scand. 2012;126:229–37.
28. Boon AJ, Tans JT, Delwel EJ, et al. Dutch normal-pressure hydrocephalus study: prediction of outcome after shunting by resistance to outflow of cerebrospinal fluid. J Neurosurg. 1997;87(5):687–93.

29. Børgesen SE, Albeck MJ, Gjerris F, Czosnyka M, Laniewski P. Computerized infusion test compared to steady pressure constant infusion test in measurement of resistance to CSF outflow. Acta Neurochir (Wien). 1992;119(1–4):12–6.
30. Meyer JS, Kitagawa Y, Tanahashi N, et al. Pathogenesis of normal-pressure hydrocephalus—preliminary observations. Surg Neurol. 1985;23:121–33.
31. Vorstrup S, Christensen J, Gjerris F, Sorensen PS, Thomsen AM, Paulson OB. Cerebral blood flow in patients with normal-pressure hydrocephalus before and after shunting. J Neurosurg. 1987;66:379–87.
32. Ziegelitz D, Arvidsson J, Hellström P, Tullberg M, Wikkelsø C, Starck G. In patients with idiopathic normal pressure hydrocephalus postoperative cerebral perfusion changes measured by dynamic susceptibility contrast magnetic resonance imaging correlate with clinical improvement. J Comput Assist Tomogr. 2015;39:531–40.
33. Mascalchi M, Filippi M, Floris R, Fonda C, Gasparotti R, Villari N. Diffusion-weighted MR of the brain: methodology and clinical application. Radiol Med. 2005;109(3):155–97.

10

Inhibition of ADAM10 promotes the clearance of Aβ across the BBB by reducing LRP1 ectodomain shedding

B. Shackleton[1,2*], F. Crawford[1,2] and C. Bachmeier[1,2]

Abstract

Background: Transport across the blood–brain barrier (BBB) is an important mediator of beta-amyloid (Aβ) accumulation in the brain and a contributing factor in the pathogenesis of Alzheimer's disease (AD). One of the receptors responsible for the transport of Aβ in the BBB is the low density lipoprotein receptor-related protein 1 (LRP1). LRP1 is susceptible to proteolytic shedding at the cell surface, which prevents endocytic transport of ligands. Previously, we reported a strong inverse correlation between LRP1 shedding in the brain and Aβ transit across the BBB. Several proteases contribute to the ectodomain shedding of LRP1 including the α-secretase, a desintegrin and metalloproteinase domain containing protein 10 (ADAM10).

Methods: The role of ADAM10 in the shedding of LRP1 and Aβ BBB clearance was assessed through pharmacological inhibition of ADAM10 in an in vitro model of the BBB and through the use of ADAM10 endothelial specific knockout mice. In addition, an acute treatment paradigm with an ADAM10 inhibitor was also tested in an AD mouse model to assess the effect of ADAM10 inhibition on LRP1 shedding and Aβbrain accumulation.

Results: In the current studies, inhibition of ADAM10 reduced LRP1 shedding in brain endothelial cultures and increased Aβ42 transit across an in vitro model of the BBB. Similarly, transgenic ADAM10 endothelial knockout mice displayed lower LRP1 shedding in the brain and significantly enhanced Aβ clearance across the BBB compared to wild-type animals. Acute treatment with the ADAM10-selective inhibitor GI254023X in an AD mouse model substantially reduced brain LRP1 shedding and increased Aβ40 levels in the plasma, indicating enhanced Aβ transit from the brain to the periphery. Furthermore, both soluble and insoluble Aβ40 and Aβ42 brain levels were decreased following GI254023X treatment, but these effects lacked statistical significance.

Conclusions: These studies demonstrate a role for ADAM10 in the ectodomain shedding of LRP1 in the brain and the clearance of Aβ across the BBB, which may provide a novel strategy for attenuating Aβ accumulation in the AD brain.

Keywords: Alzheimer's disease, A desintegrin and metalloproteinase domain containing protein 10 (ADAM10), Low density lipoprotein receptor-related protein 1 (LRP1), Blood–brain barrier (BBB), Beta-amyloid (Aβ)

Background

Alzheimer's disease is the most common cause of dementia in the elderly and is characterized, in part, by the deposition of amyloid beta (Aβ) in the brain and cerebrovasculature. The accumulation of soluble Aβ precedes the initial neurodegeneratitive and neurotoxic cascade and correlates strongly with reductions in cognitive performance [1–3]. It has been reported that the accumulation of Aβ in AD is primarily the result of inadequate Aβ elimination, with AD patients showing a 30 % reduction in the overall clearance of Aβ from the brain [4, 5]. Furthermore, in the Dutch-type mouse model of AD, the elimination of Aβ through the BBB is significantly reduced, which results in Aβ deposition along the cerebral vessels

*Correspondence: bshackleton@roskampinstitute.net
[1] The Roskamp Institute, Sarasota, FL 34243, USA

and the development of cerebral amyloid angiopathy (CAA) [6, 7].

One of the prominent mechanisms responsible for the elimination of Aβ from the brain involves transcytosis across the blood–brain barrier (BBB). The rate in which Aβ is cleared from the brain to the blood through the BBB is greater than the rate in which it can be removed via interstitial fluid bulk flow [8], likely due to the presence of various transport systems including the low density lipoprotein receptor-related protein 1 (LRP1) [9–11]. After binding to LRP1 at the abluminal surface of the brain endothelium, Aβ is transported across the BBB where it is then released into the general circulation [12, 13]. Recently, conditional endothelial LRP1 KO mice developed by Storck et al. [11] showed significant reductions in the transit of Aβ across the BBB and deficits in memory and spatial learning, highlighting the importance of BBB transport in the elimination of Aβ from the brain.

In addition to the membrane-associated protein, LRP1 also exists in a soluble form as a result of proteolytic cleavage at the surface of the cell. This soluble LRP1 fragment retains its binding capacity, but loses its ability to endocytose and transport ligands [14–16]. In line with this, recent work by our group demonstrated a strong inverse correlation between LRP1 shedding in the brain and Aβ clearance across the BBB [17], indicating that reductions in brain LRP1 shedding could promote Aβ clearance across the BBB and attenuate Aβ accumulation in the AD brain. As such, investigating the factors that regulate LRP1 shedding in the brain may provide therapeutic opportunities to lower Aβ burden and modulate the AD phenotype. One of the enzymes implicated in LRP1 ectodomain shedding is the α-secretase, ADAM10 (a desintegrin and metalloproteinase domain containing protein 10), [18]. The following studies examined the influence of ADAM10 on LRP1 shedding in vitro and in vivo and the evaluated the impact of ADAM10 modulation on Aβ clearance across the BBB.

Methods

Animals

ADAM10 endothelial KO mice were kindly provided, by Dr. Carl Blobel (Hospital for Special Surgery, New York, NY), Dr. B. De Strooper (VIB Center for the biology of Disease, Leuven, Belgium) and Dr. P. Saftig (Institute of Biochemistry, CAU Kiel, Germany). These mice were generated by crossing ADAM10 flox/flox mice [19] with Tie2-Cre transgenic mice that use the endothelial specific promoter Tie2 to drive the expression of Cre recombinase [20] to produce ADAM10 flox/flox/Tie2-Cre mice. The ADAM10 endothelial KO mice lack ADAM10 expression in the endothelial cells [21]. Wild Type mice on a C57BL/6 background were used as control animals. To evaluate the effect of ADAM10 modulation in an animal model of AD, we utilized transgenic mice overexpressing the human APP695 sw mutation and the presenilin-1 mutation M1 46L (PSAPP) which results in the overproduction of human Aβ [22]. All mice were group housed in a temperature and humidity controlled environment on a 12 h light/dark cycle with free access to food and water. All experiments involving animals were approved by the Institutional Animal Care and Use Committee of the Roskamp Institute.

Preparation of Aβ42 peptides

Using a standard protocol to limit aggregation, both human recombinant Aβ42 and fluorescein labeled Aβ42 were solubilized in 1,1,1,3,3,3-hexafluoro-2-propanol to acquire a monomeric/dimeric sample and minimize the formation of β-sheet structures as we previously described [23].

In vitro LRP1 shedding

Human Brain Microvessel endothelial cells (HBMECs) (ScienCell, USA) were seeded at 50,000 cells per cm^2 onto fibronectin-coated 6-well plates as previously described by our group [24]. When approximately 90 % confluent, cells were treated with Aβ42 (2 μM) or both Aβ42 and the ADAM10-selective inhibitor GI254023X (1 μM) (Sigma-Aldrich, USA) and incubated at 37 °C for 48 h. Our previous work demonstrated that 2 μM Aβ significantly induced LRP1 shedding in the absence of any overt cellular toxicity [25]. After the 48 h incubation, the extracellular media was collected and the level of soluble LRP1 was assessed using an ELISA for LRP1 (Cat# SEB010Hu, Cedar Lane Labs, USA).

Aβ transit across an in vitro BBB model

The impact of ADAM10 on Aβ42 transcytosis was assessed using an in vitro BBB model previously described by our group [24]. HBMECs were seeded onto fibronectin-coated 24-well membrane inserts forming a polarized monolayer representing the BBB. Aβ transcytosis across the BBB was assessed by exposing the basolateral side ("brain") to 2 μM fluorescein-Aβ42 (rPeptide, USA) and treating the apical side ("blood") with the ADAM10-selective inhibitor GI254023X (0.1–1 μM). After 60 min of incubation at 37 °C, samples were collected from the apical compartment to assess the basolateral-to-apical transcytosis of fluorescein-Aβ across the BBB model. To ensure Aβ42 or GI254023X treatment did not disrupt the integrity of the BBB monolayer, we examined the effect of Aβ and GI254023X on the permeability of the paracellular marker, 10 kDa Lucifer yellow-dextran.

Brain LRP1 shedding and Aβ BBB clearance in vivo

To determine the role of ADAM10 in the clearance of Aβ42 from the brain to the periphery, we examined the appearance of human Aβ42 in the plasma after intracranial Aβ administration as previously described by our group [24, 26]. Briefly, wild-type and ADAM10 endothelial KO mice (16–24 weeks of age) were anesthetized via inhalation using a 3 % isoflurane/oxygen mix. While under anesthesia, 3 μl of human Aβ42 (1 mM) was bilaterally injected into the caudate putamen of the brain (0.5 mm anterior to the bregma and 2 mm lateral to the midline at a depth of 3 mm below the skull surface). Ten minutes after the intracerebral injections, the mice were euthanized and the plasma and brain tissue were collected. Plasma samples were analyzed for human Aβ42 using an ELISA (Invitrogen, USA). Mouse brains were homogenised in 12 ml of ice cold Hanks Balances Salt Solution (HBSS) with a Dounce Homogenizer. For collection of the soluble brain fraction (i.e., non cell-associated), samples were centrifuged at 6000*g* for 15 min to remove intact cells, cell associated proteins and non-soluble components. The levels of LRP1 in the soluble fraction were measured in the supernatant using a LRP1 ELISA (Cat# SEB010Hu, Cedar Lane Labs, USA) and normalized to the total protein content in the brain homogenate as determined by the bicinchoninic acid (BCA) protein assay (Thermo Scientific, USA). Soluble LRP1 levels were expressed as ng of LRP1 per mg protein.

Aβ, soluble LRP1 and sAPPα levels in PSAPP mice following ADAM10 inhibition

PSAPP mice at 35 weeks of age were injected intraperitoneally with 200 mg/kg of GI254023X or vehicle (DMSO) once per day for 5 consecutive days. At this age, PSAPP mice display elevated levels of Aβ peptides in the brain [22]. This treatment regime has previously been shown to effectively inhibit ADAM10 activity in mice and was well tolerated with no adverse effects reported [27]. One hour after the final injection, the mice were euthanatized and plasma and brain tissue were collected. The right hemisphere was used to examine the levels of soluble and insoluble Aβ40 and Aβ42 in the brain. Briefly, the hemispheres were homogenized by sonication in 700 μl lysis buffer [M-PER + 1 % EDTA +0.2 % PMSF (Thermo Scientific, USA)] supplemented with Halt protease and phosphatase inhibitor cocktail (Thermo Scientific, USA) on ice before centrifugation at 14000*g* for 30 min at 4 °C. 100 μl of the resulting supernatant was mixed with 5 M guanidine in TRIS buffer resulting in the guanidine soluble (GS) fraction. For the guanidine insoluble (GI) fraction, 100 μl of the guanidine stock was combined with the original tissue pellet. Both GS and GI fractions were subsequently incubated at room temperature for 1 h and were mixed every 15 min. All samples were stored at −80 °C prior to analysis. Quantification of Aβ40 and Aβ42 in the GS, GI, and plasma fractions was determined using an ELISA for human Aβ40 and Aβ42 (Invitrogen, USA) and expressed as ng of Aβ per μg total protein. The left hemisphere was used to examine the levels of soluble LRP1 in the brain. Here, the hemisphere was homogenized using a Dounce homogenizer in ice cold in HBSS using the same procedure as the in vivo LRP1 shedding studies above. LRP1 levels in the soluble brain fraction and plasma were assessed using a mouse ELISA for LRP1 (Cedar Lane Labs, USA). Soluble brain LRP1 was normalized to the total protein content in the brain homogenate as determined by the BCA protein assay (Thermo Scientific, USA). Soluble brain LRP1 levels were expressed as ng of LRP1 per mg protein. Plasma LRP1 levels were expressed as ng/ml. In addition, sAPPα levels were examined in the brain homogenate of these same animals using an ELISA for sAPPα (IBL international, USA). The sAPPα levels were normalized to the total protein content in the brain homogenate as determined by the BCA protein assay and expressed as ng of sAPPα per mg protein.

Statistical analysis

Statistical analyses were performed using a one-way ANOVA followed by Tukey's post hoc analysis (GraphPad Prism 5, GraphPad Software Inc., USA). Moreover, where only 2 groups were compared, unpaired t tests were used to evaluate statistical significance.

Results

LRP1 shedding and Aβ BBB transit in vitro

Exposure of HBMECs to Aβ42 induced a significant increase in the extracellular shedding of LRP1 compared to control conditions (twofold) (Fig. 1). Treatment with the ADAM10 inhibitor GI254023X completely abrogated the effect of Aβ42 on shedding as extracellular LRP1 levels in the presence of GI254023X were the same as that observed under control conditions. The transcytosis of fluorescein-Aβ across an in vitro BBB model was increased following GI254023X treatment in a dose dependent manner (Fig. 2). Significant increases were observed at concentrations higher than 1 μM GI254023X showing effects of 1.25-fold or greater. Of note, no significant difference was observed between control conditions and any of the GI254023X concentrations on the BBB permeability of the paracellular marker Lucifer yellow-dextran, indicating the treatment conditions did not impact BBB integrity (data not shown).

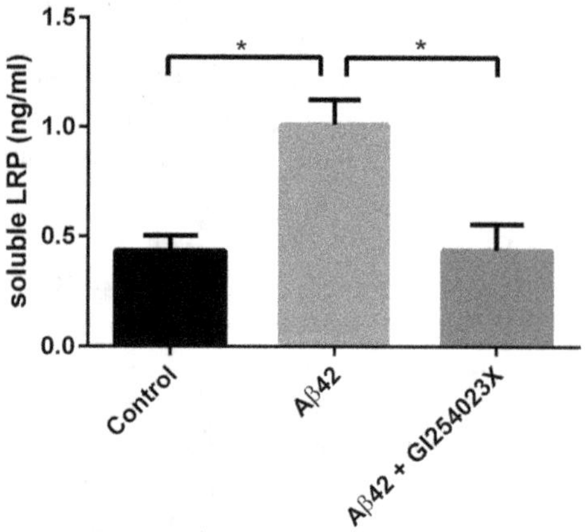

Fig. 1 LRP1shedding in human brain endothelial cells (HBMEC) following ADAM10 inhibition. HBMEC monolayers were exposed to human Aβ42 (2 μM) alone, Aβ42 (2 μM) and the ADAM10 inhibitor GI254023X (1 μM) for 48 h at 37 °C. LRP shedding was assessed by examining LRP content in the extracellular media using an LRP1 ELISA. Values represent mean ± SEM (n = 3) and are expressed as ng of extracellular LRP1 per ml of media. $^{*}p < 0.05$ as determined by one-way ANOVA followed by Tukey's post hoc analysis

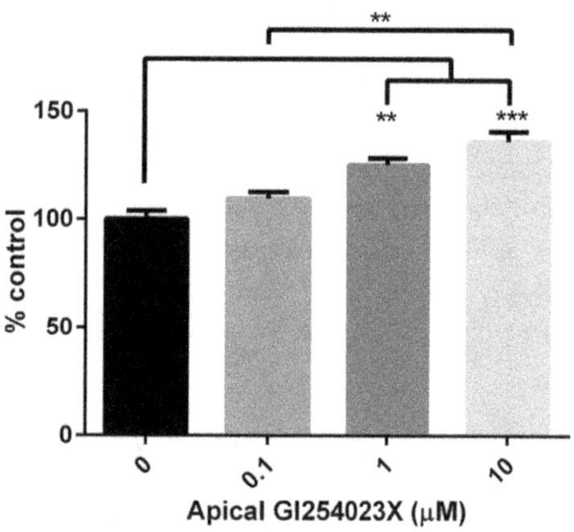

Fig. 2 Fluorescin-Aβ42 transit across an in vitro BBB model following ADAM10 inhibition. Fluorescin-Aβ42 (2 μM) was exposed to the basolateral ("brain") side of the in vitro BBB model, while various concentrations of the ADAM10 inhibitor GI254023X (0, 0.1, 1, and 10 μM) were exposed to the apical ("blood") compartment. Following incubation at 37 °C, samples were collected from the basolateral compartment at 60 min to assess the basolateral-to-apical transcytosis of fluorescin-Aβ42 across the BBB model. Values represent mean ± SEM (n = 3) and are expressed as the percentage change from control conditions. $^{*}p < 0.05$; $^{**}p < 0.01$; $^{***}p < 0.001$ as determined by one-way ANOVA followed by Tukey's post hoc analysis

Brain LRP1 shedding and Aβ BBB clearance in vivo

LRP1 levels in the soluble brain fraction of ADAM10 endothelial KO mice were lower than that observed in wild-type animals (Fig. 3a), although this effect did not achieve statistical significance. However, Aβ clearance across the BBB was significantly greater in ADAM10 endothelial KO mice compared to wild-type animals resulting in an increase of approximately 1.75-fold (Fig. 3b).

ADAM10 inhibition in PSAPP mice

To evaluate the impact of ADAM10 inhibition on Aβ tissue levels and LRP1 shedding in the brain in an AD animal model, PSAPP mice were treated with the ADAM10-selective inhibitor GI254023X. The level of soluble LRP1 in the brain was significantly lower in the GI254023X-treated mice compared to the vehicle control animals (a reduction of 60 %) (Fig. 4a). In the periphery, LRP1 levels in the plasma were not significantly different when comparing treated and control animals (Fig. 4b). To assess the effect of ADAM10 inhibition on the α-secretase cleavage of APP, the levels of sAPPα in the brain were examined following GI254023X treatment. No significant difference in the level of sAPPα in the brain was detected between GI254023X-treated mice and the control group (Fig. 5). To investigate the impact of ADAM10 inhibition on the levels of Aβ40 and Aβ42 in the plasma and whole brain homogenate of PSAPP mice. GI254023X administration significantly increased the levels of Aβ40 in the plasma (1.45-fold) compared to vehicle-treated mice, while the effect of GI254023X on Aβ42 plasma levels was not significant (Fig. 6a, b). In addition, treatment with the ADAM10 inhibitor reduced both soluble and insoluble Aβ40 (Fig. 7a, b) (1.15- and 1.20-fold respectively) and Aβ42 (Fig. 7c, d) (1.25 and 1.20-fold respectively) levels in the brain compared to vehicle-treated animals, although these values did not reach statistical significance. It should also be noted that this GI254023X treatment regimen was well tolerated as the treated animals did not display any overt changes in appearance, behavior, or weight loss.

Discussion

Dysfunction within the cerebrovascular system is now recognized as a major contributory factor in the development of AD [28]. It has been suggested that the excessive accumulation of Aβ in the AD brain may be due to aberrant Aβ elimination [29, 30] as several studies have identified reduced brain Aβ clearance in AD patients and AD animal models [5, 7]. More specifically, an important component in the removal of Aβ from the brain involves cerebrovascular transport across the BBB. Prior studies have shown that reduced levels of the receptors that transport Aβ in brain endothelia, such as LRP1, results in decreased Aβ clearance across the BBB, elevated Aβ burden in the brain, and aggravated memory and learning deficits [11, 29]. In normal aging and AD, LRP1 expression is diminished in the brain vasculature [10, 31–33]

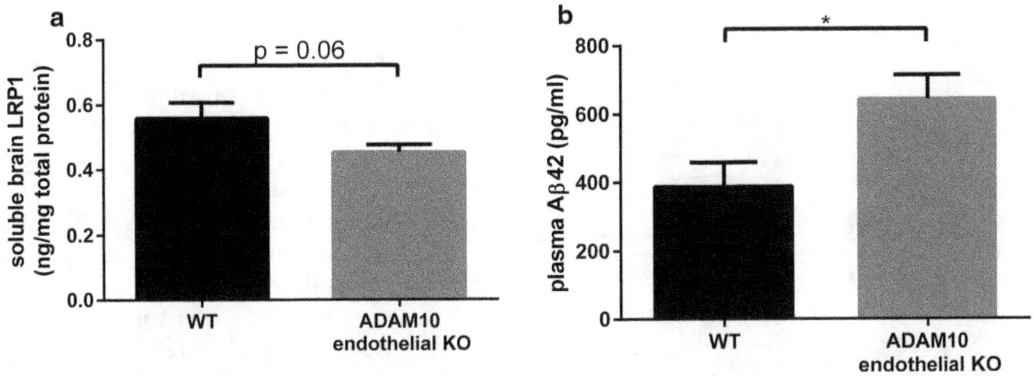

Fig. 3 LRP1 shedding in the brain and Aβ clearance across the BBB. Human Aβ42 (1 mM) was intracranially injected into ADAM10 endothelial KO and wild-type mice. Ten minutes after the injection, the brain and plasma were collected. The soluble fraction of the brain was probed for **a** LRP1 using an ELISA, while the plasma was probed for **b** Aβ42 using an ELISA. Values represent mean ± SEM (n = 8) and are expressed as amount of LRP1 per mg total protein or amount of Aβ42 per ml. Statistical analyses were performed using an unpaired t test

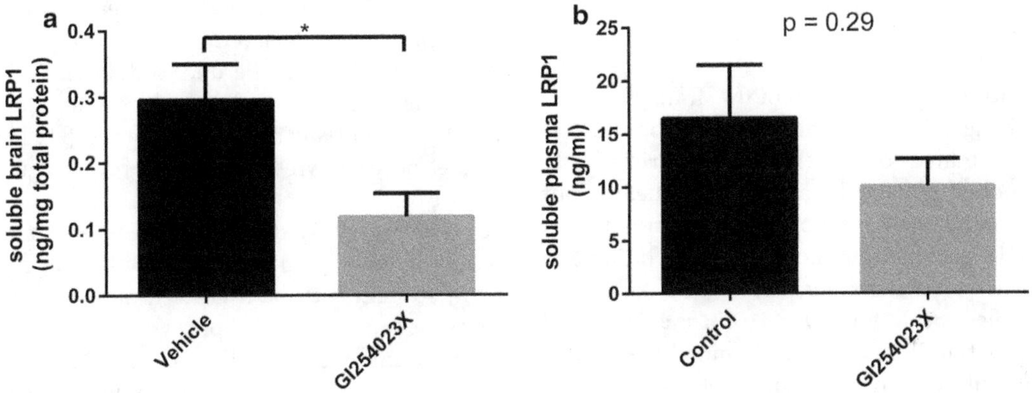

Fig. 4 LRP1 shedding brain and plasma following ADAM10 modulation in a mouse model of AD. The ADAM10 inhibitor GI254023X (200 mg/kg) or vehicle (DMSO) was administered via intraperitoneal injection once per day for five consecutive days to PSAPP mice (35 weeks of age). One hour after the final injection, the brains and plasma was collected and the soluble brain fraction **a** and the plasma **b** was probed for LRP using an ELISA. Values represent mean ± SEM (n = 8–9 [soluble brain LRP1] or 5 [soluble plasma LRP1]) and are expressed as the amount of LRP per mg total protein or per ml. *p < 0.05 as determined by an unpaired t test

and correlates with Aβ accumulation in the brain and cerebrovasculature [13, 32]. In addition, the expression of LRP1 can be affected by a variety of upstream events such as the promoter methylation status, which controls the generation of LRP1 mRNA [34]. Previously it has been shown that promoting LRP1 expression enhances the cellular uptake of Aβ [35] and facilitates Aβ clearance from the brain extracellular space [36]. Our previous work shows LRP1 is susceptible to ectodomain shedding, a process that inactivates the transport capabilities of the receptor, which results in reduced Aβ clearance across the BBB [17]. The current studies evaluated a treatment strategy targeting LRP1 shedding in the brain as a novel means to promote Aβ BBB clearance and attenuate Aβ accumulation in the AD brain.

Previous investigations have implicated the α-secretase enzyme, ADAM10, in the ectodomain shedding of LRP1 [18, 37]. In the present studies, we found that inhibition of ADAM10 effectively reduced LRP1 shedding and increased Aβ transit across an in vitro model of the BBB. This was supported by our in vivo studies in which ADAM10 endothelial KO mice displayed less LRP1 shedding in the brain in conjunction with increased Aβ clearance across the BBB compared to wild-type animals. However, the reduced shedding of brain LRP1 in the ADAM10 endothelial KO group did not reach statistical significance when compared to wild-type mice. This may not be all that unexpected as there are number of cell types in the brain that express LRP1 in addition to brain endothelia. As our analytical approach assessed LRP1

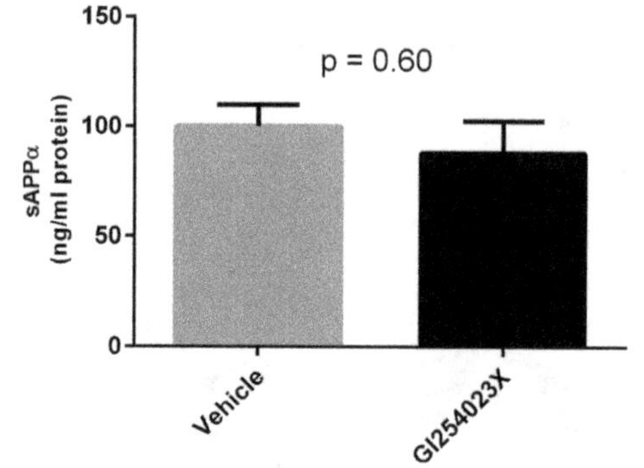

Fig. 5 Levels of sAPPα in the brain following ADAM10 modulation in a mouse model of AD. PSAPP mice (35 weeks of age) were treated in an acute 5-day treatment paradigm with ADAM10 inhibitor GI254023X (200 mg/kg) or vehicle (DMSO) which were administered via intraperitoneal injection. One hour after the final treatment, the brains were collected and sAPPα in the whole brain homogenate was probed using an sAPPα ELISA. Values represent mean ± SEM (n = 8–9) and are expressed as the amount of sAPPα per mg total protein. Statistical significance determined by an unpaired t test

levels in the entire soluble fraction of the brain, endothelial-specific changes in LRP1 shedding may be difficult to capture with so many other cells types contributing to the soluble pool of LRP in the brain. Nevertheless, our findings in vitro and in vivo demonstrate that modulation of the ADAM10 enzyme minimizes LRP1 shedding and facilitates Aβ clearance across the BBB.

As we identified a role for ADAM10 in mediating Aβ clearance across the BBB, we next examined the impact of ADAM10 inhibition on Aβ tissue levels in an animal model of AD. Using an acute 5-day treatment paradigm with the ADAM10-selective inhibitor GI254023X in PSAPP mice, we observed a substantial decrease in LRP1 shedding in the brain compared to vehicle-treated animals. Moreover, as previous studies have reported that soluble LRP1 levels in the plasma can facilitate Aβ removal from the brain by acting as a peripheral sink [12], we investigated LRP1 levels in the plasma following GI254023X administration. Soluble LRP1 levels in the plasma were found not to be significantly different between treated and control animals. However, we did find that The decrease in soluble LRP1 in the brain following treatment with GI254023X coincided with a significant increase in plasma Aβ40 levels. As such, we propose that inhibition of ADAM10 facilitates Aβ40 transit from the brain to the periphery (via reduced LRP shedding at the BBB), resulting in the elevated Aβ40 plasma levels we observed. However, no significant changes in plasma Aβ42 levels were detected following GI254023X treatment. A potential explanation for the disparity we observed in the BBB clearance between Aβ40 and Aβ42 may be due to differences in the transport rates for these species. A recent report indicated LRP1 preferentially clears Aβ40 over Aβ42 [11] and prior studies have shown that the rate of Aβ40 transport across the BBB is more than twice that observed for Aβ42 [8, 38]. Nevertheless, the increased levels of Aβ40 in the plasma following ADAM10 inhibition suggest this treatment strategy may be used to facilitate the transit of Aβ from the brain to the periphery.

To examine the impact of ADAM10 inhibition on Aβ levels in the brain, we examined both soluble and insoluble Aβ following GI254023X treatment in PSAPP

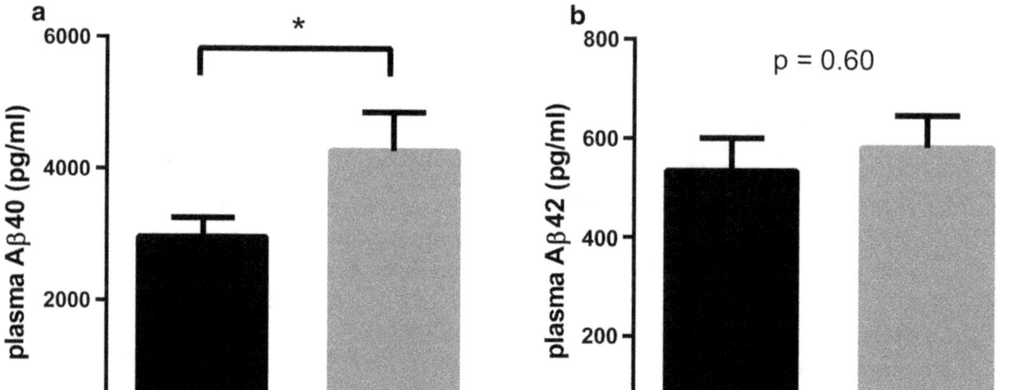

Fig. 6 Aβ plasma levels following ADAM10 modulation in a mouse model of AD. The ADAM10 inhibitor GI254023X (200 mg/kg) or vehicle (DMSO) was administered via intraperitoneal injection once per day for five consecutive days to PSAPP mice (35 weeks of age). One hour after the final injection, the plasma was collected and probed for **a** Aβ40 and **b** Aβ42 by ELISA. Values represent mean ± SEM (n = 8–9) and are expressed as the amount of Aβ40 or Aβ42 per ml of plasma. Statistical analyses were performed using an unpaired t test

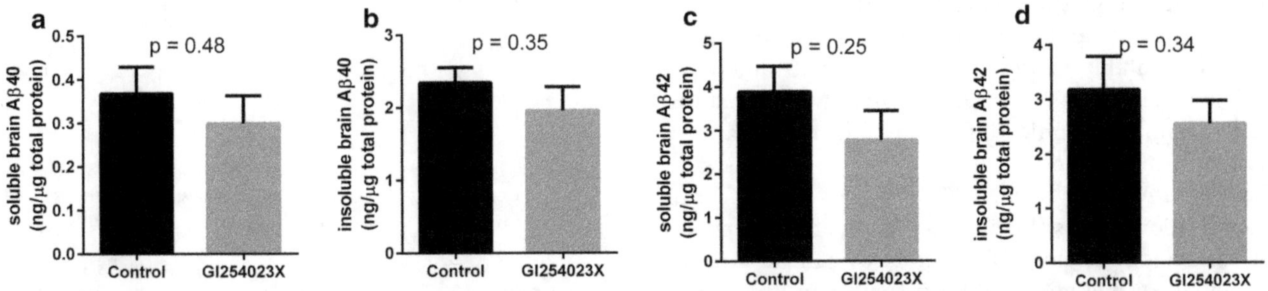

Fig. 7 Brain Aβ levels following ADAM10 modulation in a mouse model of AD. Following a 5 day treatment of PSAPP mice (35 weeks of age) with the ADAM10 inhibitor GI254023X (200 mg/kg) or vehicle (DMSO), levels of soluble and insoluble Aβ40 and Aβ42 were measured in the brain using an Aβ40 or Aβ42 ELISA (**a–d**). Values represent mean ± SEM (n = 8–9) and are expressed as the amount of Aβ40 or Aβ42 per μg of total protein. Statistical analyses were performed using an unpaired t test

animals. While we observed reductions in both soluble and insoluble Aβ40 and Aβ42 in the brain following GI254023X treatment, none of these effects were statistically significant. It is unclear why this treatment paradigm did not modulate Aβ levels in the brain more effectively. Both our prior work [17] and our current findings demonstrate a strong relationship between brain LRP1 shedding and Aβ clearance across the BBB. GI254023X treatment in the PSAPP mice reduced LRP1 shedding in the brain by 60 %, however, this effect did not translate to significant changes in Aβ levels in the brain. It may be that such an acute treatment paradigm (5 days) is not sufficient to demonstrably lower Aβ levels in the brain, and that a more chronic treatment paradigm is necessary. Another possible explanation for our observations is that LRP1 expression is known to be lower in AD patients [13, 39] and AD animals, including the PSAPP mice used in the current studies [40]. Exposure of brain vascular cells to high levels of Aβ for a prolonged period has previously been shown to reduce the expression of LRP1 [39]. In our study, the PSAPP mice were tested at an age when extensive Aβ pathology is present [22, 41]. As such, the total LRP1 population may be depleted to such an extent that any improvements in BBB LRP1 shedding to promote Aβ elimination would still prove insufficient. Therefore, this therapeutic approach may be more impactful if used earlier in the disease process when a greater density of LRP1 receptors is available for therapeutic targeting. Further evaluation of this treatment protocol and the feasibility of targeting LRP1 sheddase enzymes in AD are certainly warranted.

A primary concern in targeting an enzyme like ADAM10, especially in AD, is the potential impact on other substrates that are metabolized by ADAM10. ADAM10 is one of the α-secretases which processes APP through the non-amyloidogenic pathway, resulting in the formation of sAPPα while at the same time avoiding the production of Aβ peptides. As such, inhibition of this pathway could facilitate Aβ synthesis and potentially exacerbate Aβ burden in the AD brain. Our data suggests this is not the case, as Aβ levels in the brain did not increase upon ADAM10 inhibition, but in fact decreased. To ascertain whether GI254023X treatment influenced the α-secretase pathway specifically, we measured sAPPα levels in the brain and found no difference between GI254023X-treated animals and the vehicle control group. These data indicate ADAM10 can be modulated to reduce LRP1 shedding in the brain without affecting the α-secretase cleavage of APP. One explanation for this may be the presence of other α-secretase enzymes, which process APP when ADAM10 is diminished or absent. To this point, it was previously found that sAPPα formation was preserved in fibroblast cells derived from ADAM10-deficient animals [42]. It has also been reported that other members of the α-secretase family such as ADAM9 and ADAM17 are able to compensate for reductions in ADAM10 activity [42, 43]. Alternatively, other studies have reported a significant change in sAPPα production or increase in Aβ when ADAM10 was absent or diminished, suggesting a lack of compensation by other α-secretases [19, 44–46]. Nevertheless, our studies demonstrate that targeting the ADAM10 enzyme can effectively reduce LRP1 shedding in the cerebrovasculature without impacting APP proteolysis.

Conclusions

Previously, our work demonstrated a strong inverse correlation between LRP1 shedding in the brain and Aβ clearance across the BBB. In the present studies, we show that modulation of the ADAM10 enzyme can effectively reduce LRP1 shedding and promote Aβ transport out of the brain. In an AD mouse model, acute treatment with an ADAM10 inhibitor substantially lowered LRP1 brain shedding and increased the appearance of Aβ40 in the plasma, indicating enhanced Aβ transit from the brain to the periphery. Alternatively, while ADAM10 inhibition decreased both Aβ40 and Aβ42 brain levels in the AD mice, these values were not statistically significant, indicating a more chronic treatment paradigm may be necessary to observe demonstrable changes in Aβ brain burden. Nevertheless, while further interrogation of this therapeutic approach is necessary, our findings indicate LRP1 sheddases can be targeted to facilitate Aβ elimination from the brain, providing a novel therapeutic strategy to mitigate Aβ accumulation in the AD brain.

Abbreviations

ADAM10: a desintegrin and metalloproteinase domain containing protein 10; AD: Alzheimer's disease; APP: amyloid precursor protein; Aβ: beta-amyloid; BBB: blood–brain barrier; CAA: cerebral amyloid angiopathy; LRP1: low density lipoprotein receptor-related protein 1.

Authors' contributions

BS: design, data processing and analysis, interpretation of data, manuscript drafting, revision, and finalising; FC: conception and design, interpretation of data; CB: conception and design, data processing and analysis, interpretation of data, manuscript drafting, revision and finalising. All authors read and approved the final manuscript.

Author details

[1] The Roskamp Institute, Sarasota, FL 34243, USA. [2] The Open University, Milton Keynes, Buckinghamshire MK7 6AA, UK.

Acknowledgements

The authors would like to thank Dr. Carl Blobel (Hospital for Special Surgery, New York, NY), Dr. B. De Strooper (VIB Center for the biology of Disease, Leuven, Belgium) and Dr. P. Saftig (Institute of Biochemistry, CAU Kiel, Germany) for their generosity in supplying the ADAM10 endothelial KO mice used in this study.

Competing interests

The authors declare that they have no competing interests.

Funding

This research was supported by the Roskamp Foundation and the National Institute on Aging of the National Institutes of Health under award number R01AG041971 (awarded to Bachmeier). Additional support was provided by the Roskamp Foundation. The content is solely the responsibility of the authors and does not necessarily represent the official views of the National Institutes of Health.

References

1. Lue L-F, Kuo Y-M, Roher AE, Brachova L, Shen Y, Sue L, et al. Soluble amyloid β peptide concentration as a predictor of synaptic change in Alzheimer's disease. Am J Pathol. 1999;155:853–62.
2. LaFerla FM, Green KN, Oddo S. Intracellular amyloid-β in Alzheimer's disease. Nat Rev Neurosci. 2007;8:499–509.
3. Nordberg A. Amyloid imaging in Alzheimer's disease. Curr Opin Neurol. 2007;20:398–402.
4. Bateman RJ, Munsell LY, Morris JC, Swarm R, Yarasheski KE, Holtzman DM. Human amyloid-beta synthesis and clearance rates as measured in cerebrospinal fluid in vivo. Nat Med. 2006;12:856–61.
5. Mawuenyega KG, Sigurdson W, Ovod V, Munsell L, Kasten T, Morris JC, et al. Decreased clearance of CNS amyloid-beta in Alzheimer's disease. Science. 2010;330:1774.
6. Ellis RJ, Olichney JM, Thal LJ, Mirra SS, Morris JC, Beekly D, et al. Cerebral amyloid angiopathy in the brains of patients with Alzheimer's disease: the CERAD experience, Part XV. Neurology. 1996;46:1592–6.
7. Monro OR, Mackic JB, Yamada S, Segal MB, Ghiso J, Maurer C, et al. Substitution at codon 22 reduces clearance of Alzheimer's amyloid-β peptide from the cerebrospinal fluid and prevents its transport from the central nervous system into blood. Neurobiol Aging. 2002;23:405–12.
8. Bell RD, Sagare AP, Friedman AE, Bedi GS, Holtzman DM, Deane R, et al. Transport pathways for clearance of human Alzheimer's amyloid β-peptide and apolipoproteins E and J in the mouse central nervous system. J Cereb Blood Flow Metab. 2007;27:909–18.
9. Li Y, Lu W, Marzolo MP, Bu G. Differential functions of members of the low density lipoprotein receptor family suggested by their distinct endocytosis rates. J Biol Chem. 2001;276:18000–6.
10. Kanekiyo T, Liu C-C, Shinohara M, Li J, Bu G. LRP1 in brain vascular smooth muscle cells mediates local clearance of Alzheimer's amyloid-β. J Neurosci. 2012;32:16458–65.
11. Storck SE, Meister S, Nahrath J, Meißner JN, Schubert N, Di Spiezio A, et al. Endothelial LRP1 transports amyloid-β1–42 across the blood-brain barrier. J Clin Invest. 2015;126(1):123–36.
12. Sagare A, Deane R, Bell RD, Johnson B, Hamm K, Pendu R, et al. Clearance of amyloid-beta by circulating lipoprotein receptors. Nat Med. 2007;13:1029–31.
13. Shibata M, Yamada S, Kumar SR, Calero M, Bading J, Frangione B, et al. Clearance of Alzheimer's amyloid-β1-40 peptide from brain by LDL receptor-related protein-1 at the blood-brain barrier. J Clin Invest. 2000;106:1489–99.
14. Quinn KA, Grimsley PG, Dai Y-P, Tapner M, Chesterman CN, Owensby DA. Soluble low density lipoprotein receptor-related protein (LRP) circulates in human plasma. J Biol Chem. 1997;272:23946–51.
15. Grimsley PG, Quinn KA, Owensby DA. Soluble low-density lipoprotein receptor-related protein. Trends Cardiovasc Med. 1998;8:363–8.
16. Qiu Z, Strickland DK, Hyman BT, Rebeck GW. Elevation of LDL receptor-related protein levels via ligand interactions in Alzheimer disease and in vitro. J Neuropathol Exp Neurol. 2001;60:430–40.
17. Bachmeier C, Shackleton B, Ojo J, Paris D, Mullan M, Crawford F. Apolipoprotein E isoform-specific effects on lipoprotein receptor processing. Neuromol Med. 2014;16:686–96.
18. Liu Q, Zhang J, Tran H, Verbeek MM, Reiss K, Estus S, et al. LRP1 shedding in human brain: roles of ADAM10 and ADAM17. Mol Neurodegener. 2009;4:17.
19. Jorissen E, Prox J, Bernreuther C, Weber S, Schwanbeck R, Serneels L, et al. The disintegrin/metalloproteinase ADAM10 is essential for the establishment of the brain cortex. J Neurosci. 2010;30:4833–44.
20. Kisanuki YY, Hammer RE, Miyazaki J, Williams SC, Richardson JA, Yanagisawa M. Tie2-Cre transgenic mice: a new model for endothelial cell-lineage analysis in vivo. Dev Biol. 2001;230:230–42.
21. Glomski K, Monette S, Manova K, De Strooper B, Saftig P, Blobel CP. Deletion of Adam10 in endothelial cells leads to defects in organ-specific vascular structures. Blood. 2011;118:1163–74.
22. McGowan E, Sanders S, Iwatsubo T, Takeuchi A, Saido T, Zehr C, et al. Amyloid phenotype characterization of transgenic mice overexpressing both mutant amyloid precursor protein and mutant presenilin 1 transgenes. Neurobiol Dis. 1999;6:231–44.
23. Paris D, Ait-Ghezala G, Mathura VS, Patel N, Quadros A, Laporte V, et al. Anti-angiogenic activity of the mutant Dutch A(beta) peptide on human brain microvascular endothelial cells. Brain Res Mol Brain Res. 2005;136:212–30.
24. Bachmeier C, Mullan M, Paris D. Characterization and use of human brain microvascular endothelial cells to examine β-amyloid exchange in the blood-brain barrier. Cytotechnology. 2010;62:519–29.
25. Bachmeier C, Paris D, Beaulieu-Abdelahad D, Mouzon B, Mullan M, Crawford F. A multifaceted role for apoE in the clearance of beta-amyloid across the blood-brain barrier. Neurodegener Dis. 2013;11:13–21.
26. Paris D, Bachmeier C, Patel N, Quadros A, Volmar C-H, Laporte V, et al. Selective antihypertensive dihydropyridines lower Aβ accumulation by targeting both the production and the clearance of A? Across the blood–brain barrier. Mol Med. 2011;17:149–62.

27. Inoshima N, Wang Y, Wardenburg JB. Genetic requirement for ADAM10 in severe staphylococcus aureus skin infection. J Invest Dermatol. 2012;132:1513–6.
28. Erickson MA, Banks WA. Blood–brain barrier dysfunction as a cause and consequence of Alzheimer's disease. J Cereb Blood Flow Metab. 2013;33:1500–13.
29. Jaeger LB, Dohgu S, Hwang MC, Farr SA, Murphy MP, Fleegal-DeMotta MA, et al. Testing the neurovascular hypothesis of Alzheimer's disease: LRP-1 antisense reduces blood–brain barrier clearance, increases brain levels of amyloid-β protein, and impairs cognition. J Alzheimers Dis. 2009;17:553–70.
30. Hardy J, Selkoe DJ. The amyloid hypothesis of Alzheimer's disease: progress and problems on the road to therapeutics. Science. 2002;297:353–6.
31. Kang DE, Pietrzik CU, Baum L, Chevallier N, Merriam DE, Kounnas MZ, et al. Modulation of amyloid β-protein clearance and Alzheimer's disease susceptibility by the LDL receptor-related protein pathway. J Clin Invest. 2000;106:1159–66.
32. Donahue JE, Flaherty SL, Johanson CE, Iii JAD, Silverberg GD, Miller MC, et al. RAGE, LRP-1, and amyloid-beta protein in Alzheimer's disease. Acta Neuropathol. 2006;112:405–15.
33. Silverberg GD, Messier AA, Miller MC, Machan JT, Majmudar SS, Stopa EG, et al. Amyloid efflux transporter expression at the blood–brain barrier declines in normal aging. J Neuropathol Exp Neurol. 2010;69:1034–43.
34. Xing P, Liao Z, Ren Z, Zhao J, Song F, Wang G, et al. Roles of low-density lipoprotein receptor-related protein 1 in tumors. Chin. J. Cancer [Internet]. 2016 [cited 2016 Jul 24]; 35. http://www.ncbi.nlm.nih.gov/pmc/articles/PMC4704379/.
35. Moon JH, Kim HJ, Yang AH, Kim HM, Lee B-W, Kang ES, et al. The effect of rosiglitazone on LRP1 expression and amyloid β uptake in human brain microvascular endothelial cells: a possible role of a low-dose thiazolidinedione for dementia treatment. Int J Neuropsychopharmacol. 2012;15:135–42.
36. Kim J, Castellano JM, Jiang H, Basak JM, Parsadanian M, Pham V, et al. Overexpression of low-density lipoprotein receptor in the brain markedly inhibits amyloid deposition and increases extracellular A beta clearance. Neuron. 2009;64:632–44.
37. Selvais C, Gaide Chevronnay HP, Lemoine P, Dedieu S, Henriet P, Courtoy PJ, et al. Metalloproteinase-dependent shedding of low-density lipoprotein receptor-related protein-1 ectodomain decreases endocytic clearance of endometrial matrix metalloproteinase-2 and -9 at menstruation. Endocrinology. 2009;150:3792–9.
38. Ji Y, Permanne B, Sigurdsson EM, Holtzman DM, Wisniewski T. Amyloid\ beta40/42 clearance across the blood-brain barrier following intra-ventricular injections in wild-type, apoE knock-out and human apoE3 or E4 expressing transgenic mice. J Alzheimers Dis. 2001;3:23–30.
39. Deane R, Wu Z, Sagare A, Davis J, Yan SD, Hamm K, et al. LRP/amyloid β-peptide interaction mediates differential brain efflux of Aβ isoforms. Neuron. 2004;43:333–44.
40. Van Uden E, Carlson G, St. George-Hyslop P, Westaway D, Orlando R, Mallory M, et al. Aberrant presenilin-1 expression downregulates LDL receptor-related protein (LRP): is LRP central to Alzheimer's disease pathogenesis? Mol Cell Neurosci. 1999;14:129–40.
41. Holcomb L, Gordon MN, McGowan E, Yu X, Benkovic S, Jantzen P, et al. Accelerated Alzheimer-type phenotype in transgenic mice carrying both mutant amyloid precursor protein and presenilin 1 transgenes. Nat Med. 1998;4:97–100.
42. Hartmann D, de Strooper B, Serneels L, Craessaerts K, Herreman A, Annaert W, et al. The disintegrin/metalloprotease ADAM 10 is essential for Notch signalling but not for α-secretase activity in fibroblasts. Hum Mol Genet. 2002;11:2615–24.
43. Asai M, Hattori C, Szabó B, Sasagawa N, Maruyama K, Tanuma S, et al. Putative function of ADAM9, ADAM10, and ADAM17 as APP alpha-secretase. Biochem Biophys Res Commun. 2003;301:231–5.
44. Postina R, Schroeder A, Dewachter I, Bohl J, Schmitt U, Kojro E, et al. A disintegrin-metalloproteinase prevents amyloid plaque formation and hippocampal defects in an Alzheimer disease mouse model. J Clin Invest. 2004;113:1456–64.
45. Kuhn P-H, Wang H, Dislich B, Colombo A, Zeitschel U, Ellwart JW, et al. ADAM10 is the physiologically relevant, constitutive?-secretase of the amyloid precursor protein in primary neurons. EMBO J. 2010;29:3020–32.
46. Suh J, Choi SH, Romano DM, Gannon MA, Lesinski AN, Kim DY, et al. ADAM10 missense mutations potentiate β-amyloid accumulation by impairing prodomain chaperone function. Neuron. 2013;80:385–401.

11

Nonsurgical therapy for hydrocephalus: a comprehensive and critical review

Marc R. Del Bigio[1*] and Domenico L. Di Curzio[2]

Abstract

Pharmacological interventions have been tested experimentally and clinically to prevent hydrocephalus and avoid the need for shunting beginning in the 1950s. Clinical trials of varied quality have not demonstrated lasting and convincing protective effects through manipulation of cerebrospinal fluid production, diuresis, blood clot fibrinolysis, or manipulation of fibrosis in the subarachnoid compartment, although there remains some promise in the latter areas. Acetazolamide bolus seems to be useful for predicting shunt response in adults with hydrocephalus. Neuroprotection in the situation of established hydrocephalus has been tested experimentally beginning more recently. Therapies designed to modify blood flow or pulsation, reduce inflammation, reduce oxidative damage, or protect neurons are so far of limited success; more experimental work is needed in these areas. As has been recommended for preclinical studies in stroke and brain trauma, stringent conditions should be met for preclinical studies in hydrocephalus.

Keywords: Brain, Cerebrospinal fluid, Clinical trials, Diuretic, Drug therapy, Fibrinolysis, Hydrocephalus, Inflammation, Intracranial hemorrhage, Neuroprotective

Background

Hydrocephalus was defined by Rekate as "an active distension of the ventricular system of the brain resulting from inadequate passage of cerebrospinal fluid (CSF) from its point of production within the cerebral ventricles to its point of absorption into the systemic circulation" [1]. Although all do not accept this definition, it has helped to guide an expert consensus opinion that most forms of hydrocephalus can be classified according to an identifiable anatomical site of CSF flow obstruction or impairment [2]. There is currently no definitive cure. Most patients are managed by shunting using a silicone tube and valve system, where CSF is diverted from the cerebral ventricles to another body site [3]. Treatment by shunting is associated with frequent complications, particularly obstruction and infection in young infants, which add to morbidity and mortality. In a large population-based analysis in California (1990–2000), the cumulative 5-year complication rate was approximately 48 % in children and 27 % in adults [4]. A recent pediatric study showed a 33 % shunt failure in 3 years [5]. Surgical alternatives to ventriculo-peritoneal shunting, such as endoscopic third ventriculostomy (ETV), have become popular. In controlled trials, ETV has reasonable efficacy in pediatric hydrocephalus particularly for aqueduct stenosis [6, 7]. ETV requires more robust evidence for routine use in adult normal pressure hydrocephalus (NPH) [8]. Lumboperitoneal shunting also shows some promise in NPH [9].

Because of the potential for complications, neurosurgeons may be hesitant to operate on young (especially preterm) infants with hydrocephalus. However, enlarging ventricles and delayed shunting might be associated with progressive brain damage [10]. For more than six decades, researchers have been trying to develop nonsurgical means for management of hydrocephalus. Three main categories of treatment have been explored in animal models and, in some situations, hydrocephalic patients. These include reducing CSF production, reducing the inflammatory and fibrotic processes that occur following brain hemorrhage or meningitis, and "protection" of brain cells and axons after ventriculomegaly has developed. The latter is envisioned as a supplemental

*Correspondence: marc.delbigio@umanitoba.ca
[1] Department of Pathology, University of Manitoba; Children's Hospital Research Institute of Manitoba, Diagnostic Services Manitoba, 401 Brodie Centre, 715 McDermot Avenue, Winnipeg, MB R3E 3P5, Canada

intervention that would allow a safe delay in surgical shunting of hydrocephalus.

The purpose of this review is to summarize and evaluate research concerning pharmacological therapies for hydrocephalus. The goal is to be comprehensive with an explanation of the rationale in animal experiments and a careful consideration of the earliest and the most definitive clinical trials. The review is organized in respect to the pathophysiologic factors involved in the development of hydrocephalus, specifically CSF production, CSF pathway obstruction (inflammation, fibrosis), and brain damage. Because some aspects of the pathogenesis of hydrocephalic brain damage are very similar to those that occur in cerebral ischemia (stroke) and brain trauma, evaluation of preclinical research should be similarly robust. Therefore, the quality of preclinical research studies related to brain protection will be judged using guidelines originally proposed by the Stroke Therapy Academic Industry Roundtable group [11, 12] and adopted by brain trauma investigators [13].

Methods

The senior author beginning c2000 has collected literature related to this topic. This was supplemented by structured searches in PubMed and GoogleScholar using the main term "hydrocephalus" along with key words "anti-inflammatory, diuretic, drug therapy, drug effects, fibrinolysis, inhibitor, neuroprotective, osmotic, pharmacology, randomized, steroid". Titles and abstracts were reviewed to ensure that the main topic was hydrocephalus. There is considerable overlap with the literature concerning brain or subarachnoid hemorrhage; only papers related to CSF flow or ventricular enlargement are addressed here. Relevant manuscripts were read in detail, and additional publications that had not been identified in the search were sought from the bibliographies (especially pre-1960, a period when works are less comprehensively recorded in PubMed). There were no time limits imposed; historical context is considered important. Considering the paucity of modern randomized trials in humans, this review is not meant as a meta-analysis; there are no specific exclusion criteria. In general, the sections are organized to separate the historical and experimental background from the pediatric and adult clinical studies, although this is not always possible. Treatments for shunt infection are not included. Detailed consideration of the pharmacodynamics of the drugs is beyond the scope of the review, although they will be mentioned when relevant to the interpretation of selected experiments. Some of the pharmacologic factors were described in a previous review [14]; details of the pharmacodynamics are beyond the scope of this review.

Results

Cerebrospinal fluid production and brain fluids

Readers are referred to other reviews for comprehensive considerations of choroid plexus function including CSF production [15–17], flow of brain fluids through intercellular and paravascular compartments [18–21], and CSF absorption [22, 23].

Osmotic agents and CSF pressure

One of the first pharmacologic attempts to manage hydrocephalus was by Marriott who, in 1924, reported that the diuretic agent theobromin sodio salicylate stabilized the head size of six infants with progressive hydrocephalus [24]. In the 1950s and early 1960s, when shunt therapy was emerging, drug therapies for hydrocephalus were directed at reducing CSF production or dehydrating the brain by diuresis. Typically, an appropriate physiological response in normal animals was sufficient rationale for testing of a drug in hydrocephalic humans. An excellent pharmacologic review of these agents was previously published [14].

Isosorbide, a dihydric alcohol derived from sorbitol that functions as an osmotic diuretic, is the best studied in hydrocephalus. Oral isosorbide transiently reduced the CSF pressure in healthy adult dogs [25]. A similar reduction in ventricular CSF pressure was demonstrated in 14 hydrocephalic children, although a rebound above the baseline was reported in 5/10 children who received multiple doses [26]. In what were described as preliminary experiments, 45 hydrocephalic patients (newborn to 62 years, median age 1 month) received 1–3 g/kg orally up to six times per day for 1–54 days (median 4 days) and were monitored for benefits defined as reduced CSF pressure or head size; 53/97 treatment episodes had some benefit and 26/97 had adverse effects [27–29]. Subsequently, Lorber conducted uncontrolled trials of isosorbide in infants with many forms of hydrocephalus; he eventually concluded that it was an effective adjunct for temporarily controlling intracranial pressure (ICP) prior to shunting, but not a replacement for surgery except perhaps in a minority of infants with myelomeningocele [30–33]. A controlled study of children with myelomeningocele two decades later compared 14 treated with isosorbide and 17 managed without the drug. Although isosorbide allowed delay of the surgical closure, there was no difference in need for shunting; furthermore, side effects led the authors to conclude that it has no role in management of these children [34].

Glycerol, a trivalent sugar alcohol, was known as a diuretic agent since the early 1900s [35]. As an oral osmotic agent, it was shown to reduce intracranial pressure in adults with brain tumors and was suggested as a possible agent for managing hydrocephalus [36]. However, a few small, uncontrolled trials did not support its use. Glycerol had no effect in four premature infants with posthemorrhagic hydrocephalus [37] and did not alleviate hydrocephalus in adults with metastatic brain cancer [38]. Although not a therapeutic effect, NPH patients who displayed an increase in cerebral blood flow (CBF) after glycerol administration tended to have a favorable response to shunt surgery [39]. Other sugar alcohols, mannitol and erythritol, transiently decreased ICP in adult hydrocephalic dogs following intravenous administration [40]. Although used widely for temporary management of elevated ICP in situations of brain swelling, mannitol has seldom been used except in adults with acute hydrocephalus caused by intracerebral hemorrhage [41]. In two chronically hydrocephalic children mannitol or urea transiently reduced ICP, however there was a rebound above baseline pressure [26].

Interference with CSF production

Because CSF dynamics are affected in obstructive forms of hydrocephalus, beginning in the 1950s and 1960s researchers have sought to treat hydrocephalus by reducing CSF production.

Acetazolamide

Acetazolamide, a carbonic anhydrase inhibitor, decreases CSF flow and ICP in rabbits and cats [42–44]. This was initially thought to be a diuretic and natriuretic effect through inhibition of carbonic anhydrase in the kidneys. However, later it was determined that choroid plexus has high levels of carbonic anhydrase and acetazolamide causes direct inhibition of CSF production. More recently, acetazolamide was also shown to inhibit aquaporin-mediated water conductance through several molecular pathways [45]. Acetazolamide was shown to reduce the lateral ventricle size of young adult rats, 1 day following injection of thrombin into the ventricle [46, 47]; however, ventricular enlargement was minimal in controls and the survival time too brief to be meaningful. Veterinary use of acetazolamide in hydrocephalus dogs is not beneficial [48].

Acetazolamide in hydrocephalic children

In trials beginning 1956, Elvidge and coworkers found that oral acetazolamide improved the clinical condition of a hydrocephalic child who was suffering from numerous shunt complications; vasopressin had no beneficial effect [49]. Benefit was also reported anecdotally and in small trials by others [50–55]. However, detailed physiologic studies on humans showed inconsistent reductions in CSF production [56]. By the late 1960s, it had become apparent that the therapeutic effect of acetazolamide in hydrocephalic children was negligible [57, 58].

Acetazolamide in hydrocephalic adults

Despite failed use in children, acetazolamide was proposed as an alternative to shunting for adults with NPH [59]. Although there was no persisting effect on ICP, the transient reduction in ICP following an acetazolamide bolus was shown to be predictive of good response to shunting in NPH patients [60]. Normal people have a transient increase in CBF (measured by first-pass radionuclide angiography) in response to a bolus; people with NPH have an impaired cerebrovascular response [61] and a blunted response was reported to be predictive of good response to shunting [62]. The poor increase in CBF following acetazolamide is thought to indicate a low capacity for vasodilation in the hydrocephalic brain, possibly due to compression of blood vessels [63]. In 5/8 NPH patients, administration of oral acetazolamide (125–375 mg/day) was associated with a decrease in the periventricular hyperintensities seen on magnetic resonance (MR) imaging [64] and an increase in CBF measured using MR arterial spin labeling [65]. There remains limited interest in the use of acetazolamide for treatment of idiopathic intracranial hypertension [66, 67].

Furosemide/acetazolamide combination in hydrocephalic children

Furosemide is a diuretic agent that inhibits the Na–K–2Cl symporter located in the distal tubules of kidney. Furosemide has minimal effect on CSF formation in healthy cats and dogs [44, 68], but CSF formation was reduced in preterm rabbits and in adult rabbits, albeit much less potently than acetazolamide [69, 70]. Vinas mentioned use of furosemide in management of a hydrocephalic child [71]. Chaplin and coworkers claimed to have arrested the progression of hydrocephalus in 4/7 infants with posthemorrhagic hydrocephalus by repeated CSF drainage and administration of oral acetazolamide and furosemide [72]. Shinnar et al. [73] gave the drug combination to 49 hydrocephalic children; they reported a 57 % success rate (avoidance of shunt) in non-myelomeningocele patients but only 26 % success in infants with myelomeningocele. An uncontrolled trial conducted from 1982–86 also hinted at benefit [74, 75]. A randomized control trial of the acetazolamide/furosemide combination for premature infants with posthemorrhagic ventricular dilatation was conducted from 1992–96. Unfortunately it failed to show benefit [76–78]. This trial was criticized for its failure to prove a solid rationale and safety background before starting [79].

Other ion channel blockers

Other drugs that block ion channels have been tested in small numbers of hydrocephalic patients. Digoxin, an inhibitor of Na–K–ATPase, reduces CSF production in humans at doses that are not cardiotoxic [80]. Digoxin was reported to reduce CSF production in three hydrocephalic children [81], but in three hydrocephalic infants it failed to prevent enlargement of the head [82]. Triamterene is a diuretic drug that blocks the epithelial sodium channel (ENaC). Three adults (age 25–76 years) with chronic hydrocephalus had resolution of symptoms during a 3–12 week treatment with triamterene [83]. Antagonists to the transient receptor potential vanilloid 4 (TRPV4), a gated divalent cation channel highly expressed by choroid plexus [84], have also been proposed as a treatment for hydrocephalus [85], but there are no published data supporting the concept.

Glucocorticoids

Steroids, in particular the glucocorticoids, have been used for decades with variable benefit in a range of neurological disorders associated with raised ICP. In healthy rabbits, betamethasone reduced CSF production after 5 days [86]. In normal dogs and in dogs with kaolin-induced hydrocephalus, intravenous dexamethasone or methylprednisolone caused a 40 % reduction in CSF flow for approximately 6 h, in the absence of diuresis or changes in blood pressure [87, 88]. The effect is through specific binding to the mineralocorticoid receptor (NR3C2; nuclear receptor subfamily 3 group C member 2) on choroid plexus epithelial cells, with subsequent regulation of several functions [89]. In 13 shunted hydrocephalic children with symptomatic slit ventricle syndrome, dexamethasone was associated with temporary relief of symptoms, although 9/13 required subsequent surgical intervention [90]. In the context of hydrocephalus, corticosteroids have also been used as a possible way to reduce the fibrosis in the subarachnoid compartment (see below).

Choroid plexus destruction

Surgical ablation of the choroid plexus as a means to control hydrocephalus was proposed by Dandy [91]. Using modern surgical techniques in combination with endoscopic third ventriculostomy, Warf has shown that this approach can be successful in selected cases less than 1-year age [92]. Non-surgical means of destroying the choroid plexus have also been attempted. In the 1970s, several groups of investigators injected radioactive agents into the ventricles of cats and dogs with kaolin-induced hydrocephalus. Gold-198 in colloidal form caused necrosis of the choroid plexus and reduced CSF production [93–95]. Rhenium-188 [96] and technetium-99 m [97] were not effective in similar model systems. Intraventricular injection of radioactive chromic phosphate-phosphorus-32 into four hydrocephalic infants was reported to arrest head growth, but long-term results were not presented [98]. Likely due to the high potential for side effects, others have not pursued this approach.

Destruction of choroid plexus by ricin toxin-conjugated to antibodies that bind to the epithelial cells was tested in culture and was proposed as a means for managing hydrocephalus [99, 100]. However, there are no published experiments using animal models.

Summary of CSF modulation for managing hydrocephalus

Reduction of brain water with osmotic agents and inhibition of choroid plexus ion channels provide transient reductions in the ICP or CSF pressure of hydrocephalic children and adults. However, no lasting effects have been demonstrated in published clinical trials, although recent work in NPH suggests that there might be a role for acetazolamide at least as a test agent to predict response to shunting [101]. Considering that the half-life of acetazolamide is 4 h, divided dosing regimens might be needed to achieve optimal effectiveness. Conceivably, highly selective inhibition of choroid plexus ion channels that are not present in other epithelia (e.g. kidney) might be associated with fewer side effects and might work in situations where obstructions to CSF flow are only partial. It will likely be difficult to avoid toxicity in non-surgical ablation approaches.

Cerebrospinal fluid pathway modulation

CSF pathway inflammation and fibrosis

One of the general features of hydrocephalus is a relative restriction of CSF movement (bulk flow or pulsatile movement) along its anatomical route [2]. Circumstances that can lead to restrictions include intraventricular hemorrhage, subarachnoid hemorrhage, or infection (e.g. meningitis); all are associated with secondary inflammation and fibrosis in the CSF pathways, especially the subarachnoid compartment [102]. In children, intraventricular hemorrhage and bacterial meningitis are associated with meningeal fibrosis, which obliterates the subarachnoid space [103, 104]. In adults with subarachnoid hemorrhage, inflammation occurs within the arachnoid villi during the first week and is followed by proliferation of arachnoid cap cells [105] and collagen production [106]. Enzymatic dissolution of the intraventricular or subarachnoid blood collections, interference with the inflammatory process, and interference with the production of extracellular matrix molecules are approaches that have been explored as ways to reduce the likelihood of developing hydrocephalus.

Enzymatic dissolution of intracranial blood collections in animals

Tissue plasminogen activator (tPA) is a serine proteinase that binds to fibrin in clotted blood and converts plasminogen to plasmin, thereby initiating fibrinolysis and dissolution of the blood clot. Urokinase (or urokinase-type plasminogen activator/uPA) is a proteolytic enzyme present in urine, blood, and extracellular matrix; it is also capable of activating plasminogen and it can digest extracellular matrix proteins [107]. Streptokinase is a bacterial enzyme capable of cleaving plasminogen, although it is less discriminate and can activate plasminogen that is not associated with blood clots [108]. Thrombolytic therapies for ischemic stroke were first pursued in the 1970s; intravascular recombinant tPA is an important intervention for some adults with early ischemic stroke [109]. However, tPA can have adverse effects in the brain parenchyma [110].

Experimental brain hemorrhage models have been used to determine if these agents can accelerate clot lysis and reduce the subsequent development of hydrocephalus. In dogs with experimental subarachnoid hemorrhage, intrathecal urokinase reduced fibrosis in the intracranial subarachnoid compartment at 3 weeks and 3 months [111]. The number of subarachnoid macrophages was greater following urokinase than in control dogs [112]. In dogs with experimental intraventricular hemorrhage (IVH), urokinase effectively lysed the blood clot in 3–6 days (vs. 38–65 days in controls); only 2/10 treated dogs (compared to 9/10 control dogs) developed progressive hydrocephalus [113]. Cats that were treated with an infusion of intrathecal tPA 1 day after the intracisternal blood injection did not develop hydrocephalus at 7 days [114]. Pigs with experimental IVH had more rapid resolution of the blood clot and reduction in the ventricle size at 1 week after treatment with tPA, although the control animals had reached comparable ventricle size by 6 weeks [115, 116]. In the collagenase model of intracerebral hemorrhage in young adult rats, infusion of urokinase or tPA into the lateral ventricle for 1 h beginning 3 h after collagenase was associated with reduced ventricle size measured by MRI after 3 days. However, only urokinase was associated with improved behavioral outcome [117].

Thrombolytic agents in children with posthemorrhagic hydrocephalus

Pediatric clinical trials in the 1990s initially showed some promise for prevention of post-hemorrhagic hydrocephalus through use of several thrombolytic agents. Premature infants with IVH (n = 18 vs. 39 controls, nonrandomized) were treated with intraventricular urokinase for 7 days; they were reported to have a lower requirement for shunting than historical controls (37 vs. 92 %) [118, 119]. In a pilot study, six premature infants with IVH, ventricular dilation, and head enlargement (>2 cm per week) despite diuretic therapy and serial lumbar punctures received intraventricular urokinase for 3 days. Although the intraventricular clot decreased in size and there were no apparent side effects, all infants required a shunt. The authors concluded that late initiation of urokinase was ineffective in this situation [120]. Following the observation that CSF plasminogen levels were low in premature infants with IVH [121], Whitelaw and coworkers administered intraventricular bolus of recombinant tPA to 22 infants with post-hemorrhagic hydrocephalus; among the 21 survivors, 12 did not require a shunt [122]. A phase 1 clinical trial then showed that 17/23 survivors did not require a CSF shunt [123]. However, a multicenter randomized trial of 70 infants showed that intraventricular tPA and CSF washing (drainage, irrigation, and fibrinolytic therapy; DRIFT) did not reduce shunt surgery or death and was potentially associated with secondary intraventricular hemorrhage [124]. Although the immediate results did not look favorable, a 2-year follow-up of surviving children from the DRIFT trial indicated that treatment was associated with a reduction of severe cognitive disability [125], but this did not correlate with any improvement in brain volume measured by MRI [126].

During this same period, nine preterm infants received intraventricular infusion of streptokinase for 12–72 h without major adverse events [127]. A randomized case-control trial conducted 1992–1994 included six infants who received intraventricular streptokinase for 4 days. Although fibrin degradation products were significantly elevated and blood clot reabsorption occurred after infusion, there was no difference in the number of children who required shunting (3/5 survivors in each group); the authors concluded that they could "not recommend fibrinolytic intraventricular infusion as a routine treatment" [128]. Another prospective case control trial of six treated and six untreated infants also led to the conclusion that streptokinase should not be used in this situation [129]. In 1999, the authors of an excellent review of the five small case series published to that time concluded, "While there is insufficient evidence to justify any claim that fibrinolytic therapy is safe and effective, there is also insufficient evidence to justify discarding this form of treatment as ineffective or unsafe" [130]. Systematic reviews of the randomized trials show no support for intraventricular streptokinase treatment after intraventricular hemorrhage in premature infants [131].

Thrombolytic agents in adults with posthemorrhagic hydrocephalus

Similar clinical approaches have been used with varied success in adults with hydrocephalus following IVH or subarachnoid hemorrhage. Among six adults with severe IVH who received intraventricular urokinase for 7 days, 5/6 had a good or excellent outcome, while only two required shunting for hydrocephalus [132]. A small randomized trial of adults with IVH showed a lower mortality and slightly lower likelihood of need for shunt (3/9 vs. 2/4), but a high incidence of very poor neurological outcome among survivors (7/10) [133]. A retrospective study of 14 adults with spontaneous IVH and hydrocephalus treated with intraventricular urokinase from 2002–2005, suggested that the therapy was safe; in comparison to historical controls, it seemed to be associated with reduced mortality and reduced incidence of ventricular drain obstruction [134]. Wang advocated for intrathecal administration of urokinase to treat acute hydrocephalus in adults [135]. A pilot experiment in adults with IVH showed that intraventricular tPA was associated with reduction of intraventricular blood and normalization of ventricular size within 1–2 days [136]. In an uncontrolled trial, adults with intracerebral hemorrhage and hydrocephalus exhibited rapid resolution of the hematoma when tPA was infused into the ventricle; compared to the historical controls, tPA infusion combined with lumbar drainage seemed to reduce the need for CSF shunting (33 vs. 3 %) [137, 138]. High dose tPA (4 mg tPA every 12 h to a maximum cumulative dose of 20 mg tPA) was associated with more rapid clot resolution from the lateral ventricles but not the third or fourth ventricles [139]. In 2007–2008, 41 subarachnoid hemorrhage patients received intraventricular tPA for 5–7 days. In comparison to historical controls, tPA recipients had fewer days in severe vasospasm and the incidence of hydrocephalus requiring shunt was also lower (18 vs. 43 %) [140]. A randomized double blind trial testing the value of intraventricular tPA for adults with IVH was underway in 2015 [141]; interim analysis showed that the rate of rebleeding was not a major risk [142]. Unfortunately, the need for a shunt to treat hydrocephalus is not one of the planned outcome criteria.

Summary of blood clot lysis for hydrocephalus

In general, animal and human studies (both pediatric and adult) show that enzymatic blood clot lysis accelerates the resolution of the blood collection, but offers no long-term protection against the development of hydrocephalus [143, 144]. Authors of a systematic review concluded "intraventricular thrombolytic agents including tPA, urokinase, or streptokinase are not recommended as methods to reduce the need for shunt placement in premature infants with [posthemorrhagic hydrocephalus" (high clinical certainty) [145]. Similarly, a meta-analysis of trials on adult patients with aneurysmal IVH concluded "intraventricular rt-PA has no significant efficacy on the long-term functional recovery" [146]. A more recent trial found that intraventricular tPA had no effect on the need for CSF shunt dependency or the functional outcome of adults with endovascular-treated aneurysmal SAH [147]. Recent data suggest that the sudden release of blood breakdown products by fibrinolysis might fail to protect against hydrocephalus because inflammation is increased by rapid blood clot lysis [148]. Nevertheless, there remains the possibility that tPA in children with posthemorrhagic hydrocephalus might offer some long-term benefits unrelated to the development of ventriculomegaly.

Experimental interference with inflammation in the meninges

There is a clear association between inflammation in the CSF pathways and subsequent development of hydrocephalus. Therefore, anti-inflammatory agents have been tested experimentally to prevent post-meningitis and post-hemorrhagic hydrocephalus. Rabbits with meningitis caused by *S. pneumoniae* develop increased resistance to CSF outflow. If they are treated with methylprednisolone within 1 day after the bacterial inoculation, CSF outflow is normalized, likely due to decreased inflammation [149]. Adult rabbits develop hydrocephalus following intraventricular blood injections repeated over a 2-week period. Those that received concurrent intramuscular methylprednisolone had significantly reduced severity of hydrocephalus, but intraventricular methylprednisolone caused ventricular enlargement in 35 % of rabbits [150]. A detailed study of post-hemorrhage fibrosis in the subarachnoid compartment of dogs with autologous blood injection into the cisterna magna showed that intrathecal dexamethasone did not significantly alter the fibrosis at 3 weeks or 3 months [151]; the ventricle size was not measured in these dogs.

Anti-inflammatory agents in humans with meningitis

In humans, high quality randomized trials of corticosteroid therapy for acute bacterial meningitis show significantly reduced hearing loss and neurological sequelae, although there are no specific data concerning development of hydrocephalus [152]. A recent retrospective study of adults with bacterial meningitis suggests that increased brain ventricle size in the acute phase of bacterial meningitis is associated with increased mortality [153]. A meta-analysis of clinical trials using corticosteroids to treat tuberculosis meningitis indicated a marginal benefit with reduction of death and disabling residual neurological deficit amongst survivors [154], but the likelihood of developing hydrocephalus was not changed [155, 156]. However, a recent randomized study of children with tuberculous meningitis suggested that high dose prednisolone (4 mg/kg/day over 4 weeks vs. 2 mg/kg/day) might be associated with increased risk of hydrocephalus [157]. A rare congenital autoimmune disease called chronic infantile neurologic, cutaneous, articular (CINCA) syndrome is characterized by neonatal-onset chronic meningitis; a single child who developed hydrocephalus was successfully managed with anakinra, a recombinant interleukin-1-receptor antagonist [158].

Role of transforming growth factor beta in the development of subarachnoid fibrosis

Considering the marginal successes of blood lysis and anti-inflammatory agents for managing hydrocephalus, a more targeted molecular approach seems worth considering. Transforming growth factor beta (TGF-β) is a growth factor released from platelets at sites of blood clotting whereupon it regulates proliferation of fibroblasts (and other cell types), as well as the synthesis of extracellular matrix proteins. In 1994, high levels of TGF-β1 in the CSF of adults with subarachnoid hemorrhage were shown to be associated with enlargement of the cerebral ventricles [159, 160]. A similar association was later shown in premature infants with IVH [161, 162]. However, it must be noted that recent data obtained from a CSF assay study failed to support a critical role for TGF β1 and TGF β2 in the development of posthemorrhagic hydrocephalus in adults [163].

In neonatal rats with intraventricular blood injection, TGF-β1, TGF-β2, and TGF-β3 are increased, although only the latter was associated with enlarged ventricles and only TGF-β1 was restricted to the meninges. This was accompanied by deposition of fibronectin, laminin, and vitronectin in brain tissue [164]. In animal experiments, injection of TGF-β1 into the subarachnoid compartment of 10-day old mice caused hydrocephalus [165, 166] as a consequence of progressive fibrosis in the leptomeninges [167]. Intracerebroventricular infusion of recombinant human hepatocyte growth factor, which antagonizes the fibrosis-inducing effect of TGF-β1, for 7 or 14 days, improved the memory, ventricle size, CSF flow, and meningeal fibrosis in mice with TGF-β1 injection-induced hydrocephalus [168].

Transgenic mice with TGF-β1 overexpression linked to the glial fibrillary acidic protein (GFAP) promoter in astrocytes develop hydrocephalus with no obstructions in the ventricular system [169, 170]. These mice have increased cellularity and obstruction to CSF flow in the subarachnoid compartment, and they develop enlarged ventricles beginning at postgestation day 15 [171–173].

Interference with the TGF-β1 pathway has been explored as a means to treat or prevent experimental hydrocephalus. Seven-day-old rats with post-IVH hydrocephalus were randomized to receive the drugs pirfenidone or losartan, which have been shown to reduce TGF-β expression and decrease inflammatory fibrosis in lungs and other organs. After 14 days treatment, neither drug had a beneficial effect on ventricle size or behavior [174]. Infusion of thrombin into the subarachnoid compartment of adult rats mimics some of the changes that occur after subarachnoid hemorrhage, including increased expression of TGF-β1 and meningeal collagen accumulation. Administration of the TGF-β1 inhibitor SB-431542 into the cisterna magna prior to thrombin injection blocked the collagen accumulation at 10 and 20 days [175].

Three-week old rats received subarachnoid injections of kaolin with or without infusions of decorin, a small proteoglycan that can bind TGF-β1. There was good evidence that the decorin-treated rats had reduced inflammation and fibrosis in the subarachnoid compartment [176]. However, the fact that treatment began before the onset of hydrocephalus and the large number of exclusions from the decorin group makes this an interesting proof-of-principle only. A follow-up experiment by the same group is planned with delayed (1 week) initiation of decorin treatment (personal communication; Dr. P. McAllister September 2015). Another group used a subarachnoid model in 6-week-old rats; the rats received intracisternal injection of decorin immediately before blood injection followed by intracerebroventricular injection of decorin 10 days later. The treated rats convincingly had inhibited up-regulation of TGF-β1, reduced collagen, reduced ventricle size, and improved cognitive outcome [177].

The TGF-β and Wnt signaling pathways converge through the Smad/YAP complex, which translocates to the nucleus to activate various genes related to fibrosis [178]. Ventricle size and reactive astroglial changes were measured in adult rats following injection of kaolin into the lateral ventricle. If sFRP-1, a Wnt inhibitor, was added to the kaolin, the ventricle enlargement was less severe and the GFAP expression was reduced in periventricular regions of unspecified location [179]. Although not measured directly, inhibition of the Wnt signaling cascade might alleviate development of hydrocephalus by reducing fibrosis.

Young adult mice with kaolin-induced hydrocephalus were maintained on tap water or deuterium water beginning 7 days prior to kaolin. The stated rationale was previous evidence that deuterium could inhibit cell proliferation and fibrosis in vitro. After 4 weeks, the treated rats had ventricles of normal size, reduced collagen on extracted tissue sections, and reduced TGF-β1 immunoreactivity in posterior fossa compared to untreated hydrocephalic rats [180]. This demonstration of a seemingly miraculous treatment had several shortcomings; the most important being the failure to demonstrate that kaolin was actually delivered into the subarachnoid compartment. Finally, 7-day rats with periventricular hemorrhage induced by intracerebral injection of collagenase received the TGF receptor 1 inhibitor SD208 daily for 3 days, beginning 1 h or 3 days after collagenase injection. SD208 reduced the adverse behavioral effects, weight loss, and associated brain injury [181]. However, considering that the ventricular enlargement was unilateral and apparently due to brain atrophy, this experiment should not be considered evidence for treatment of hydrocephalus.

In summary, antagonism of the TGF-β1 pathway has excellent rationale for prevention of post-hemorrhagic or post-meningitis hydrocephalus, but more preclinical experimentation is required.

Deferoxamine for preventing fibrosis

Deferoxamine is a chelating agent that binds free ferric iron (Fe^{3+}). It is used effectively in a variety of diseases associated with blood breakdown; it can prevent fibrosis by attenuating oxidative stress and the subsequent inflammatory cascade [182]. There are promising experimental data for treatment of intracerebral hemorrhage [183]. Ventricular enlargement was studied after fluid percussion brain injury in adult rats. Deferoxamine was administered beginning 2 h after injury and the brains were studied at 1 day. Deferoxamine was associated with normalized ventricle size and upregulation of heme oxygenase 1 [184]. In another lab, young adult rats received unilateral injection of autologous whole blood or ferric chloride ($FeCl_3$) into the lateral ventricle. Intraperitoneal deferoxamine was administered beginning immediately afterward and then for 7 days; the brains were examined at 1 or 4 weeks. Blood or $FeCl_3$ caused enlarged ventricles and deferoxamine treatment prevented ventricle enlargement [185, 186]. The authors discussed neuroprotective properties and anti-fibrotic properties of the agent, but did not directly study the meningeal compartment.

Reversing accumulation of extracellular matrix molecules in the subarachnoid compartment

As with any wound healing processes, hyaluronic acid and a variety of proteoglycans are produced in the first few days after a hemorrhagic or inflammatory process. Several weeks are necessary before collagen, which is more permanent, is produced [187, 188]. These fibrosis-associated molecules seemed a reasonable target, albeit a late one, for modulation in hydrocephalus. A variety of purified enzymes, including the matrix metalloproteinases (MMP), are capable of degrading a variety of extracellular matrix molecules.

In a rabbit model of IVH, ventricular enlargement occurs. Single intracerebroventricular injection of chondroitinase ABC, which digests a variety of proteoglycans, did not reduce the ventriculomegaly, although it should be noted that the subarachnoid compartment was not studied directly [189].

In a few small case series, animal-derived hyaluronidase was administered intrathecally on a weekly basis for several weeks to children with tuberculous meningitis and hydrocephalus. One of the earliest trials suggested that hyaluronidase was superior to shunt surgery [190]. A later trial showed improved level of consciousness but no overall improvement in comparison to CSF shunting [191]. One report claimed that hyaluronidase offered mild transient benefit in three children with myelomeningocele [192]. However, the largest published trial showed that hyaluronidase was associated with reduced intracranial pressure but no change in ventricle size in 12/17 children with tuberculosis-associated hydrocephalus [193]; it is considered of historical interest only [194].

The MMP are a family of diverse enzymes capable of degrading a variety of extracellular matrix molecules. In experimental hydrocephalus, adult rats had elevated MMP9 in the CSF after intraventricular kaolin injection [195] while transgenic mice with TGF-β overexpression have reduced MMP9 mRNA and activity [196]. MMPs were assayed in the CSF of 13 premature children with posthemorrhagic hydrocephalus, 10 infants with non-hemorrhagic hydrocephalus, and 10 controls. Pro-MMP9 was found to be elevated in the CSF in 9/13 infants that did not require a shunt and the authors speculated that modulation of MMP9 activity might be a therapeutic strategy worth testing [197, 198]. However, inspection of their data shows that two children with very high levels skewed the MMP9 level.

Cerebral blood flow and pulsation in hydrocephalus

Diminished regional blood flow, particularly in the cerebral white matter, is well documented in pediatric and adult hydrocephalus [199, 200]. It is not entirely clear if this is a purely mechanical phenomenon that results from distorted or compressed blood vessels, or if there is a dysregulation due to altered innervation or local cell interactions. Regardless of the cause, hypoxia likely contributes to the pathogenesis of axon damage [201, 202]. Many adults with NPH have arterial hypertension and cerebrovascular disease [203, 204]. These epidemiologic data suggest that pre-existing vascular disease can aggravate the brain dysfunction associated with hydrocephalus or that the abnormal blood pressure can contribute to the development of ventriculomegaly. The role of vascular pulsations as mechanical contributor to ventricular enlargement is currently of great interest [205, 206]. A seldom-cited case report of an infant with hydrocephalus suggested that bilateral common carotid artery ligation was associated with reduced intracranial pulsation and stabilization of head size [207].

Vasoactive drugs in experimental hydrocephalus

Using the 3-week rat model of kaolin-induced hydrocephalus we demonstrated several aspects of the axonal damage that suggested a possible role for activation of proteolytic enzymes by intracellular calcium [208]. Based on that information, hydrocephalic rats were treated by continuous administration of the calcium channel blocker nimodipine for 2 weeks, beginning 2 weeks after induction of hydrocephalus (i.e. beginning at 5 weeks age). Nimodipine treatment prevented the declines in motor and cognitive behavior that were observed in untreated control rats, and although the degree of ventricular enlargement was equal, the corpus callosum was thicker in the treated rats [209]. We later showed that Mg^{++} (delivered as $MgSO_4$), a Ca^{++} competitor, had a similar but weaker protective effect [210]. However, when nimodipine or Mg^{++} was administered to 1-week rats, there was no protective effect and the side effects were more substantial [211]. Recent experiments from our lab showed that both agents, at the doses that were protective, have significant vasoactive effects in rats; these include decreased systemic arterial blood pressure, decreased cerebral perfusion and intracerebral pulse pressure, but no change in CBF (unpublished work; Shulyakov and Del Bigio, in preparation). We went on to test $MgSO_4$ in a ferret model of hydrocephalus [212]; two-week ferrets received kaolin injections and beginning 2 weeks later received MgSO4 by parenteral injections. Although they had significant side effects (lethargy), there was no evidence for protection at the behavioral, structural, or biochemical level (Di Curzio, Turner-Brannen, Mao, Del Bigio; manuscript submitted). We are planning a ferret experiment with nimodipine is planned to determine if the protection is reproducible in a gyrencephalic animal with hydrocephalus.

Vasoactive drugs in humans with hydrocephalus

One group treated 18 hydrocephalic infants with oral isosorbide dinitrate, a nitrate vasodilator (8 mg/kg/day; for 1–25 months, median 3 months) [213]; the authors seem to have mistakenly equated this drug with the osmotic agent isosorbide. They considered the treatment useful because only 2/10 posthemorrhagic cases required shunting (versus 5/5 myelomeningocele cases).

Eight adults with NPH underwent blood pressure monitoring during administration of the calcium channel blocker nimodipine, which is commonly used for treatment of hypertension. Four hours after nimodipine, the mean arterial blood pressure was lower, the ICP was slightly higher, and overall there was no change in cerebral perfusion pressure (estimated from the arterio-venous oxygen difference) [214]. The antihypertensive agent ketanserin was administered to eight patients with NPH as a single bolus; it caused a decrease in blood pressure without altering ICP of CBF [215]. These studies prove nothing in the context of managing hydrocephalus, although it does suggest that nimodipine should be safe.

Greitz suggested that selective venous constriction, for example using dihydroergotamine, might modulate the intravascular dynamics, although it should be noted that his logic was not entirely clear ("Venous constriction would result in dilatation of the venous side of the capillary, decrease of the microvascular resistance, opening up of the microcirculation and reduced intracranial pressure") [216]. This approach has never been tested experimentally. Dihydroergotamine causes contraction of isolated human cortical arteries and veins [217], but it has no effect on CBF in normal adults [218]. It can reduce intracranial pressure in patients with traumatic brain injury [219], while it may be associated with increased intracranial pressure in brain tumor patients, possibly due to loss of autoregulation [220]. Based on these contradictory data, pursuing dihydroergotamine as a therapy for hydrocephalus seems unwise.

Vascular endothelial growth factor (VEGF) in hydrocephalus

VEGF is one of the best-known promoters of angiogenesis and vascular survival. It also plays a role in vascular permeability factor, and it may also provide direct trophic support to neurons [221]. Because of the known vascular and CBF alterations in hydrocephalic brains, VEGF is a logical target for investigation. VEGF function is mediated through specific receptors in the brain [222]. In a dog model of chronic hydrocephalus, significant decreases in frontal cortex VEGFR-2 were reported; VEGF was not altered in tissue, but it increased in the CSF [223]. In the same dogs, VEGFR-2 increased in the hippocampus; this corresponded to increased blood vessel density, which was not seen in frontal cerebrum [224]. This is of interest because typically the hippocampus sustains only minimal direct damage in hydrocephalic brains (although there is considerable damage to the connecting pathways) [225]. The authors suggested that modulation of VEGF and its receptor might be a useful therapy for the chronic brain hypoxia that occurs in hydrocephalus [226]. Moderate arm exercise in adults with chronic hydrocephalus was associated with elevated VEGF in the CSF [227].

In contradiction to the potential protective function of VEGF, another research group reported increased CSF levels of VEGF in children and young adults with hydrocephalus. They then infused VEGF into the cerebral ventricles of non-hydrocephalic rats and found that the ventricles were enlarged. Simultaneous infusion of bevacizumab, an antagonist of VEGF, prevented this enlargement [228]. The authors devised an extremely complicated postulate in which the VEGF interacts with VEGFR-2 on ependymal cells leading to dysfunction of fluid regulation and ultimately to hydrocephalus [229].

Thus, we have a situation where one group of investigators suggests that VEGF/VEGFR-2 alterations are secondary to hydrocephalus and represent a beneficial adaptation to chronic hypoxia, while another group claims that VEGF causes ventriculomegaly. This is a subject that needs clarification before drug interventions are tested in humans.

Brain protection in hydrocephalus

Hydrocephalus is associated with gradual destruction of periventricular white matter leading to a disconnection syndrome. In the circumstance of the immature brain, hydrocephalus also interferes with developmental processes including cell genesis and myelination [201, 230]. In the situation of progressive ventricular enlargement wherein shunt therapy is likely necessary, drugs might be used to protect the brain temporarily prior to shunting. Considering the overlap in pathophysiology between hydrocephalus, stroke, and trauma, it is anticipated that candidates from the latter two diseases should be considered for protecting the hydrocephalic brain. In neonatal hypoxic-ischemic brain injury, a variety of potential early therapeutics have broadly been categorized into anti-oxidative, anti-inflammatory, anti-apoptotic, and anti-excitotoxic mechanisms, with melatonin and erythropoietin covering multiple mechanisms [231]. Additional file 1: Table 1 summarizes the experiments conducted to date in hydrocephalic animals including the rationale, strengths, and weaknesses.

Anti-inflammatory interventions and microglia

Microglial and astroglial activation occurs in animals and humans with hydrocephalus [232, 233]. Microglial response is reported to contribute to brain damage in many disorders [234], although microglial activation might also have beneficial effects [235, 236]. Nevertheless, until the damage-benefit balance related to microglia is settled, anti-inflammatory interventions could be considered in the treatment of hydrocephalus.

Minocycline is a semi-synthetic tetracycline derivative with anti-inflammatory properties. It appears to be protective in a range of animal neurological disorders as well as human stroke [237, 238]. Intraperitoneal administration of minocycline to H-Tx rats with congenital hydrocephalus from postnatal day 15 to day 21 was associated with increased cortical thickness (ventricle size was not measured) and reduced cerebral immunolabeling for Iba-1 (a microglial marker) and GFAP (an astrocyte marker) [239]. Young adult rats with kaolin-induced hydrocephalus were given minocycline from day 15 to day 21 after kaolin. Treated rats had reduced progression of the ventricle size and reduced Iba-1 and GFAP in the brain [240]. In 7-day-old rats that had intracerebral hemorrhage induced with collagenase injection, minocycline treatment administered daily for 5 days beginning immediately was also associated with improved behavioral outcome and less severe ventricular enlargement at 28 days [241]. Although minocycline seems promising, the main side effect of tooth discoloration must be considered in the pediatric population [242].

Transgenic mice with hydrocephalus secondary to TGF-β overexpression were administered the non-steroidal anti-inflammatory agents ibuprofen or pioglitazone, a peroxisome proliferator-activated receptor-γ agonist, from 2 to 4 months age. Although both suppressed activation of microglia (based upon cellular hypertrophy), neither drug had an effect on thioflavin S staining of amyloid in cerebral blood vessels and pioglitazone aggravated the ventriculomegaly (ventricle size was not measured in the ibuprofen recipients) [243]. It is not clear, however, that thioflavin S staining is a good outcome measure in young rats.

Adult rabbits were treated 1 day after intracisternal kaolin injection with a single dose of infliximab, a monoclonal antibody that binds to tumor necrosis factor-alpha (TNF), which is an important mediator of inflammatory responses that is produced by microglia. After 2 weeks, blood and CSF levels of TNF were reduced in treated rabbits, although ICP was not different between the groups. After sacrifice the only histological evaluation was terminal deoxynucleotidyl transferase-mediated dUTP nick end labeling (TUNEL) in the optic disc, optic radiation, and the lateral geniculate body; treated rabbits had fewer labeled cells with microglial morphology in the two latter locations [244]. Unfortunately, this experiment is very difficult to interpret because the ventricle size was not measured at any time and the significance of microglial death in the optic pathway is of unknown significance.

Antioxidative interventions

Numerous animal experiments and investigations of human CSF indicate that hydrocephalus is associated with oxidative and nitrosylative cell responses and damage, likely secondary to the chronic hypoxia [245, 246]. In 3-week rats with kaolin-induced hydrocephalus, epigallocatechin gallate derived from green tea and N-acetylcystein [sic] were both shown to reduce brain tissue malondialdehyde, one of the end products of lipid peroxidation [247, 248]. However, the biochemical assay was the sole outcome parameter (ventricle size was not measured) so the value of these interventions is unclear. Two-week old rats received daily melatonin injections for 4 weeks beginning immediately after intracisternal kaolin injection. Nitric oxide content was not significantly changed and glutathione was almost normalized in the choroid plexus of hydrocephalic animals [249]. However, ventricle size was assessed only qualitatively by inspection of the midsagittal slice, and the histologic interpretation of the choroid plexus is not convincing. Beginning 2 weeks after kaolin injection into 3-week-old rats, we administered an oral mixture of antioxidants (alpha-tocopherol, L-ascorbic acid, coenzyme Q10, reduced glutathione, and reduced lipoic acid) for 2 weeks. We detected no therapeutic effect on the analysis of behavior, brain structure, or biochemical content; of uncertain significance, we observed that the canola oil carrier normalized anti-oxidant capacity of the brain tissue [250]. Catechin polyphenols present in the leaves of *Camellia sinensis* are potent antioxidants. Seven-day-old rats were injected with kaolin and received extracts of *C. sinensis* daily beginning 2 days later. Although there was no behavioral protection and the ventricle size was not measured, treated rats had thicker corpus callosum at 10 days age (but not 21 days age) and had a significant reduction in the reactive astrocytes [251]. Using a similar protocol, the same group is currently doing a study with edaravone (30 mg/kg; Luiza da Silva Lopes, unpublished work), which is a free radical scavenger that appears to have some benefit in adults with acute ischemic stroke [252]. Adult rats received intraventricular injection of autologous whole blood; those that received simultaneous edaravone had less brain edema and less tissue malondialdehyde on day 1 and improved memory on day 28 [253].

Neuron and axon protection

Periventricular axons sustain most of the damage in hydrocephalic brains with secondary retrograde degenerative changes in some neuron populations [201, 230]. Memantine, a non-competitive NMDA receptor antagonist, protects neurons and axons in a variety of animal models [254]. One day after kaolin injection, 3-week old rats began receiving memantine daily for 2 weeks. Low resolution MRI verified the presence of hydrocephalus at the end of the study. Histologic counts indicated reduced neurons in the hippocampus of hydrocephalic rats, and partial recovery in the CA1 and CA2 (but not CA3) sectors of memantine-treated rats [255]. It should be noted that in other rodent hydrocephalus studies, hippocampal neurons are reported to be spared or show various secondary abnormalities due to deafferentation [256–258]. Memantine or an herbal medicine, Morinda citrifolia, were given to adult rabbits for 2 weeks beginning immediately after intracisternal kaolin injection; brain tissue around the fourth ventricle was analyzed by immunostaining for activated caspase-3 as a measure of cell death. The authors reported that memantine aggravated cell death while the herbal therapy was neutral with respect to hydrocephalus [259]. This experiment is flawed because the fourth ventricle size was not reported, the presence of kaolin in the immediate vicinity was not documented, and the caspase 3 immunostaining is not convincing. The lead author's group is planning to test memantine in young hydrocephalic rats and measure behavioral, structural, and biochemical outcomes (experiment scheduled for early 2016).

Based on prior reports of axon protection in traumatic brain injury models, we treated 3-week-old hydrocephalic rats with tacrolimus, cyclosporine A, or calpain inhibitor I; there was no statistically significant protection in regard to behavior, brain structure or brain composition in any of the experiments [260]. In the same model system, we found no evidence for protection using the sodium channel-blocking agents mexiletine and riluzole [261].

Cerebral stimulants

Considerable experimental work [201] and many assays of human CSF [262] have showed that the monoamine neurotransmitter systems are disturbed in hydrocephalus. These correlate with some of the functional disturbances seen in hydrocephalic patients. A monoamine oxidase inhibitor, bifemelane, used as an antidepressant and "cerebral metabolic activator" tended to normalize norepinephrine and serotonin levels (albeit with wide variance) in the striatum and cerebral cortex of young adult rats with kaolin-induced hydrocephalus [263]. Several case reports of hydrocephalic patients treated with a variety of similar agents have been published. Methylphenidate, which is widely used for treatment of attention deficit hyperactivity disorder and which acts by blocking the dopamine and norepinephrine transporters, was administered to a single NPH patient (20 mg) in a double blind cross-over trial after she had been shunted; the drug as associated with improved cognitive performance and reduced apathy [264]. In another case report, a single NPH patient with depression responded well to twice-daily oral doses of 10 mg methylphenidate [265].

In two separate reports, two people with hydrocephalus and akinetic mutism (that persisted after shunt revision) responded well to bromocriptine and ephedrine [266, 267]; the former is a dopamine agonist and the latter is a sympathomimetic amine that increases the activity of norepinephrine. Finally, an unshunted 19 year-old with severe hydrocephalus and aggressive self-injurious behavior responded well to trazodone (200 mg/day) [268], which is an antidepressant of the serotonin antagonist and reuptake inhibitor class.

Although entirely anecdotal, this avenue of therapy seems open for further investigation.

Protection of the developing brain in early-onset hydrocephalus

A poorly studied aspect of hydrocephalus-associated brain damage is that due to disruption of the periventricular germinal matrix [269], which is the zone of proliferating cells that gives rise to neuron and glial precursors during human fetal life (or during the postnatal life of extremely premature infants).

In an elegant experiment, embryonic mice received injections of blood plasma, blood serum, or lysophosphatidic acid (LPA; which is a normal component of blood plasma) into the lateral ventricle on in utero day 13.5. These (but not red blood cells) caused severe hydrocephalus, which was progressive for at least 30 days after birth. The authors identified damage to the germinal cells along the ventricle wall and occlusion of the third ventricle as the cause of hydrocephalus. Pharmacological blockade with Ki16425, a receptor antagonist of LPA1 and LPA3, prevented the hydrocephalus [270]. The pathologic features in this mouse model resemble those in human fetal hydrocephalus caused by cryptic hemorrhage [271] and prematurity associated germinal matrix hemorrhage [272]. LPA from blood is postulated to disrupt the germinal zone. More experimental work is needed to determine if this can be developed into a practical clinical therapy for premature infants with intraventricular hemorrhage [273].

The H-Tx rat has inherited hydrocephalus that is caused by aqueduct stenosis, which develops around 18 days gestation [274]. The genetic cause of this partially penetrant disorder is not yet known [275]. Maternal administration (subcutaneous) of folic acid aggravates the incidence of hydrocephalus while a mixture of folinic acid and tetrahydrofolate significantly reduces the incidence of hydrocephalus. Various experiments led to the conclusion that folate imbalance is responsible for the defects that lead to this form of early-onset hydrocephalus [276].

Cell transplantation

Although cell transplantation is not, strictly speaking, a non-surgical intervention, it is mentioned here because it is not a shunt intervention. In one experiment, the serotoninergic innervation was destroyed by injection of the toxin 5,7-dehydroxytriptamine into brains of young adult rats, which were then rendered hydrocephalic by injection of kaolin. After 2 weeks, brain cells from 14-day gestation rat embryos were transplanted into the hippocampus; transplanted cells were detected by immunohistochemistry 4 weeks later. In the few animals studied, surviving cells were identified; the authors simply concluded that the hydrocephalic brain is capable of accepting transplanted cells [277]. Intracerebral transplantation of human umbilical cord mesenchymal stem cells was reported in a pair of experiments. Four-day-old rats received bilateral injections of maternal blood into the lateral ventricles, 2 days later MRI was used to evaluate the ventricle size, and then rats were randomized to receive intraventricular stem cells or fibroblasts or vehicle. By 32 days age, stem cell recipients (but not those in the other groups) had attenuation of the ventricle size as well as improved behavior, reduced brain cell death, and reduced reactive astroglial change. Reduced quantity of periventricular microglia and reduced levels of pro-inflammatory cytokines in the CSF and periventricular brain tissue led the authors to speculate that the mesenchymal stem cells reduced the hemorrhage-associated inflammation [278, 279], but this mechanism was not proved.

Conclusions

Hydrocephalus can be modeled in a wide range of animal species by injection of blood or kaolin into the CSF pathway, or by genetic manipulation [280]. Many of the models reflect the pathogenesis of hydrocephalus in human disorders. Several pharmacologic interventions appear to alleviate experimental hydrocephalus over relatively short terms (i.e. weeks). Manipulation of water balance or CSF production by osmotic agents or ion channel antagonists also works transiently in humans. However, poorly controlled clinical studies and rare randomized trials show no overall benefit in the management of hydrocephalic patients. CBF response to acetazolamide challenge appears to have a role as a test for predicting shunt responsiveness in adults with NPH. There may be some opportunity for revisiting acetazolamide with proper dosing in accordance with its pharmacodynamics or development of agents that more selectively inhibit the choroid plexus.

Fibrinolytic agents that hasten the resolution of intraventricular or subarachnoid blood collections do not clearly prevent the development of hydrocephalus in infants or adults. A European survey conducted in 2010 indicated that there remains no consensus on the treatment of infants with post hemorrhagic hydrocephalus;

only a small minority of neonatal care centers (6 %) was using fibrinolytic agents [281, 282]. Nevertheless, attenuation of the iron toxicity (e.g. with deferoxamine) remains a potential target for reduction of the inflammatory and fibrotic reactions that block the CSF pathways after hemorrhage or meningitis. Targeted molecular manipulation of the cellular mechanisms that lead to fibrosis in the leptomeninges (e.g. of TGF beta or pathways) might reduce obstruction to CSF flow through the subarachnoid compartment, thereby preventing the development of hydrocephalus. Once the reactive extracellular matrix molecules are established in the subarachnoid compartment, opportunities for digesting them seem limited.

Modulation of cerebral blood flow through vasoactive agents also seems sensible, but this work remains in the preclinical status. Use of cerebral stimulants to augment compromised neurotransmitter systems is wide open for investigation. Brain protection is also in the early preclinical stages. Minocycline, which acts through multiple molecular routes [283], shows early promise. Anti-oxidant therapies have typically been unsuccessful, or the experiments are limited by drug administration in a clinically irrelevant manner or by inadequate outcome analysis.

Perhaps surprising, some multifunctional agents that have progressed into clinical trials have not been tested in hydrocephalus. Erythropoietin is a multifunctional molecule that is neuroprotective through its receptor (EpoR) and has systemic anti-inflammatory and angiogenic effects that can reduce brain injury. Several randomized trials are underway to determine its effect in preterm infants [284]. A retrospective analysis of extremely low birth weight infants treated with erythropoietin from 1993 to 1998 indicated that hydrocephalus requiring shunting occurred in 4.5 % of treated survivors and 7.0 % of controls [285]. Other less well-studied agents (e.g. ginsenoside [286]) also deserve attention.

Brain protection has been the Holy Grail for thousands of stroke and trauma experiments, and has almost always failed in translation to the clinical setting [13, 287–291]. Those interested in hydrocephalus must take great care in the preclinical development of proposed therapies. Based upon recommendations from the stroke and brain trauma literature [11–13], we must design robust experiments including the following considerations: (a) the chosen animal model of hydrocephalus must have validity with respect to the human situation of interest (rodent models may be useful for screening but verification should be performed in a larger animal with gyrencephalic brain and voluminous white matter); (b) ventricle size should be measured before and after the intervention (preferably using in vivo imaging); (c) drug assignments should be randomized or organized to ensure that groups are comparable; (d) evaluations must be conducted by blinded investigators; (e) the primary outcome measures must be pre-determined; (f) outcome measures should include a combination of morphological, behavioral, and biochemical parameters; (g) drug administration should mimic the timing, delivery route, and dosage feasible in humans; careful attention must be paid to the pharmacokinetic properties of agents to be tested to ensure an optimal response; blood brain barrier permeability must also be considered because, in general, the blood brain barrier is intact in the hydrocephalic brain [292]; (h) drug administration should not involve pre-ventriculomegaly administration except as proof-of-principle (unless the agent is being used to prevent hydrocephalus in high risk situations); (i) statistical assessment of outcomes should use appropriate corrections for multiple comparisons; (j) candidate drugs should work in multiple species and in multiple laboratories before testing in humans. Unlike stroke and trauma in which most of the damage is initiated within the first few minutes, hydrocephalus is progressive; therefore, in the absence of a shunt intervention or in the circumstance of chronic static hydrocephalus, long-term outcomes may not be possible.

Despite over 5 decades research, no compelling nonsurgical therapies have been developed for hydrocephalus. However, there remain several targets for prevention of hydrocephalus or as a complement to shunting. Ultimately, high quality preclinical experiments should be used to design clinical trials for premature neonates and adults in which ventricle size and need for shunting are included among the main outcome measures. Complex experiments testing augmented recovery or regeneration after shunting have not been attempted, but may be needed to address the clinical fact that some patients ultimately do need a shunt.

Abbreviations

CA: cornu ammonis; CSF: cerebrospinal fluid; ETV: endoscopic third ventriculostomy; GFAP: glial fibrillary acidic protein; ICP: intracranial pressure; IVH: intraventricular hemorrhage; LPA: lysophosphatidic acid; MMP: matrix metalloproteinase; NPH: normal pressure hydrocephalus; TGF-β: transforming growth factor beta; TNF: tumor necrosis factor; tPA: tissue plasminogen activator; TUNEL: terminal deoxynucleotidyl transferase-mediated dUTP nick end labeling; VEGF: vascular endothelial growth factor.

Authors' contributions

DB wrote the main text. DC wrote the section on Brain Protection and designed the Tabular evaluation of experiments. Both authors reviewed the final version. Both authors read and approved the final manuscript.

Author details

[1] Department of Pathology, University of Manitoba; Children's Hospital Research Institute of Manitoba, Diagnostic Services Manitoba, 401 Brodie Centre, 715 McDermot Avenue, Winnipeg, MB R3E 3P5, Canada. [2] Department of Human Anatomy and Cell Science, University of Manitoba, Winnipeg, Canada.

Acknowledgements

Dr. Del Bigio holds the Canada Research Chair in Developmental Neuropathology (funded by the Canadian Institutes of Health Research). Mr. Di Curzio is funded by a studentship from Research Manitoba.

Competing interests

The authors declare that they have no competing interests. Dr. Del Bigio has in the past (>3 years ago) received consultant fees for shunt development projects from Heyer–Schulte Neurocare, Johnson and Johnson Professional Inc. (Codman), and Medtronic.

References

1. Rekate HL. A contemporary definition and classification of hydrocephalus. Semin Pediatr Neurol. 2009;16:9–15.
2. Rekate HL. A consensus on the classification of hydrocephalus: its utility in the assessment of abnormalities of cerebrospinal fluid dynamics. Childs Nerv Syst. 2011;27:1535–41.
3. Aschoff A, Kremer P, Hashemi B, Kunze S. The scientific history of hydrocephalus and its treatment. Neurosurg Rev. 1999;22:67–93.
4. Wu Y, Green NL, Wrensch MR, Zhao S, Gupta N. Ventriculoperitoneal shunt complications in California: 1990–2000. Neurosurgery. 2007;61:557–562, discussion 562–3.
5. Riva-Cambrin J, Kestle JR, Holubkov R, Butler J, Kulkarni AV, Drake J, Whitehead WE, Wellons JC 3rd, Shannon CN, Tamber MS, Limbrick DD, Jr., Rozzelle C, Browd SR, Simon TD: Risk factors for shunt malfunction in pediatric hydrocephalus: a multicenter prospective cohort study. J Neurosurg Pediatr. 2015;1–9.
6. Limbrick DD Jr, Baird LC, Klimo P Jr, Riva-Cambrin J, Flannery AM, Pediatric Hydrocephalus Systematic R, Evidence-Based Guidelines Task F. Pediatric hydrocephalus: systematic literature review and evidence-based guidelines. Part 4: Cerebrospinal fluid shunt or endoscopic third ventriculostomy for the treatment of hydrocephalus in children. J Neurosurg Pediatr. 2014;14(Suppl 1):30–4.
7. Rasul FT, Marcus HJ, Toma AK, Thorne L, Watkins LD. Is endoscopic third ventriculostomy superior to shunts in patients with non-communicating hydrocephalus? A systematic review and meta-analysis of the evidence. Acta Neurochir (Wien). 2013;155:883–9.
8. Tudor KI, Tudor M, McCleery J, Car J. Endoscopic third ventriculostomy (ETV) for idiopathic normal pressure hydrocephalus (iNPH). Cochrane Database Syst Rev. 2015;7:CD010033.
9. Kazui H, Miyajima M, Mori E, Ishikawa M, Investigators S. Lumboperitoneal shunt surgery for idiopathic normal pressure hydrocephalus (SINPHONI-2): an open-label randomised trial. Lancet Neurol. 2015;14:585–94.
10. Del Bigio MR, Kanfer JN, Zhang YW. Myelination delay in the cerebral white matter of immature rats with kaolin-induced hydrocephalus is reversible. J Neuropathol Exp Neurol. 1997;56:1053–66.
11. Fisher M, Feuerstein G, Howells DW, Hurn PD, Kent TA, Savitz SI, Lo EH. Update of the stroke therapy academic industry roundtable preclinical recommendations. Stroke. 2009;40:2244–50.
12. (STAIR) STAIR. Recommendations for standards regarding preclinical neuroprotective and restorative drug development. Stroke. 1999;30:2752–8.
13. Diaz-Arrastia R, Kochanek PM, Bergold P, Kenney K, Marx CE, Grimes CJ, Loh LT, Adam LT, Oskvig D, Curley KC, Salzer W. Pharmacotherapy of traumatic brain injury: state of the science and the road forward: report of the Department of Defense Neurotrauma Pharmacology Workgroup. J Neurotrauma. 2014;31:135–58.
14. Poca MA, Sahuquillo J. Short-term medical management of hydrocephalus. Expert Opin Pharmacother. 2005;6:1525–38.
15. Spector R, Keep RF, Snodgrass SR, Smith QR, Johanson CE. A balanced view of choroid plexus structure and function: focus on adult humans. Exp Neurol. 2015;267:78–86.
16. Lun MP, Monuki ES, Lehtinen MK. Development and functions of the choroid plexus-cerebrospinal fluid system. Nat Rev Neurosci. 2015;16:445–57.
17. Damkier HH, Brown PD, Praetorius J. Cerebrospinal fluid secretion by the choroid plexus. Physiol Rev. 2013;93:1847–92.
18. Nagelhus EA, Ottersen OP. Physiological roles of aquaporin-4 in brain. Physiol Rev. 2013;93:1543–62.
19. Bulat M, Klarica M. Recent insights into a new hydrodynamics of the cerebrospinal fluid. Brain Res Rev. 2011;65:99–112.
20. Jessen NA, Munk AS, Lundgaard I, Nedergaard M. The glymphatic system: a beginner's guide. Neurochem Res. 2015;40:2583.
21. Brinker T, Stopa E, Morrison J, Klinge P. A new look at cerebrospinal fluid circulation. Fluids Barriers CNS. 2014;11:10.
22. Hladky SB, Barrand MA. Mechanisms of fluid movement into, through and out of the brain: evaluation of the evidence. Fluids Barriers CNS. 2014;11:26.
23. Carare RO, Hawkes CA, Weller RO. Afferent and efferent immunological pathways of the brain. Anatomy, function and failure. Brain Behav Immun. 2014;36:9–14.
24. Marriott WM. The use of theobromin sodio salicylate (diuretin) in the treatment of hydrocephalus. Am J Dis Child. 1924;28:479–83.
25. Wise BL, Mathis JL, Wright JH. Experimental use of isosorbide: an oral osmotic agent to lower cerebrospinal pressure and reduce brain bulk. J Neurosurg. 1966;25:183–8.
26. Hayden PW, Foltz EL, Shurtleff DB. Effect of on oral osmotic agent on ventricular fluid pressure of hydrocephalic children. Pediatrics. 1968;41:955–67.
27. Shurtleff DB, Hayden PW. The treatment of hydrocephalus with isosorbide, and oral hyperosmotic agent. J Clin Pharmacol New Drugs. 1972;12:108–14.
28. Shurtleff DB, Hayden PW, Weeks R, Laurence KM. Temporary treatment of hydrocephalus and myelodysplasia with isosorbide: preliminary report. J Pediatr. 1973;83:651–7.
29. Hayden PW, Shurtleff DB. The medical management of hydrocephalus. Dev Med Child Neurol Suppl. 1972;27:52–8.
30. Lorber J. The use of isosorbide in the treatment of hydrocephalus. Dev Med Child Neurol Suppl. 1972;27:87–93.
31. Lorber J. Isosorbide in the medical treatment of infantile hydrocephalus. J Neurosurg. 1973;39:702–11.
32. Lorber J. Isosorbide in treatment of infantile hydrocephalus. Arch Dis Child. 1975;50:431–6.
33. Lorber J, Salfield S, Lonton T. Isosorbide in the management of infantile hydrocephalus. Dev Med Child Neurol. 1983;25:502–11.
34. Liptak GS, Gellerstedt ME, Klionsky N. Isosorbide in the medical management of hydrocephalus in children with myelodysplasia. Dev Med Child Neurol. 1992;34:150–4.
35. Johnson V, Carlson AJ, Johnson A. Studies on the physiological action of glycerol on the animal organism. Am J Physiol. 1933;103:517–34.
36. Cantore G, Guidetti B, Virno M. Oral glycerol for the reduction of intracranial pressure. J Neurosurg. 1964;21:278–83.
37. Hill A, Volpe JJ. Normal pressure hydrocephalus in the newborn. Pediatrics. 1981;68:623–9.
38. Yamanaka R, Koga H, Yamamoto Y, Yamada S, Sano T, Fukushige T. Characteristics of patients with brain metastases from lung cancer in a palliative care center. Support Care Cancer. 2011;19:467–73.
39. Shimoda M, Oda S, Shibata M, Masuko A, Sato O. Change in regional cerebral blood flow following glycerol administration predicts. Clinical result from shunting in normal pressure hydrocephalus. Acta Neurochir (Wien). 1994;129:171–6.
40. Mase M, Ueda Y, Nagai H. Effect of NIK-242 inj. (20 % erythritol) on intracranial pressure in dogs with acute obstructive hydrocephalus. No To Shinkei. 1990;42:79–85.
41. Diringer MN, Edwards DF, Zazulia AR. Hydrocephalus: a previously unrecognized predictor of poor outcome from supratentorial intracerebral hemorrhage. Stroke. 1998;29:1352–7.

42. Tschirgi RD, Frost RW, Taylor JL. Inhibition of cerebrospinal fluid formation by a carbonic anhydrase inhibitor, 2-acetylamino-1,3,4-thiadiazole-5-sulfonamide (diamox). Proc Soc Exp Biol Med. 1954;87:373–6.
43. Maren TH, Robinson B. The pharmacology of acetazolamide as related to cerebrospinal fluid and the treatment of hydrocephalus. Bull Johns Hopkins Hosp. 1960;106:1–24.
44. Domer FR. Effects of diuretics on cerebrospinal fluid formation and potassium movement. Exp Neurol. 1969;24:54–64.
45. Swenson ER: Pharmacology of acute mountain sickness: old drugs and newer thinking. J Appl Physiol 2016;120:204–15.
46. Gao F, Liu F, Chen Z, Hua Y, Keep RF, Xi G. Hydrocephalus after intraventricular hemorrhage: the role of thrombin. J Cereb Blood Flow Metab. 2014;34:489–94.
47. Gao F, Zheng M, Hua Y, Keep RF, Xi G. Acetazolamide attenuates thrombin-induced hydrocephalus. Acta Neurochir Suppl. 2016;121:373–7.
48. Kolecka M, Ondreka N, Moritz A, Kramer M, Schmidt MJ. Effect of acetazolamide and subsequent ventriculo-peritoneal shunting on clinical signs and ventricular volumes in dogs with internal hydrocephalus. Acta Vet Scand. 2015;57:49.
49. Elvidge AR, Branch CL, Thompson GB. Observations in a case of hydrocephalus treated with Diamox. J Neurosurg. 1957;14:628–38.
50. Ricci G, Copaitich T. Trial acetazolamide therapy of hydrocephalus in tuberculous meningitis. Clin Ter. 1959;16:20–32.
51. Huttenlocher PR. Treatment of hydrocephalus with acetazolamide: results in 15 cases. J Pediatr. 1965;66:1023–30.
52. Birzis L, Carter CH, Maren TH. Effects of acetazolamide on CSF pressure and electrolytes in hydrocephalus. Neurology. 1958;8:522–8.
53. Mercuri E, Faundez JC, Cowan F, Dubowitz L. Acetazolamide without frusemide in the treatment of post-haemorrhagic hydrocephalus. Acta Paediatr. 1994;83:1319–21.
54. Miner ME. Acetazolamide treatment of progressive hydrocephalus secondary to intraventricular hemorrhage in a preterm infant. Childs Nerv Syst. 1986;2:105–6.
55. Nalin A, Gatti G: Effects of treatment with acetazolamide (Diamox) in cases of non tumourous hydrocephalus early diagnosed and controlled by encephalography. Acta Univ Carol Med Monogr. 1976:170–3.
56. Cutler RW, Page L, Galicich J, Watters GV. Formation and absorption of cerebrospinal fluid in man. Brain. 1968;91:707–20.
57. Schain RJ. Carbonic anhydrase inhibitors in chronic infantile hydrocephalus. Am J Dis Child. 1969;117:621–5.
58. Mealey J Jr, Barker DT. Failure of oral acetazolamide to avert hydrocephalus in infants with myelomeningocele. J Pediatr. 1968;72:257–9.
59. Aimard G, Vighetto A, Gabet JY, Bret P, Henry E. Acetazolamide: an alternative to shunting in normal pressure hydrocephalus? Preliminary results. Rev Neurol (Paris). 1990;146:437–9.
60. Miyake H, Ohta T, Kajimoto Y, Deguchi J. Diamox challenge test to decide indications for cerebrospinal fluid shunting in normal pressure hydrocephalus. Acta Neurochir (Wien). 1999;141:1187–93.
61. Chang CC, Kuwana N, Ito S, Ikegami T. Impairment of cerebrovascular reactivity to acetazolamide in patients with normal pressure hydrocephalus. Nuclear Med Commun. 2000;21:139–41.
62. Chang CC, Asada H, Mimura T, Suzuki S. A prospective study of cerebral blood flow and cerebrovascular reactivity to acetazolamide in 162 patients with idiopathic normal-pressure hydrocephalus. J Neurosurg. 2009;111:610–7.
63. Yamada SM, Masahira N, Kawanishi Y, Fujimoto Y, Shimizu K. Preoperative acetazolamide SPECT is useful for predicting outcome of shunt operation in idiopathic normal pressure hydrocephalus patients. Clin Nucl Med. 2013;38:671–6.
64. Alperin N, Oliu CJ, Bagci AM, Lee SH, Kovanlikaya I, Adams D, Katzen H, Ivkovic M, Heier L, Relkin N. Low-dose acetazolamide reverses periventricular white matter hyperintensities in iNPH. Neurology. 2014;82:1347–51.
65. Ivkovic M, Reiss-Zimmermann M, Katzen H, Preuss M, Kovanlikaya I, Heier L, Alperin N, Hoffmann KT, Relkin N. MRI assessment of the effects of acetazolamide and external lumbar drainage in idiopathic normal pressure hydrocephalus. Fluids Barriers CNS. 2015;12:9.
66. Supuran CT. Acetazolamide for the treatment of idiopathic intracranial hypertension. Expert Rev Neurother. 2015;15:851–6.
67. Piper RJ, Kalyvas AV, Young AM, Hughes MA, Jamjoom AA, Fouyas IP. Interventions for idiopathic intracranial hypertension. Cochrane Database Syst Rev. 2015;8:CD003434.
68. Miller TB, Wilkinson HA, Rosenfeld SA, Furuta T. Intracranial hypertension and cerebrospinal fluid production in dogs: effects of furosemide. Exp Neurol. 1986;94:66–80.
69. McCarthy KD, Reed DJ. The effect of acetazolamide and furosemide on cerebrospinal fluid production and choroid plexus carbonic anhydrase activity. J Pharmacol Exp Ther. 1974;189:194–201.
70. Lorenzo AV, Hornig G, Zavala LM, Boss V, Welch K. Furosemide lowers intracranial pressure by inhibiting CSF production. Z Kinderchir. 1986;41(Suppl 1):10–2.
71. Vinas F, De Cabrera C, De Vinas MS. Tratamiento de la hidrocefalia con un derivado del acido sulfamoilantranilico. Comunicacion previa. Prensa Med Argent. 1967;54:496–9.
72. Chaplin ER, Goldstein GW, Myerberg DZ, Hunt JV, Tooley WH. Posthemorrhagic hydrocephalus in the preterm infant. Pediatrics. 1980;65:901–9.
73. Shinnar S, Gammon K, Bergman EW Jr, Epstein M, Freeman JM. Management of hydrocephalus in infancy: use of acetazolamide and furosemide to avoid cerebrospinal fluid shunts. J Pediatr. 1985;107:31–7.
74. Libenson MH, Kaye EM, Rosman NP, Gilmore HE. Acetazolamide and furosemide for posthemorrhagic hydrocephalus of the newborn. Pediatr Neurol. 1999;20:185–91.
75. Pouplard F, Pineau P. Use of acetazolamide in external hydrocephalus in infants. Ann Pediatr (Paris). 1990;37:310–2.
76. Kennedy CR, Ayers S, Campbell MJ, Elbourne D, Hope P, Johnson A. Randomized, controlled trial of acetazolamide and furosemide in posthemorrhagic ventricular dilation in infancy: follow-up at 1 year. Pediatrics. 2001;108:597–607.
77. International PHVD Drug Trial Group. International randomised controlled trial of acetazolamide and furosemide in posthaemorrhagic ventricular dilatation in infancy. Lancet. 1998;352:433–40.
78. Whitelaw A, Kennedy CR, Brion LP: Diuretic therapy for newborn infants with posthemorrhagic ventricular dilatation. Cochrane Database Syst Rev. 2001:CD002270.
79. Hack M, Cohen AR. Acetazolamide plus furosemide for periventricular dilatation: lessons for drug therapy in children. Lancet. 1998;352:418–9.
80. Neblett CR, Waltz TA Jr, McNeel DP, Harrison GM. Effect of cardiac glycosides on human cerebrospinal-fluid production. Lancet. 1972;2:1008–9.
81. Allonen H, Anderson KE, Iisalo E, Kanto J, Stromblad LG, Wettrell G. Passage of digoxin into cerebrospinal fluid in man. Acta Pharmacol Toxicol (Copenh). 1977;41:193–202.
82. Bass NH, Fallstrom SP, Lundborg P. Digoxin-induced arrest of the cerebrospinal fluid circulation in the infant rat: implications for medical treatment of hydrocephalus during early postnatal life. Pediatr Res. 1979;13:26–30.
83. Penisson-Besnier I, Cesbron JG, L'Heveder G, Laine-Cessac P, Dubas F. Efficacy of triamterene in hydrocephalus in adults. Presse Med. 1993;22:224–5.
84. Narita K, Sasamoto S, Koizumi S, Okazaki S, Nakamura H, Inoue T, Takeda S. TRPV4 regulates the integrity of the blood-cerebrospinal fluid barrier and modulates transepithelial protein transport. FASEB J. 2015;29:2247–59.
85. Gattone V, Blazer-Yost B: Use of TRPV4 antagonists to ameliorate hydrocephalus and related materials and methods. WO 2014089013 A1. USA: Indiana University Research And Technology Corporation; 2014.
86. Lindvall-Axelsson M, Hedner P, Owman C. Corticosteroid action on choroid plexus: reduction in Na+ –K+ –ATPase activity, choline transport capacity, and rate of CSF formation. Exp Brain Res. 1989;77:605–10.
87. Weiss MH, Nulsen FE. The effect of glucocorticoids on CSF flow in dogs. J Neurosurg. 1970;32:452–8.
88. Sato O. The effect of dexamethasone on cerebrospinal fluid production rate in the dog. No To Shinkei. 1967;19:485–92.
89. Gomez-Sanchez CE, de Rodriguez AF, Romero DG, Estess J, Warden MP, Gomez-Sanchez MT, Gomez-Sanchez EP. Development of a panel of monoclonal antibodies against the mineralocorticoid receptor. Endocrinology. 2006;147:1343–8.
90. Fattal-Valevski A, Beni-Adani L, Constantini S. Short-term dexamethasone treatment for symptomatic slit ventricle syndrome. Childs Nerv Syst. 2005;21:981–4.
91. Dandy WE. Extirpation of the choroid plexus of the lateral ventricles in communicating hydrocephalus. Ann Surg. 1918;68:569–79.
92. Warf BC. Comparison of endoscopic third ventriculostomy alone and combined with choroid plexus cauterization in infants younger than

1 year of age: a prospective study in 550 African children. J Neurosurg. 2005;103:475–81.
93. Weiss MH, Roessmann U. Radioactive tissue changes induced to control experimental hydrocephalus. J Neurosurg. 1972;36:266–9.
94. Weiss MH, Nulsen FE, Kaufman B. Selective radionecrosis of the choroid plexus for control of experimental hydrocephalus. J Neurosurg. 1972;36:270–5.
95. Rish BL, Meacham WF. Experimental study of the intraventricular instillation of radioactive gold. J Neurosurg. 1967;27:15–20.
96. Bardfeld PA, Shulman K. Rhenium-188 therapy of experimental hydrocephalus. Exp Neurol. 1976;50:777–85.
97. Bernstein GA, Fingerhut AG, Becker D. Pertechnetate in the treatment of hydrocephalus. J Nuc Med. 1969;10:322.
98. Christensen J. Gonzalez Toledo EC: Radioisotope treatment of hydrocephalus. Preliminary report. Arch Fund Roux Ocefa. 1971;5:87–8.
99. Surash S, Nemeth P, Chakrabarty A, Chumas P. The conjugation of an AQP1-directed immunotoxin in the study of site-directed therapy within the CNS. Childs Nerv Syst. 2011;27:811–8.
100. Timothy J, Chumas P, Chakrabarty A, Drake JM, Morrison E. Destruction of choroid plexus cells in vitro: a new concept for the treatment of hydrocephalus? Neurosurgery. 2004;54:727–32.
101. Halperin JJ, Kurlan R, Schwalb JM, Cusimano MD, Gronseth G, Gloss D. Practice guideline: idiopathic normal pressure hydrocephalus: response to shunting and predictors of response: report of the guideline development, dissemination, and implementation subcommittee of the American academy of neurology. Neurology. 2015;85:2063–71.
102. Strahle J, Garton HJ, Maher CO, Muraszko KM, Keep RF, Xi G. Mechanisms of hydrocephalus after neonatal and adult intraventricular hemorrhage. Transl Stroke Res. 2012;3:25–38.
103. Berman PH, Banker BQ. Neonatal meningitis. A clinical and pathological study of 29 cases. Pediatrics. 1966;38:6–24.
104. Cherian S, Whitelaw A, Thoresen M, Love S. The pathogenesis of neonatal post-hemorrhagic hydrocephalus. Brain Pathol. 2004;14:305–11.
105. Massicotte EM, Del Bigio MR. Human arachnoid villi response to subarachnoid hemorrhage: possible relationship to chronic hydrocephalus. J Neurosurg. 1999;91:80–4.
106. Sajant J, Heikkinen E, Majamaa K. Rapid induction of meningeal collagen synthesis in the cerebral cisternal and ventricular compartments after subarachnoid hemorrhage. Acta Neurochir (Wien). 2001;143:821–6.
107. Pepper MS. Role of the matrix metalloproteinase and plasminogen activator-plasmin systems in angiogenesis. Arterioscler Thromb Vasc Biol. 2001;21:1104–17.
108. Keramati M, Mianroodi RA, Memarnejadian A, Mirzaie A, Sazvari S, Aslani MM, Roohvand F. Towards a superior streptokinase for fibrinolytic therapy of vascular thrombosis. Cardiovasc Hematol Agents Med Chem. 2013;11:218–29.
109. Gurman P, Miranda OR, Nathan A, Washington C, Rosen Y, Elman NM. Recombinant tissue plasminogen activators (rtPA): a review. Clin Pharmacol Ther. 2015;97:274–85.
110. Lemarchant S, Docagne F, Emery E, Vivien D, Ali C, Rubio M. tPA in the injured central nervous system: different scenarios starring the same actor? Neuropharmacology. 2012;62:749–56.
111. Julow J. Prevention of subarachnoid fibrosis after subarachnoid haemorrhage with urokinase. Scanning electron microscopic study in the dog. Acta Neurochir (Wien). 1979;51:51–63.
112. Julow J, Ishii M, Iwabuchi T. Scanning electron microscopy of the subarachnoid macrophages after subarachnoid haemorrhage, and their possible role in the formation of subarachnoid fibrosis. Acta Neurochir (Wien). 1979;50:273–80.
113. Pang D, Sclabassi RJ, Horton JA. Lysis of intraventricular blood clot with urokinase in a canine model: Part 3. Effects of intraventricular urokinase on clot lysis and posthemorrhagic hydrocephalus. Neurosurgery. 1986;19:553–72.
114. Brinker T, Seifert V, Dietz H. Subacute hydrocephalus after experimental subarachnoid hemorrhage: its prevention by intrathecal fibrinolysis with recombinant tissue plasminogen activator. Neurosurgery. 1992;31:306–11.
115. Mayfrank L, Kissler J, Raoofi R, Delsing P, Weis J, Kuker W, Gilsbach JM. Ventricular dilatation in experimental intraventricular hemorrhage in pigs. Characterization of cerebrospinal fluid dynamics and the effects of fibrinolytic treatment. Stroke. 1997;28:141–8.
116. Mayfrank L, Kim Y, Kissler J, Delsing P, Gilsbach JM, Schroder JM, Weis J. Morphological changes following experimental intraventricular haemorrhage and intraventricular fibrinolytic treatment with recombinant tissue plasminogen activator. Acta Neuropathol. 2000;100:561–7.
117. Gaberel T, Montagne A, Lesept F, Gauberti M, Lemarchand E, Orset C, Goulay R, Bertrand T, Emery E, Vivien D. Urokinase versus Alteplase for intraventricular hemorrhage fibrinolysis. Neuropharmacology. 2014;85:158–65.
118. Hudgins RJ, Boydston WR, Hudgins PA, Adler SR. Treatment of intraventricular hemorrhage in the premature infant with urokinase. A preliminary report. Pediatr Neurosurg. 1994;20:190–7.
119. Hudgins RJ, Boydston WR, Hudgins PA, Morris R, Adler SM, Gilreath CL. Intrathecal urokinase as a treatment for intraventricular hemorrhage in the preterm infant. Pediatr Neurosurg. 1997;26:281–7.
120. Hansen AR, Volpe JJ, Goumnerova LC, Madsen JR. Intraventricular urokinase for the treatment of posthemorrhagic hydrocephalus. Pediatr Neurol. 1997;17:213–7.
121. Whitelaw A, Mowinckel MC, Abildgaard U. Low levels of plasminogen in cerebrospinal fluid after intraventricular haemorrhage: a limiting factor for clot lysis? Acta Paediatr. 1995;84:933–6.
122. Whitelaw A, Saliba E, Fellman V, Mowinckel MC, Acolet D, Marlow N. Phase I study of intraventricular recombinant tissue plasminogen activator for treatment of posthaemorrhagic hydrocephalus. Arch Dis Child Fetal Neonatal Ed. 1996;75:F20–6.
123. Whitelaw A, Pople I, Cherian S, Evans D, Thoresen M. Phase 1 trial of prevention of hydrocephalus after intraventricular hemorrhage in newborn infants by drainage, irrigation, and fibrinolytic therapy. Pediatrics. 2003;111:759–65.
124. Whitelaw A, Evans D, Carter M, Thoresen M, Wroblewska J, Mandera M, Swietlinski J, Simpson J, Hajivassiliou C, Hunt LP, Pople I. Randomized clinical trial of prevention of hydrocephalus after intraventricular hemorrhage in preterm infants: brain-washing versus tapping fluid. Pediatrics. 2007;119:e1071.
125. Whitelaw A, Jary S, Kmita G, Wroblewska J, Musialik-Swietlinska E, Mandera M, Hunt L, Carter M, Pople I. Randomized trial of drainage, irrigation and fibrinolytic therapy for premature infants with posthemorrhagic ventricular dilatation: developmental outcome at 2 years. Pediatrics. 2010;125:e852–8.
126. Jary S, De Carli A, Ramenghi LA, Whitelaw A. Impaired brain growth and neurodevelopment in preterm infants with posthaemorrhagic ventricular dilatation. Acta Paediatr. 2012;101:743–8.
127. Whitelaw A, Rivers RP, Creighton L, Gaffney P. Low dose intraventricular fibrinolytic treatment to prevent posthaemorrhagic hydrocephalus. Arch Dis Child. 1992;67:12–4.
128. Luciano R, Velardi F, Romagnoli C, Papacci P, De Stefano V, Tortorolo G. Failure of fibrinolytic endoventricular treatment to prevent neonatal post-haemorrhagic hydrocephalus. A case-control trial. Childs Nerv Syst. 1997;13:73–6.
129. Yapicioglu H, Narli N, Satar M, Soyupak S, Altunbasak S. Intraventricular streptokinase for the treatment of posthaemorrhagic hydrocephalus of preterm. J Clin Neurosci. 2003;10:297–9.
130. Haines SJ, Lapointe M. Fibrinolytic agents in the management of posthemorrhagic hydrocephalus in preterm infants: the evidence. Childs Nerv Syst. 1999;15:226–34.
131. Whitelaw A, Odd D. Intraventricular streptokinase after intraventricular hemorrhage in newborn infants. Cochrane Database Syst Rev. 2007;4:CD000498.
132. Todo T, Usui M, Takakura K. Treatment of severe intraventricular hemorrhage by intraventricular infusion of urokinase. J Neurosurg. 1991;74:81–6.
133. Tung MYY, Ong PL, Seow WT, Tan KK. A study on the efficacy of intraventricular urokinase in the treatment of intraventricular haemorrhage. Br J Neurosurg. 1998;12:234–9.
134. Torres A, Plans G, Martino J, Godino O, Garcia I, Gracia B, Acebes JJ. Fibrinolytic therapy in spontaneous intraventricular haemorrhage: efficacy and safety of the treatment. Br J Neurosurg. 2008;22:269–74.
135. Wang B, Huang Q, Liu H, Yang H: Intrathecal injection of urokinase: a promising therapeutic method for acute hydrocephalus? Med Hypotheses. 2009;74:955.

136. Mayfrank L, Lippitz B, Groth M, Bertalanffy H, Gilsbach JM. Effect of recombinant tissue plasminogen activator on clot lysis and ventricular dilatation in the treatment of severe intraventricular haemorrhage. Acta Neurochir (Wien). 1993;122:32–8.
137. Staykov D, Huttner HB, Struffert T, Ganslandt O, Doerfler A, Schwab S, Bardutzky J. Intraventricular fibrinolysis and lumbar drainage for ventricular hemorrhage. Stroke. 2009;40:3275–80.
138. Staykov D, Huttner HB, Lunkenheimer J, Volbers B, Struffert T, Doerfler A, Ganslandt O, Juettler E, Schwab S, Bardutzky J. Single versus bilateral external ventricular drainage for intraventricular fibrinolysis in severe ventricular haemorrhage. J Neurol Neurosurg Psychiatry. 2010;81:105–8.
139. Staykov D, Wagner I, Volbers B, Huttner HB, Doerfler A, Schwab S, Bardutzky J. Dose effect of intraventricular fibrinolysis in ventricular hemorrhage. Stroke. 2011;42:2061–4.
140. Ramakrishna R, Sekhar LN, Ramanathan D, Temkin N, Hallam D, Ghodke BV, Kim LJ. Intraventricular tissue plasminogen activator for the prevention of vasospasm and hydrocephalus after aneurysmal subarachnoid hemorrhage. Neurosurgery. 2010;67:110–7.
141. Ziai WC, Tuhrim S, Lane K, McBee N, Lees K, Dawson J, Butcher K, Vespa P, Wright DW, Keyl PM, Mendelow AD, Kase C, Wijman C, Lapointe M, John S, Thompson R, Thompson C, Mayo S, Reilly P, Janis S, Awad I, Hanley DF, Investigators CI. A multicenter, randomized, double-blinded, placebo-controlled phase III study of Clot Lysis Evaluation of Accelerated Resolution of Intraventricular Hemorrhage (Clear III). Int J Stroke. 2014;9:536–42.
142. Dey M, Stadnik A, Riad F, Zhang L, McBee N, Kase C, Carhuapoma JR, Ram M, Lane K, Ostapkovich N, Aldrich F, Aldrich C, Jallo J, Butcher K, Snider R, Hanley D, Ziai W, Awad IA, Investigators CIT. Bleeding and infection with external ventricular drainage: a systematic review in comparison with adjudicated adverse events in the ongoing Clot Lysis Evaluating Accelerated Resolution of Intraventricular Hemorrhage Phase III (CLEAR-III IHV) trial. Neurosurgery. 2015;76:291–300 **(discussion 301)**.
143. Whitelaw A, Aquilina K. Management of posthaemorrhagic ventricular dilatation. Arch Dis Child Fetal Neonatal Ed. 2012;97:F229–3.
144. Shooman D, Portess H, Sparrow O. A review of the current treatment methods for posthaemorrhagic hydrocephalus of infants. Cerebrospinal Fluid Res. 2009;6:1.
145. Mazzola CA, Choudhri AF, Auguste KI, Limbrick DD Jr, Rogido M, Mitchell L, Flannery AM. Pediatric hydrocephalus: systematic literature review and evidence-based guidelines Part 2 Management of posthemorrhagic hydrocephalus in premature infants. J Neurosurg Pediatr. 2014;14(Suppl 1):8–23.
146. Shi L, Xu L, Shi L, Brandon D, Chen S, Zhang J: Intraventricular recombinant tissue plasminogen activator in treatment of aneurysmal intraventricular hemorrhage: a meta-analysis. Curr Drug Targets 2015 [Epub ahead of print].
147. Gerner ST, Kuramatsu JB, Abel H, Kloska SP, Lucking H, Eyupoglu IY, Doerfler A, Schwab S, Huttner HB. Intraventricular fibrinolysis has no effects on shunt dependency and functional outcome in endovascular-treated aneurysmal SAH. Neurocrit Care. 2014;21:435–43.
148. Kramer AH, Jenne CN, Zygun DA, Roberts DJ, Hill MD, Holodinsky JK, Todd S, Kubes P, Wong JH. Intraventricular fibrinolysis with tissue plasminogen activator is associated with transient cerebrospinal fluid inflammation: a randomized controlled trial. J Cereb Blood Flow Metab. 2015;35:1241–8.
149. Scheld WM, Dacey RG, Winn HR, Welsh JE, Jane JA, Sande MA. Cerebrospinal fluid outflow resistance in rabbits with experimental meningitis. Alterations with penicillin and methylprednisolone. J Clin Invest. 1980;66:243–53.
150. Wilkinson HA, Wilson RB, Patel PP, Esmaili M. Corticosteroid therapy of experimental hydrocephalus after intraventricular-subarachnoid haemorrhage. J Neurol Neurosurg Psychiatry. 1974;37:224–9.
151. Julow J. The influence of dexamethasone on subarachnoid fibrosis after subarachnoid haemorrhage Scanning electron microscopic study in the dog. Acta Neurochir (Wien). 1979;51:43–51.
152. Brouwer MC, McIntyre P, Prasad K, van de Beek D. Corticosteroids for acute bacterial meningitis. Cochrane Database Syst Rev. 2015;9:CD004405.
153. Sporrborn JL, Knudsen GB, Solling M, Seieroe K, Farre A, Lindhardt BO, Benfield T, Brandt CT. Brain ventricular dimensions and relationship to outcome in adult patients with bacterial meningitis. BMC Infect Dis. 2015;15:367.
154. Critchley JA, Young F, Orton L, Garner P. Corticosteroids for prevention of mortality in people with tuberculosis: a systematic review and meta-analysis. Lancet Infect Dis. 2013;13:223–37.
155. Prasad K, Singh MB: Corticosteroids for managing tuberculous meningitis. *Cochrane Database Syst Rev* 2008:CD002244.
156. Schoeman JF, Van Zyl LE, Laubscher JA, Donald PR. Effect of corticosteroids on intracranial pressure, computed tomographic findings, and clinical outcome in young children with tuberculous meningitis. Pediatrics. 1997;99:226–31.
157. Shah I, Meshram L. High dose versus low dose steroids in children with tuberculous meningitis. J Clin Neurosci. 2014;21:761–4.
158. Rigante D, Ansuini V, Caldarelli M, Bertoni B, La Torraca I, Stabile A. Hydrocephalus in CINCA syndrome treated with anakinra. Childs Nerv Syst. 2006;22:334.
159. Kitazawa K, Tada T. Elevation of transforming growth factor-beta 1 level in cerebrospinal fluid of patients with communicating hydrocephalus after subarachnoid hemorrhage. Stroke. 1994;25:1400–4.
160. Douglas MR, Daniel M, Lagord C, Akinwunmi J, Jackowski A, Cooper C, Berry M, Logan A. High CSF transforming growth factor beta levels after subarachnoid haemorrhage: association with chronic communicating hydrocephalus. J Neurol Neurosurg Psychiatry. 2009;80:545–50.
161. Whitelaw A, Christie S, Pople I. Transforming growth factor-beta1: a possible signal molecule for posthemorrhagic hydrocephalus? Pediatr Res. 1999;46:576–80.
162. Heep A, Stoffel-Wagner B, Bartmann P, Benseler S, Schaller C, Groneck P, Obladen M, Felderhoff-Mueser U. Vascular endothelial growth factor and transforming growth factor-beta1 are highly expressed in the cerebrospinal fluid of premature infants with posthemorrhagic hydrocephalus. Pediatr Res. 2004;56:768–74.
163. Kaestner S, Dimitriou I. TGF beta1 and TGF beta2 and their role in posthemorrhagic hydrocephalus following SAH and IVH. J Neurol Surg A Cent Eur Neurosurg. 2013;74:279–84.
164. Cherian S, Thoresen M, Silver IA, Whitelaw A, Love S. Transforming growth factor-betas in a rat model of neonatal posthaemorrhagic hydrocephalus. Neuropathol Appl Neurobiol. 2004;30:585–600.
165. Kanaji M, Tada T, Kobayashi S. A murine model of communicating hydrocephalus: role of TGF-beta1. J Clin Neurosci. 1997;4:51–6.
166. Tada T, Kanaji M, Kobayashi S. Induction of communicating hydrocephalus in mice by intrathecal injection of human recombinant transforming growth factor-beta 1. J Neuroimmunol. 1994;50:153–8.
167. Nitta J, Tada T. Ultramicroscopic structures of the leptomeninx of mice with communicating hydrocephalus induced by human recombinant transforming growth factor-beta 1. Neurol Med Chir (Tokyo). 1998;38:819–24.
168. Tada T, Zhan H, Tanaka Y, Hongo K, Matsumoto K, Nakamura T. Intraventricular administration of hepatocyte growth factor treats mouse communicating hydrocephalus induced by transforming growth factor beta1. Neurobiol Dis. 2006;21:576–86.
169. Galbreath E, Kim SJ, Park K, Brenner M, Messing A. Overexpression of TGF-beta 1 in the central nervous system of transgenic mice results in hydrocephalus. J Neuropathol Exp Neurol. 1995;54:339–49.
170. Wyss-Coray T, Feng L, Masliah E, Ruppe MD, Lee HS, Toggas SM, Rockenstein EM, Mucke L. Increased central nervous system production of extracellular matrix components and development of hydrocephalus in transgenic mice overexpressing transforming growth factor-beta 1. Am J Pathol. 1995;147:53–67.
171. Moinuddin SM, Tada T. Study of cerebrospinal fluid flow dynamics in TGF-beta 1 induced chronic hydrocephalic mice. Neurol Res. 2000;22:215–22.
172. Hayashi N, Leifer DW, Cohen AR. Chronologic changes of cerebral ventricular size in a transgenic model of hydrocephalus. Pediatr Neurosurg. 2000;33:182–7.
173. Cohen AR, Leifer DW, Zechel M, Flaningan DP, Lewin JS, Lust WD. Characterization of a model of hydrocephalus in transgenic mice. J Neurosurg. 1999;91:978–88.
174. Aquilina K, Hobbs C, Tucker A, Whitelaw A, Thoresen M. Do drugs that block transforming growth factor beta reduce posthaemorrhagic ventricular dilatation in a neonatal rat model? Acta Paediatr 2008;97:1181–6.

175. Li T, Zhang P, Yuan B, Zhao D, Chen Y, Zhang X. Thrombin-induced TGF-beta1 pathway: a cause of communicating hydrocephalus post subarachnoid hemorrhage. Int J Mol Med. 2013;31:660–6.
176. Botfield H, Gonzalez AM, Abdullah O, Skjolding AD, Berry M, McAllister JP 2nd, Logan A. Decorin prevents the development of juvenile communicating hydrocephalus. Brain. 2013;136:2842–58.
177. Yan H, Chen Y, Li L, Jiang J, Wu G, Zuo Y, Zhang JH, Feng H, Yan X, Liu F. Decorin alleviated chronic hydrocephalus via inhibiting TGF-beta1/Smad/CTGF pathway after subarachnoid hemorrhage in rats. Brain Res. 2016;1630:241–53.
178. Piersma B, Bank RA, Boersema M. Signaling in fibrosis: tGF-beta, WNT, and YAP/TAZ converge. Front Med. 2015;2:59.
179. Xu H, Xu B, Wang Z, Tan G, Shen S. Inhibition of Wnt/beta-catenin signal is alleviated reactive gliosis in rats with hydrocephalus. Childs Nerv Syst. 2015;31:227.
180. Hatta J, Hatta T, Moritake K, Otani H. Heavy water inhibiting the expression of transforming growth factor-beta1 and the development of kaolin-induced hydrocephalus in mice. J Neurosurg. 2006;104:251–8.
181. Manaenko A, Lekic T, Barnhart M, Hartman R, Zhang JH. Inhibition of transforming growth factor-beta attenuates brain injury and neurological deficits in a rat model of germinal matrix hemorrhage. Stroke. 2014;45:828–34.
182. Darwish SF, El-Bakly WM, El-Naga RN, Awad AS, El-Demerdash E. Antifibrotic mechanism of deferoxamine in concanavalin A induced-liver fibrosis: impact on interferon therapy. Biochem Pharmacol. 2015;98:231–42.
183. Belur PK, Chang JJ, He S, Emanuel BA, Mack WJ. Emerging experimental therapies for intracerebral hemorrhage: targeting mechanisms of secondary brain injury. Neurosurg Focus. 2013;34:E9.
184. Zhao J, Chen Z, Xi G, Keep RF, Hua Y. Deferoxamine attenuates acute hydrocephalus after traumatic brain injury in rats. Transl Stroke Res. 2014;5:586–94.
185. Meng H, Li F, Hu R, Yuan Y, Gong G, Hu S, Feng H. Deferoxamine alleviates chronic hydrocephalus after intraventricular hemorrhage through iron chelation and Wnt1/Wnt3a inhibition. Brain Res. 2015;1602:44–52.
186. Chen Q, Tang J, Tan L, Guo J, Tao Y, Li L, Chen Y, Liu X, Zhang JH, Chen Z, Feng H. Intracerebral hematoma contributes to hydrocephalus after intraventricular hemorrhage via aggravating iron accumulation. Stroke. 2015;46:2902.
187. Aya KL, Stern R. Hyaluronan in wound healing: rediscovering a major player. Wound Repair Regen. 2014;22:579–93.
188. Sonnemann KJ, Bement WM. Wound repair: toward understanding and integration of single-cell and multicellular wound responses. Annu Rev Cell Dev Biol. 2011;27:237–63.
189. Vinukonda G, Zia MT, Bhimavarapu BB, Hu F, Feinberg M, Bokhari A, Ungvari Z, Fried VA, Ballabh P. Intraventricular hemorrhage induces deposition of proteoglycans in premature rabbits, but their in vivo degradation with chondroitinase does not restore myelination, ventricle size and neurological recovery. Exp Neurol. 2013;247:630–44.
190. Gourie-Devi M, Satish P. Hyaluronidase as an adjuvant in the treatment of cranial arachnoiditis (hydrocephalus and optochiasmatic arachnoiditis) complicating tuberculous meningitis. Acta Neurol Scand. 1980;62:368–81.
191. Bhagwati SN, George K. Use of intrathecal hyaluronidase in the management of tuberculous meningitis with hydrocephalus. Childs Nerv Syst. 1986;2:20–5.
192. Gegalian L. Use of hyaluronidase in the central nervous system. Surg Neurol. 1979;12:3–5.
193. Schoeman J, Donald P, van Zyl L, Keet M, Wait J. Tuberculous hydrocephalus: comparison of different treatments with regard to ICP, ventricular size and clinical outcome. Dev Med Child Neurol. 1991;33:396–405.
194. Garg RK, Paliwal V, Malhotra HS. Tuberculous optochiasmatic arachnoiditis: a devastating form of tuberculous meningitis. Expert Rev Anti Infect Ther. 2011;9:719–29.
195. Zhang S, Chen D, Huang C, Bao J, Wang Z. Expression of HGF, MMP-9 and TGF-beta1 in the CSF and cerebral tissue of adult rats with hydrocephalus. Int J Neurosci. 2013;123:392–9.
196. Zechel J, Gohil H, Lust WD, Cohen A. Alterations in matrix metalloproteinase-9 levels and tissue inhibitor of matrix metalloproteinases-1 expression in a transforming growth factor-beta transgenic model of hydrocephalus. J Neurosci Res. 2002;69:662–8.
197. Okamoto T, Takahashi S, Nakamura E, Nagaya K, Hayashi T, Shirai M, Fujieda K. Increased expression of matrix metalloproteinase-9 and hepatocyte growth factor in the cerebrospinal fluid of infants with posthemorrhagic hydrocephalus. Early Hum Dev. 2010;86:251–4.
198. Okamoto T, Takahashi S, Nakamura E, Nagaya K, Hayashi T, Shirai M, Fujieda K. Matrix metalloproteinases in infants with posthemorrhagic hydrocephalus. Early Hum Dev. 2008;84:137–9.
199. Yeom KW, Lober RM, Alexander A, Cheshier SH, Edwards MS. Hydrocephalus decreases arterial spin-labeled cerebral perfusion. Am J Neuroradiol. 2014;35:1433–9.
200. Owler BK, Pickard JD. Normal pressure hydrocephalus and cerebral blood flow: a review. Acta Neurol Scand. 2001;104:325–42.
201. Del Bigio MR. Neuropathology and structural changes in hydrocephalus. Dev Disabil Res Rev. 2010;16:16–22.
202. Del Bigio MR. Morphology of astroglial swelling in culture and in the edematous brain: an adaptive response to a disturbed microenvironment. In: Fedoroff S, Juurlink BHJ, Doucette R, editors. Biology and pathology of astrocyte-neuron interactions. New York: Plenum Press; 1993. p. 347–58.
203. Krauss JK, Regel JP, Vach W, Droste DW, Borremans JJ, Mergner T. Vascular risk factors and arteriosclerotic disease in idiopathic normal-pressure hydrocephalus of the elderly. Stroke. 1996;27:24–9.
204. Boon AJ, Tans JT, Delwel EJ, Egeler-Peerdeman SM, Hanlo PW, Wurzer HA, Hermans J. Dutch Normal-Pressure Hydrocephalus Study: the role of cerebrovascular disease. J Neurosurg. 1999;90:221–6.
205. Wagshul ME, Eide PK, Madsen JR. The pulsating brain: a review of experimental and clinical studies of intracranial pulsatility. Fluids Barriers CNS. 2011;8:5.
206. Park EH, Dombrowski S, Luciano M, Zurakowski D, Madsen JR. Alterations of pulsation absorber characteristics in experimental hydrocephalus. J Neurosurg Pediatr. 2010;6:159–70.
207. Fuller CK. Some observations on chronic hydrocephalus with report of a case apparently arrested. Can Med Assoc J. 1927;17:675–7.
208. Del Bigio MR. Calcium-mediated proteolytic damage in white matter of hydrocephalic rats? J Neuropathol Exp Neurol. 2000;59:946–54.
209. Del Bigio MR, Massicotte EM. Protective effect of nimodipine on behavior and white matter of rats with hydrocephalus. J Neurosurg. 2001;94:788–94.
210. Khan OH, Enno T, Del Bigio MR. Magnesium sulfate therapy is of mild benefit to young rats with kaolin-induced hydrocephalus. Pediatr Res. 2003;53:970–6.
211. Khan OH, McPhee LC, Moddemann LN, Del Bigio MR. Calcium antagonism in neonatal rats with kaolin-induced hydrocephalus. J Child Neurol. 2007;22:1161–6.
212. Di Curzio DL, Buist RJ, Del Bigio MR. Reduced subventricular zone proliferation and white matter damage in juvenile ferrets with kaolin-induced hydrocephalus. Exp Neurol. 2013;248:112–28.
213. Nieto Barrera M, Candau Fernandez Mensaque R, Rufo Campos M, Rodriguez Criado G, Barrionuevo Gallo B. El tratamiento de la hidrocefalia infantil con dinitrato de isosorbide [Treatment of infantile hydrocephalus with isosorbide dinitrate]. An Esp Pediatr. 1977;10:843–56.
214. Schmidt JF, Albeck M, Gjerris F. The effect of nimodipine on ICP and CBF in patients with normal-pressure hydrocephalus. Acta Neurochir (Wien). 1990;102:11–3.
215. Olsen KS, Albeck M, Agerlin N, Schmidt JF. The effect of ketanserin on ICP and CBF in patients with normal-pressure hydrocephalus. J Neurosurg Anesthesiol. 1996;8:216–9.
216. Greitz D, Greitz T, Hindmarsh T. A new view on the CSF-circulation with the potential for pharmacological treatment of childhood hydrocephalus. Acta Paediatr. 1997;86:125–32.
217. Nilsson F, Nilsson T, Edvinsson L, Bjorkman S, Nordstrom CH. Effects of dihydroergotamine and sumatriptan on isolated human cerebral and peripheral arteries and veins. Acta Anaesthesiol Scand. 1997;41:1257–62.
218. Andersen AR, Tfelt-Hansen P, Lassen NA. The effect of ergotamine and dihydroergotamine on cerebral blood flow in man. Stroke. 1987;18:120–3.
219. Asgeirsson B, Grande PO, Nordstrom CH, Messeter K, Sjoholm H. Cerebral haemodynamic effects of dihydroergotamine in patients

with severe traumatic brain lesions. Acta Anaesthesiol Scand. 1995;39:922–30.
220. Bundgaard H, von Oettingen G, Jorgensen HA, Jensen K, Cold GE. Effects of dihydroergotamine on intracranial pressure, cerebral blood flow, and cerebral metabolism in patients undergoing craniotomy for brain tumors. J Neurosurg Anesthesiol. 2001;13:195–201.
221. Licht T, Keshet E. Delineating multiple functions of VEGF-A in the adult brain. Cell Mol Life Sci. 2013;70:1727–37.
222. Wittko-Schneider IM, Schneider FT, Plate KH. Brain homeostasis: VEGF receptor 1 and 2-two unequal brothers in mind. Cell Mol Life Sci. 2013;70:1705–25.
223. Yang J, Dombrowski SM, Deshpande A, Krajcir N, Luciano MG. VEGF/VEGFR-2 changes in frontal cortex, choroid plexus, and CSF after chronic obstructive hydrocephalus. J Neurol Sci. 2010;296:39–46.
224. Deshpande A, Dombrowski SM, Leichliter A, Krajcir N, Zingales N, Inoue M, Schenk S, Fukamachi K, Luciano MG. Dissociation between vascular endothelial growth factor receptor-2 and blood vessel density in the caudate nucleus after chronic hydrocephalus. J Cereb Blood Flow Metab. 2009;29:1806–15.
225. Del Bigio MR, Wilson MJ, Enno T. Chronic hydrocephalus in rats and humans: white matter loss and behavior changes. Ann Neurol. 2003;53:337–46.
226. Dombrowski SM, Deshpande A, Dingwall C, Leichliter A, Leibson Z, Luciano MG. Chronic hydrocephalus-induced hypoxia: increased expression of VEGFR-2+ and blood vessel density in hippocampus. Neuroscience. 2008;152:346–59.
227. Yang J, Shanahan KJ, Shriver LP, Luciano MG: Exercise-induced changes of cerebrospinal fluid vascular endothelial growth factor in adult chronic hydrocephalus patients. J Clin Neurosci. 2015, in press.
228. Shim JW, Sandlund J, Han CH, Hameed MQ, Connors S, Klagsbrun M, Madsen JR, Irwin N. VEGF, which is elevated in the CSF of patients with hydrocephalus, causes ventriculomegaly and ependymal changes in rats. Exp Neurol. 2013;247:703–9.
229. Shim JW, Sandlund J, Madsen JR. VEGF: a potential target for hydrocephalus. Cell Tissue Res. 2014;358:667–83.
230. Del Bigio MR. Neuropathological changes caused by hydrocephalus. Acta Neuropathol (Berl). 1993;85:573–85.
231. Wu Q, Chen W, Sinha B, Tu Y, Manning S, Thomas N, Zhou S, Jiang H, Ma H, Kroessler DA, Yao J, Li Z, Inder TE, Wang X. Neuroprotective agents for neonatal hypoxic-ischemic brain injury. Drug Discov Today. 2015;20:1372.
232. Deren KE, Packer M, Forsyth J, Milash B, Abdullah OM, Hsu EW, McAllister JP 2nd. Reactive astrocytosis, microgliosis and inflammation in rats with neonatal hydrocephalus. Exp Neurol. 2010;226:110–9.
233. Ulfig N, Bohl J, Neudorfer F, Rezaie P. Brain macrophages and microglia in human fetal hydrocephalus. Brain Dev. 2004;26:307–15.
234. Marin-Teva JL, Cuadros MA, Martin-Oliva D, Navascues J. Microglia and neuronal cell death. Neuron Glia Biol. 2011;7:25–40.
235. Graeber MB, Streit WJ. Microglia: biology and pathology. Acta Neuropathol. 2010;119:89–105.
236. Fernandes A, Miller-Fleming L, Pais TF. Microglia and inflammation: conspiracy, controversy or control? Cell Mol Life Sci. 2014;71:3969–85.
237. Li C, Yuan K, Schluesener H. Impact of minocycline on neurodegenerative diseases in rodents: a meta-analysis. Rev Neurosci. 2013;24:553–62.
238. Kohler E, Prentice DA, Bates TR, Hankey GJ, Claxton A, van Heerden J, Blacker D. Intravenous minocycline in acute stroke: a randomized, controlled pilot study and meta-analysis. Stroke. 2013;44:2493–9.
239. McAllister JP 2nd, Miller JM. Minocycline inhibits glial proliferation in the H-Tx rat model of congenital hydrocephalus. Cerebrospinal Fluid Res. 2010;7:7.
240. Xu H, Tan G, Zhang S, Zhu H, Liu F, Huang C, Zhang F, Wang Z. Minocycline reduces reactive gliosis in the rat model of hydrocephalus. BMC Neurosci. 2012;13:148.
241. Guo J, Chen Q, Tang J, Zhang J, Tao Y, Li L, Zhu G, Feng H, Chen Z. Minocycline-induced attenuation of iron overload and brain injury after experimental germinal matrix hemorrhage. Brain Res. 2015;1594:115–24.
242. Sanchez AR, Rogers RS 3rd, Sheridan PJ. Tetracycline and other tetracycline-derivative staining of the teeth and oral cavity. Int J Dermatol. 2004;43:709–15.
243. Lacombe P, Mathews PM, Schmidt SD, Breidert T, Heneka MT, Landreth GE, Feinstein DL, Galea E. Effect of anti-inflammatory agents on transforming growth factor beta over-expressing mouse brains: a model revised. J Neuroinflammation. 2004;1:11.
244. Kurt G, Cemil B, Borcek AO, Borcek P, Akyurek N, Sepici A, Ceviker N. Infliximab administration reduces neuronal apoptosis on the optic pathways in a rabbit hydrocephalus model: a preliminary report. Br J Neurosurg. 2010;24:275–9.
245. Del Bigio MR, Khan OH, da Silva Lopes L, Juliet PA. Cerebral white matter oxidation and nitrosylation in young rodents with kaolin-induced hydrocephalus. J Neuropathol Exp Neurol. 2012;71:274–88.
246. Tarnaris A, Watkins LD, Kitchen ND. Biomarkers in chronic adult hydrocephalus. Cerebrospinal Fluid Res. 2006;3:11.
247. Etus V, Gazioglu N, Belce A. N-acetylcystein reduces cerebral lipid peroxidation in a rat model of infantile hydrocephalus. J Neurol Sci (Turk). 2001;18:2.
248. Etus V, Altug T, Belce A, Ceylan S. Green tea polyphenol (-)-epigallocatechin gallate prevents oxidative damage on periventricular white matter of infantile rats with hydrocephalus. Tohoku J Exp Med. 2003;200:203–9.
249. Turgut M, Erdogan S, Ergin K, Serter M. Melatonin ameliorates blood-brain barrier permeability, glutathione, and nitric oxide levels in the choroid plexus of the infantile rats with kaolin-induced hydrocephalus. Brain Res. 2007;1175:117–25.
250. Di Curzio DL, Turner-Brannen E, Del Bigio MR. Oral antioxidant therapy for juvenile rats with kaolin-induced hydrocephalus. Fluids Barriers CNS. 2014;11:23.
251. Catalao CH, Correa DA, Saito ST, Lopes LD. Camellia sinensis neuroprotective role in experimentally induced hydrocephalus in Wistar rats. Childs Nerv Syst. 2013;30:591.
252. Feng S, Yang Q, Liu M, Li W, Yuan W, Zhang S, Wu B, Li J: Edaravone for acute ischaemic stroke. Cochrane Database Syst Rev. 2011:CD007230.
253. Chen Z, Zhang J, Chen Q, Guo J, Zhu G, Feng H. Neuroprotective effects of edaravone after intraventricular hemorrhage in rats. NeuroReport. 2014;25:635–40.
254. Wenk GL, Parsons CG, Danysz W. Potential role of N-methyl-D-aspartate receptors as executors of neurodegeneration resulting from diverse insults: focus on memantine. Behav Pharmacol. 2006;17:411–24.
255. Cabuk B, Etus V, Bozkurt SU, Sav A, Ceylan S. Neuroprotective effect of memantine on hippocampal neurons in infantile rat hydrocephalus. Turk Neurosurg. 2011;21:352–8.
256. Taveira KV, Carraro KT, Catalao CH, Lda Lopes S. Morphological and morphometric analysis of the hippocampus in Wistar rats with experimental hydrocephalus. Pediatr Neurosurg. 2012;48:163–7.
257. Shim I, Ha Y, Chung JY, Lee HJ, Yang KH, Chang JW. Association of learning and memory impairments with changes in the septohippocampal cholinergic system in rats with kaolin-induced hydrocephalus. Neurosurgery. 2003;53:416–25.
258. Ding Y, McAllister JP II, Yao B, Yan N, Canady AI. Neuron tolerance during hydrocephalus. Neuroscience. 2001;106:659–67.
259. Kokturk S, Ceylan S, Etus V, Yasa N, Ceylan S. *Morinda citrifolia* L. (noni) and memantine attenuate periventricular tissue injury of the fourth ventricle in hydrocephalic rabbits. Neural Regen Res. 2013;8:773–82.
260. Khan OH, Enno T, Del Bigio MR. Tacrolimus and cyclosporine A are of no benefit to young rats with kaolin-induced hydrocephalus. Pediatr Neurosurg. 2003;39:309–13.
261. Del Bigio MR, Wang X, Wilson MJ. Sodium channel-blocking agents are not of benefit to rats with kaolin-induced hydrocephalus. Neurosurgery. 2002;51:460–7.
262. Malm J, Kristensen B, Ekstedt J, Wester P. CSF concentration gradients of monoamine metabolites in patients with hydrocephalus. J Neurol Neurosurg Psychiatr. 1994;57:1026–33.
263. Miyake H, Eghwrudjakpor P, Sakamoto T, Kurisaka M, Mori K. Neurotransmitter changes in hydrocephalus: effects of cerebral metabolic activator on kaolin-induced hydrocephalus. In: Matsumoto S, Tamaki N, editors. Hydrocephalus: pathogenesis and treatment. Tokyo: Springer-Verlag; 1991. p. 68–74.
264. Keenan S, Mavaddat N, Iddon J, Pickard JD, Sahakian BJ. Effects of methylphenidate on cognition and apathy in normal pressure hydrocephalus: a case study and review. Br J Neurosurg. 2005;19:46–50.

265. Wheeler GA, Young SA. Use of methylphenidate in a case of mild, inoperative, idiopathic, normal pressure hydrocephalus. Gen Hosp Psychiatry. 1994;16:361–3.
266. Anderson B. Relief of akinetic mutism from obstructive hydrocephalus using bromocriptine and ephedrine. Case report. J Neurosurg. 1992;76:152–5.
267. Mateo-Sierra O, Gutierrez FA, Fernandez-Carballal C, Pinilla D, Mosqueira B, Iza B, Carrillo R. Akinetic mutism related to hydrocephalus and cerebellar surgery treated with bromocriptine and ephedrine. A pathophysiological review. Neurocirugia (Astur). 2005;16:134–141; discussion 141.
268. Mashiko H, Yokoyama H, Matsumoto H, Niwa S. Trazodone for aggression in an adolescent with hydrocephalus. Psychiatry Clin Neurosci. 1996;50:133–6.
269. Owen-Lynch PJ, Draper CE, Mashayekhi F, Bannister CM, Miyan JA. Defective cell cycle control underlies abnormal cortical development in the hydrocephalic Texas rat. Brain. 2003;126:623–31.
270. Yung YC, Mutoh T, Lin ME, Noguchi K, Rivera RR, Choi JW, Kingsbury MA, Chun J. Lysophosphatidic Acid signaling may initiate fetal hydrocephalus. Sci Transl Med. 2011;3:99ra87.
271. Lategan B, Chodirker BN, Del Bigio MR. Fetal hydrocephalus caused by cryptic intraventricular hemorrhage. Brain Pathol. 2010;20:391–8.
272. Del Bigio MR. Cell proliferation in human ganglionic eminence and suppression after prematurity-associated haemorrhage. Brain. 2011;134:1344–61.
273. Stoddard NC, Chun J. Promising pharmacological directions in the world of lysophosphatidic acid signaling. Biomol Ther (Seoul). 2015;23:1–11.
274. Jones HC, Bucknall RM. Inherited prenatal hydrocephalus in the H-Tx rat: a morphological study. Neuropathol Appl Neurobiol. 1988;14:263–74.
275. Jones HC, Depelteau JS, Carter BJ, Lopman BA, Morel L. Genome-wide linkage analysis of inherited hydrocephalus in the H-Tx rat. Mamm Genome. 2001;12:22–6.
276. Cains S, Shepherd A, Nabiuni M, Owen-Lynch PJ, Miyan J. Addressing a folate imbalance in fetal cerebrospinal fluid can decrease the incidence of congenital hydrocephalus. J Neuropathol Exp Neurol. 2009;68:404–16.
277. Tsubokawa T, Katayama Y, Miyazaki S, Ogawa H, Kawamata T, Iwasaki M, Sako Y. Raphe-cell transplantation into the hippocampus of the hydrocephalic rat brain. Brain Inj. 1988;2:67–74.
278. Ahn SY, Chang YS, Sung DK, Sung SI, Yoo HS, Lee JH, Oh WI, Park WS. Mesenchymal stem cells prevent hydrocephalus after severe intraventricular hemorrhage. Stroke. 2013;44:497.
279. Ahn SY, Chang YS, Sung DK, Sung SI, Yoo HS, Im GH, Choi SJ, Park WS. Optimal route for mesenchymal stem cells transplantation after severe intraventricular hemorrhage in newborn rats. PLoS One. 2015;10:e0132919.
280. Del Bigio MR. Future directions for therapy of childhood hydrocephalus: a view from the laboratory. Pediatr Neurosurg. 2001;34:172–81.
281. Brouwer AJ, Brouwer MJ, Groenendaal F, Benders MJ, Whitelaw A, de Vries LS. European perspective on the diagnosis and treatment of posthaemorrhagic ventricular dilatation. Arch Dis Child Fetal Neonatal Ed. 2012;97:F50–5.
282. Brouwer AJ, Groenendaal F, Benders MJ, de Vries LS. Early and late complications of germinal matrix-intraventricular haemorrhage in the preterm infant: what is new? Neonatology. 2014;106:296–303.
283. Garrido-Mesa N, Zarzuelo A, Galvez J. Minocycline: far beyond an antibiotic. Br J Pharmacol. 2013;169:337–52.
284. Juul SE, Pet GC. Erythropoietin and neonatal neuroprotection. Clin Perinatol. 2015;42:469–81.
285. Neubauer AP, Voss W, Wachtendorf M, Jungmann T. Erythropoietin improves neurodevelopmental outcome of extremely preterm infants. Ann Neurol. 2010;67:657–66.
286. Ye R, Zhao G, Liu X. Ginsenoside Rd for acute ischemic stroke: translating from bench to bedside. Expert Rev Neurother. 2013;13:603–13.
287. Del Zoppo GJ. Why do all drugs work in animals but none in stroke patients? 1. Drugs promoting cerebral blood flow. J Intern Med. 1995;237:79–88.
288. Grotta J. Why do all drugs work in animals but none in stroke patients? 2. Neuroprotective therapy. J Intern Med. 1995;237:89–94.
289. Dirnagl U. Bench to bedside: the quest for quality in experimental stroke research. J Cereb Blood Flow Metab. 2006;26:1465–78.
290. O'Collins VE, Macleod MR, Donnan GA, Horky LL, van der Worp BH, Howells DW. 1,026 experimental treatments in acute stroke. Ann Neurol. 2006;59:467–77.
291. Tosetti P, Hicks RR, Theriault E, Phillips A, Koroshetz W, Draghia-Akli R, Workshop P. Toward an international initiative for traumatic brain injury research. J Neurotrauma. 2013;30:1211–22.
292. Del Bigio MR, Slobodian I, Schellenberg AE, Buist RJ, Kemp-Buors TL. Magnetic resonance imaging indicators of blood-brain barrier and brain water changes in young rats with kaolin-induced hydrocephalus. Fluids Barriers CNS. 2011;8:22.

12

Hyperdynamic CSF motion profiles found in idiopathic normal pressure hydrocephalus and Alzheimer's disease assessed by fluid mechanics derived from magnetic resonance images

Ken Takizawa[1], Mitsunori Matsumae[1*], Naokazu Hayashi[1], Akihiro Hirayama[1], Satoshi Yatsushiro[2,3] and Kagayaki Kuroda[2,3]

Abstract

Background: Magnetic resonance imaging (MRI) does not only ascertain morphological features, but also measures physiological properties such as fluid velocity or pressure gradient. The purpose of this study was to investigate cerebrospinal fluid (CSF) dynamics in patients with morphological abnormalities such as enlarged brain ventricles and subarachnoid spaces. We used a time-resolved three dimensional phase contrast (3D-PC) MRI technique to quantitatively evaluate CSF dynamics in the Sylvian aqueduct of healthy elderly individuals and patients with either idiopathic normal pressure hydrocephalus (iNPH) or Alzheimer's disease (AD) presenting with ventricular enlargement.

Methods: Nineteen healthy elderly individuals, ten iNPH patients, and seven AD patients (all subjects ≥ 60 years old) were retrospectively evaluated 3D-PC MRI. The CSF velocity, pressure gradient, and rotation in the Sylvian aqueduct were quantified and compared between the three groups using Kolmogorov–Smirnov and Mann–Whitney U tests.

Results: There was no statistically significant difference in velocity among the three groups. The pressure gradient was not significantly different between the iNPH and AD groups, but was significantly different between the iNPH group and the healthy controls ($p < 0.001$), and similarly, between the AD group and the healthy controls ($p < 0.001$). Rotation was not significantly different between the iNPH and AD groups, but was significantly different between the iNPH group and healthy controls ($p < 0.001$), and similarly, between the AD group and the healthy controls ($p < 0.001$).

Conclusions: Quantitative analysis of CSF dynamics with time resolved 3D-PC MRI revealed differences and similarities in the Sylvian aqueduct between healthy elderly individuals, iNPH patients, and AD patients. The results showed that CSF motion is in a hyperdynamic state in both iNPH and AD patient groups compared to healthy elderly individuals, and that iNPH patients and AD patients display similar CSF motion profiles.

Keywords: Idiopathic normal pressure hydrocephalus, Alzheimer's disease, Cerebrospinal fluid, Magnetic resonance imaging, Fluid dynamics

*Correspondence: mike@is.icc.u-tokai.ac.jp
[1] Department of Neurosurgery, Tokai University School of Medicine, 143 Shimokasuya, Isehara, Kanagawa 2591193, Japan
Full list of author information is available at the end of the article

Background

The Cerebrospinal fluid (CSF) removes unnecessary substances and heat produced by metabolic activity from the brain parenchyma [1]. Therefore, understanding CSF dynamics is important for evaluating intracranial changes, pathological analysis, and treatment management of idiopathic normal pressure hydrocephalus (iNPH) and Alzheimer's disease (AD) patients. Lately, noninvasive techniques using magnetic resonance imaging (MRI) have become prevalent in the analysis of CSF motion dynamics, and researchers commonly use phase contrast (PC) MR images to understand CSF physiology [2–6]. In the present study, we analyzed CSF motion using PC. Specifically, we used a time-resolved three-dimensional PC (3D-PC) MRI acquisition where the time dimension is added to the anterior–posterior, right–left, and head-foot dimensions in order to quantify and analyze CSF motion in elderly healthy individuals, idiopathic normal pressure hydrocephalus (iNPH) patients, and Alzheimer's disease (AD) patients. In two-dimensional imaging, CSF velocity can only be calculated in-plane. Using 3D-PC, CSF motion can be calculated in three dimensions, and therefore the pressure gradient and rotation of the CSF motion can be measured in addition to velocity. Understanding fluid dynamics is important to determine the pressure gradient and rotation. CSF motion in elderly groups has only been investigated in a small number of studies and there is no consensus on the characteristics of CSF motion in AD patients [3, 7, 8]. In the iNPH study, CSF motion appears to be hyper dynamic [3, 9, 10]. The aim of this study was to compare the CSF dynamics of healthy elderly volunteers with those of AD and iNPH patients.

Methods

This study was conducted with informed consent from volunteers and patients after explaining the purpose of the study in accordance with the ethics regulations of the authors' affiliated institution.

Patients

The patient's characteristics are shown in Table 1. The subjects included seven AD patients (age range 66–89 years), ten iNPH patients (age range 67–87 years), and nineteen healthy elderly volunteers (age range 67–80 years). The iNPH group was selected in accordance with the guidelines outlined by the Japanese Society of Normal Pressure Hydrocephalus [11] and consisted of patients who displayed at least one symptom of the classical medical triad (gait disturbance, cognitive dysfunction, or urinary incontinence) and presented an enlargement of the anterior lateral ventricle horn with an Evans ratio ≥ 0.3, narrowing of high convexity subarachnoid space, and enlargement of the Sylvian fissure [12]. Eight out of ten iNPH patients received a shunting procedure: six received a ventriculo-peritoneal shunt and two patients a lumbo-peritoneal shunt. Gait disturbance improved in all patients, cognitive function improved in four patients, and urinary dysfunction improved in six patients after the shunting procedure. The AD group included individuals with probable AD according to the criteria delineated by the National Institute of Neurological and Communicative Diseases and Stroke/ Alzheimer's Disease and Related Disorders Association [13]. The healthy elderly control group was selected from volunteers recruited at our institution that did not have a history of central nervous system disorders, did not exhibit neurological abnormalities upon examination by neurologists or neurosurgeons, and did not present abnormalities on neurological and standard MRI.

Table 1 Characteristics of the group

	iNPH	AD	Control
Number of subjects	10	7	19
Mean age	73	77	74
Age range	67–87	66–89	67–80
Female	5	5	12

MRI acquisition

A 1.5 Tesla MRI scanner with an eight-channel phased array head and neck surface coil (Gyroscan; Philips, Best, Netherlands) was used. A time resolved 3D-PC MRI sequence was used, providing a 4D velocity field. Flow-encoding directions were head–foot, right–left, and anterior–posterior. A dynamic cine image of one cardiac cycle was created by imaging 32 phases per heartbeat (without interpolation), synchronized with the heartbeat. The imaging parameters were: repetition time, 9.8–16.4 ms; echo time, 6.6–6.7 ms; flip angle, 20°; field of view, 22 × 22 for females and 32 × 32 cm^2 for males; velocity encoding, 5 cm/s for volunteers, 30 cm/s for AD and iNPH patients; acquisition matrix, 1.96 × 1.96 × 1.96 mm^3 (isotropic); sensitivity encoding factor of 2. Ten slices per volume were acquired, using 4–8 pixels to calculate the velocity and pressure gradient, and 12–20 pixels for the rotation. The acquisition time for this sequence was on average 32 min, depending on heart rate. The trigger for timing the 3D-PC was the peripheral pulse, measured from a finger.

Image processing

Pressure gradients were calculated from the velocity data using Navier–Stokes equations. Color-coded CSF velocity vectors, pressure gradients, and rotations were overlaid on T_2-weighted images. All processing was performed on a workstation (Power Mac Pro, Quad-Core Intel Xeon; Apple Inc., Cupertino, CA, USA) with our in-house software, written in Matlab (R2012b; Mathworks, Natick, MA, USA). Regions of interest (ROIs) at both the entry point and outlet point of the Sylvian aqueduct were drawn on sagittal images by the researchers, including a neurosurgery specialist, using an in-house mouse-operated graphical user interface. Partial volume effects caused by the relatively large voxel size (approximately 2 mm) used can lead to segmentation errors on T_2-weighted images. Therefore, a "spatial-based fuzzy clustering" segmentation method [14] was used to reduce partial volume effects.

The principle of this study was based on obtaining velocity and rotation in three-dimensional space (anterior–posterior, right–left, and head–foot directions) using the PC technique. The pressure gradient was then calculated from these velocity data using Navier–Stokes equations. Further details of this method can be found elsewhere [4].

Statistical analysis

CSF velocity and pressure gradient data calculated from the ROIs were represented as box plots. CSF velocities and pressure gradients were compared between groups as nonparametric data using Kolmogorov–Smirnov and

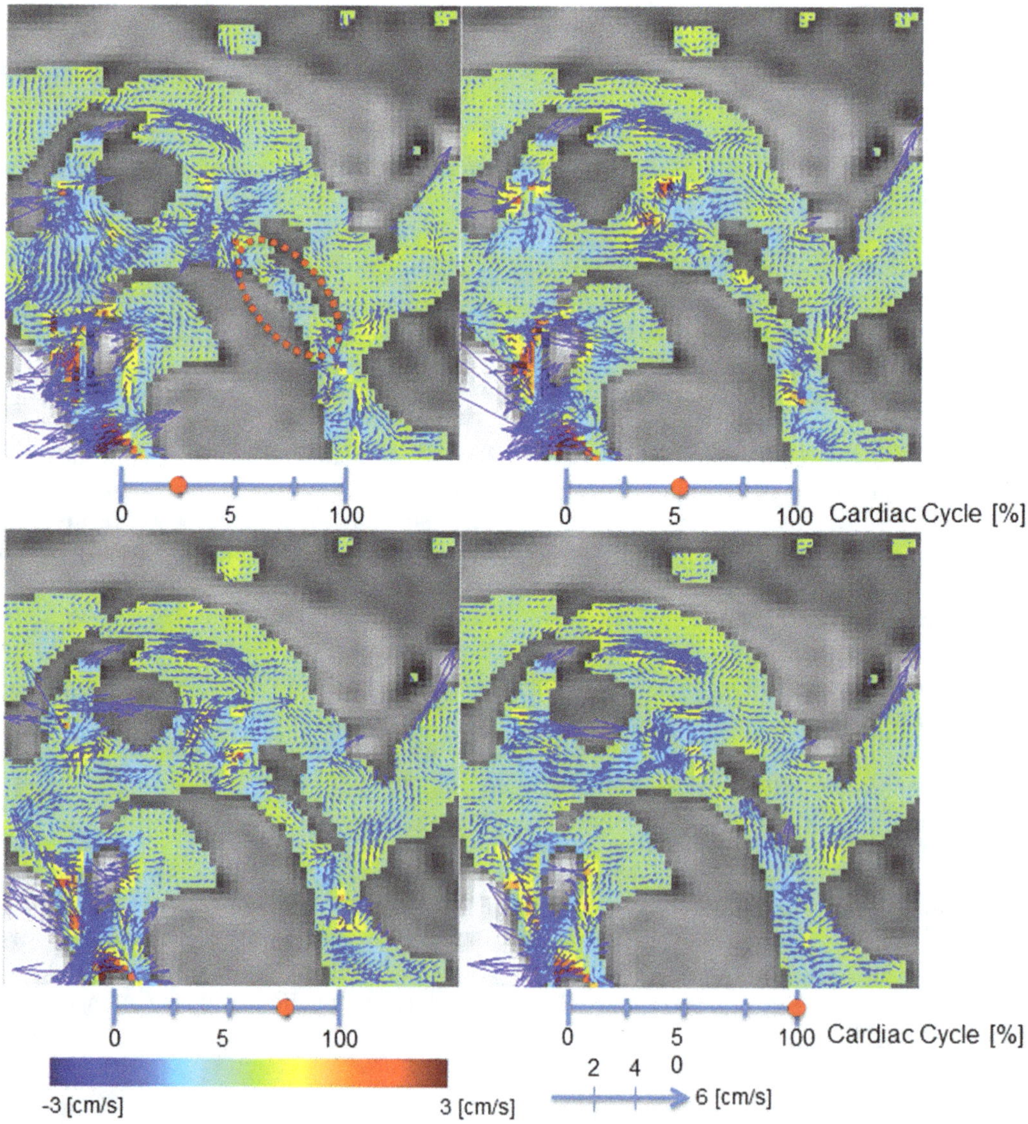

Fig. 1 Velocity mapping of the volunteer by 3D-PC at 4 different stages of the cardiac cycle. In-plane velocities were visualized using vectors and through-plane velocities were visualized using colors. The color-coded CSF velocity field vector was then superimposed onto T_2-weighted images of the stationary tissues. Red circle indicates Sylvian aqueduct

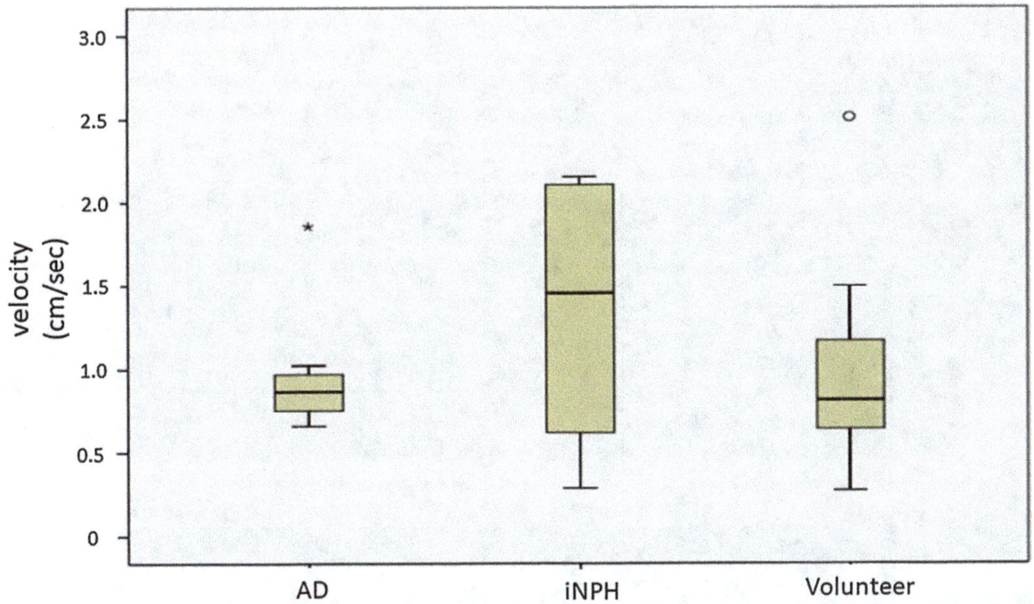

Fig. 2 Box plots of velocity in the Sylvian aqueduct for AD patients, iNPH patients, and healthy elderly volunteers. There were no statistically significant differences between the patient groups and volunteer group. AD Alzheimer's disease, iNPH idiopathic normal pressure hydrocephalus outside values are indicated by a small "o" and far-out values are indicated by an asterisk

Mann–Whitney U tests. All statistical analyses were conducted using SPSS software version 13 (SPSS Japan Inc., Tokyo).

Results

Comparison of velocity between AD patients, iNPH patients, and healthy elderly volunteers

Figure 1 shows velocity images for a 67 year old male volunteer. Figure 2 shows the calculated velocity in the Sylvian aqueduct of AD patients, iNPH patients, and healthy elderly volunteers. There was no statistically significant difference ($p = 0.380$) between the AD (median = 0.868 cm/s) and iNPH groups (median = 1.452 cm/s). Similarly, there were no significant differences ($p = 0.912$) between the AD and healthy controls (median = 0.801 cm/s) or between the iNPH and healthy controls ($p = 0.271$).

Comparison of pressure gradient between AD patients, iNPH patients, and healthy elderly volunteers

Figure 3 shows pressure gradient images for a 67-year-old male volunteer. Figure 4 shows the pressure gradient in the Sylvian aqueduct of AD patients, iNPH patients, and healthy elderly volunteers. The median pressure gradients for each group were: 426.6 Pa/m for the AD group, 473.8 Pa/m for iNPH group, and 117.8 Pa/m for the healthy elderly group. Both the AD and iNPH groups had significantly greater pressure gradients in the Sylvian aqueduct compared to the healthy controls ($p < 0.001$ for both comparisons). There was no significant difference between the AD and iNPH groups ($p = 0.696$).

Comparison of rotation between AD patients, iNPH patients, and healthy elderly volunteers

Figure 5 shows rotation images for a 67-year-old male volunteer. Figure 6 shows the rotation in the Sylvian aqueduct of AD patients, iNPH patients, and healthy elderly volunteers. There was no significant difference ($p = 0.845$) between the AD (median = 10.243 cycle/s cm^2) and iNPH groups (median = 9.159 cycle/s cm^2). Both the AD and iNPH groups had greater rotation compared to the healthy elderly group (median = 3.447 cycle/s cm^2, $p < 0.001$ for both comparisons).

Discussion

In the present study, we assessed three elements that describe CSF motion (CSF velocity, pressure gradient, and rotation) in the Sylvian aqueduct, using a time resolved 3D-PC MRI sequence and compared these between AD patients, iNPH patients, and healthy elderly volunteers. Although previous studies have investigated the physiology and pathology of AD and iNPH patients, few reports have analyzed CSF dynamics using MR, particularly in AD patients. Moreover, apart from one preliminary study [3], no other studies have shown that the pressure gradient is elevated in iNPH patients compared to healthy elderly controls, and our present report is the

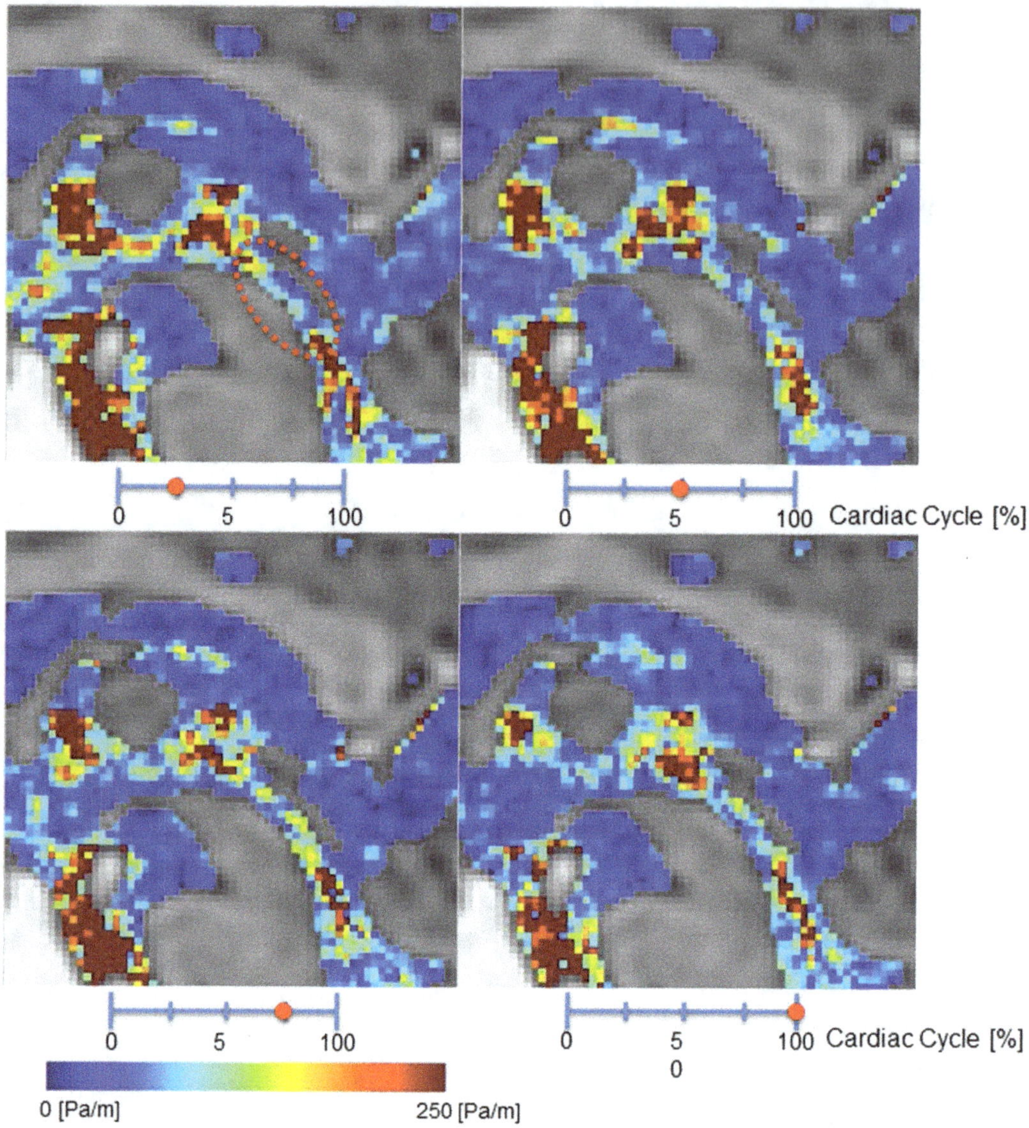

Fig. 3 Pressure gradient color mapping of the volunteer by 3D-PC at 4 stages of the cardiac cycle. The intensity of the pressure gradient was indicated using a color scale. The color-coded CSF pressure gradient were then superimposed onto T_2-weighted images of the stationary tissues. Red circle indicates Sylvian aqueduct

first to investigate the pressure gradient in AD patients. Therefore, the present study analyzed the components of fluid dynamics such as velocity, pressure gradient, and rotation, in order to better understand the pathology of a disease that also presents as a similar enlargement of CSF spaces.

The results showed that CSF velocity was not statistically significantly different between the AD and iNPH patient groups and healthy elderly volunteers. However, pressure gradient and rotation were significantly greater in AD and iNPH patient groups compared to the healthy elderly group. Pressure gradient was determined using the Navier–Stokes equations, consisting of acceleration, convection, and viscosity terms. We hypothesized that CSF viscosity and convection, as well as the anatomical morphology of the Sylvian aqueduct are not significantly different between the AD and iNPH patient groups and the healthy elderly group. This would mean that only acceleration has a significant effect on the pressure gradients of CSF, with acceleration increases resulting in pressure gradient increases. In other words, the AD and iNPH patient groups had greater CSF flow acceleration compared to the healthy controls, and this consequently influenced the pressure gradient. Furthermore,

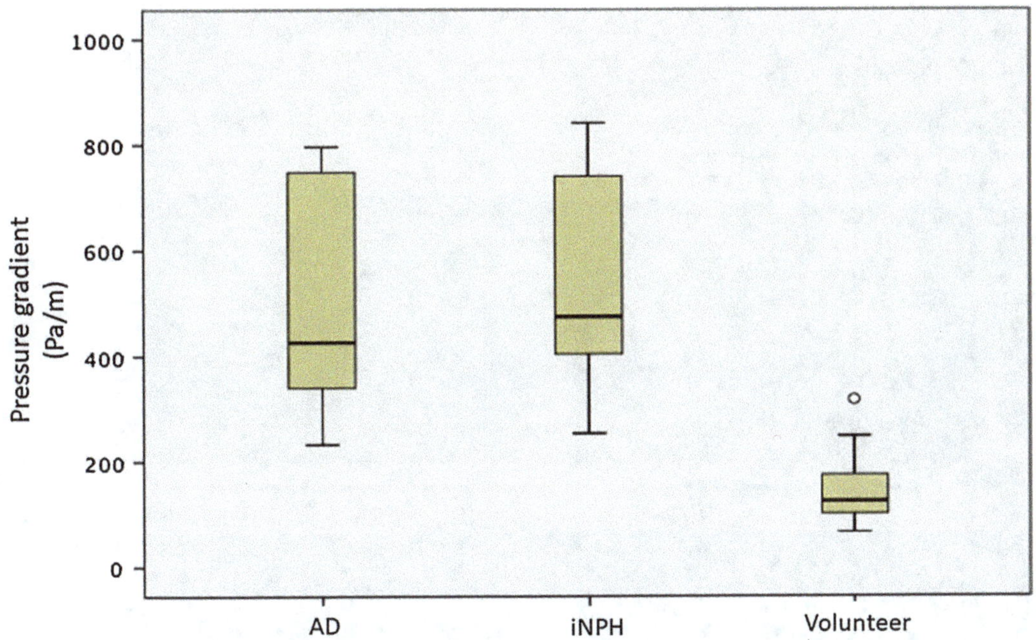

Fig. 4 Box plots of pressure gradients in the Sylvian aqueduct between AD patients, iNPH patients, and healthy elderly volunteers. Both the AD and iNPH groups had significantly greater pressure gradients compared to the volunteer group. AD Alzheimer's disease, iNPH idiopathic normal pressure hydrocephalus outside values are indicated by a small "o"

large velocity changes may lead to a disturbance in CSF motion, inducing turbulence in the Sylvian aqueduct, and this may have also been reflected in the large differences in rotation. Thus, it appears that CSF dynamics are in a hyper-dynamic state in both the AD and iNPH patient groups. The details of the relationship between pressure gradient and or velocity compared with rotation is described elsewhere [15]. To the best of our knowledge, this is the first study to report CSF rotation in AD and iNPH patients. Moreover, apart from one preliminary study [3], no other studies have shown that the pressure gradient is elevated in iNPH patients compared to healthy elderly controls, and our present report is the first to investigate the pressure gradient in AD patients. On the other hand, there are various PC MRI studies that have shown that the CSF flow in iNPH patients is in a hyper-dynamic state, which is in accordance with our results. Specifically, it has been shown that mean CSF flow is greater in iNPH but not AD patients compared to healthy controls [7, 10], CSF motion increases in iNPH patients [16], and stroke volume increases in iNPH patients [9, 17, 18]. However, it is not currently possible to use markers such as stroke volume [8] to distinguish between iNPH and AD. Also, we have compared the result of preoperative CSF dynamics and postoperative surgical results in iNPH group. Due to the limited number of patients, we currently could not differentiate between shunt responders and shunt non-responders.

These results pose the question as to why CSF is in a hyper-dynamic state in our patients compared to the healthy elderly group. A decrease in brain volume due to aging or AD leads to a relative increase in ventricular volume and subarachnoid space leading to a general increase in CSF volume, and this consequently increases the space available for free CSF motion. It is unlikely that this increased freedom leads to pressure gradient elevation, rotation increase, or turbulence. On the contrary, it would most likely decrease pressure gradient and rotation. If so, the most probable factor inducing elevated CSF pressure gradients and increased rotation would be the restriction in CSF motion due to decreased compliance in the cerebrospinal cavity that surrounds the subarachnoid space and ventricles. Mase and colleagues reported that iNPH patients had lower compliance compared to patients with ventricular dilatation or asymptomatic ventricular dilatation and healthy volunteers [19–21]. On the other hand, Edwards et al. described that the compliance of spinal subarachnoid space (especially dural sac) has a large effect on the compliance of overall CSF, indicating that degenerative diseases of the spinal cord induce decreased compliance [22]. Studies using mathematical models showed that decreased compliance is a significant element in ventricle enlargement [23, 24], and simulations using these models are extremely easy to understand. These results all indicated that decreased compliance in the CSF environment is important in

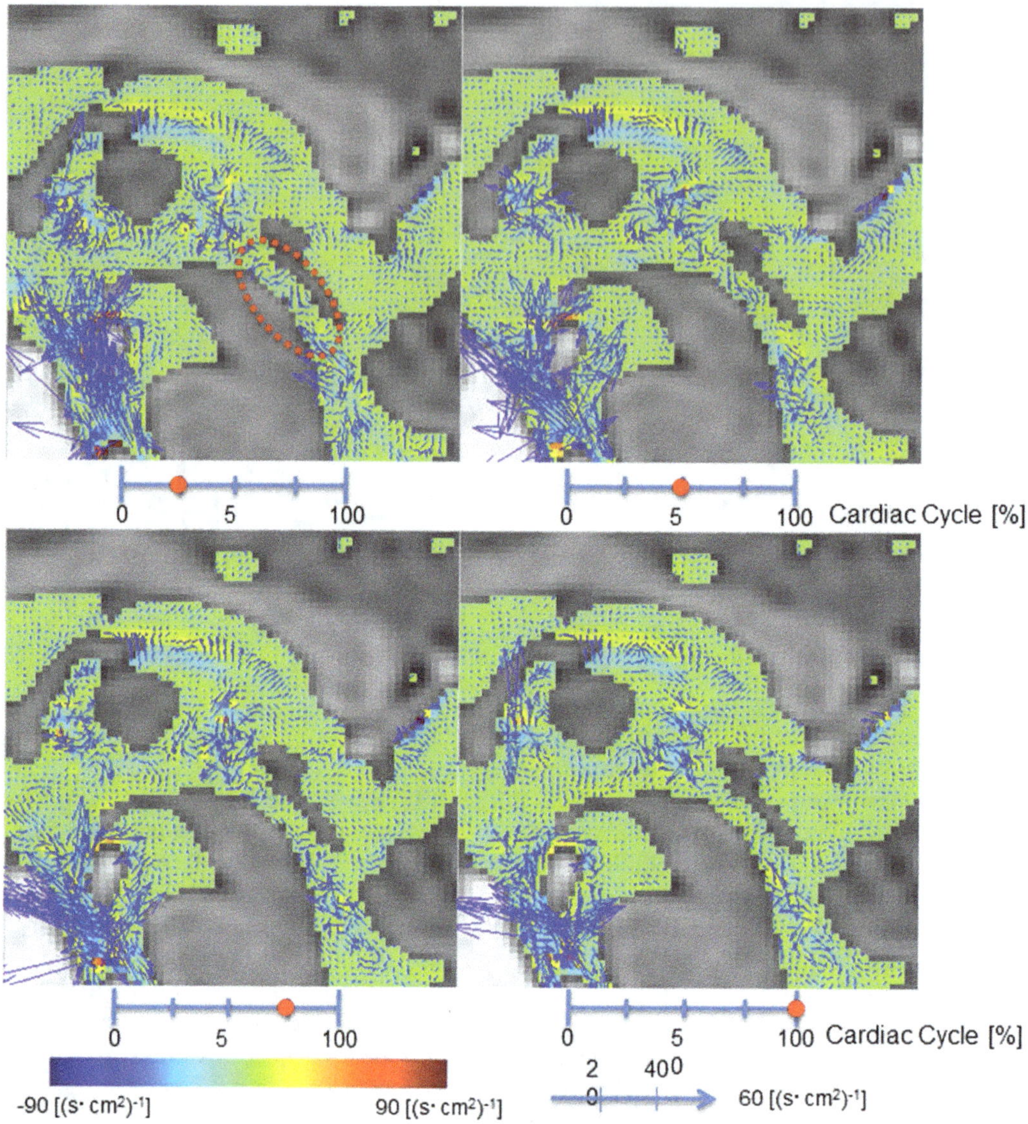

Fig. 5 Rotation mapping of the volunteer by 3D-PC at 4 stages of the cardiac cycle. In-plane rotations were visualized using vectors and through-plane rotations were visualized using colors. The color-coded CSF rotation field vector was then superimposed onto T_2-weighted images of the stationary tissues. Red circle indicates Sylvian aqueduct

diseases such as iNPH that are associated with enlarged ventricles. Furthermore, Bateman et al. investigated compliance in iNPH and AD groups and found that iNPH patients had significantly lower compliance compared to healthy volunteers and that the AD group had a compliance that was midway between the healthy volunteers and the iNPH group [25], corroborating the presence of decreased compliance in iNPH patients and suggesting that further investigations are required for AD patients. Based on these reports, it seems likely that the increased CSF pressure gradient and rotation in the Sylvian aqueduct of iNPH patients are due to decreased compliance in the cerebrospinal cavity. This is presumably the case in AD patients who also exhibit increased CSF pressure gradients and rotation in the Sylvian aqueduct.

In the above section, we discussed the common pathological state between iNPH and AD based on the fluid dynamics analysis of CSF. Regarding the discrimination of iNPH and AD, there are some contradictory findings in brain tissue biopsy [26, 27] and examinations using CSF biomarkers may not be able to differentiate between these groups [28]. This indicated that there are overlaps between iNPH and AD in addition to the pathological condition assessed based on the fluid dynamics analysis

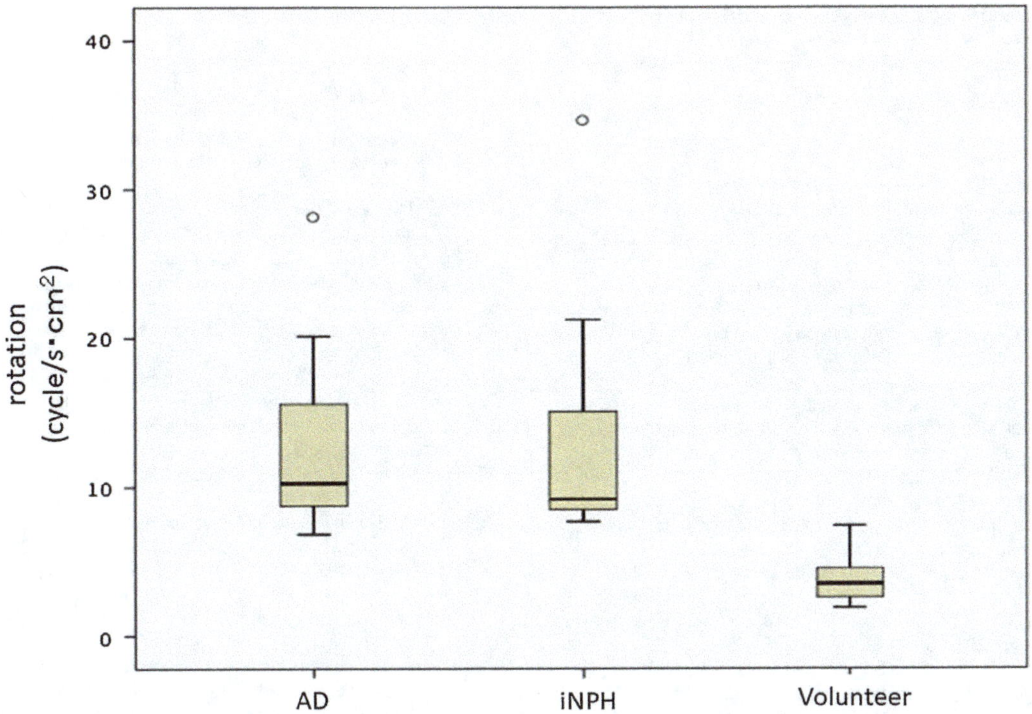

Fig. 6 Box plots of rotation in the Sylvian aqueduct between AD patients, iNPH patients, and healthy elderly volunteers. Both the AD and iNPH groups had greater rotation compared to the volunteer group. AD: Alzheimer's disease, iNPH idiopathic normal pressure hydrocephalus outside values are indicated by a small "o"

of CSF we reported in the present study. Therefore, it can be concluded that there is not currently a suitable method to distinctly classify iNPH and AD.

A limitation of the present technique is that this quantitative measurements based on the PC technique can only measure fluid velocity with 10% accuracy [29], especially for small voxel size.

Conclusions

In the present study, we quantitatively analyzed time-resolved 3D-PC MRI data of the Sylvian aqueduct in iNPH and AD patients, and healthy elderly volunteers. The 3D-PC method is useful to understand CSF dynamics in AD, iNPH, and healthy elderly volunteers. As iNPH and AD patients show a different CSF motion profile from that of healthy elderly individuals, it suggests that there is a difference in compliance between the patient groups and healthy controls.

Abbreviations

CSF: cerebrospinal fluid; MRI: magnetic resonance imaging; PC: phase contrast; 3D-PC: three-dimensional phase contrast; iNPH: idiopathic normal pressure hydrocephalus; AD: Alzheimer's disease.

Authors' contributions

KT carried out patient and volunteer data collection, statistical analysis, and drafted the manuscript. MM carried out patient and volunteer data collection, statistical analysis, and drafted the manuscript. NH and AH carried out patient and volunteer data collection. SY carried out patient and volunteer data collection, and statistical analysis. KK participated in the coordination of the study. All authors read and approved the final manuscript.

Author details

[1] Department of Neurosurgery, Tokai University School of Medicine, 143 Shimokasuya, Isehara, Kanagawa 2591193, Japan. [2] Course of Science and Technology, Graduate School of Science and Technology, Tokai University, 4-1-1 Kitakaname, Hiratsuka, Kanagawa 2591292, Japan. [3] Department of Biological Engineering, Tokai University, School of Biological Engineering, 4-1-1 Kitakaname, Hiratsuka, Kanagawa 2591292, Japan.

Acknowledgements

The authors would like to thank the patients with AD referred from the Department of Neurology in Tokai University Hospital, as well as the volunteers that participated in the study.

Competing interests

Kagayaki Kuroda is an employ of the Bioview Inc. Other authors have no financial conflicts or any interest with any commercial product used in this study or any substantial relationship with an entity that may impact or benefit from the conclusions of this research.

Funding

This study was supported in part by the Research and Study Project of Tokai University Educational System General Research Organization, and Health and Labor Sciences Research grants from the Japanese government for research on rare and intractable disease.

References

1. Matsumae M, Sato O, Hirayama A, Hayashi N, Takizawa K, Atsumi H, Sorimachi T. Research into the physiology of cerebrospinal fluid reaches a new horizon: intimate exchange between cerebrospinal fluid and interstitial fluid may contribute to maintenance of homeostasis in the central nervous system. Neurol Med Chir (Tokyo). 2016;56:416–41.
2. Hirayama A, Matsumae M, Yatsushiro S, Abdulla A, Atsumi H, Kuroda K. Visualization of pulsatile CSF motion around membrane-like structures with both 4d velocity mapping and time-SLIP technique. Magn Reson Med Sci. 2015;14:263–73.
3. Hayashi N, Matsumae M, Yatsushiro S, Hirayama A, Abdullah A, Kuroda K. Quantitative analysis of cerebrospinal fluid pressure gradients in healthy volunteers and patients with normal pressure hydrocephalus. Neurol Med Chir (Tokyo). 2015;55:657–62.
4. Matsumae M, Hirayama A, Atsumi H, Yatsushiro S, Kuroda K. Velocity and pressure gradients of cerebrospinal fluid assessed with magnetic resonance imaging. J Neurosurg. 2014;120:218–27.
5. Alperin N, Hushek SG, Lee SH, Sivaramakrishnan A, Lichtor T. MRI study of cerebral blood flow and CSF flow dynamics in an upright posture: the effect of posture on the intracranial compliance and pressure. Acta Neurochir Suppl. 2005;95:177–81.
6. Bradley WG Jr. CSF flow in the brain in the context of normal pressure hydrocephalus. AJNR Am J Neuroradiol. 2015;36:831–8.
7. Luetmer PH, Huston J, Friedman JA, Dixon GR, Petersen RC, Jack CR, McClelland RL, Ebersold MJ. Measurement of cerebrospinal fluid flow at the cerebral aqueduct by use of phase-contrast magnetic resonance imaging: technique validation and utility in diagnosing idiopathic normal pressure hydrocephalus. Neurosurgery. 2002;50:534–43 **(discussion 543–534)**.
8. Bateman GA, Levi CR, Schofield P, Wang Y, Lovett EC. The pathophysiology of the aqueduct stroke volume in normal pressure hydrocephalus: can co-morbidity with other forms of dementia be excluded? Neuroradiology. 2005;47:741–8.
9. El Sankari S, Gondry-Jouet C, Fichten A, Godefroy O, Serot JM, Deramond H, Meyer ME, Baledent O. Cerebrospinal fluid and blood flow in mild cognitive impairment and Alzheimer's disease: a differential diagnosis from idiopathic normal pressure hydrocephalus. Fluids Barriers CNS. 2011;8:12.
10. Aslan K, Tokatlioglu O, Aydin R, Polat AV, Incesu L. Normal pressure hydrocephalus versus atrophic dilatation to distinguish and predict the benefits of surgical intervention with a phase-contrast MRI technique. Turk Neurosurg. 2014;24:525–31.
11. Mori E, Ishikawa M, Kato T, Kazui H, Miyake H, Miyajima M, Nakajima M, Hashimoto M, Kuriyama N, Tokuda T, et al. Guidelines for management of idiopathic normal pressure hydrocephalus: second edition. Neurol Med Chir (Tokyo). 2012;52:775–809.
12. Hashimoto M, Ishikawa M, Mori E, Kuwana N. Diagnosis of idiopathic normal pressure hydrocephalus is supported by MRI-based scheme: a prospective cohort study. Cerebrospinal Fluid Res. 2010;7:18.
13. McKhann G, Drachman D, Folstein M, Katzman R, Price D, Stadlan EM. Clinical diagnosis of Alzheimer's disease: report of the NINCDS-ADRDA work group under the auspices of Department of Health and Human Services Task Force on Alzheimer's Disease. Neurology. 1984;34:939–44.
14. Abdullah A, Hirayama A, Yatsushiro S, Matsumae M, Kuroda K. Cerebrospinal fluid image segmentation using spatial fuzzy clustering method with improved evolutionary expectation maximization. Conf Proc IEEE Eng Med Biol Soc. 2013;2013:3359–62.
15. Feynman R. Leighton R. Sands M: The Feynman lectures on physics. Addison Wesley Longman; 1970. p. 2.
16. Schroth G, Klose U. MRI of CSF flow in normal pressure hydrocephalus. Psychiatry Res. 1989;29:289–90.
17. Scollato A, Tenenbaum R, Bahl G, Celerini M, Salani B, Di Lorenzo N. Changes in aqueductal CSF stroke volume and progression of symptoms in patients with unshunted idiopathic normal pressure hydrocephalus. AJNR Am J Neuroradiol. 2008;29:192–7.
18. Daouk J, Chaarani B, Zmudka J, Capel C, Fichten A, Bouzerar R, Gondry-Jouet C, Jouanny P, Baledent O. Relationship between cerebrospinal fluid flow, ventricles morphology, and DTI properties in internal capsules: differences between Alzheimer's disease and normal-pressure hydrocephalus. Acta Radiol. 2014;55:992–9.
19. Mase M, Miyati T, Kasai H, Demura K, Osawa T, Hara M, Shibamoto Y, Yamada K. Noninvasive estimation of intracranial compliance in idiopathic NPH using MRI. Acta Neurochir Suppl. 2008;102:115–8.
20. Miyati T, Mase M, Kasai H, Hara M, Yamada K, Shibamoto Y, Soellinger M, Baltes C, Luechinger R. Noninvasive MRI assessment of intracranial compliance in idiopathic normal pressure hydrocephalus. J Magn Reson Imaging. 2007;26:274–8.
21. Kan H, Miyati T, Mase M, Osawa T, Ohno N, Kasai H, Arai N, Kawano M, Shibamoto Y. Dynamic state of water molecular displacement of the brain during the cardiac cycle in idiopathic normal pressure hydrocephalus. Comput Med Imaging Graph. 2015;40:88–93.
22. Edwards RJ, Dombrowski SM, Luciano MG, Pople IK. Chronic hydrocephalus in adults. Brain Pathol. 2004;14:325–36.
23. Egnor M, Zheng L, Rosiello A, Gutman F, Davis R. A model of pulsations in communicating hydrocephalus. Pediatr Neurosurg. 2002;36:281–303.
24. Wilkie KP, Nagra G, Johnston M. A mathematical analysis of physiological and molecular mechanisms that modulate pressure gradients and facilitate ventricular expansion in hydrocephalus. Int J Numer Anal Model B. 2012;316:65–81.
25. Bateman GA, Loiselle AM. Can MR measurement of intracranial hydrodynamics and compliance differentiate which patient with idiopathic normal pressure hydrocephalus will improve following shunt insertion? Acta Neurochir (Wien). 2007;149:455–62 **(discussion 462)**.
26. Savolainen S, Paljarvi L, Vapalahti M. Prevalence of Alzheimer's disease in patients investigated for presumed normal pressure hydrocephalus: a clinical and neuropathological study. Acta Neurochir (Wien). 1999;141:849–53.
27. Golomb J, Wisoff J, Miller DC, Boksay I, Kluger A, Weiner H, Salton J, Graves W. Alzheimer's disease comorbidity in normal pressure hydrocephalus: prevalence and shunt response. J Neurol Neurosurg Psychiatry. 2000;68:778–81.
28. Graff-Radford NR. Alzheimer CSF biomarkers may be misleading in normal-pressure hydrocephalus. Neurology. 2014;83:1573–5.
29. Tang C, Blatter DD, Parker DL. Accuracy of phase-contrast flow measurements in the presence of partial-volume effects. J Magn Reson Imaging. 1993;3:377–85.

13

Cerebral hypoxia/ischemia selectively disrupts tight junctions complexes in stem cell-derived human brain microvascular endothelial cells

Shyanne Page, Alli Munsell and Abraham J. Al-Ahmad*

Abstract

Background: Cerebral hypoxia/ischemia (H/I) is an important stress factor involved in the disruption of the blood–brain barrier (BBB) following stroke injury, yet the cellular and molecular mechanisms on how the human BBB responds to such injury remains unclear. In this study, we investigated the cellular response of the human BBB to chemical and environmental H/I in vitro.

Methods: In this study, we used immortalized hCMEC/D3 and IMR90 stem-cell derived human brain microvascular endothelial cell lines (IMR90-derived BMECs). Hypoxic stress was achieved by exposure to cobalt chloride ($CoCl_2$) or by exposure to 1 % hypoxia and oxygen/glucose deprivation (OGD) was used to model ischemic injury. We assessed barrier function using both transendothelial electrical resistance (TEER) and sodium fluorescein permeability. Changes in cell junction integrity were assessed by immunocytochemistry and cell viability was assessed by trypan-blue exclusion and by MTS assays. Statistical analysis was performed using one-way analysis of variance (ANOVA).

Results: $CoCl_2$ selectively disrupted the barrier function in IMR90-derived BMECs but not in hCMEC/D3 monolayers and cytotoxic effects did not drive such disruption. In addition, hypoxia/OGD stress significantly disrupted the barrier function by selectively disrupting tight junctions (TJs) complexes. In addition, we noted an uncoupling between cell metabolic activity and barrier integrity.

Conclusions: In this study, we demonstrated the ability of IMR90-derived BMECs to respond to hypoxic/ischemic injury triggered by both chemical and environmental stress by showing a disruption of the barrier function. Such disruption was selectively targeting TJ complexes and was not driven by cellular apoptosis. In conclusion, this study suggests the suitability of stem cell-derived human BMECs monolayers as a model of cerebral hypoxia/ischemia in vitro.

Background

The blood–brain barrier (BBB), a component of the neurovascular unit, constitutes a crucial biological barrier in the maintenance of brain homeostasis by restricting the diffusion of solutes and toxins to brain parenchyma. The presence of such barrier is supported by brain microvascular endothelial cells (BMECs), which are present in the cerebral microvasculature. BMECs provide both a physical (tight junctions complexes) and a chemical barrier (drug and nutrient transporters), which tightly regulate the diffusion of small molecules between the blood and brain. However, the integrity of the BBB is compromised in several neurological diseases including multiple sclerosis [1], neurodegenerative diseases [2–5], and stroke [1, 6, 7].

Stroke constitutes the fifth leading cause of death in industrialized countries and is a leading cause of disability [8]. The majority of stroke events are classified as an ischemic, marked by an abrupt decreased perfusion in a

*Correspondence: abraham.al-ahmad@ttuhsc.edu
Department of Pharmaceutical Sciences, School of Pharmacy, Texas Tech University Health Sciences Center, 1300 South Coulter Street, Amarillo, TX, USA

defined brain region, resulting in an impairment of both oxygen and nutrient supply. This ultimately leads to the onset of a cerebral hypoxic/ischemic (H/I) injury.

BMECs are the first cell type of the neurovascular to sense hypoxia and respond to such injury by disrupting barrier function. Such disruption will eventually lead to a vascular leakage. The mechanisms by which H/I impacts barrier function have been extensively studied in rodents and non-human primates [9–17], yet the literature showing similar outcomes at the human BBB remains unclear.

In this study, we investigated the effect of H/I on a stem cell-derived model of the human BBB using the IMR90-c4 induced pluripotent stem cell line [18–21] and compared their response to hCMEC/D3, an immortalized human BMEC line commonly used in the literature [22].

Methods

Cell culture

hCMEC/D3 cell line [22] was purchased from Millipore (EMD Millipore, Billerica, MA, USA) and maintained following established manufacturer protocol. IMR90-c4 induced pluripotent stem cell (iPSC) cell line [18] was purchased from WiCell (WiCell, Madison, WI). IMR90-c4 iPS cell line was maintained in mTeSR1 (Stem Cell Technologies, Vancouver, BC, USA) and grown on hPSC-qualified Matrigel (Corning Inc., Corning, NY, USA). The IMR90 cell line was differentiated into BMECs (iPSC-BMECs) following the differentiation protocol established by Lippmann and colleagues [20, 21] and summarized in Additional file 1: Figure S1. In brief, cells were seeded at 20,000 cells/cm^2 5 days before differentiation and maintained in mTeSR medium. Five days after seeding, BMECs differentiation was set using unconditioned maturation medium (UMM) following the same composition as previously described: DMEM/F12 with 15 mM HEPES supplemented with 20 % KO serum replacement, 1 % MEM non-essential aminoacids, and 0.5 % Glutamax I, (ThermoFisher, Waltham, MA, USA) and 0.1 mM β-mercaptoethanol (Sigma-Aldrich, St Louis, MO, USA) for 6 days. After such differentiation, IMR90-derived BMECs were incubated in presence EC differentiation medium (EC serum free medium (ThermoFisher), supplemented with 1 % platelet-poor derived plasma serum (ThermoFisher), 20 μg/mL human basic fibroblast growth factor (R&D Systems) and 10 μM all-trans retinoic acid (Sigma-Aldrich) for 2 days. After 8 days of differentiation, cells were enzymatically dissociated and seeded at a density of 10^6 cells/cm^2 on 12-well Transwell polyester cell culture inserts (0.4 μm pore size) coated with collagen from human placenta (Sigma-Aldrich) and fibronectin from bovine plasma (Sigma-Aldrich) at concentrations of 80 and 20 μg/cm^2. After 24 h (day 9), BMECs were maintained in EC differentiation medium containing only 1 % platelet-poor plasma-derived serum. All experiments were carried out 48 h after seeding.

Barrier function

Cells were grown on 12-well Transwell polyester membranes (Corning Inc.) coated with 30 μg/cm^2 collagen I (Sigma-Aldrich, St Louis, MO, USA) or with 80 μg/cm^2 collagen supplemented with 20 μg/cm^2 fibronectin (Sigma-Aldrich) mixture to allow hCMEC/D3 and IMR90-derived BMECs to attach respectively. Monolayer tightness was assessed by measuring transendothelial electrical resistance (TEER) using an EVOM STX2 chopstick electrode (World Precision Instruments, Sarasota, FL, USA). Paracellular permeability was assessed in monolayers by measuring the diffusion profile of 1 μM of sodium fluorescein (Sigma-Aldrich) using the clearance method described by Perriere and colleagues [23]. Fluorescence was assessed using a Synergy MX2 ELISA plate reader (Bio-Tek Instruments, Burlington, VT, USA). Average TEER and permeability values of both monolayers can be found in Table 1. TEER and permeability values from untreated monolayers were used to normalize experimental values expressed as % of control. Untreated group experimental values were arbitrarily set to 100 % control.

Cobalt chloride and hypoxic treatment

Cobalt chloride ($CoCl_2$, MP Biomedicals, Santa Ana, CA, USA) was freshly dissolved in complete cell medium at a stock concentration of 100 mM and further dissolved to achieve the concentrations of 10, 30 and 100 μM. Cells were incubated in presence of $CoCl_2$ for 24 h. For the hypoxic experiments, cell medium was replaced with fresh medium and cells were incubated in a normobaric hypoxic C-chamber (Biospherix, Laconia, NY, USA) set at 1 % O_2, 5 % CO_2 and maintained at 37 °C for 6 or 24 h. In experiments involving oxygen deprivation (OD), cell medium was replaced with Dulbecco's Modified Eagle Medium (DMEM) containing 1 g/L D-glucose and 1 %

Table 1 Biological values of hCMEC/D3 and IMR90-derived BMECs under resting conditions

Cell type	hCMEC/D3	IMR90-derived BMECs
Cell density (× 10^3 cells/cm^2)	128 ± 21	98 ± 19
TEER (Ω cm^2)	40 ± 14	392 ± 113
Pe fluorescein (10^{-4} cm/min)	19 ± 8	2.44 ± 1.12
Metabolic activity (OD 490 nm)	1.26 ± 0.45	0.89 ± 0.34

Average cell density, TEER, fluorescein permeability (Pe) and metabolic activity (MTS absorbance at 490 nm wavelength). Mean ± SD, n = 18 for TEER and Pe values platelet-poor derived serum (Alfa Aesar, Ward Hill, MA, USA). In GD and OGD experiments, glucose-free and pyruvate-free DMEM were used instead of DMEM containing 1 g/L D-glucose.

Immunocytochemistry

Cells were grown to confluence on 48-well coated plates and quickly washed with ice-cold phosphate buffered saline (PBS) solution and fixed with either 4 % paraformaldehyde (Electron Microscopy Sciences, Hatfield, PA, USA) or cold methanol (ThermoFisher) and processed as previously described [20, 21].

Cell density and viability assay

Cell density was assessed on monolayers by Trypan-blue exclusion based assay. In brief, monolayers were briefly washed with ice-cold PBS and incubated in presence of accutase (corning) or 0.25 % trypsin–EDTA (ThermoFisher) for 5 min followed by a centrifugation at 1000 rpms for 5 min. Cells were resuspended in 0.5 mL PBS and counted using a Countess II automated cell counter (ThermoFisher). Cell viability was assessed by MTS-based CellTiter 96® Aqueous (Promega, Madison, WI, USA). After treatment, cells grown on 96-well plates were incubated in presence of MTS reagent for 1 h. Absorbance was measured at 490 nm and corrected against unconditioned medium containing the same amount of MTS. Absorbance values from all samples were normalized against their respective control samples.

Statistics

All experiments were performed using cells coming from at least three independent experiments (distinct cell passages, each experiment was performed with two technical replicates). Statistical analysis was performed using one-way ANOVA followed by a post hoc analysis using Dunnett's test with the control group as the reference group. P values lesser or equal to 0.05 were considered statistically significant.

Results

$CoCl_2$ induces barrier disruption in IMR90-derived BMECs but not in hCMEC/D3 monolayers

In order to demonstrate the suitability of IMR90-derived BMECs (iPSC-BMECs) as an in vitro model of cerebral hypoxia/ischemia, it is important to show that such cells can respond to known hypoxic stimuli. Thus, we first assessed the cellular response of iPSC-BMEC monolayers to chemical hypoxia (Fig. 1) by exposing them to different concentrations of cobalt chloride ($CoCl_2$), a common hypoxia-mimetic chemical used in various cell types [9, 24–29]. We compared iPSC-BMECs response to hCMEC/D3 cell monolayers, a human brain microvascular endothelial cell line commonly used in the literature [22, 30–32]. It should be noted that these cell monolayers have lower baseline TEERs and higher sodium fluorescein permeabilities that the iPSC-BMEC monolayers (Table 1).

Upon exposure of 24 h to $CoCl_2$, there was a decrease in the iPSC-BMECs barrier function as noted by a significant decrease in TEER (Fig. 1a) in cells treated with $CoCl_2$ at 30 and 100 μM. However, hCMEC/D3 failed to display any changes in barrier function even when exposed at 100 μM (a dose known to trigger a barrier breakdown in rat brain endothelial cell monolayers [9]). To further confirm this observation, we investigated changes in sodium fluorescein permeability in both iPSC-BMECs monolayers and hCMEC/D3 following $CoCl_2$ treatment (Fig. 1b). As observed in our previous experiment, $CoCl_2$ treatment affected the barrier integrity in iPSC-BMECs at 30 and 100 μM, with a 3- to 4-fold increase in paracellular permeability to sodium fluorescein compared to untreated cells.

$CoCl_2$ treatment differentially affects cell density and metabolism in hCMEC/D3 and IMR90-derived BMEC monolayers

Because $CoCl_2$ treatment can induce cell apoptosis in various mammalian cell lines [33–36], we investigated changes in cell viability following $CoCl_2$ treatment using MTS and Trypan-blue exclusion assays (Fig. 1c, d). After 24 h of $CoCl_2$ treatment, we did not note a significant decrease in hCMEC/D3 cell density (Fig. 1c). However, we noted a 50 % decrease in cell density only in iPSC-BMEC group exposed to 100 μM, suggesting a detrimental effect of $CoCl_2$ on the monolayer integrity. However, no change in hCMEC/D3 cell monolayer density was observed, even at the highest $CoCl_2$ concentration.

Attempts to use trypan blue exclusion assay only provided information on adherent cells remaining after $CoCl_2$ treatment. Furthermore, the additional mechanical stress applied to assess cell viability in non-adherent cells using such method may also interfere with the method accuracy. Therefore, we consider such method not suited for cytotoxic assays. Notably, tetrazolium-based cytotoxic assays directly assess changes in mitochondrial activity and can be directly applied to adherent and non-adherent cells. Therefore, we investigated changes in cell viability following $CoCl_2$ treatment using an MTS-based assay (Fig. 1d), an assay commonly used to assess cytotoxicity by measuring changes in cell metabolic activity [37]. Notably, we did not notice changes in cell viability in iPSC-BMEC monolayers following exposure to $CoCl_2$ compared to control. We even noted an increase in cell viability following 30 μM and 100 μM treatment. In contrast, we noted a dose-dependent decrease in cell viability

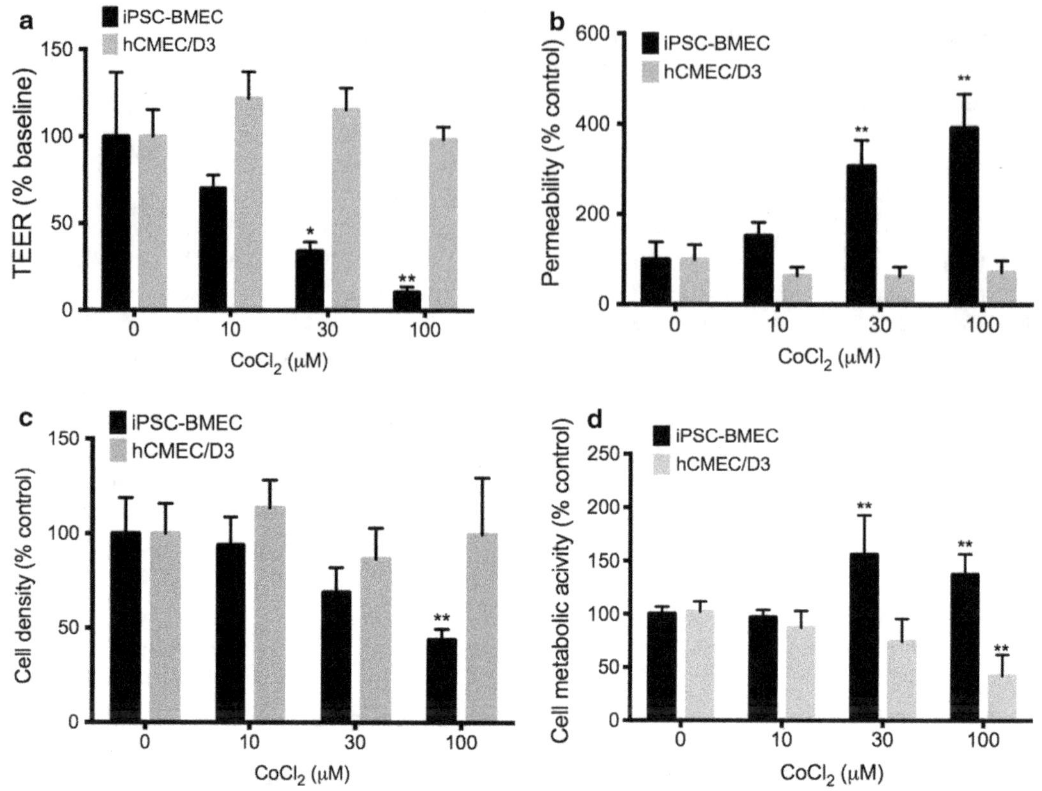

Fig. 1 Cobalt chloride induces barrier disruption in iPSC-derived BMECs but not in hCMEC/D3 monolayers. Cells were treated with cobalt chloride ($CoCl_2$) for 24 h and were compared to untreated cell monolayers. Changes in the monolayer integrity were assessed by TEER (**a**) and by sodium fluorescein (**b**). Note the decrease in barrier function in IMR90-derived BMECs (iPSC-BMEC) versus the hCMEC/D3 monolayers. **c** Cobalt chloride induced decrease in adherent cell density in iPSC-BMEC at high concentrations (100 μM). * and ** denotes $P < 0.05$ and $P < 0.01$ versus control (untreated) groups. **d** Metabolic activity following treatment with $CoCl_2$ did not induce cell toxicity in IMR90-derived BMECs, as we noted no decrease versus control group. Mean ± SD, n = 3 for each group, * and ** denotes $P < 0.05$ and $P < 0.01$ versus control (untreated) groups

in hCMEC/D3 monolayer with a 50 % decrease in cell metabolism.

To further understand how $CoCl_2$ impacted barrier function in iPSC-BMECs, we investigated changes in cell junction integrity by immunocytochemistry (Fig. 2). At 30 μM, we observed alterations in the distribution of tight junction complexes (claudin-5 and occludin) with a loss of immunostaining at the cell borders and a relocalization into cell cytoplasm. Surprisingly, such relocalization was not observed in adherens junction complexes (PECAM-1 and β-catenin). Taken together, these observations are consistent with observations in RBE4 monolayers [9] and suggest the ability of IMR90-derived BMECs to respond to hypoxic stimulus in similar fashion to rodent-based in vitro models.

Hypoxia induces barrier disruption in both IMR90-derived BMECs and hCMEC/D3 cell monolayers

Hypoxia-induced BBB disruption is a well-established phenomenon reported in both in vitro and in vivo models [9, 38–44]. Therefore, we assessed the ability of both IMR90-derived BMECs and hCMEC/D3 to respond to hypoxic stress by exposing our monolayers to 1 % O_2 for 6 or 24 h (Fig. 3).

Acute (6 h) hypoxic stress resulted in significant decrease of over 70 % in TEER in hCMEC/D3 monolayers (Fig. 3a), whereas IMR90-derived BMECs showed only a mild decrease. However, such changes in TEER were not reflected in changes in vascular permeability, as we noted no significant increase in sodium fluorescein permeability (Fig. 3b).

In contrast, prolonged hypoxic (24 h) injury resulted in loss of barrier function in both IMR90-derived BMECs and hCMEC/D3, as we observed a 50 % decrease in TEER (Fig. 3a) and a 2.5-fold increase in fluorescein permeability (Fig. 3b) compared to normoxic monolayers. These results suggest the ability of the monolayers to respond to hypoxia similarly to the existing literature.

To further understand how hypoxia affects the barrier function, we investigated changes in cell junction complexes in IMR90-derived BMECs by immunocytochemistry (Fig. 3c). After 24 h of hypoxia, we did not

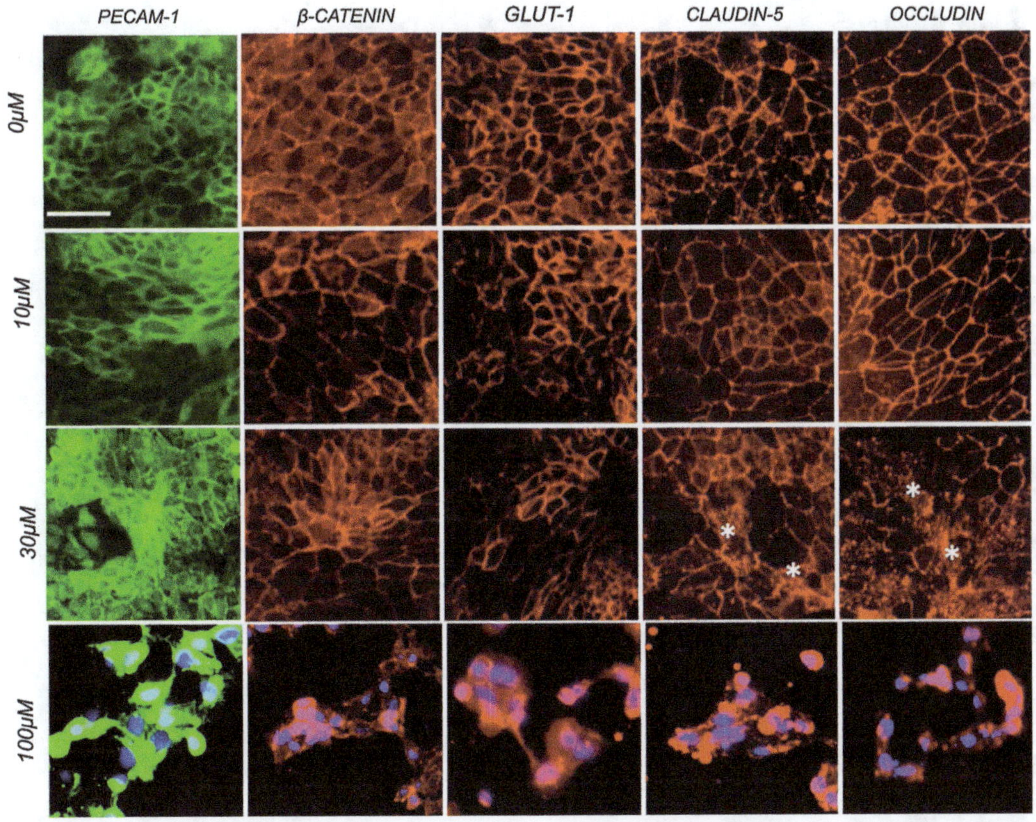

Fig. 2 Cobalt-chloride treatment impact monolayer integrity in iPSC-derived BMECs. Representative immunocytochemistry micrograph pictures of IMR90-derived BMECs monolayers in presence of $CoCl_2$. Cells were treated with different $CoCl_2$ concentrations. Note the presence of irregular patterning in TJ proteins (claudin-5 and occludin) as marked by asterisks at 30 μM treatment and a complete disruption at 100 μM. *Scale bar* = 20 μm

observe any changes in adherens junction (PECAM-1 and β-catenin) complexes. However, we noted changes in tight junction (claudin-5 and occludin) complexes with a discontinuous staining pattern. Finally, we assessed by MTS whether this insult impacted cell viability (Fig. 3d). Following 24 h of hypoxic stress, we did not find any significant changes in cell metabolic activity, as the average metabolic activity was 80 and 70 % of the normoxic levels in IMR90-derived BMECs and hCMEC/D3 monolayers, respectively. In conclusion, our data demonstrate that IMR90-derived BMECs, as well as hCMEC/D3 cell monolayers, actively respond to hypoxia by disruption of their barrier function. Such disruption appears driven by alterations in the tight junction complexes rather than cell death.

Oxygen-glucose deprivation impairs barrier function in both IMR90-derived BMECs and hCMEC/D3 monolayers

Next, we investigated how hypoxia/aglycemia affected the barrier function in our human models of the BBB by exposing our cells to hypoxia, aglycemia or to oxygen-glucose deprivation (OGD) stress (Fig. 4). Interestingly, incubation in glucose-deprived medium (GD) for 24 h resulted in a significant decrease in TEER (~50 %) in both hCMEC/D3 and IMR90-derived BMEC monolayers (Fig. 4) but failed to show any significant increase in cell permeability to sodium fluorescein (Fig. 4b) suggesting that aglycemia alone was not sufficient to induce BBB disruption. On the other hand, hypoxia (OD) was capable of inducing BBB disruption, as we noted a significant decrease in TEER and an increase in when fluorescein permeability. However, we observed the maximum disruption cells were subjected to both oxygen and glucose deprivation (OGD), as noted by the lowest TEER values (20 % of control) and highest permeability values to fluorescein (5-fold increase).

Following such observations, we investigated changes in cell junction complexes in IMR90-derived BMECs following OGD stress by immunocytochemistry (Fig. 4c). OGD stress was capable of altering adherens junction complexes (as noted by a decrease in VE-cadherin immunoreactivity) but more importantly, we noted a complete loss of immunoreactivity for tight junction complex proteins.

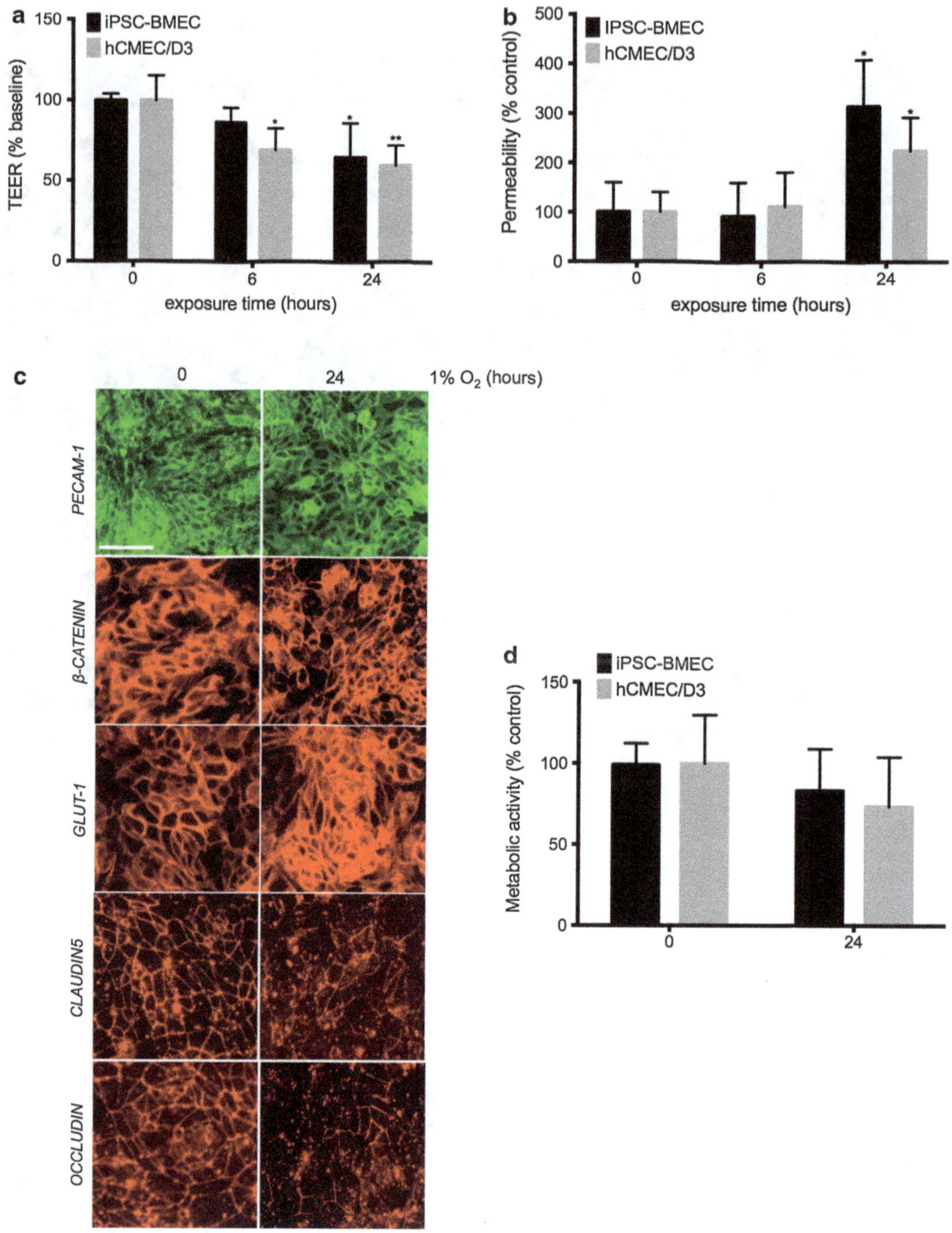

Fig. 3 Prolonged Hypoxia impairs the barrier function in both cell monolayers. TEER (**a**) and sodium fluorescein (**b**) permeability values in both iPSC-BMECs and hCMEC/D3 cell monolayers following exposure to hypoxia for 6 and 24 h. Note the early onset of hypoxia-induced barrier disruption in hCMEC/D3 at 6 h as indicated by TEER compared to IMR90-derived BMECs, with a significant decrease at 24 h. Hypoxia-induced paracellular permeability however was only observed after 24 h in both groups. **c** Immunocytochemistry profile of IMR90-derived BMECs following exposure to hypoxia (1 % O_2) for 24 h. Note the decreased immunoreactivity of claudin-5 and occludin following hypoxia, whereas no changes where noted in other cell junction proteins (β-catenin and PECAM-1). *Scale bar* = 20 μm. **d** Cell metabolic activity as measured by MTS assay. Following hypoxic incubation, MTS was added to the cell conditioned medium and incubated for 1 h before readout. Mean ± SD, n = 3 for each group. * and ** denotes $P < 0.05$ and $P < 0.01$ to controls (labeled as 0 h) respectively

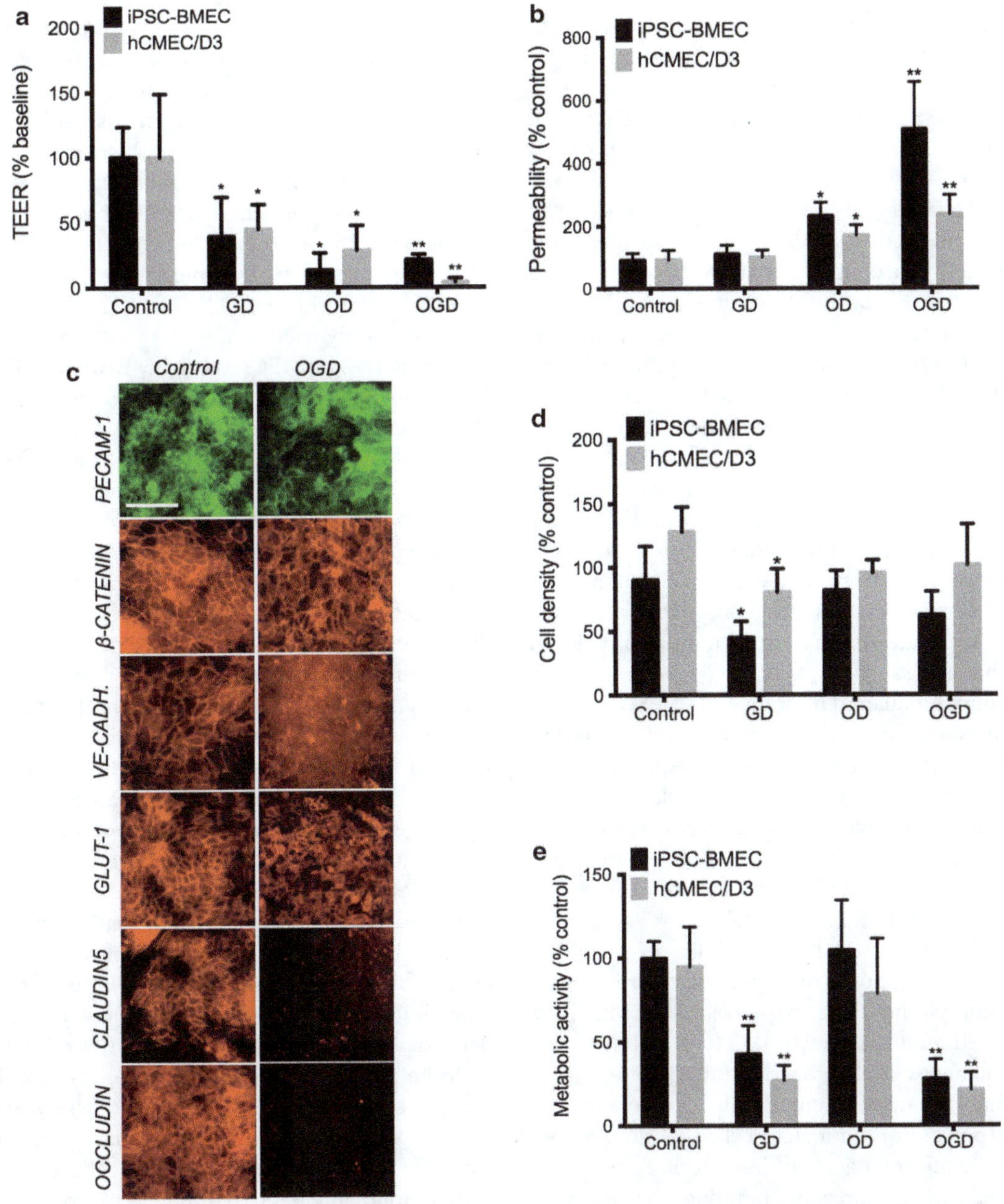

Fig. 4 OGD induced barrier disruption in human BMECs.TEER (**a**) and sodium fluorescein (**b**) permeability values in both iPSC-BMECs and hCMEC/D3 cell monolayers following aglycemic (GD), hypoxic (OD) and oxygen-glucose deprivation (OGD) stress. Cells incubated in DMEM with glucose under normoxia served as control. Note the increase in fluorescein permeability following OD and OGD stress. **c** Representative immunocytochemistry pictures in iPSC-derived BMECs monolayers following 24 h of OGD stress. Note the overall degradation in cell junctions, with a quasi-disappearance in TJ complexes immunoreactivity. *Scale bar* = 20 μm. **d** IMR90-derived BMECs and hCMEC/D3 average cell density following treatment with aglycemia, hypoxia or OGD stress. Notably, aglycemia (GD) showed the lowest cell density in both cell monolayers. **e** Cell metabolic activity following 24 h of treatment. After 24 h of treatment, MTS reagent was added to conditioned cell medium and allowed to further incubate for 1 h. Mean ± SD, n = 3 for each group. * and ** denotes $P < 0.05$ and $P < 0.01$ to controls (DMEM with glucose, normoxia) respectively

Taken together, loss of tight junction complexes during OGD stress may be a contributor to the BBB disruption.

As changes in cell density and viability may impact the barrier integrity during injury, we investigated changes in cell density by trypan-blue exclusion assay (Fig. 4d). Interestingly, we noted a significant decrease in cell density after aglycemic treatment in both IMR90-derived BMECs and in hCMEC/D3 monolayers. However, we did not notice a significant decrease in cell density following hypoxia and OGD stress (two conditions shown to have an impact on the barrier function). Furthermore, we observed a similar outcome when we measured changes in cell viability by MTS assay (Fig. 4e). Aglycemia decreased metabolic activity level by 60 % compared to controls in both monolayers. However, hypoxia (OD) alone showed no differences compared to controls. Finally, cells exposed to OGD stress showed only 15–20 % of the metabolic activity observed in the control group. Taken together, our study demonstrates that both IMR90-derived BMECs and hCMEC/D3 respond to OGD stress with disrupted barrier function. However, we noted an uncoupling between BBB barrier function and cell density/cell metabolic activity following hypoxic or aglycemic treatment.

Discussion

Stroke constitutes the fifth leading cause of death and it is a major cause of disability in the United States. Although important efforts have been made to identify therapeutics capable of improving outcome in stroke patients, the ability to translate findings from animal models to patients has had little success.

Human Induced pluripotent stem cells (iPSCs) based in vitro models of the neurovascular unit (integrating BMECs, astrocytes and neurons) may help provide a screening platform to improve such translation. However, pluripotent stem cells are also highly hypoxic tolerant [45], therefore questioning the suitability of stem-cell based models for understanding the effects of hypoxic/ischemic injury in vitro.

In this study, we investigated the ability of stem cell derived BMECs to respond to hypoxic/ischemic injury in vitro by comparing their response to hCMEC/D3, an immortalized adult human BMEC line [22]. We first investigated changes in the barrier function following $CoCl_2$ treatment, a chemical commonly used to simulate a hypoxic response in mammalian cells [25, 26, 28, 29]. We noted a significant decrease in barrier function in IMR90-derived BMECs and a loss of monolayer integrity. Such results are in agreement with a previous study by Engelhardt and colleagues [9]. In that study, the authors observed that $CoCl_2$ was capable of significantly decreasing barrier function in RBE4 cells monolayers as early as 6 h. In contrast to their findings, we observed a significant decrease in the barrier function only after 24 h in IMR90-derived BMECs. Surprisingly, we did not observe a response in hCMEC/D3 monolayers following $CoCl_2$ exposure, with no changes in barrier function compared to untreated groups.

A difference in response to $CoCl_2$ between the two monolayers might be explained by differences in oxygen sensing, as $CoCl_2$ exerts its activity through the activation of the hypoxia-induced factor (HIF)-1 pathway. Such differences maybe also inherent to the nature of the hCMEC/D3 cells, as Patak and colleagues reported an absence of up-regulation in ABCB1 and ABCC1 expression following hypoxic stress [46]. We are currently investigating such dimorphism in oxygen sensing between these two cells by comparing HIF-1α expression at protein levels and VEGF production.

Following these observations, we investigated the cellular response to environmental hypoxia by incubating cells in the presence of 1 % O_2, a gas phase concentration commonly used in the literature. In our study, both IMR90-derived BMECs and hCMEC/D3 cells responded to prolonged hypoxic injury in vitro with decreased barrier function. Furthermore, IMR90-derived BMECs displayed alterations in tight junction complex distribution similar to previous reports [9]. However, oxygen-glucose deprivation (OGD) stress was necessary to achieve a major barrier disruption in both IMR90-derived BMECs and hCMEC/D3 cells. Such disruption was marked by the greatest decrease in TEER and highest increase in fluorescein permeability.

This dramatic decrease in barrier function was likely due to a major disruption in tight junction complex integrity, as we noted a significant decrease in immunoreactivity of both claudin-5 and occludin in IMR90-derived BMECs. We speculate such decreased immunoreactivity may be indicative of a cleavage of such proteins by a select number of matrix metalloproteinases (MMPs), in particular by MMP-2 and MMP-9 [47–49].

In addition to changes in barrier function due to changes in MMP activity, we also speculate that impaired energy production during hypoxic/ischemic injury may contribute to barrier disruption. A recent study by Vandekeere and colleagues suggests ATP production in brain endothelial cell metabolism is driven by glycolysis under aerobic conditions [50]. MTS-based assays are designed to measure changes in mitochondrial hydrogenase activity [51]. Thus, we were expecting little change in MTS activity following hypoxic/OGD stress in our model. Surprisingly, we noted no changes in MTS activity in hypoxic cells. Such results were consistent with a recent study published by Ogunshola and colleagues [10], in which no significant changes in cell metabolism were observed following prolonged hypoxia.

Interestingly, we noted changes in cell density following $CoCl_2$ treatment as well as during glucose deprivation. Although a decrease in cell density was accompanied by an increase in permeability following $CoCl_2$ treatment, we did not observe such phenomenon in glucose-deprived cells.

Finally, we observed a conundrum between metabolic activity and barrier function in BMECs, in particular between hypoxic and aglycemic treatments. Decreased cell metabolism in aglycemic cells was not accompanied by decreased barrier function, whereas we noted a loss of barrier function was not accompanied by a decrease in cell metabolism. Such data suggests that tight junction disruption following hypoxia may not be due to energy deficiency, but also suggests that IMR90-derived BMECs may utilize other nutrients to maintain mitochondrial activity through some anaploretic reactions (in particular glutamine). Thus, we are currently investigating how hypoxia/OGD stress influences energy production in BMECs; in particular we are investigating how such stress influences changes in glycolysis and oxidative phosphorylation mechanism.

Conclusions

In summary, this study demonstrates the suitability of stem cell-derived in vitro model of the human BBB as an in vitro model for H/I. This model may effectively complement existing in vivo models and help improve the identification of novel therapeutics capable of fighting H/I-induced BBB disruption following stroke.

Abbreviations

BBB: blood-brain barrier; BMECs: brain microvascular endothelial cells; DMEM: Dulbecco's modified eagle medium; GD: glucose deprivation; H/I: hypoxia-ischemia; OD: oxygen deprivation; OGD: oxygen-glucose deprivation; PBS: phosphate-buffered saline solution; TEER: transendothelial electrical resistance; TJ: tight junctions.

Authors' contributions

AA has designed and contributed in the experimental design, performed some of the experiments and analyzed the results and edited the manuscript and figures. SP and AM have contributed in the experimental design and equally contributed in the experiments. SP has contributed in the analysis and the redaction of the manuscript. All authors read and approved the final manuscript.

Competing interests

The authors declare that they have no competing interests.

Funding

This research funding was supported by institutional support to AA.

References

1. Lopes Pinheiro MA, Kooij G, Mizee MR, Kamermans A, Enzmann G, Lyck R, et al. Immune cell trafficking across the barriers of the central nervous system in multiple sclerosis and stroke. Biochim Biophys Acta. 2015;1862(3):461–71.
2. Duits FH, Hernandez-Guillamon M, Montaner J, Goos JD, Montanola A, Wattjes MP, et al. Matrix metalloproteinases in Alzheimer's disease and concurrent cerebral microbleeds. J Alzheimers Dis. 2015;48(3):711–20.
3. Drouin-Ouellet J, Sawiak SJ, Cisbani G, Lagace M, Kuan WL, Saint-Pierre M, et al. Cerebrovascular and blood-brain barrier impairments in Huntington's disease: potential implications for its pathophysiology. Ann Neurol. 2015;78(2):160–77.
4. Qosa H, Abuasal BS, Romero IA, Weksler B, Couraud PO, Keller JN, et al. Differences in amyloid-beta clearance across mouse and human blood-brain barrier models: kinetic analysis and mechanistic modeling. Neuropharmacology. 2014;79:668–78.
5. Garbuzova-Davis S, Sanberg PR. Blood-CNS Barrier Impairment in ALS patients versus an animal model. Front Cell Neurosci. 2014;8:21.
6. Shah K, Abbruscato T. The role of blood-brain barrier transporters in pathophysiology and pharmacotherapy of stroke. Curr Pharm Des. 2014;20(10):1510–22.
7. Jickling GC, Liu D, Stamova B, Ander BP, Zhan X, Lu A, et al. Hemorrhagic transformation after ischemic stroke in animals and humans. J Cereb Blood Flow Metab. 2014;34:185–99.
8. Go AS, Mozaffarian D, Roger VL, Benjamin EJ, Berry JD, Blaha MJ, et al. Heart disease and stroke statistics–2014 update: a report from the American Heart Association. Circulation. 2014;129:e28–292.
9. Engelhardt S, Al-Ahmad AJ, Gassmann M, Ogunshola OO. Hypoxia selectively disrupts brain microvascular endothelial tight junction complexes through a hypoxia-inducible factor-1 (HIF-1) dependent mechanism. J Cell Physiol. 2014;229(8):1096–105.
10. Engelhardt S, Huang SF, Patkar S, Gassmann M, Ogunshola OO. Differential responses of blood-brain barrier associated cells to hypoxia and ischemia: a comparative study. Fluids Barriers CNS. 2015;12:4.
11. Al Ahmad A, Gassmann M, Ogunshola OO. Involvement of oxidative stress in hypoxia-induced blood-brain barrier breakdown. Microvasc Res. 2012;84(2):222–5.
12. Lee B, Clarke D, Al Ahmad A, Kahle M, Parham C, Auckland L, et al. Perlecan domain V is neuroprotective and proangiogenic following ischemic stroke in rodents. J Clin Investig. 2011;121(8):3005–23.
13. Al Ahmad A, Gassmann M, Ogunshola OO. Maintaining blood-brain barrier integrity: pericytes perform better than astrocytes during prolonged oxygen deprivation. J Cell Physiol. 2009;218(3):612–22.
14. Abbruscato TJ, Davis TP. Combination of hypoxia/aglycemia compromises in vitro blood-brain barrier integrity. J Pharmacol Exp Ther. 1999;289:668–75.
15. Yamagata K, Tagami M, Takenaga F, Yamori Y, Itoh S. Hypoxia-induced changes in tight junction permeability of brain capillary endothelial cells are associated with IL-1beta and nitric oxide. Neurobiol Dis. 2004;17:491–9.
16. Brown RC, Davis TP. Hypoxia/aglycemia alters expression of occludin and actin in brain endothelial cells. Biochem Biophys Res Commun. 2005;327:1114–23.
17. Culot M, Mysiorek C, Renftel M, Roussel BD, Hommet Y, Vivien D, et al. Cerebrovascular protection as a possible mechanism for the protective effects of NXY-059 in preclinical models: an in vitro study. Brain Res. 2009;1294:144–52.
18. Yu J, Vodyanik MA, Smuga-Otto K, Antosiewicz-Bourget J, Frane JL, Tian S, et al. Induced pluripotent stem cell lines derived from human somatic cells. Science. 2007;318(5858):1917–20.
19. Wilson HK, Canfield SG, Hjortness MK, Palecek SP, Shusta EV. Exploring the effects of cell seeding density on the differentiation of human pluripotent stem cells to brain microvascular endothelial cells. Fluids Barriers CNS. 2015;12:13.
20. Lippmann ES, Al-Ahmad A, Azarin SM, Palecek SP, Shusta EV. A retinoic acid-enhanced, multicellular human blood-brain barrier model derived from stem cell sources. Sci Rep. 2014;4:4160.
21. Lippmann ES, Azarin SM, Kay JE, Nessler RA, Wilson HK, Al-Ahmad A, et al. Derivation of blood-brain barrier endothelial cells from human pluripotent stem cells. Nat Biotechnol. 2012;30(8):783–91.
22. Weksler BB, Subileau EA, Perriere N, Charneau P, Holloway K, Leveque M, et al. Blood-brain barrier-specific properties of a human adult brain endothelial cell line. FASEB J. 2005;19:1872–4.
23. Perriere N, Demeuse P, Garcia E, Regina A, Debray M, Andreux JP, et al. Puromycin-based purification of rat brain capillary endothelial cell cultures. Effect on the expression of blood-brain barrier-specific properties. J Neurochem. 2005;93(2):279–89.
24. Guo L, Lan J, Lin Y, Guo P, Nie Q, Mao Q, et al. Hypoxia/ischemia up-regulates Id2 expression in neuronal cells in vivo and in vitro. Neurosci Lett. 2013;554:88–93.

25. Gotoh M, Sano-Maeda K, Murofushi H, Murakami-Murofushi K. Protection of neuroblastoma Neuro2A cells from hypoxia-induced apoptosis by cyclic phosphatidic acid (cPA). PLoS ONE. 2012;7(12):e51093.
26. Wang B, Zou Y, Yuan ZL, Xiao JG. Genistein suppressed upregulation of vascular endothelial growth factor expression by cobalt chloride and hypoxia in rabbit retinal pigment epithelium cells. J Ocul Pharmacol Ther. 2003;19(5):457–64.
27. Bernaudin M, Bellail A, Marti HH, Yvon A, Vivien D, Duchatelle I, et al. Neurons and astrocytes express EPO mRNA: oxygen-sensing mechanisms that involve the redox-state of the brain. Glia. 2000;30:271–8.
28. Wang GL, Jiang BH, Rue EA, Semenza GL. Hypoxia-inducible factor 1 is a basic-helix-loop-helix-PAS heterodimer regulated by cellular O2 tension. Proc Natl Acad Sci USA. 1995;92:5510–4.
29. Minchenko A, Bauer T, Salceda S, Caro J. Hypoxic stimulation of vascular endothelial growth factor expression in vitro and in vivo. Lab Invest. 1994;71:374–9.
30. Naik P, Cucullo L. In vitro blood-brain barrier models: current and perspective technologies. J Pharm Sci. 2012;101:1337–54.
31. Poller B, Gutmann H, Krahenbuhl S, Weksler B, Romero I, Couraud PO, et al. The human brain endothelial cell line hCMEC/D3 as a human blood-brain barrier model for drug transport studies. J Neurochem. 2008;107:1358–68.
32. Cucullo L, Couraud PO, Weksler B, Romero IA, Hossain M, Rapp E, et al. Immortalized human brain endothelial cells and flow-based vascular modeling: a marriage of convenience for rational neurovascular studies. J Cereb Blood Flow Metab. 2008;28(2):312–28.
33. Hartwig K, Fackler V, Jaksch-Bogensperger H, Winter S, Furtner T, Couillard-Despres S, et al. Cerebrolysin protects PC12 cells from CoCl2-induced hypoxia employing GSK3 beta signaling. Int J Dev Neurosci. 2014;38:52–8.
34. Guan D, Su Y, Li Y, Wu C, Meng Y, Peng X, et al. Tetramethylpyrazine inhibits CoCl2 -induced neurotoxicity through enhancement of Nrf2/GCLc/GSH and suppression of HIF1alpha/NOX2/ROS pathways. J Neurochem. 2015;134(3):551–65.
35. Huang CY, Hsieh YL, Ju DT, Lin CC, Kuo CH, Liou YF, et al. Attenuation of magnesium sulfate on CoCl(2)-induced cell death by activating ERK1/2/MAPK and inhibiting HIF-1alpha via mitochondrial apoptotic signaling suppression in a neuronal cell line. Chin J Physiol. 2015;58(4):244–53.
36. Mo SJ, Hong J, Chen X, Han F, Ni Y, Zheng Y, et al. VEGF-mediated NF-kappaB activation protects PC12 cells from damage induced by hypoxia. Neurosci Lett. 2016;610:54–9.
37. Sumantran VN. Cellular chemosensitivity assays: an overview. Methods Mol Biol. 2011;731:219–36.
38. Ogunshola OO, Al Ahmad A. HIF-1 at the blood-brain barrier: a mediator of permeability? Special topic: the many faces of hypoxia HIF-1 at the blood-brain barrier. High Alt Med Biol. 2012;13:153–61.
39. Zhu H, Wang Z, Xing Y, Gao Y, Ma T, Lou L, et al. Baicalin reduces the permeability of the blood-brain barrier during hypoxia in vitro by increasing the expression of tight junction proteins in brain microvascular endothelial cells. J Ethnopharmacol. 2011;141:714–20.
40. Yan J, Zhou B, Taheri S, Shi H. Differential effects of HIF-1 inhibition by YC-1 on the overall outcome and blood-brain barrier damage in a rat model of ischemic stroke. PLoS ONE. 2011;6:e27798.
41. Kimura K, Teranishi S, Kawamoto K, Nishida T. Protective effect of dexamethasone against hypoxia-induced disruption of barrier function in human corneal epithelial cells. Exp Eye Res. 2011;92:388–93.
42. Lochhead JJ, McCaffrey G, Quigley CE, Finch J, DeMarco KM, Nametz N, et al. Oxidative stress increases blood-brain barrier permeability and induces alterations in occludin during hypoxia-reoxygenation. J Cereb Blood Flow Metab. 2010;30:1625–36.
43. Natah SS, Srinivasan S, Pittman QJ, Zhao Z, Dunn JF. Effects of acute hypoxia and hyperthermia on the permeability of the blood brain barrier in adult rats. J Appl Physiol. 2009;107(4):1348–56.
44. McCaffrey G, Willis CL, Staatz WD, Nametz N, Quigley CA, Hom S, et al. Occludin oligomeric assemblies at tight junctions of the blood-brain barrier are altered by hypoxia and reoxygenation stress. J Neurochem. 2009;110:58–71.
45. Semenza GL. Dynamic regulation of stem cell specification and maintenance by hypoxia-inducible factors. Mol Aspects Med. 2015;47:15–23.
46. Patak P, Jin F, Schafer ST, Metzen E, Hermann DM. The ATP-binding cassette transporters ABCB1 and ABCC1 are not regulated by hypoxia in immortalised human brain microvascular endothelial cells. Exp Transl Stroke Med. 2011;3:12.
47. Cunningham LA, Wetzel M, Rosenberg GA. Multiple roles for MMPs and TIMPs in cerebral ischemia. Glia. 2005;50:329–39.
48. Yang T, Roder KE, Abbruscato TJ. Evaluation of bEnd5 cell line as an in vitro model for the blood-brain barrier under normal and hypoxic/aglycemic conditions. J Pharm Sci. 2007;96:3196–213.
49. Yang Y, Rosenberg GA. Blood-brain barrier breakdown in acute and chronic cerebrovascular disease. Stroke. 2011;42:3323–8.
50. Vandekeere S, Dewerchin M, Carmeliet P. Angiogenesis revisited: an overlooked role of endothelial cell metabolism in vessel sprouting. Microcirculation. 2015;22(7):509–17.
51. Berg K, Hansen MB, Nielsen SE. A new sensitive bioassay for precise quantification of interferon activity as measured via the mitochondrial dehydrogenase function in cells (MTT-method). APMIS. 1990;98(2):156–62.

14

Growth-factor reduced Matrigel source influences stem cell derived brain microvascular endothelial cell barrier properties

Ronak Patel and Abraham J. Alahmad*

Abstract

Background: Patient-derived induced pluripotent stem cells (iPSCs) are an innovative source as an in vitro model for neurological diseases. Recent studies have demonstrated the differentiation of brain microvascular endothelial cells (BMECs) from various stem cell sources, including iPSC lines. However, the impact of the culturing conditions used to maintain such stem cell pluripotency on their ability to differentiate into BMECs remains undocumented. In this study, we investigated the effect of different sources of Matrigel and stem cell maintenance medium on BMEC differentiation efficiency.

Methods: The IMR90-c4 iPSC line was maintained on mTeSR1 or in essential-8 (E-8) medium on growth factor-reduced (GFR) Matrigel from three different manufacturers. Cells were differentiated into BMECs following published protocols. The phenotype of BMEC monolayers was assessed by immunocytochemistry. Barrier function was assessed by transendothelial electrical resistance (TEER) and permeability to sodium fluorescein, whereas the presence of drug efflux pumps was assessed by uptake assay using fluorescent substrates.

Results: Stem cell maintenance medium had little effect on the yield and barrier phenotype of IMR90-derived BMECs. The source of GFR-Matrigel used for the differentiation process significantly impacted the ability of IMR90-derived BMECs to form tight monolayers, as measured by TEER and fluorescein permeability. However, the Matrigel source had minimal effect on BMEC phenotype and drug efflux pump activity.

Conclusion: This study supports the ability to differentiate BMECs from iPSCs grown in mTeSR1 or E-8 medium and also suggests that the origin of GFR-Matrigel has a marked inpact on BMEC barrier properties.

Keywords: Stem cells, Blood–brain barrier, Matrigel, Barrier function, Drug transporters

Background

The blood–brain barrier (BBB), or neurovascular unit, provides a stable and defined microenvironment for the central nervous system (CNS). Among the different types of cells forming the BBB, brain microvascular endothelial cells (BMECs) provide both a physical and chemical barrier, tightly regulating the diffusion of water, ions and lipophilic compounds into the CNS [1–4].

In vitro models of the BBB are valuable tools for drug discovery research as they provide an insight into the diffusion profile of existing and prospective drug candidates targeting the CNS [2, 5]. However, the current use of in vitro models of the human BBB based on primary cultures and immortalized cell lines remains hampered by their limited barrier tightness [6].

Recently, several studies have documented success in differentiating BMECs from stem cell sources, including human pluripotent stem cells such as embryonic stem cells (hESCs), hematopoietic stem cells (HSCs) and induced pluripotent stem cells (iPSCs) [7–10]. Such stem cell-derived BMECs share similarities with established models including the expression of tight

*Correspondence: abraham.al-ahmad@ttuhsc.edu
Department of Pharmaceutical Sciences, School of Pharmacy, Texas Tech University Health Sciences Center, 1300 South Coulter Street, Amarillo, TX 79106, USA

junction proteins, the formation of a tight monolayer and the expression of functional drug transporters. Several parameters have been described as important for the generation of human pluripotent stem cell-derived BMECs in order to achieve barrier tightness suitable for drug permeability screening. These include cell density [11], the addition of retinoic acid [7], and co-culture with astrocytes and neurons [7, 8]. However, the ability to translate the differentiation protocol for patient-derived iPSCs may be hampered by variations in stem cell maintenance protocols. For instance, human pluripotent stem cells (hPSCs) grown and maintained in a feeder-free system are routinely grown on growth factor reduced (GFR) Matrigel- or vitronectin-N (VTN)-coated tissue culture plastic surfaces [12, 13], supplemented with mTeSR1 or essential 8 medium (E8) [12, 13]. GFR Matrigel constitutes a complex extracellular matrix (ECM) mixture secreted by Engelbreth–Holm–Swarm mouse sarcoma cells with an approximate composition of 60 % laminin, 30 % collagen IV and 8 % entactin as well as other undefined ECM components [14]. Because of its complexity, Matrigel remains undefined and may constitute a source of variability that can impact hPSC-derived BMEC differentiation efficacy [15]. However, the effect of other culturing conditions (ECMs and media) on the outcome of hPSC-derived BMEC differentiation remains undocumented. In this study, we investigated the effects of different ECMs and stem cell maintenance medium on IMR90-c4 human iPSC line, a cell line with a highly-documented BMEC differentiation profile.

Methods

The undifferentiated IMR90 (IMR90-c4) iPSC line [13] (WiCell, Madison, WI, USA) was maintained in mTeSR (mTeSR1, Stem Cell Technologies, Vancouver BC, Canada) or in essential-8 medium (E-8, ThermoFisher, Waltham, MA, USA) on hESC-qualified GFR-Matrigel (C-Matrigel, Corning, Corning, NY, USA) [13].

Undifferentiated IMR90-c4 iPSC colonies were routinely maintained on 6-well tissue culture plates (Corning) coated with C-Matrigel in presence of mTeSR1 or E-8 medium. Prior to differentiation, cells were dissociated as single cells using Accutase cell detachment solution (Corning) and seeded at a seeding density of 8×10^3 cells/cm^2 (B-Matrigel) or 20×10^3 cells/cm^2 on tissue culture plates (Corning). Plates were coated with one of the following hESC-qualified GFR-Matrigels at a concentration 8.3 μg/cm^2 for B-Matrigel, (BD Biosciences, Fairleigh, NJ, USA) and T-Matrigel, (Trevigen, Gaithersburg, MD, USA) or at a dilution indicated by the manufacturer for C-Matrigel; L-Matrigel, and Vitronectin (ThermoFisher, Waltham, MA, USA). This study was conducted with at least two distinct ECM batches serial numbers. After 5 days of culture, IMR90 iPSCs became differentiated into BMECs as previously reported [7, 11]. In brief, cells were maintained in unconditioned medium (UM; DMEM/F12 with 15 mM HEPES supplemented with 20 % KO serum replacement, 1 % MEM non-essential aminoacids, and 0.5 % Glutamax I, ThermoFisher) and 0.1 mM β-mercaptoethanol (Sigma-Aldrich, St Louis, MO, USA) for six consecutive days, with the medium replaced daily. After 6 days of differentiation, IMR90-derived BMECs were further matured in EC differentiation medium (EC serum free medium (ThermoFisher), supplemented with 1 % platelet-poor derived plasma serum (ThermoFisher), 20 μg/mL human basic fibroblast growth factor (R&D Systems) and 10 μM all-trans retinoic acid (Sigma-Aldrich) for 2 days. After 8 days of differentiation, cells were enzymatically dissociated and seeded at a density of 10^6 cells/cm^2 on 12-well transwell polyester cell culture inserts (0.4 μm pore size) coated with collagen from human placenta (Sigma-Aldrich) and fibronectin from bovine plasma (Sigma-Aldrich) at concentrations of 80 and 20 μg/cm^2 respectively as previously published [7, 11]. After 24 h (day 9), BMECs were maintained in EC differentiation medium containing only 1 % platelet-poor plasma-derived serum. On day 10, 48 h after seeding, transendothelial electrical resistance (TEER) was assessed using an EVOM STX2 chopstick electrode (World Precision Instruments, Sarasota, FL, USA) and by measuring permeability (Pe) to sodium fluorescein solution (1 μg/mL, Sigma-Aldrich) using the clearance slope method as previously reported [7, 11, 16].

The immunostaining procedure on fixed cells was identical to that previously published [7, 11]. Cells were visualized on an Olympus IX81 inverted epifluorescence microscope. Photomicrographs were acquired using Slidebook 4.5 (Intelligent Imaging Innovation, Denver, CO, USA) and processed with ImageJ (NIH, Bethesda, MD, USA).

Drug efflux pump activity was assessed using the same accumulation assays as previously reported [7, 11]. In brief, BMECs monolayers were incubated in presence of 10 μM Rhodamine 123 and 10 μM BODIPY-FL prazosin (Sigma-Aldrich), 5 μM doxorubicin or 10 μM CM-DCFDA for 1 h at 37 °C. For experiments involving inhibitors, cells were pre-incubated in presence of cyclosporine A (CsA), 5 μM, Ko143, 1 μM, or MK571, 10 μM (Sigma-Aldrich) for 1 h prior to the experiment and maintained during the whole procedure. Cells were washed with ice-cold PBS and lysed using RIPA extraction buffer (ThermoFisher). The fluorescence of the cell extract was assessed using a fluorescent plate reader (SynergyMX2, BioTek, Burlington, VT, USA). Raw fluorescence units (RFU) were adjusted to the cell extract protein concentration (as determined by BCA assay) to determine the drug uptake (expressed as RFU/μg protein). The drug uptake in untreated (without inhibitors) monolayers was arbitrarily set at 100 % and identified as control. The drug uptake in treated monolayers (with pharmacological inhibitors) was normalized to their respective controls, as previously published [7, 11].

Data are expressed as mean ± SD from a minimum of six experiments (two distinct ECM batches, three distinct differentiation passages for each batch. For each passage, experiments were done with two technical duplicates). Statistical analysis was performed using one-way ANOVA using Prism 6.0 statistical package (Graphpad Software, La Jolla, CA, USA).

Results

Experiments using mTeSR medium

We first investigated the impact of different Matrigel sources on undifferentiated IMR90 stem cell growth and maintenance in mTeSR medium at a seeding density of 20 × 10^3 cells/cm^2 (Fig. 1a). In our hands, IMR90 iPSC colonies grown on B-Matrigel, L-Matrigel and T-Matrigel showed similar doubling times (27.28, 26.69 and 24.49 h respectively), however IMR90 cells grown on C-Matrigel showed a much slower growth rate, with an average doubling time of 42.30 h. We found that culturing IMR90 iPSCs on C-Matrigel and T-Matrigel with a starting seeding cell density of 8 × 10^3 cells/cm^2 as previously reported [11], failed to achieve a complete differentiation and we noted a significant cell loss after 3–4 days of growth in unconditioned medium (UM, data not shown). A satisfactory differentiation was only achieved when we set our seeding cell density at 20 × 10^3 cells/cm^2 and allowed our colonies to grow for 5 days. At this seeding density, the yield (calculated as the number of cells harvested at day 8 of differentiation versus the initial seeding density at day 0) was approximately 26.92 ± 4.69-fold increase in B-Matrigel group, but was lower in C- and T-Matrigel, with increases of 6.30 ± 1.32 and 4.03 ± 1.32-fold, respectively (Fig. 1b). Upon purification, we noted a homogenous BMEC cell monolayer in all three groups, as these cells expressed markers representative of the vascular endothelial lineage (PECAM-1, VE-cadherin), and also the expression of BBB markers (GLUT1, claudin-5, occludin), consistent with the existing literature (Fig. 1c) [7, 8, 11]. Taken together, our data suggest that Matrigel from different sources may affect the outcome in terms of BMEC differentiation and yield.

Next, we assessed the barrier properties of such monolayers in monocultures by measuring both transendothelial electrical resistance (TEER) and paracellular permeability to sodium fluorescein (NaF). On B-Matrigel, IMR90 showed TEER (Fig. 2a) values of 1332 ± 558 Ω cm^2. In contrast, BMECs differentiated on

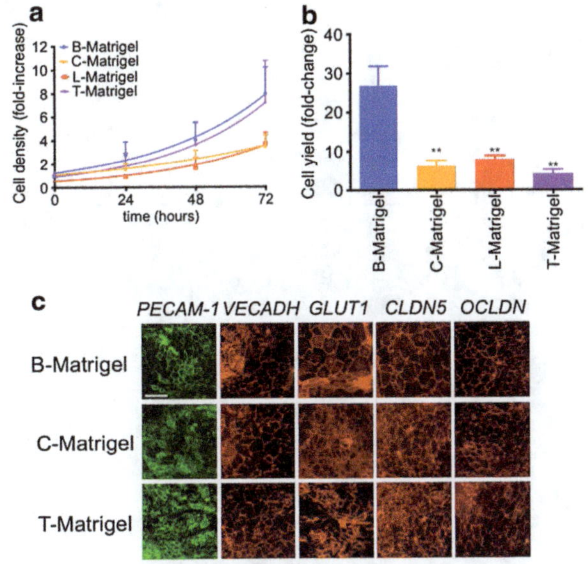

Fig. 1 Effects of Matrigel origin on IMR90 iPS cell growth and BMEC differentiation using mTeSR medium. **a** Undifferentiated IMR90 cells maintained in mTeSR were dissociated as single cells seeded on Matrigel from BD Biosciences (B-Matrigel, *blue*), from Corning (C-Matrigel, *orange*), from ThermoFisher (L-Matrigel, *red*) or from Trevigen (T-Matrigel, *purple*) at 20 × 10^3 cells/cm^2. After 24, 48 and 72 h following cell seeding, IMR90 iPSC colonies were dissociated and counted using a cell hemocytometer and Trypan blue exclusion assay. **b** BMEC yield after 8 days of differentiation obtained by calculating the ratio of cell density at 8 days of differentiation versus the initial cell density seeded at day 0, ** denotes $P < 0.01$ in comparison to B-Matrigel. **c** Representative immunostained micrographs of PECAM-1, VE-cadherin, Glut-1 Claudin 5 and Occludin expression in purified BMEC monolayers 48 h post-purification. *Note* the formation of a monolayer as marked by defined tight junction complexes in one focal plane and the absence of junctional cellular overlap. *Scale bar* = 20 μm

C-Matrigel displayed a much lower TEER and the average electrical resistance measured was 424.3 ± 205.1 Ω cm^2. Finally, on T-Matrigel we noted showed TEER values of 1439 ± 281.4 Ω cm^2. Using a different technique to confirm such differences in the barrier function, we measured changes in paracellular permeability using sodium fluorescein (NaF) as a paracellular marker (Fig. 2b). In our hands, we noted permeability (Pe) values of 0.44 × 10^{-4} cm/min on monolayers differentiated on B-Matrigel. Cells differentiated on C-Matrigel showed a tenfold higher permeability, with an average Pe value of 4.20 × 10^{-4} cm/min, whereas cells grown on T-Matrigel had a Pe value of 1.57 × 10^{-4} cm/min.

In addition, we investigated the expression (Fig. 2c) and activity (Fig. 3) of P-glycoprotein (P-gp), breast cancer resistant protein (BCRP) and multidrug resistant protein (MRP) by immunocytochemistry and by drug accumulation assay, respectively. In our hands, all groups had

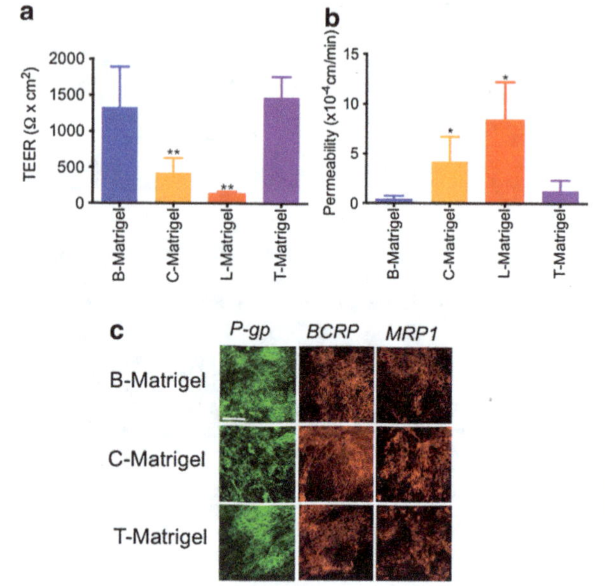

Fig. 2 Matrigel origin impacts BMECs barrier properties. **a**, **b** TEER and sodium fluorescein permeabilities in IMR90-derived BMECs differentiated on B-, C- or T-Matrigel. *Note* the degraded barrier function of cells grown on C-Matrigel compared to the two other groups. * and ** denotes $P < 0.05$ and $P < 0.01$ in comparison to B-Matrigel. **c** Representative immunostained micrographs of P-gp, BCRP and MRP1 expression in purified BMECs monolayers. *Scale bar* = 40 µm

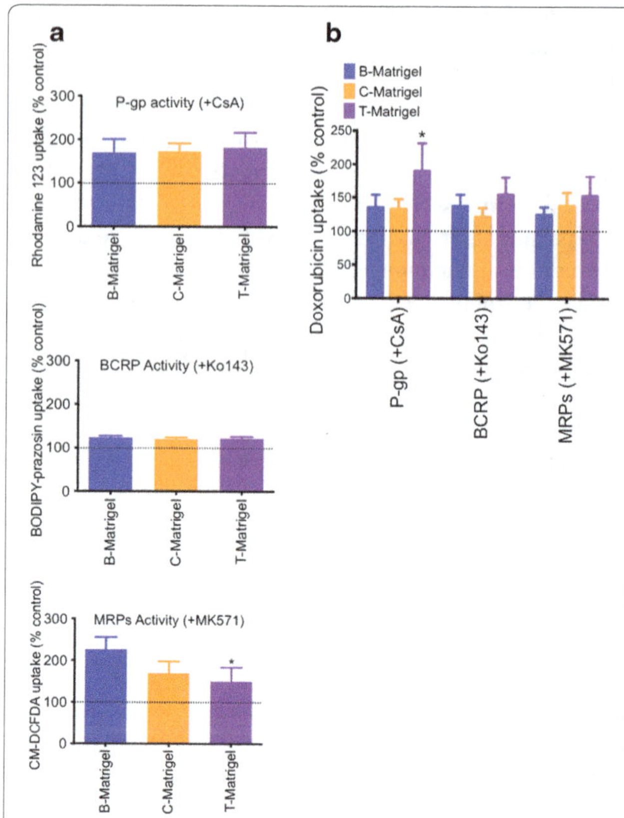

Fig. 3 Matrigel origin has a minor impact on BMECs drug efflux activity. **a** Drug uptake of rhodamine 123, BODIPY FL-prazosin and CM-DCFDA in presence of 5 µM cyclosporine A (CsA, P-gp inhibitor), 1 µM Ko143 (BCRP inhibitor) or 10 µM MK571 (pan-MRP inhibitor), respectively. Fluorescence values in controls (no inhibitor) were arbitrarily set to 100 %, * and ** denote $P < 0.05$ and $P < 0.01$ in comparison to B-Matrigel. **b** Doxorubicin accumulation profile in presence of CsA, Ko143 or MK571. Doxorubicin net uptake was calculated as previously described

positive expression for P-gp, BCRP and MRP1 (Fig. 2c); all three proteins were detected in our monolayers and this was consistent with the existing literature [7, 8, 11]. We did not notice any dramatic differences in immunoreactivity between the three groups. Thus we consider there are similar protein expression levels in all groups. To demonstrate that Matrigel had little effect on drug efflux pump activity, we assessed changes in efflux activity by measuring, in the presence or absence of inhibitors, uptake of rhodamine 123, FL-BODIPY prazosin, and CM-DCFDA as these fluorescent dyes are known substrates for P-gp [17], BCRP [18–20] and MRPs [21], respectively (Fig. 3). The net uptake (the difference in fluorescence between untreated group designated 100 %, and inhibitor-treated group), was not significantly different for P-gp-mediated efflux between the groups (Fig. 3a, upper panel). However, we noted a 1.7 fold increase in uptake of rhodamine 123 following inhibition with 5 µM CsA: this increase was consistent with the previous literature [7, 8, 11]. A similar outcome was observed in the net uptake of FL-BODIPY prazosin following inhibition with Ko143 (Fig. 3a, middle panel). However, we noted a slight but significant difference in net uptake of CM-DCFDA in that cells grown on B-Matrigel showed a 2.3 fold-increase in uptake in presence of MK571 compared to control, whereas cells grown on T-Matrigel showed only a 1.6 fold-increase in uptake compared to control (Fig. 3a, lower panel). Because such substrates are not exclusive to their efflux pumps and may interact with other efflux pumps, we further confirmed the presence of efflux pump activity using doxorubicin, a substrate for all three pumps (Fig. 3b). With the exception of a twofold increase in doxorubicin net uptake following CsA treatment in the T-Matrigel group, we did not notice any significant differences in the net uptake between the different Matrigel groups. We noted an increase of 1.3 to 1.4-fold compared to control, which is consistent with previous literature [7]. In conclusion, the source of Matrigel influenced the barrier outcome in IMR90-derived BMECs in terms of barrier tightness but not in terms of drug efflux-mediated transport.

Experiments using essential-8 medium

Because GFR-Matrigel from different sources displayed variable outcomes on IMR90 differentiation into BMECs, and also that the production of B-Matrigel has been discontinued, we investigated alternative culturing conditions that can circumvent these issues. In particular, we investigated the possibility to change the BMEC differentiation protocol using defined conditions with, E-8 medium and two additional ECMs, vitronectin and L-Matrigel (Fig. 4). Undifferentiated IMR90 iPSCs grown on C-Matrigel in presence of E-8 medium (Fig. 4a, orange line), showed a doubling time similar to mTeSR (26.72 and 27.28 h respectively), as well as cells grown on Geltrex [L-Matrigel (red line), 20.31 h] and Vitronectin-N [Vitronectin (green line), 29.69 h]. However, cells grown on T-Matrigel (purple line) in combination with E-8 medium displayed a much reduced growth rate compared to mTeSR with an average doubling time of 41.05 h. By maintaining the same seeding density as previously mentioned, we obtained after 8 days of differentiation an average BMEC yield (Fig. 4b) of 15.45 ± 9.08 and 14.66 ± 8.78-fold increase in cells grown in C-Matrigel and T-Matrigel respectively. Surprisingly, cells grown on L-Matrigel or on Vitronectin were incapable of reaching a yield that was higher than twofold. Next we compared the average barrier function of these monolayers by measuring changes in TEER and permeability (Fig. 4c, d). Maintenance of IMR90 iPSCs in E-8 did not interfere with the BMEC barrier tightness, as we noted TEER values (305.4 ± 85.09 and 1254 ± 523.7 Ω cm^2) and permeability (3.66 ± 1.20 and 0.54 ± 0.13 × 10^{-4} cm/min) for C and T-Matrigels, similar to those reported in IMR90 iPSCs maintained in mTeSR media. However, cells differentiated on L-Matrigel and Vitronectin showed poor barrier properties, as noted by lower TEER (169.0 ± 32.86 and 23.75 ± 16.99 Ω cm^2) and higher permeabilities (5.76 ± 1.05 and 9.50 ± 2.90 × 10^{-4} cm/min). Finally, we investigated changes in drug efflux activity by measuring changes in rhodamine 123, FL-BODIPY prazosin and CM-DCFDA uptake in cells grown on both C- and T-Matrigel (Fig. 5). We observed similar trends to cells maintained in mTeSR prior to differentiation (Fig. 5a), although the net uptake values for each pumps were

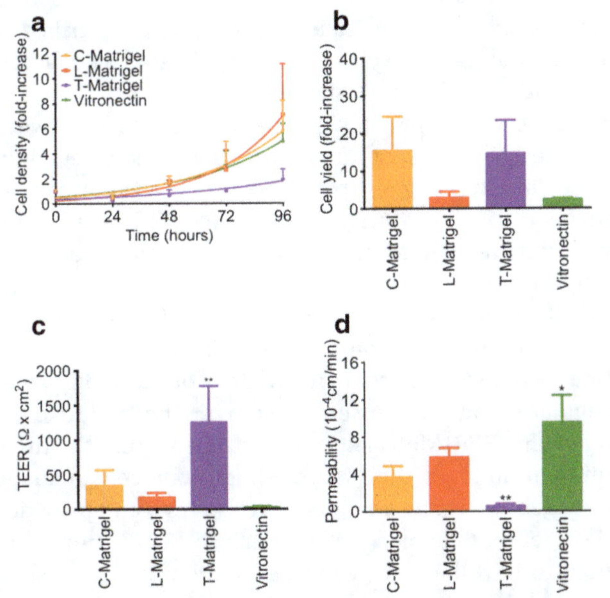

Fig. 4 Essential-8 medium does not impact BMECs differentiation. **a** IMR90 iPSC growth curve on C-Matrigel (*orange*), L-Matrigel (*red*), T-Matrigel (*purple*) or vitronectin (*green*)-coated surfaces. IMR90 iPSCs were seeded as single cells at day 0 at a density of 20 × 10^3 cells/cm^2 on the different types of matrices and maintained in E-8 medium. At each timepoint (day), IMR90 iPSC colonies were dissociated as single cells using Accutase and counted with a cell hemocytometer using 0.4 % Trypan blue as an exclusion dye. **b** Cell yield at day 8 of differentiation. Cell yield was determined by dividing average density at day 8 of differentiation by the initial cell seeding density at day 0. **c**, **d** TEER and sodium fluorescein permeability values on purified iPSC-derived BMECs monolayers 48 h after purification. *Note* the poor barrier properties in cells differentiated on Geltrex (L-Matrigel) or on vitronectin-N (vitronectin), * and ** denote $P < 0.05$ and $P < 0.01$ in comparison to C-Matrigel

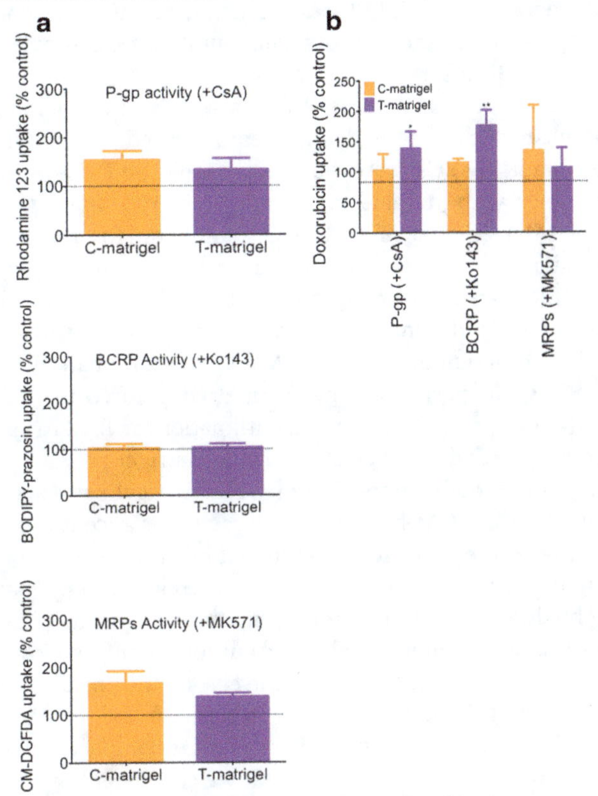

Fig. 5 Essential-8 medium. **a** Drug uptake profile of rhodamine 123, BODIPY-prazosin and CM-DCFDA in presence of CsA, Ko143 or MK571. Drug uptakes of the same efflux substrates in absence of inhibitors were used as controls. Fluorescence in controls was arbitrarily set to 100 %. **b** Doxorubicin drug uptake profile in presence of CsA, Ko143 or MK571, * and ** denote $P < 0.05$ and $P < 0.01$ in comparison to C-Matrigel

slightly lower than IMR90 iPSCs maintained in mTeSR. Such decreased drug efflux pump activity was also observed in the net uptake of doxorubicin (Fig. 5b), especially in cells differentiated on C-Matrigel. In conclusion, our data suggest that the nature of the medium used in maintenance of pluripotent stem cells has little impact on the differentiation process. However, the replacement of Matrigel by a defined ECM has a detrimental effect on BMEC differentiation.

Discussion

In the last few years, in vitro models based on patient-derived iPSCs have gained a sizable momentum in modeling neurodegenerative disorders and certain types of epilepsies [22–25]. More recently, the publication of stem cell-based models of the human BBB brought a complementary approach to other in vitro models based on human primary cultures or on the hCMEC/D3 immortalized cell line [7–9, 11, 26–29]. Such patient-specific and disease-specific sources of cells may provide a valuable tool in modeling the impact of genetic disorders at the BBB and lead to a better understanding of how such disorders may result in the dysfunction of one or several components of the neurovascular unit (e.g. astrocytes, neurons, BMECs).

In their previous studies, Shusta and colleagues have established the method and demonstrated the ability to obtain BMECs from both embryonic and iPS stem cell lines with variable outcomes [7, 8, 11]. They used GFR-Matrigel and mTeSR as a foundation for the differentiation. In this study, we investigated the impact of GFR-Matrigel from different sources and xeno-free culturing conditions (E-8 medium and Vitronectin) on BMEC differentiation using IMR90-c4, a human iPSC line [13]. In particular, the main driving force for our study was primed by the discontinuation of B-Matrigel production and its replacement by C-Matrigel.

Although the composition of GFR-Matrigel suggests a reduction in ECM-bound growth factors, a recent comparative proteomic study conducted by Hughes and colleagues between conventional and GFR-Matrigel has highlighted notable differences in their chemical composition [15]. Interestingly, the authors identified over 400 peptides that were exclusively found inside the GFR-Matrigel and they also found signatures of proteins found naturally in cytoplasmic or nuclear compartments. Based on this study and our data, we can speculate that Matrigel composition may make an important contribution to BMEC differentiation. We speculate that cell-ECM interactions with integrins maybe an important driving force in this differentiation process, as we were not able to obtain any satisfactory differentiation when cells were grown on vitronectin-N. However, we cannot exclude the presence of non-ECM factors (e.g. growth factors) retained by the GFR-Matrigel that may influence such differentiation.

An interesting feature observed in our study was the notable decrease in barrier tightness when cells were grown on C-Matrigel. On this ECM, differentiating iPSC colonies failed to form neural tracts as observed by Shusta and colleagues [7, 8, 11]. Indeed, IMR90 differentiating colonies on this substrate showed a macroscopical profile similar to the low-density (10×10^3 cells/cm^2) group described by Wilson et al. [11], although we initiated our differentiation at a much higher cell density (100×10^3 cells/cm^2). Barrier properties from BMEC monolayers differentiated in C-Matrigel shared similar values to BMECs purified from the low-density group, as marked by low TEER values (~300 Ω cm^2). Notably such values coincide with those reported in the seminal study by Lippmann et al. [8], in which BMEC differentiation was performed in absence of retinoic acid (RA). RA has been documented as a barrier inducer in hCMEC/D3 cell monolayers [30], yet the induction range was much more modest compared to IMR90-derived BMECs. We speculate that in our model, neuron progenitors described in such neural tracts might be secreting RA-induced factors resulting in the barrier tightening.

Finally, we observed significant differences between matrices in terms of undifferentiated stem cell doubling time thus suggesting differences in growth factors intrinsic to GFR-Matrigel sources. GFR-Matrigel differs from regular Matrigel by an additional treatment with ammonium sulfate. Such treatment results in the reduction of growth factors bound to the extracellular matrix components contained within the Matrigel [31]. Thus, we speculate that one source of variability may originate from this essential step in the manufacturing of the GFR-Matrigel. In this study, among the three different manufacturers providing stem cell qualified Matrigel, only one manufacturer (Trevigen) provided Matrigel that enabled IMR90-derived BMEC monocultures to have barrier properties similar to the existing literature.

Conclusion

This study confirms the ability to differentiate iPSC-derived BMECs from the IMR90-c4 cells as previously reported. Whereas the effect of stem cell maintenance medium has little impact on BMEC differentiation, variations in the production and manufacturing of GFR-Matrigel raised important issues that should foster further research. A transition from empirically-formulated ECMs into a highly-defined synthetic scaffold would ensure consistent BMEC differentiation using a xeno-free, growth factor-independent medium.

Authors' contributions

RP carried out the experiments involving E-8 medium, AJA carried out the experiments involving mTeSR1 medium. AJA conceived and designed the experiments. AJA drafted the manuscript. Both authors read and approved the final manuscript.

Acknowledgements

This study was funded by institutional funds and by a BD Biosciences Stem Cell Award to AA.

Competing interests

The authors declare that they have no competing interests.

References

1. Blanchette M, Daneman R. Formation and maintenance of the BBB. Mech Dev. 2015. doi:10.1016/j.mod.2015.07.007.
2. Palmiotti CA, Prasad S, Naik P, Abul KM, Sajja RK, Achyuta AH, et al. In vitro cerebrovascular modeling in the 21st century: current and prospective technologies. Pharm Res. 2014;31(12):3229–50. doi:10.1007/s11095-014-1464-6.
3. Obermeier B, Daneman R, Ransohoff RM. Development, maintenance and disruption of the blood–brain barrier. Nat Med. 2013;19(12):1584–96. doi:10.1038/nm.3407.
4. Abbott NJ. Blood–brain barrier structure and function and the challenges for CNS drug delivery. J Inherit Metab Dis. 2013;36(3):437–49. doi:10.1007/s10545-013-9608-0.
5. Wilhelm I, Krizbai IA. In vitro models of the blood–brain barrier for the study of drug delivery to the brain. Mol Pharm. 2014;11(7):1949–63. doi:10.1021/mp500046f.
6. Shawahna R, Decleves X, Scherrmann J-M. Hurdles with using in vitro models to predict human blood–brain barrier drug permeability: a special focus on transporters and metabolizing enzymes. Curr Drug Metab. 2013;14:120–36.
7. Lippmann ES, Al-Ahmad A, Azarin SM, Palecek SP, Shusta EV. A retinoic acid-enhanced, multicellular human blood–brain barrier model derived from stem cell sources. Sci Rep. 2014;4:4160. doi:10.1038/srep04160.
8. Lippmann ES, Azarin SM, Kay JE, Nessler RA, Wilson HK, Al-Ahmad A, et al. Derivation of blood–brain barrier endothelial cells from human pluripotent stem cells. Nat Biotechnol. 2012;30(8):783–91. doi:10.1038/nbt.2247.
9. Cecchelli R, Aday S, Sevin E, Almeida C, Culot M, Dehouck L, et al. A stable and reproducible human blood–brain barrier model derived from hematopoietic stem cells. PLoS One. 2014;9(6):e99733. doi:10.1371/journal.pone.0099733.
10. Zhao Z, Sagare AP, Ma Q, Halliday MR, Kong P, Kisler K, et al. Central role for PICALM in amyloid-beta blood–brain barrier transcytosis and clearance. Nat Neurosci. 2015;18(7):978–87. doi:10.1038/nn.4025.
11. Wilson HK, Canfield SG, Hjortness MK, Palecek SP, Shusta EV. Exploring the effects of cell seeding density on the differentiation of human pluripotent stem cells to brain microvascular endothelial cells. Fluids Barriers CNS. 2015;12:13. doi:10.1186/s12987-015-0007-9.
12. Chen G, Gulbranson DR, Hou Z, Bolin JM, Ruotti V, Probasco MD, et al. Chemically defined conditions for human iPSC derivation and culture. Nat Methods. 2011;8(5):424–9. doi:10.1038/nmeth.1593.
13. Yu J, Vodyanik MA, Smuga-Otto K, Antosiewicz-Bourget J, Frane JL, Tian S, et al. Induced pluripotent stem cell lines derived from human somatic cells. Science. 2007;318(5858):1917–20. doi:10.1126/science.1151526.
14. Emonard H, Grimaud JA, Nusgens B, Lapiere CM, Foidart JM. Reconstituted basement-membrane matrix modulates fibroblast activities in vitro. J Cell Physiol. 1987;133(1):95–102. doi:10.1002/jcp.1041330112.
15. Hughes CS, Postovit LM, Lajoie GA. Matrigel: a complex protein mixture required for optimal growth of cell culture. Proteomics. 2010;10(9):1886–90. doi:10.1002/pmic.200900758.
16. Perriere N, Demeuse P, Garcia E, Regina A, Debray M, Andreux JP, et al. Puromycin-based purification of rat brain capillary endothelial cell cultures. Effect on the expression of blood–brain barrier-specific properties. J Neurochem. 2005;93(2):279–89. doi:10.1111/j.1471-4159.2004.03020.x.
17. Wang Q, Yang H, Miller DW, Elmquist WF. Effect of the p-glycoprotein inhibitor, cyclosporin A, on the distribution of rhodamine-123 to the brain: an in vivo microdialysis study in freely moving rats. Biochem Biophys Res Commun. 1995;211:719–26.
18. Ni Z, Bikadi Z, Shuster DL, Zhao C, Rosenberg MF, Mao Q. Identification of proline residues in or near the transmembrane helices of the human breast cancer resistance protein (BCRP/ABCG2) that are important for transport activity and substrate specificity. Biochemistry. 2011;50(37):8057–66. doi:10.1021/bi200573t.
19. Cygalova LH, Hofman J, Ceckova M, Staud F. Transplacental pharmacokinetics of glyburide, rhodamine 123, and BODIPY FL prazosin: effect of drug efflux transporters and lipid solubility. J Pharmacol Exp Ther. 2009;331(3):1118–25. doi:10.1124/jpet.109.160564.
20. Robey RW, Honjo Y, van de Laar A, Miyake K, Regis JT, Litman T, et al. A functional assay for detection of the mitoxantrone resistance protein, MXR (ABCG2). Biochim Biophys Acta. 2001;1512(2):171–82.
21. Miranda CL, Reed RL, Kuiper HC, Alber S, Stevens JF. Ascorbic acid promotes detoxification and elimination of 4-hydroxy-2(E)-nonenal in human monocytic THP-1 cells. Chem Res Toxicol. 2009;22(5):863–74. doi:10.1021/tx900042u.
22. Parent JM, Anderson SA. Reprogramming patient-derived cells to study the epilepsies. Nat Neurosci. 2015;18(3):360–6. doi:10.1038/nn.3944.
23. Zeng X, Hunsberger JG, Simeonov A, Malik N, Pei Y, Rao M. Concise review: modeling central nervous system diseases using induced pluripotent stem cells. Stem Cells Transl Med. 2014;3(12):1418–28. doi:10.5966/sctm.2014-0102.
24. Broccoli V, Giannelli SG, Mazzara PG. Modeling physiological and pathological human neurogenesis in the dish. Front Neurosci. 2014;8:183. doi:10.3389/fnins.2014.00183.
25. Beevers JE, Caffrey TM, Wade-Martins R. Induced pluripotent stem cell (iPSC)-derived dopaminergic models of Parkinson's disease. Biochem Soc Trans. 2013;41(6):1503–8. doi:10.1042/BST20130194.
26. Poller B, Gutmann H, Krahenbuhl S, Weksler B, Romero I, Couraud PO, et al. The human brain endothelial cell line hCMEC/D3 as a human blood–brain barrier model for drug transport studies. J Neurochem. 2008;107:1358–68.
27. Cucullo L, Couraud PO, Weksler B, Romero IA, Hossain M, Rapp E, et al. Immortalized human brain endothelial cells and flow-based vascular modeling: a marriage of convenience for rational neurovascular studies. J Cereb Blood Flow Metab. 2008;28(2):312–28. doi:10.1038/sj.jcbfm.9600525.
28. Cecchelli R, Berezowski V, Lundquist S, Culot M, Renftel M, Dehouck M-P, et al. Modelling of the blood–brain barrier in drug discovery and development. Nat Rev Drug Discov. 2007;6:650–61. doi:10.1038/nrd2368.
29. Weksler BB, Subileau EA, Perriere N, Charneau P, Holloway K, Leveque M, et al. Blood–brain barrier-specific properties of a human adult brain endothelial cell line. FASEB J. 2005;19:1872–4. doi:10.1096/fj.04-3458fje.
30. Mizee MR, Wooldrik D, Lakeman KA, van het Hof B, Drexhage JA, Geerts D, et al. Retinoic acid induces blood–brain barrier development. J Neurosci. 2013;33(4):1660–71. doi:10.1523/JNEUROSCI.1338-12.2013.
31. Vukicevic S, Kleinman HK, Luyten FP, Roberts AB, Roche NS, Reddi AH. Identification of multiple active growth factors in basement membrane Matrigel suggests caution in interpretation of cellular activity related to extracellular matrix components. Exp Cell Res. 1992;202(1):1–8.

15

Cerebrospinal fluid (CSF) biomarkers of iron status are associated with CSF viral load, antiretroviral therapy, and demographic factors in HIV-infected adults

Stephanie M. Patton[1*†], Quan Wang[2], Todd Hulgan[3], James R. Connor[1], Peilin Jia[4], Zhongming Zhao[4], Scott L. Letendre[5], Ronald J. Ellis[6], William S. Bush[7], David C. Samuels[8], Donald R. Franklin[5], Harpreet Kaur[9], Jennifer Iudicello[10], Igor Grant[10] and Asha R. Kallianpur[9,11†]

Abstract

Background: HIV-associated neurocognitive disorder (HAND) remains common, despite antiretroviral therapy (ART). HIV dysregulates iron metabolism, but cerebrospinal fluid (CSF) levels of iron and iron-transport proteins in HIV-infected (HIV+) persons are largely unknown. The objectives of this study were to characterize CSF iron-related biomarkers in HIV+ adults and explore their relationships to known predictors of HAND.

Methods: We quantified total iron, transferrin and heavy-chain (H)-ferritin by immunoassay in CSF sampled by lumbar puncture in 403 HIV+ participants in a multi-center, observational study and evaluated biomarker associations with demographic and HIV-related correlates of HAND [e.g., age, sex, self-reported race/ethnicity, ART, and detectable plasma virus and CSF viral load (VL)] by multivariable regression. In a subset (N = 110) with existing CSF: serum albumin (Q_{Alb}) measurements, Q_{Alb} and comorbidity severity were also included as covariates to account for variability in the blood–CSF-barrier.

Results: Among 403 individuals (median age 43 years, 19% women, 56% non-Whites, median nadir CD4+ T cell count 180 cells/μL, 46% with undetectable plasma virus), men had 25% higher CSF transferrin (median 18.1 vs. 14.5 μg/mL), and 71% higher H-ferritin (median 2.9 vs. 1.7 ng/mL) than women (both *p*-values $\leq$0.01). CSF iron was 41% higher in self-reported Hispanics and 27% higher in (non-Hispanic) Whites than in (non-Hispanic) Blacks (median 5.2 and 4.7 μg/dL in Hispanics and Whites, respectively, vs. 3.7 μg/dL in Blacks, both $p \leq 0.01$); these findings persisted after adjustment for age, sex, and HIV-specific factors. Median H-ferritin was 25% higher ($p < 0.05$), and transferrin 14% higher ($p = 0.06$), in Whites than Blacks. Transferrin and H-ferritin were 33 and 50% higher, respectively, in older (age > 50 years) than in younger persons (age $\leq$ 35 years; both $p < 0.01$), but these findings lost statistical significance in subset analyses that adjusted for Q_{Alb} and comorbidity. After these additional adjustments, associations were observed for CSF iron and transferrin with race/ethnicity as well as CSF VL, for transferrin with sex and ART, and for H-ferritin with plasma virus detectability and significant comorbidity (all $p < 0.05$).

Conclusions: CSF iron biomarkers are associated with demographic factors, ART, and CSF VL in HIV+ adults. Future studies should investigate a role for CNS iron dysregulation, to which an altered blood-CSF barrier may contribute, in HAND.

Keywords: Iron transport, Cerebrospinal fluid, HIV, Transferrin, H-ferritin, HIV-associated neurocognitive disorders

*Correspondence: spatton@hmc.psu.edu; smp11@psu.edu
†Stephanie M. Patton and Asha R. Kallianpur contributed equally to this work
[1] Department of Neurosurgery, Penn State Hershey Medical Center, 500 University Drive, Mailbox H110, Hershey, PA 17033, USA
Full list of author information is available at the end of the article

Background

HIV affects an estimated 40 million people worldwide [1], and owing to the success of combination antiretroviral therapy (ART) in suppressing viral replication, this population is aging [2–4]. An increasing number of chronic disease complications, such as HIV-associated neurocognitive disorders (HAND), are therefore the focus of current efforts to improve quality of life for HIV-infected (HIV+) individuals. HAND remains disturbingly common despite ART, for reasons that are only partially understood, occurring in 30–60% of unselected HIV+ persons, even when the virus is undetectable [5, 6]. Intensive research has suggested many possible mechanisms and etiologies for HAND, including persistent low-level immune activation and inflammation within the central nervous system (CNS) [4, 7, 8], comorbid conditions [9], and accelerated aging [10], but few of these mechanisms are directly actionable, and effective interventions remain elusive. Risk factors for HAND include the nadir CD4+ T-cell count, indicating the depth of immunosuppression achieved during the course of HIV disease, older age at seroconversion, anemia, delay in initiating ART, and the presence of HIV RNA in the CSF and plasma, as well as comorbidity [11–14]. Anemia is prevalent in HIV infection, even when the virus is undetectable during successful ART, and it has been consistently associated with increased morbidity and mortality in HIV infection in retrospective and prospective studies [15]. In addition, the possibility that CNS toxicity due to ART contributes to HAND remains a matter of debate; certain antiretroviral drugs such as zidovudine (ZDV) have well-described effects on iron transport and frequently cause anemia, and others may exhibit neurotoxicity [14, 16, 17]. Female sex appears also to be associated with higher susceptibility to HAND, but women have been underrepresented in prior HIV studies, and factors unrelated to HIV infection may also explain this finding [18–20]. Finally, HIV+ persons of Hispanic ethnicity experience an increased risk of neurocognitive decline, possibly due in part to reduced or delayed access to health care [13, 18, 21–23].

Iron homeostasis is essential for normal brain function: iron is required for the synthesis of monoamine neurotransmitters, for mitochondrial function, myelin synthesis, and the catalytic function of a large number of metabolic enzymes [4, 24]. Alterations in brain iron content and distribution (e.g., excess iron deposition) have long been associated with complex neurodegenerative disorders such as Parkinson's disease, Alzheimer's disease, and amyotrophic lateral sclerosis (ALS) [25]. Neurocognitive impairment has also been reported in the restless leg syndrome (RLS), in which brain iron deficiency contributes to dopaminergic dysfunction within the brain [26]. It has been challenging to determine the extent to which iron plays a pathogenic as opposed to a bystander role in these conditions, but evidence is accumulating in favor of the former [27–30]. An extensive literature has established that peripheral iron deficiency also leads to reduced cognitive performance and behavioral disturbances, which in children and adolescents may be long-lasting and not fully reversible upon iron repletion [31–33]. Despite the known importance of iron to brain health, iron and iron transport proteins in the CSF have been measured only anecdotally in small numbers of HIV-negative persons with specific neurodegenerative conditions, or in healthy controls [34–38]. CNS iron homeostasis has not been adequately investigated in HIV+ individuals with or without HAND, either by measurement of iron or iron-related biomarkers in CSF, or indirectly, by iron-sensitive neuroimaging [4, 39, 40].

Transferrin, the chief iron-transporter in the circulation, binds and transports ferric iron in a soluble, nonreactive state to metabolically active cells throughout the body, whereupon transferrin-bound iron is internalized by receptor-mediated endocytosis [41]. Transferrin is synthesized and secreted by the choroid plexus and is also produced by oligodendrocytes; it is the chief mode of delivery of iron to neurons [42]. Ferritin, the principal intracellular iron-storage molecule in tissues, is frequently elevated in HIV+ persons, possibly reflecting a prolonged acute-phase inflammatory response [43, 44]. Ferritin comprises varying proportions of heavy (iron-avid) and light (relatively iron-poor) chains (H- and L-ferritin, respectively), depending on the tissue of origin. H-ferritin is the predominant form in the CNS, and it delivers iron to oligodendrocytes via the Tim-2 receptor [45, 46]. Iron delivery by H-ferritin to other cell types has also been suggested [47]. Serum ferritin levels generally rise, and transferrin levels fall, with increasing systemic iron stores; the reverse changes occur in functionally iron-deficient states [41, 43]. Both transferrin and H-ferritin can be influenced by inflammatory stimuli, such as infection or comorbid conditions [48, 49]. The synthesis, transport, and regulation of iron, transferrin, and ferritin within the CNS are incompletely understood and the subject of ongoing investigation [24] In contrast to many other serum proteins, levels of these iron-related proteins in CSF have often been reported not to correlate with those in the peripheral circulation, and the brain is well buffered against systemic iron deficiency or excess [50]. Although a number of studies have examined peripheral (serum or plasma) iron biomarkers in HIV infection as a factor in disease outcomes [51–54], CSF levels of iron, transferrin, and H-ferritin remain inadequately characterized from an epidemiological perspective [55, 56].

Serum is the most convenient source for routine, noninvasive testing of iron parameters, but the CSF is more likely to provide an accurate reflection of iron transport in the CNS. There is also considerable precedent for the use of CSF biomarkers as surrogate markers of iron metabolism and/or neuronal injury in the brain [57–59]. Recent studies have documented selective prioritization and partitioning of iron across different tissues in the anemic state, for example, and thus, blood indices may not reflect CNS iron depletion [60, 61]. Another advantage of CSF as the biological medium for estimating CNS iron status is that CSF is sequestered behind both the blood–brain barrier (BBB) and blood–CSF barrier. This isolation from the periphery permits measurement of iron and iron-management proteins at least in part derived from or in equilibrium with the brain parenchyma and specific to the CNS, potentially reflecting unique aspects of iron transport within that compartment.

It is of interest to evaluate associations of known predictors of neurocognitive decline in HIV infection with levels of CSF iron and iron-transport proteins, because such associations would suggest a possible novel role for dysregulation of iron metabolism or iron transport pathways in the pathogenesis of HAND that might be targeted therapeutically. Analogous approaches have proven instructive in achieving a better understanding of other chronic disease phenotypes linked to inflammation, such as cancer [62]. The purpose of this study was therefore to quantify, for the first time, iron and biomarkers of iron transport in the CSF of HIV+ persons and systematically evaluate their relationships to host factors such as age, sex, ethnicity or ancestry, and key HIV disease-related factors like ART (including ZDV use) and the presence and quantity of CSF virus.

Methods

Patient selection and CSF sampling

The CNS HIV Antiretroviral Therapy Effects Research (CHARTER) Study is an observational, prospective cohort study that enrolled ambulatory, HIV+ adults at six large U.S. Medical Centers in the U.S., including Johns Hopkins University School of Medicine (Baltimore, MD, USA), the University of California (San Diego, CA, USA), University of Texas Medical Branch (Galveston, TX, USA), Washington University School of Medicine (Saint Louis, MO, USA), University of Washington (Seattle, WA, USA), and the Icahn School of Medicine of Mount Sinai (New York, NY, USA). CHARTER was designed specifically to evaluate neurological outcomes in HIV+ individuals; hence, all participants underwent detailed neuromedical, neuropsychological, and cognitive evaluations at baseline and 6-month follow-up visits, as previously described [7]. Comorbid conditions were categorized upon careful assessment as minimal, mild or moderate, or severe by expert clinicians [6, 63].

Participants in this study of CSF iron biomarkers were selected based on availability of at least 1.0 mL of CSF at both baseline (N = 403) and 6-month (N = 100) follow-up visits. Individuals with comorbid conditions deemed by expert clinicians to be severe (conditions such as traumatic brain injury with prolonged loss of consciousness, recent stroke, or a history of developmental delay) were excluded, and the remainder were classified as having minimal or mild-moderate comorbidity following extensive chart review [6]. Basic demographic information (e.g., age, sex, self-reported race/ethnicity) and HIV disease characteristics [e.g., ART, nadir CD4+ T-cell count, and HIV RNA concentrations (viral load, VL) in plasma and CSF] were determined at the baseline visit during structured in-person interviews, when CSF was first sampled, as described in detail previously [13]. Non-Hispanic Whites of European ancestry are henceforth referred to as "Whites" and non-Hispanic Blacks, as "Blacks", to distinguish them from self-reported Hispanic individuals. Nine study participants reported their race/ethnicity as "Other" and were too few in number for subgroup analyses; therefore, race-stratified analyses included only self-reported Black, White, and Hispanic study participants.

All CHARTER study participants provided written informed consent for the study, and the CHARTER study adheres to the ethical principles set forth in the Declaration of Helsinki. The present study was also approved by the institutional review boards of all participating institutions.

CSF iron quantification

Iron content within the CSF was evaluated using the Quantichrom iron assay (BioAssay Systems, Hayward, CA, USA) and the manufacturer's protocol. Briefly, 50 μL of standards or patient CSF samples were mixed with 200 μL Quantichrom Working Reagent in a 96-well plate (in duplicate) and incubated at room temperature for 40 min. The iron concentration in experimental samples was determined by comparison of the optical density at 590 nm with the standard curve.

CSF transferrin quantification

Transferrin content within sampled CSF was determined by enzyme-linked immunosorbent assay (Human Transferrin ELISA kit (ab108902) (Abcam, Cambridge, MA, USA) performed according to the manufacturer's protocol. After the CSF was collected and centrifuged, the samples (in duplicate) were diluted 1:1000 with mix diluent. Briefly, transferrin standard or diluted CSF sample (50 μL) was added to each well and the solution was incubated for 2 h. Following incubation, the plate was washed five times with 200 μL of 1× Wash Buffer. Following the wash step, 1× Biotinylated transferrin antibody (50 μL) was added to each well and the solution was incubated for 1 h. The plate was washed again as described above. 1× SP Conjugate (50 μL) was added to each well and the solution was incubated for 30 min. The microplate was washed again as described above. Chromogen substrate (50 μL) was added to each well and the solution was incubated for 12 min. Stop solution (50 μL) was added to each well and the absorbance was read immediately on a microplate reader at 450 nm. Transferrin concentration was then determined by comparison to the standard curve.

CSF H-ferritin quantification

The H-ferritin content of CSF was determined by an enzyme-linked immunosorbent assay (Human H-ferritin ELISA kit, Abnova, Taipei, Taiwan) performed according to the supplier's instructions. Briefly, 20 μL of standards, subject samples (in duplicate), and controls were combined with 100 μL of enzyme conjugate reagent. The solution was mixed for 30 s and incubated at room temperature for 45 min. The incubation mixture was removed and the plate was rinsed five times with distilled water. The TMB Reagent (100 μL) was added into each well, the solution was mixed for 10 s, and the solution was incubated at room temperature in the dark for 20 min. Stop Solution (100 μL) was added to each well and the solution was mixed for 30 s. The ferritin concentration in the experimental samples was determined by comparison of the optical density at 450 nm with the standard curve within 15 min.

Serum iron biomarker measurement

Iron, ferritin, and transferrin were also quantified in serum using routine, commercially available, automated assays in a subset of study participants ($N = 11$) who had sufficient serum available at the 6-month follow-up visit. Circulating ferritin, which consists primarily of the L subunit, was quantified by electrochemiluminescence assay ("ECLIA"), using a biotinylated, monoclonal ferritin-specific antibody and a ruthenium-labeled monoclonal ferritin antibody to form a sandwich complex. Upon addition of streptavidin-coated microparticles, chemiluminescence emission was measured by a photomultiplier (Roche e411 immunoassay analyzer, Roche Diagnostics, Indianapolis, IN, USA) and ferritin concentration determined from a standard curve. Serum iron and transferrin were measured on a Roche c311 automated chemistry analyzer (Roche Diagnostics, Indianapolis, IN, USA), iron by a colorimetric method based on the FerroZine reaction (without deproteinization), which captures unbound and transferrin-bound iron, and transferrin by immunoturbidimetry [64].

Functional integrity of the blood–CSF barrier

As a measure of the integrity of the blood–CSF barrier, CSF and matched serum levels of albumin were quantified by the nephelometric method (Dade Behring BNII, Deerfield, IL, USA) in CHARTER study subjects, 110 of whom participated in this study, and the ratio of CSF to serum albumin (CSF: serum albumin ratio, or Q_{Alb}) was calculated as $Q_{Alb} = \text{albumin(CSF)/albumin(serum)}$ [65]. Individuals with matched CSF and serum albumin measurements from multiple visits were assigned a mean value for Q_{Alb}.

Statistical analyses

The Wilcoxon rank sum test was used to determine univariate differences in CSF iron, H-ferritin, and transferrin levels among HIV-infected individuals by demographic and clinical characteristics or factors. Spearman's *rho* values were determined for correlation between CSF iron biomarkers at baseline or at 6-months, and between CSF and corresponding serum biomarker levels at the 6-month visit in the subset with matched measurements. Unadjusted and adjusted analyses of association were performed after taking the natural logarithm of biomarker values to enforce normality, in order to fulfill the assumptions of linear regression.

Associations of each CSF biomarker with age, sex, and race/ethnicity (dichotomized as Blacks compared with Whites, Whites compared with Hispanics, or Blacks compared with Hispanics), and clinical HIV disease characteristics were individually evaluated in multivariable regression models. Clinical disease factors that were evaluated included: VL in plasma and CSF and presence or absence of detectable plasma or CSF virus, estimated duration of HIV infection (months), ART (on vs. off therapy at the time of blood sampling), current ZDV use (yes/no), nadir CD4+ T-cell count, AIDS status (yes/no), hemoglobin level, anemia status (yes/no), current alcohol use (yes/no), and comorbidity (minimal vs. mild-to-moderate). Hemoglobin, anemia status, and alcohol use showed no relationship to CSF iron biomarkers in univariate analyses and were therefore not included in models to optimize power. Regression models for iron, transferrin, and H-ferritin are presented with partial or full covariate adjustment. For CSF iron, models included the following covariates: (1) age, sex, and race/ethnicity (partial adjustment), or all of the covariates listed in (1) as well as ART (on vs. off), current ZDV use (yes vs. no), plasma VL detectability (yes vs. no), and CSF VL (full adjustment). Covariates in partially adjusted models of transferrin and H-ferritin included age, sex, race/

ethnicity, and ZDV use; ART, plasma VL detectability and CSF VL were added to fully adjusted models. *Beta*-coefficients and their 95% Confidence Intervals were estimated for associations, and two-sided *p*-values were determined. Following analyses in the entire study sample of 403 individuals, similar analyses with additional adjustment for mean Q_{Alb} were performed in the 110 individuals who had this data. All analyses were performed using STATA statistical software v10.0.

Results

CSF iron-related biomarkers in CHARTER study participants

Characteristics of the CHARTER study population at baseline are summarized in Table 1. Median CSF iron levels in this sample were 3.1 μg/dL (interquartile range or IQR 1.6–5.7 μg/dL); median transferrin levels were 17.2 μg/mL (IQR 10.3–27.6 μg/mL), and median H-ferritin levels were 2.7 ng/mL (IQR 1.4–4.2). In order to characterize demographic differences in CSF iron-related biomarkers in HIV+ persons, we measured CSF iron, transferrin, and H-ferritin in 403 cryopreserved CSF samples from CHARTER study participants collected at baseline and in 100 of the same persons at 6 months of follow-up. Within individuals, CSF iron, transferrin and ferritin levels measured at the baseline visit were correlated with levels of the same biomarkers measured at the 6-month visit (all $p < 0.01$, see Additional file 1: Figure S1 and Additional file 2: Table S1). Correlations between different iron-related biomarkers at baseline, and the same correlations at 6 months are shown in Fig. 1. CSF iron levels were weakly correlated with CSF transferrin and H-ferritin levels at baseline and 6 months (Spearman's $rho = 0.12$ and 0.24 at baseline, and $rho = 0.28$ and 0.24 at 6 months, respectively, all *p*-values <0.05). Transferrin levels in CSF were modestly correlated with H-ferritin levels at baseline ($rho = 0.37$, $p < 0.05$), but not at 6 months. Age, sex, and ZDV use did not differ between study participants sampled at baseline and 6-months. As shown in Table 2 and Fig. 2, CSF transferrin and H-ferritin levels differed significantly between men and women in the study in univariate analyses (median transferrin levels in men at the baseline visit were 18.1 vs. 14.5 μg/mL, $p < 0.05$; median H-ferritin levels were 2.9 vs. 1.7 ng/mL, $p = 1.4 \times 10^{-5}$). Significant sex differences in CSF iron content were not observed.

In order to better explore age-related differences in CSF iron measures, we evaluated CSF iron, transferrin, and H-ferritin levels in non-contiguous age groups of younger (≤35 years) and older HIV+ adults (>50 years of age) from the CHARTER Study. As shown in Table 3 and Fig. 3, 134 study participants were included in this

Table 1 Summary of demographic and HIV disease characteristics of CHARTER study participants at baseline (entry) whose iron biomarkers were measured

Variable at baseline visit	All participants N = 403
Age (years), median (IQR)	43 (39, 49)
Sex (N, % women)	78 (19)
Race/ethnicity by self-report (N, %)	
Non-Hispanic Black	174 (43.2)
Non-Hispanic White	178 (44.2)
Hispanic	42 (10.4)
Other	9 (2.2)
Estimated duration of HIV infection (months), median (IQR)	118 (57, 183)
Nadir CD4+ T-cell count, median (IQR)	180 (56, 315)
AIDS status (N, %)	245 (61)
Virus detectability in plasma (N, % >LLQ)	215 (54)
Virus detectability in CSF (N, % >LLQ)	126 (31)[a]
CSF VL (log_{10} HIV RNA copies/mL), median (IQR)	1.7 (1.7, 2.2)[a]
ZDV use (N, % yes)	79 (20)
Comorbidity (% mild to moderate)	134 (33)
Current alcohol abuse (N, % yes)	10 (2.5)
Hemoglobin, mean ± SD	14.1 ± 1.5
Anemia (N, %)	54 (14)
CSF iron (μg/dL), median (IQR)[b]	3.1 (1.6, 5.7)
CSF transferrin (μg/mL), median (IQR)[b]	17.2 (10.3, 27.6)
CSF ferritin (ng/mL), median (IQR)[b]	2.7 (1.4, 4.2)

IQR interquartile range, *LLQ* lower limit of quantitation, *CSF* cerebrospinal fluid, *VL* viral load (HIV RNA), *ZDV* zidovudine, *SD* standard deviation, *μg/ng//dL/mL* micrograms or nanograms per deciliter or milliliter

[a] Three individuals did not have CSF viral load measurements

[b] Values of zero for iron biomarkers were at or below the lower limit of detection of the assay

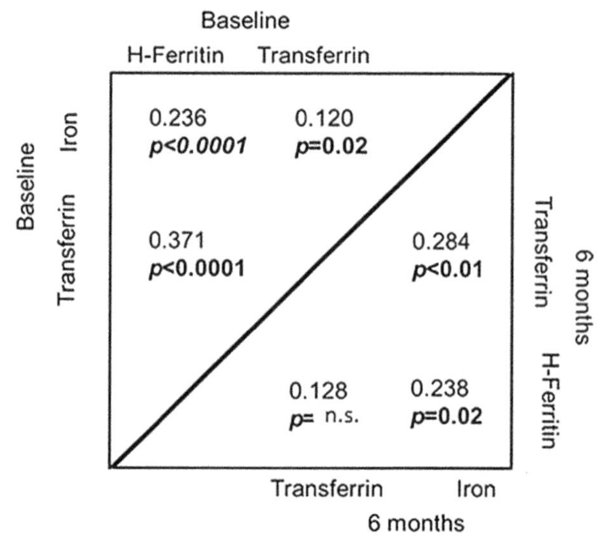

Fig. 1 Spearman correlations between different CSF iron biomarkers in CHARTER study participants at baseline and at 6 months. *p*-values <0.05 (*bolded*) are considered statistically significant

Table 2 Distributions of iron biomarkers in CSF at the baseline visit by sex [median value (interquartile range, IQR)]

CSF biomarker (units)	Men (N = 325)	Women (N = 78)	*p*-value
Iron (μg/dL)	3.25 (1.60, 5.63)	2.84 (1.60, 5.88)	n.s.
Transferrin (μg/mL)	18.07 (10.80, 28.74)	14.47 (6.99, 24.03)	*0.01*
H-ferritin (ng/mL)	2.94 (1.69, 4.55)	1.72 (0.61, 3.05)	*<0.0001*

μg/dL micrograms per deciliter, *μg/mL* micrograms per milliliter, *ng/mL* nanograms per milliliter

p-values <0.05 (italics) are statistically significant

Table 3 CSF iron biomarker distributions at baseline [median (interquartile range)] in younger as compared to older CHARTER subjects

CSF biomarker	Age ≤ 35 (N = 65)	Age > 50 (N = 69)	*p*-value
Iron (μg/dL)	3.00 (1.75, 6.37)	3.88 (2.30, 6.25)	n.s.
Transferrin (μg/mL)	14.51 (9.96, 23.16)	19.29 (13.21, 33.42)	*<0.01*
H-ferritin (ng/mL)	2.24 (1.22, 4.01)	3.37 (2.47, 5.21)	*<0.01*

comparison, which was not adjusted for other HIV-related or demographic factors. CSF transferrin and H-ferritin levels were significantly higher in older than in younger individuals in this study population (both p-values <0.01), but CSF total iron content did not differ significantly between these groups.

Since there is evidence of genetic differences among population subgroups with regard to iron metabolism [66], we also compared levels of CSF iron, transferrin, and H-ferritin between self-reported HIV+ White, Black, and Hispanic study participants and were able to discern ancestry-related differences. As shown in Table 4 and Fig. 4, differences in CSF transferrin levels did not attain statistical significance between any of these subgroups in unadjusted analyses, although self-identified Whites tended to have higher CSF transferrin levels than Blacks ($p = 0.057$). CSF H-ferritin levels were significantly lower in Blacks than in Whites ($p < 0.05$) in this HIV+ sample, however, and total iron CSF iron levels were also significantly lower in Blacks compared to either Whites or Hispanics ($p = 0.002$ and $p = 0.013$, respectively).

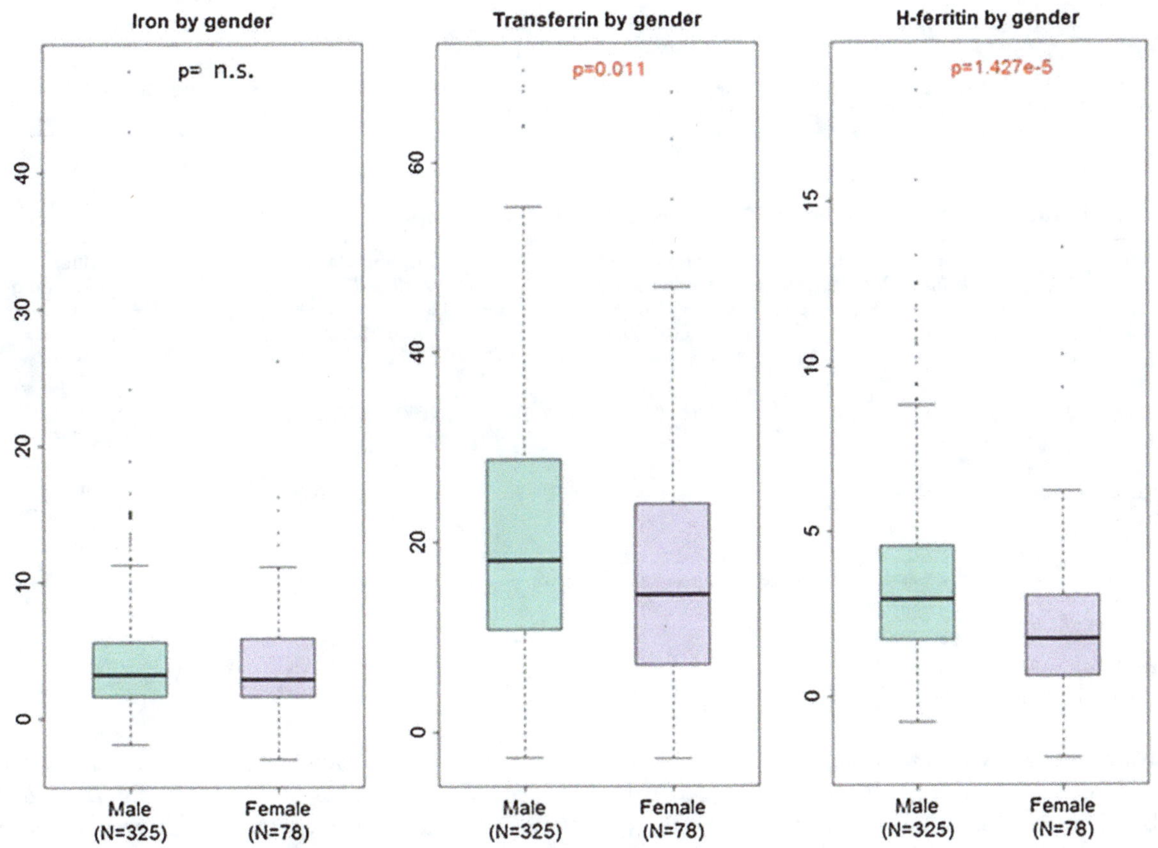

Fig. 2 Boxplots of CSF iron biomarker distribution in CHARTER participants based on sex. *p*-values <0.05 are statistically significant and indicated in *red*. Units of measurement are as follows: iron (μg/dL), transferrin (μg/mL), H-ferritin (ng/mL)

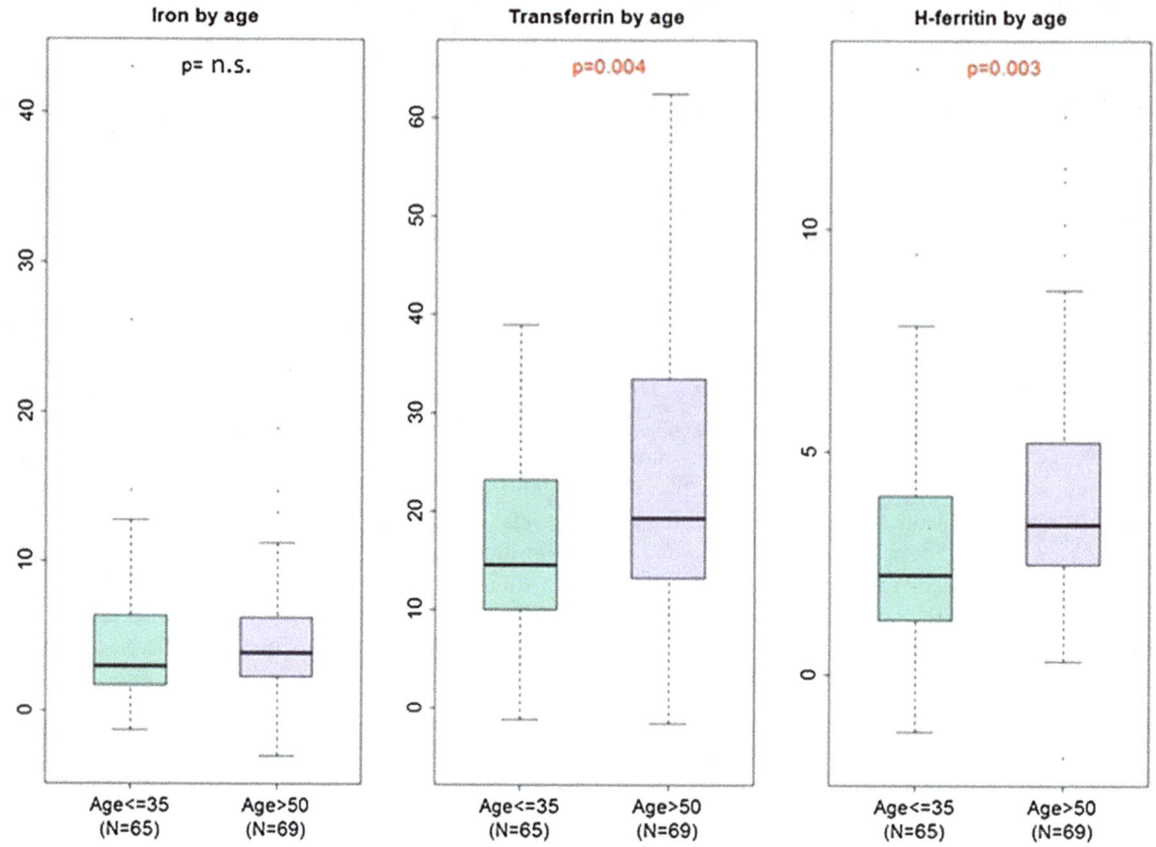

Fig. 3 Boxplots of CSF iron biomarker distributions in CHARTER subjects 35 years or younger, or older than 50 years of age. *p*-values <0.05 are indicated in *red*. Units of measurement: iron (µg/dL), transferrin (µg/mL), H-ferritin (ng/mL)

Table 4 Distributions of iron biomarkers in CSF in different CHARTER subpopulations

CSF biomarker	Whites (N = 178) *Median (IQR)*	Blacks (N = 174) *Median (IQR)*	Hispanics (N = 42) *Median (IQR)*	*p*-value, (compared groups)
Iron (µg/dL)	3.50 (2.12, 6.13)	2.60 (1.00, 4.88)	4.57 (2.00, 6.63)	*<0.01* (W/B)[a] n.s. (W/H)[b] *0.01* (H/B)[c]
Transferrin (µg/mL)	18.91 (11.26, 29.53)	16.64 (9.49, 26.63)	16.71 (10.69, 27.56)	0.06 (W/B)[a] n.s. (W/H)[b] n.s. (H/B)[c]
H-ferritin (ng/mL)	3.02 (1.44, 4.84)	2.41 (1.42, 3.86)	2.61 (1.24, 4.00)	*0.04* (W/B)[a] n.s. (W/H)[b] n.s. (H/B)[c]

Self-reported ancestry (race/ethnicity) was reported as "Other" by 9 participants (*not shown*)

p-values < 0.05 (italics) are statistically significant

[a] Self-reported whites compared to black individuals

[b] Whites compared to Hispanic individuals

[c] Hispanics compared to black individuals

In unadjusted analyses (*data not shown*), CSF iron was not associated with any HIV disease-related variables, but CSF transferrin was associated with CSF VL and current ZDV use (both *p*-values <0.05) and tended to be higher in Whites than in Blacks ($p = 0.05$); CSF H-ferritin levels showed a borderline association with plasma VL detectability ($p = 0.06$) and current ZDV use ($p = 0.05$). In order to estimate the degree of association between CSF iron biomarkers and demographic or HIV-related factors while accounting for possible confounding

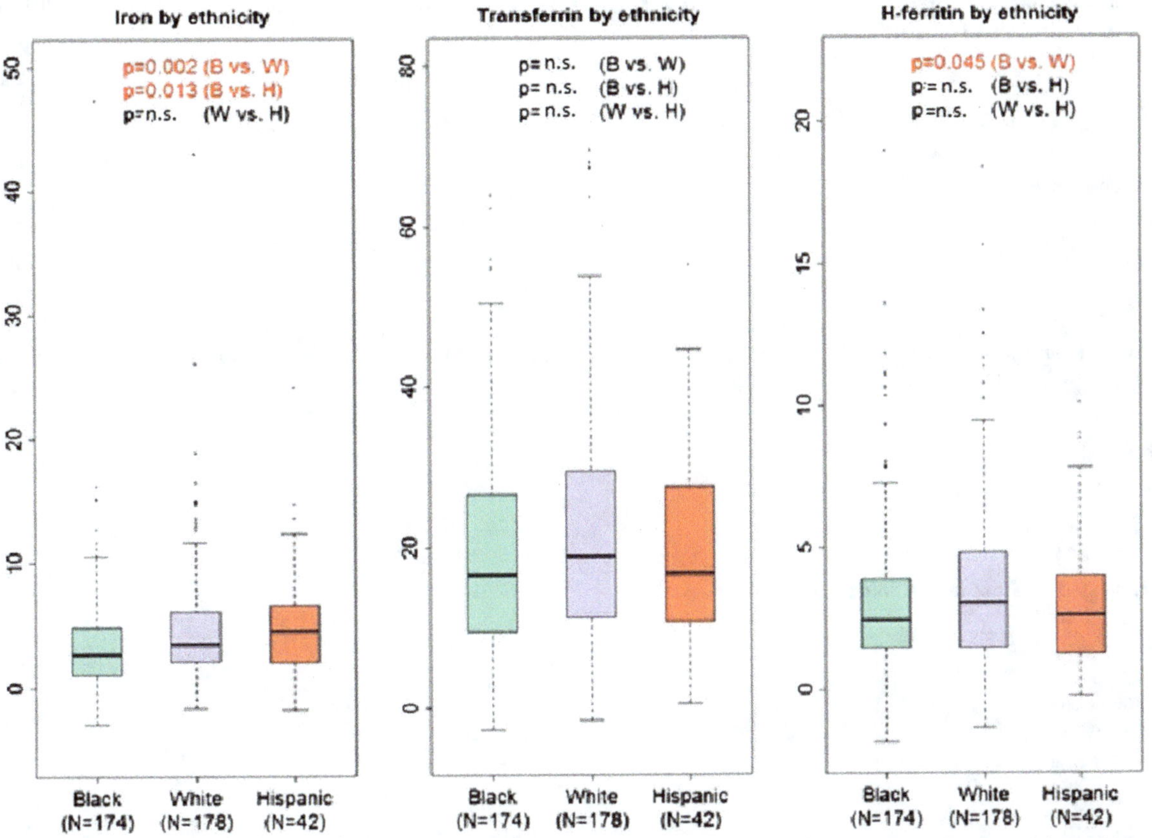

Fig. 4 Boxplots of CSF Iron biomarker distributions in CHARTER study participants based on self-reported race and ethnicity. *p*-values <0.05 are indicated in *red*. Units of measurement are as: iron (μg/dL), transferrin (μg/mL), H-ferritin (ng/mL). *B* Black, *W* White, *H* Hispanic self-reported race/ethnicity

by these factors, some of which promote inflammation, multivariable-adjusted linear regression analyses were conducted, using natural-log-transformed biomarker values to enforce normality. These results are shown in Table 5. CSF iron levels remained significantly associated with self-reported ancestry: iron levels were higher in Whites and Hispanics than in Blacks. CSF iron levels were not significantly related to plasma or CSF VL or virus detectability, current use of ART or ZDV, age, or sex in adjusted models. CSF transferrin associations with age (positive) and sex (lower levels in women, $\beta = -0.225$ [95% CI -0.445 to 0.006], $p < 0.05$) persisted following adjustment, but the association with ancestry lost significance. With regard to HIV-related factors, CSF transferrin levels remained negatively associated with ZDV use ($\beta = -0.254$ [95% CI -0.467, -0.040], $p = 0.03$) and increased with CSF VL ($\beta = 0.297$ [95% CI 0.145, 0.450], $p < 0.01$). H-ferritin levels in the CSF also remained positively associated with age and negatively associated with female sex after multivariable adjustment. Study participants with detectable plasma virus had lower CSF ferritin levels ($\beta = -0.242$ [95% CI -0.449, -0.035], $p = 0.02$), and those who were currently on ZDV also tended to have lower levels ($\beta = -0.196$ [95% CI -0.413, 0.021], $p = 0.07$); the association of transferrin with plasma VL detectability, though in the same direction, was nonsignificant. Higher H-ferritin levels were associated with increasing CSF VL ($\beta = 0.142$ [95% CI -0.002, 0.286], $p = 0.05$). Neither CSF transferrin nor H-ferritin was significantly related to race/ethnicity in multivariable-adjusted analyses. Estimates of association with age, sex, and ancestry did not appreciably change for any biomarker with full adjustment, including HIV disease factors.

In the subset of individuals in this study who had available Q_{Alb} data (N = 110), similar multivariable regression analyses were performed. In these models, Q_{Alb} as well as comorbidity were included as additional covariates to adjust for likely changes in the functional integrity of the blood-CSF barrier that occur with age as well as HIV infection, and for comorbidity-related inflammation, which can influence iron biomarkers [14]. These models are summarized in Table 6. Higher CSF iron was again significantly associated with race/ethnicity

Table 5 Multivariable-adjusted regression models associating CSF iron biomarkers with demographic and HIV disease-related factors in CHARTER study participants

Partially adjusted (age, sex, race/ethnicity)	**Multivariable-adjusted *β* (95% CI)**	***p*-value**
CSF iron		
Age	0.004 (−0.007, 0.015)	n.s.
Sex (women vs. men)	0.102 (−0.134, 0.337)	n.s.
Race/ethnicity[a]	0.104 (0.037, 0.171)	*<0.01*
W compared to B	0.329 (0.130, 0.529)	*<0.01*
W compared to H	−0.014 (−0.318, 0.289)	n.s.
H compared to B	0.327 (−0.019, 0.674)	*0.01*
Fully adjusted (age, sex, race/ethnicity, ART, ZDV use, plasma virus detectability, and CSF VL)	**Multivariable-adjusted *β*-estimate (95% CI)**	***p*-value**
CSF iron		
Detectable plasma virus (Y vs. N)	0.003 (−0.222, 0.230)	n.s.
CSF HIV RNA concentration (VL)	0.072 (−0.079, 0.223)	n.s.
ART (on vs. off)	0.141 (−0.149, 0.431)	n.s.
Current ZDV use (Y vs. N)	0.037 (−0.206, 0.280)	n.s.
Partially adjusted (age, sex, race/ethnicity, ZDV use)	**Multivariable-adjusted *β* (95% CI)**	***p*-value**
CSF transferrin		
Age	0.012 (0.001, 0.022)	*0.03*
Sex (women vs. men)	−0.225 (−0.445, 0.006)	*0.04*
Race/ethnicity[a]	0.036 (−0.025, 0.097)	n.s.
W compared to B	0.110 (−0.078, 0.297)	n.s.
W compared to H	0.103 (−0.185, 0.390)	n.s.
H compared to B	0.070 (−0.233, 0.372)	n.s.
Current ZDV use (Y vs. N)	−0.254 (−0.467, −0.040)	*0.03*
Fully adjusted (age, sex, race/ethnicity, ART, ZDV use, plasma virus detectability and CSF VL)	**Multivariable-adjusted *β* (95% CI)**	***p*-value**
CSF transferrin		
Detectable plasma virus (Y vs. N)	−0.172 (−0.376, 0.032)	n.s.
CSF HIV RNA concentration (VL)	0.297 (0.145, 0.450)	*<0.01*
ART (on vs. off)	0.153 (−0.107, 0.413)	n.s.
Partially adjusted (age, sex, race/ethnicity, ZDV use)	**Multivariable-adjusted *β* (95% CI)**	***p*-value**
CSF ferritin		
Age	0.017 (0.006, 0.027)	*<0.01*
Sex (women vs. men)	−0.324 (−0.550, −0.097)	*<0.01*
Race/ethnicity[a]	0.020 (−0.042, 0.081)	n.s.
W compared to B	0.072 (−0.121, 0.264)	n.s.
W compared to H	0.017 (−0.297, 0.332)	n.s.
H compared to B	0.049 (−0.235, 0.333)	n.s.
Current ZDV use (Y/N)	−0.196 (−0.413, 0.021)	n.s.
Fully adjusted (age, sex, race/ethnicity, ART, ZDV use, plasma virus detectability, and CSF VL)	**Multivariable-adjusted *β* (95% CI)**	***p*-value**
CSF ferritin		
Detectable plasma virus (Y vs. N)	−0.242 (−0.449, −0.035)	*0.02*

Table 5 continued

Fully adjusted (age, sex, race/ethnicity, ART, ZDV use, plasma virus detectability, and CSF VL)	Multivariable-adjusted *β* (95% CI)	*p*-value
CSF HIV RNA concentration (VL)	0.142 (−002, 0.286)	*0.05*
ART (on vs. off)	−0.017 (−0.285, 0.251)	n.s.

The natural logarithm of each biomarker variable was used in all analyses due to non-normal distributions. For each biomarker, partially and fully adjusted separate multiple linear regression models are shown, which included the covariates listed, with *β*-estimates and their 95% confidence intervals and *p*-values. *p*-values <0.05 are statistically significant

For each biomarker, significance of covariates in partially adjusted models did not change appreciably with full adjustment

W Whites, *B* Blacks, *H* Hispanics (self-reported ancestry), *VL* viral (HIV RNA) load, *ZDV* zidovudine, *ART* antiretroviral therapy, *CI* confidence interval, *CSF* cerebrospinal fluid

[a] For each dichotomous comparison by race/ethnicity (ancestry), only one ancestry term (e.g., whites compared to black individuals) was entered into the model

Table 6 Multivariable-adjusted regression models in the subset of CHARTER study participants (N = 110) who had available, matched CSF and serum albumin measurements

Iron biomarker or covariate	Multivariable-adjusted *β* (95% CI)	*p*-value
CSF iron		
Age	−0.014 (−0.055, 0.027)	n.s.
Sex (women vs. men)	0.258 (−0.347, 0.864)	n.s.
Race/ethnicity[a]	0.732 (0.108, 1.36)	*0.02*
Detectable plasma virus (Y vs. N)	0.611 (−0.022, 1.24)	0.06[b]
Log_{10} (CSF HIV RNA concentration)	−0.581 (−1.09, −0.072)	*0.03*
ART on vs. off	0.234 (−0.544, 1.01)	n.s.
Q_{Alb}	0.215 (0.023, 0.407)	*0.03*
Comorbidity (mild-moderate vs. minimal)	0.098 (−0.466, 0.661)	n.s.
CSF transferrin		
Age	0.005 (−0.016, 0.025)	n.s.
Sex (women vs. men)	−0.389 (−0.750, −0.029)	*0.03*
Race/ethnicity	−0.100 (−0.202, 0.002)	*0.06*[b]
Detectable plasma virus (Y vs. N)	−0.322 (−0.736, 0.090)	n.s.
Log_{10} (CSF HIV RNA concentration)	0.380 (0.001, 0.760)	*0.05*[c]
ART on *vs.* off	0.801 (0.067, 1.54)	*0.03*
Current ZDV use (Y vs. N)	0.009 (−0.364, 0.381)	n.s.
Q_{Alb}	0.723 (0.346, 1.10)	*<0.01*
Comorbidity (mild-moderate vs. minimal)	0.007 (−0.299, 0.313)	n.s.
CSF H-ferritin		
Age	0.734 (−0.438, 1.91)	n.s.
Sex (women *vs.* men)	0.022 (−0.482, 0.487)	n.s.
Race/ethnicity	−0.036 (−0.378, 0.305)	n.s.
Detectable plasma virus (Y vs. N)	−0.407 (−0.780, −0.033)	*0.03*
Log_{10} (CSF HIV RNA concentration)	0.277 (−0.129, 0.683)	n.s.
ART on vs. off	0.688 (−0.197,1.57)	n.s.
Q_{Alb}	0.084 (−0.006, 0.173)	n.s.
Comorbidity (mild-moderate vs. minimal)	0.416 (0.038, 0.793)	*0.03*

For each biomarker, all covariates in the regression model, including CSF: serum albumin ratio (QAlb), are shown. Biomarker values were (natural) log-transformed for all analyses

[a] Self-reported Hispanics or non-Hispanic Whites vs. Blacks

[b] *p*-value = 0.057

[c] *p*-value = 0.049

($\beta = 0.732$, $p = 0.02$; higher iron in Hispanics and Whites than in Blacks), as well as with plasma virus detectability ($\beta = 0.611$, $p = 0.05$) but lower CSF VL ($\beta = -0.511$, $p = 0.03$). Higher transferrin levels were associated with male sex ($\beta = -0.389$, $p = 0.03$), non-White race/ethnicity ($\beta = -0.100$, $p = 0.057$, and being on ART ($\beta = 0.801$, $p = 0.03$), but not with comorbidity; the associations with age and ZDV use lost significance. Finally, levels of H-ferritin in CSF were significantly higher among subjects with clinically mild-to-moderate comorbidity ($\beta = 0.416$, $p = 0.03$) and when plasma virus was undetectable ($\beta = -0.407$, $p = 0.03$); CSF VL, age, and gender were no longer significant factors, though the direction of the point estimate for age remained the same. Associations for all iron biomarkers with blood–CSF barrier integrity (mean Q_{Alb}) were statistically significant with the exception of H-ferritin (p-value = 0.07). None of the CSF iron biomarkers was associated with nadir CD4+ T-cell count, hemoglobin level, or anemia (*data not shown*).

Iron and biomarkers of iron transport were quantified in serum in 11 individuals with available serum as well as measured CSF biomarkers at 6 months, and we evaluated correlations of iron, ferritin and transferrin levels in serum to levels of the same analytes in CSF (Additional file 3: Table S2); the methods of quantification were the same. No significant correlations were observed between levels of any of these biomarkers in CSF and their corresponding serum values.

Discussion

This represents the first large study to systematically quantify levels of iron and the two major iron-transport proteins, transferrin and (H)-ferritin, in the CSF of HIV+ persons and to evaluate their associations with known predictors of neurocognitive impairment in this population. Due to the invasive nature of lumbar puncture, published data for CSF iron biomarkers have been scarce even in HIV-negative individuals, in whom data are available only in small numbers of individuals with specific disorders and at different stages of neurodegenerative disease [36, 37, 67–69]. Hence, normal variations of these biomarkers in healthy persons are also not well documented in the literature [38, 67, 70]. Our findings in over 400 clinically well-characterized HIV+ individuals demonstrate that CSF iron and transferrin are independently associated with demographic factors (race/ethnicity and/or sex) and HIV-disease-specific factors (plasma virus detectability, ART, and/or CSF VL), while CSF H-ferritin is related to comorbidity and virus detectability in plasma. Interestingly, observed differences in CSF iron by self-reported race/ethnicity parallel known differences in the risk of neurocognitive decline in HIV+ adults, with the highest levels occurring in persons of Hispanic ethnicity who also appear to be at increased risk of HAND [13]. This study provides the only available estimates of the range and degree of variability of iron biomarkers in HIV + CSF currently available, and the observed relationships to known risk factors for HAND are hypothesis-generating with regard to the potential role of iron dyshomeostasis in HIV-associated neurocognitive decline.

Both nonhuman primate and human studies have shown that systemic iron deficiency and anemia have lasting impact on brain iron homeostasis and neuronal health, influencing memory and cognition [32, 60, 71–73]. In Alzheimer's disease and ALS, both peripheral and CSF iron biomarker profiles suggest disruption of iron homeostasis with concomitant inflammation within the brain [28, 30, 34, 35]. The situation in HIV infection may be similar, with neuroinflammation due to HIV-activated macrophage–monocytes migrating across a damaged BBB triggering a reduction in iron bioavailability in the CNS that may promote neurocognitive decline. Accumulating evidence for systemic changes in iron transport by HIV [54, 74, 75], mediated at least in part by the iron-regulatory hormone hepcidin, and appearance of the virus in the CNS within days of acute infection, suggest that HIV-mediated iron dysregulation may also occur in the CNS. HIV does not infect neurons, but the virus has been shown to infect perivascular macrophages, microglia, and other supporting cells within the CNS, some of which play central roles in regulating brain iron content and distribution [4, 24, 50]. HIV infection of macrophages has also been shown to downregulate expression of the MHC-class I-like iron-regulatory protein Hfe on the macrophage cell surface via the actions of viral proteins, thereby increasing macrophage iron content to benefit viral replication [76].

In the present study, higher CSF iron content tended to be associated with detectable virus in the plasma but with lower CSF VL, when adjusting for the Q_{Alb}, a measure reflecting variability in integrity of the blood–CSF barrier. This apparent discordance suggests that either (1) more iron fails to cross the CSF–brain barrier when HIV levels in the brain or CSF are low, leading to higher levels in the CSF, or (2) higher amounts of virus in the brain or CSF are associated with greater extraction of iron from the CSF, because HIV requires iron for its replication [77]. The significantly lower CSF transferrin levels among persons of Hispanic ethnicity and non-Hispanic Whites compared to Blacks after adjustment for Q_{Alb} were also in accord with the corresponding observed CSF iron differences. Even when accounting for the effects of ZDV, an antiretroviral drug that can affect iron transport, ART was independently associated with higher CSF transferrin, raising the possibility that other commonly used antiretroviral drugs may impact transferrin levels in the CNS, possibly by inducing a functionally iron-deficient state. Initiation of ART has been temporally linked to an increase in soluble transferrin receptors, a sensitive indicator of tissue iron deficiency [78, 79]. Other mechanisms by which functional iron deficiency might be induced in the CNS during HIV infection are the depletion of cellular iron due to active viral replication and/or chronic inflammation in the brain that results in iron entrapment within supporting cells that normally deliver iron, or iron deficiency of these cells themselves [24, 76, 80]. Indeed, higher CSF VL was associated in our analyses with higher CSF transferrin levels, with and without Q_{Alb} adjustment. Interestingly, HIV+ individuals are at increased risk of RLS, a condition associated with iron deficiency in the brain [81, 82].

Although men are known to have significantly higher systemic iron stores than pre-menopausal women, differences in CSF levels of iron, transferrin, or H-ferritin levels have not been documented, and they may have clinical relevance [83]. Women were observed to have significantly lower levels of both transferrin and H-ferritin before Q_{Alb} adjustment; this association persisted following adjustment only for transferrin, and the direction of the estimate remained the same for H-ferritin although significance was lost. That higher H-ferritin levels were associated with undetectable plasma virus but a higher quantity of CSF virus suggests that induction of H-ferritin in the CNS may be a physiological (cytoprotective) response to viral compartmentalization and replication in the CNS. HIV-induced oxidative stress is manifested by upregulation of heme-oxygenase-1 in the brain [84], and the ferroxidase activity of H-ferritin has recently been shown to mediate the antioxidant activity of heme oxygenase-1 [85]. Due to its high metabolic demands, the brain also requires a steady supply of iron in non-reactive form, for energy production as well as myelin and neurotransmitter synthesis [61, 86–88]. Todorich et al. [46] previously identified H-ferritin as an important source of iron for oligodendrocytes, and although the origin of CSF iron, H-ferritin, and transferrin cannot be established in this type of study, it is possible that both proteins are upregulated in persons with suppressed viremia in an attempt to preserve iron delivery to oligodendrocytes, other supporting cells of the CNS, and neurons. Indeed, HIV infection is associated with decreased amounts of myelin or loss of myelin integrity [89–91]. One neuroimaging study that used modern, iron-sensitive techniques reported possible decreases in brain iron in HIV-infected individuals [40], and studies using diffusion tensor imaging or other modalities have consistently revealed white matter damage [40, 83]. It is not surprising that CSF H-ferritin levels were also associated with more clinically significant comorbidity, as comorbidity has emerged as a powerful predictor of neurocognitive decline and is a common correlate of chronic inflammation in HIV+ persons [92]. Mechanisms other than inflammation may also explain increases in H-ferritin in CSF, including HIV-induced changes in autophagy or even ferritinophagy [93, 94]. Finally, associations with age, a strong risk factor for HAND, with both CSF transferrin and H-ferritin were pronounced before adjusting for Q_{Alb} but lost significance after this adjustment; this begs the question whether the loss of iron regulation (or the loss of compartmentalization of iron) in the CSF due to age- or HIV-related damage to the blood–CSF barrier may in part mediate age-related neurocognitive decline.

Levels of CSF iron biomarkers in this HIV+ population were not dramatically different from levels previously reported in small numbers of healthy individuals, but the different assay methods used complicate any comparisons: CSF ferritin levels in this study were lower than levels in individuals either with or without RLS that were reported by Mizuno et al. and they were also lower than levels observed in chronic demyelinating disorders like chronic progressive multiple sclerosis [37, 38, 67]. Assays for total ferritin, rather than H-ferritin, may also have been used in previous studies. As with other intracellular microorganisms, the manipulation of cellular iron homeostasis by HIV to benefit its own replication may eventually result in altered brain iron balance (either functional iron deficiency, or iron excess in specific brain regions, or a combination of these). Significant changes in total CSF iron biomarker levels may or may not accurately reflect these regional changes. CSF iron, transferrin and ferritin did not appear to be correlated with their respective serum levels in 11 individuals with visit-matched CSF and serum samples, but the small size of the sample with both sets of measurements precludes firm conclusions. While possibly due to insufficient power, the absence of significant correlations supports the concept that levels of iron and iron transporters in the CNS are actively regulated and do not merely reflect passive influx from the circulation; this view is entirely consistent with prior studies [50]. Differences in serum and CSF assays used for iron-biomarker quantification and the fact that H-ferritin was measured in CSF, while the L subunit (iron-poor form) of ferritin predominates in serum, could also account for these differences. Relatively little is known about mechanisms controlling total or H-ferritin levels in either compartment [95].

We acknowledge the limitations of this study, including its cross-sectional design, which limits interpretation, the lack of an HIV-negative comparison group, and absence of matched serum iron biomarker data for most participants. Moderately correlated, within-individual values of iron, transferrin and H-ferritin obtained at baseline and 6 months in 100 of the study participants, however, support the use of single CSF biomarker measurements for our analyses and favor their stability in HIV+ persons over short periods of time. Regarding the lack of HIV-negative controls, we would stress that our objective was not to determine the impact of HIV on CSF iron biomarker levels, but to ascertain their associations with key demographic, HIV disease- and treatment-related predictors of neurocognitive decline, since measures of HAND are often imprecise and fluctuate in individuals over time [4]. Better knowledge of iron biomarker variability and associations with these other host factors will facilitate the design of future studies and inform the precision of predictive models. Longitudinal follow-up studies with measurements of biomarkers at more than one time-point in individual disease trajectories will be needed to clarify the temporal sequence of iron dysregulation after HIV infection, although such studies may be challenging due to the invasive nature of CSF sampling. This study provides a systematic assessment of the demographic and disease-related factors associated with CSF iron biomarker levels in HIV+ persons, laying the foundation for studies that specifically evaluate whether changes in these iron-related measures promote the development of HAND.

Conclusions

In HIV+ adults, CSF levels of iron and major biomarkers of iron-transport are independently associated with sex, self-reported race/ethnicity, ART, plasma virus detectability and/or CSF VL. Associations of CSF iron biomarkers with age, which disappeared following adjustment for a measure of blood-CSF barrier function, suggests the possibility that age- or HIV-related declines in the integrity of the blood-CSF barrier may contribute to changes in CNS iron balance as HIV+ individuals age. Furthermore, this study raises the intriguing possibility that consistent correlates of HAND such as race/ethnicity, ART, and HIV RNA in the CSF, may be linked to HAND in part via changes in CNS iron homeostasis. Additional studies, preferably including longitudinal samples and a higher number of participants over 50 years of age, as well as matched HIV-negative controls, are needed to further investigate these questions.

Abbreviations

CSF: cerebrospinal fluid; ART: antiretroviral therapy; HAND: HIV-associated neurocognitive disorder; CNS: central nervous system; HIV+: HIV-infected; ZDV: zidovudine; ALS: amyotrophic lateral sclerosis; RLS: restless leg syndrome; BBB: blood–brain barrier; VL: viral load (HIV RNA concentration); CHARTER: CNS HIV antiretroviral therapy effects research (study); IQR: interquartile range; Q_{Alb}: CSF to serum albumin ratio.

Authors' contributions

Specific contributions to this manuscript were as follows: SP performed all CSF iron, transferrin and ferritin measurements at the bench and drafted the manuscript; QW and PJ performed multivariable regression analyses; ZZ supervised all analyses and commented on the manuscript; JC assisted in study design, supervised biomarker measurement in his laboratory, and provided helpful comments on the manuscript; TH assisted in data interpretation and commented on the manuscript; RE and SL assisted in selection of CSF samples and commented on the manuscript; DF assisted in sample selection and coordinated sample shipments; WB and DC provided helpful comments on the manuscript; HK assisted in analyses and development of figures for the revised manuscript; JI helped to acquire CSF and serum albumin data and provided this quality-controlled dataset for analyses; AK conceived, designed, and implemented the study, revised the manuscript, and performed some of the statistical analyses. IG was Principal Investigator of the parent CHARTER study that provided data and samples for these analyses. Both TH and AK funded the study. Authors SP and AK contributed equally to this work. All authors read and approved the final manuscript.

Author details

[1] Department of Neurosurgery, Penn State Hershey Medical Center, 500 University Drive, Mailbox H110, Hershey, PA 17033, USA. [2] Department of Biomedical Informatics, Vanderbilt University School of Medicine, Nashville, TN, USA. [3] Department of Medicine, Vanderbilt University School of Medicine, Nashville, TN, USA. [4] School of Biomedical Informatics, The University of Texas Health Science Center at Houston, Houston, TX, USA. [5] Department of Medicine, University of California-San Diego, San Diego, CA, USA. [6] Department of Neurology, University of California-San Diego, San Diego, CA, USA. [7] Department of Epidemiology and Biostatistics, Case Western Reserve University School of Medicine, Cleveland, OH, USA. [8] Department of Molecular Physiology and Biophysics, Vanderbilt University, Nashville, TN, USA. [9] Genomic Medicine Institute, Cleveland Clinic/Lerner Research Institute, Cleveland, OH, USA. [10] Department of Psychiatry, University of California-San Diego, San Diego, CA, USA. [11] Department of Molecular Medicine, Cleveland Clinic Lerner College of Medicine of Case Western Reserve University, Cleveland, OH, USA.

Acknowledgements

The authors gratefully acknowledge the many CHARTER study participants who provided CSF and clinical data for this study, as well as the support of all CHARTER study investigators and sites.

CHARTER is affiliated with the University of California, San Diego; Johns Hopkins University; the Icahn School of Medicine of Mount Sinai; University of Texas Medical Branch, Galveston; University of Washington, Seattle; Washington University, Saint Louis, and it is headquartered at the University of California, San Diego.

Competing interests

The authors declare that they have no competing interests.

Funding

NIH R01 MH095621 and Supplemental Award NIH MH095621 04S1 (to A.R.K. and T.H.).

References

1. (UNAIDS) J.U.N.P.o.H.A., global report: UNAIDS report on the global AIDS epidemic; 2012.
2. Mateen FJ, Mills EJ. Aging and HIV-related cognitive loss. JAMA. 2012;308:349–50.
3. Wing EJ. HIV and aging. Int J Infect Dis. 2016;53:61–8.
4. Kallianpur AR, Levine AJ. Host genetic factors predisposing to HIV-associated neurocognitive disorder. Curr HIV/AIDS Rep. 2014;11:336–52.
5. So-Armah KA, Chang J, Alcorn C, Lo Re V, Baker JV, Tracy R, et al. HIV infection, antiretroviral therapy initiation and longitudinal changes in biomarkers of organ function. Curr HIV Res. 2014;12:50–9.
6. Heaton RK, Clifford DB, Franklin DR Jr, Woods SP, Ake C, Vaida F, CHARTER Group, et al. HIV-associated neurocognitive disorders persist in the era of potent antiretroviral therapy: CHARTER Study. Neurology. 2010;75:2087–96.
7. Heaton RK, Franklin DR, Ellis RJ, McCutchan JA, Letendre SL, Leblanc S, CHARTER Group, HNRC Group, et al. HIV-associated neurocognitive disorders before and during the era of combination antiretroviral therapy: differences in rates, nature, and predictors. J Neurovirol. 2011;17:3–16.

8. Angelovich TA, Hearps AC, Maisa A, Martin GE, Lichtfuss GF, Cheng WJ, et al. Viremic and virologically suppressed hiv infection increases age-related changes to monocyte activation equivalent to 12 and 4 years of aging respectively. J Acquir Immune Defic Syndr. 2015;69:11–7.
9. Tedaldi EM, Minniti NL, Fischer T. HIV-associated neurocognitive disorders: the relationship of HIV infection with physical and social comorbidities. Biomed Res Int. 2015;2015:641913.
10. Horvath S, Levine AJ. HIV-1 infection accelerates age according to the epigenetic clock. J Infect Dis. 2015;212:1563–73.
11. Ellis RJ, Badiee J, Vaida F, Letendre S, Heaton RK, Clifford D, CHARTER Group, et al. CD4 nadir is a predictor of HIV neurocognitive impairment in the era of combination antiretroviral therapy. AIDS. 2011;25:1747–51.
12. McArthur JC, Hoover DR, Bacellar H, Miller EN, Cohen BA, Becker JT, et al. Dementia in AIDS patients: incidence and risk factors. Multicenter AIDS Cohort Study. Neurology. 1993;43:2245–52.
13. Heaton RK, Franklin DR Jr, Deutsch R, Letendre S, Ellis RJ, Casaletto K, CHARTER Group, et al. Neurocognitive change in the era of HIV combination antiretroviral therapy: the longitudinal CHARTER study. Clin Infect Dis. 2015;60:473–80.
14. Kallianpur AR, Wang Q, Jia P, Hulgan T, Zhao Z, Letendre SL, CHARTER Study Group, et al. Anemia and red blood cell indices predict HIV-associated neurocognitive impairment in the highly active antiretroviral therapy era. J Infect Dis. 2016;213:1065–73.
15. Redig AJ, Berliner N. Pathogenesis and clinical implications of HIV-related anemia in 2013. Hematol Am Soc Hematol Educ Progr. 2013;2013:377–81.
16. Bozzi A, Brisdelli F, D'Alessandro AM, D'Andrea G, Lizzi AR, Rinaldi AC, et al. Effects of AZT on cellular iron homeostasis. Biometals. 2004;17:443–50.
17. D'Andrea G, Brisdelli F, Bozzi A. AZT: an old drug with new perspectives. Curr Clin Pharmacol. 2008;3:20–37.
18. Maki PM, Martin-Thormeyer E. HIV, cognition and women. Neuropsychol Rev. 2009;19:204–14.
19. Royal W 3rd, Cherner M, Burdo TH, Umlauf A, Letendre SL, Jumare J, et al. Associations between cognition, gender and monocyte activation among HIV infected individuals in Nigeria. PLoS ONE. 2016;11:e0147182.
20. Hestad KA, Menon JA, Silalukey-Ngoma M, Franklin DR Jr, Imasiku ML, Kalima K, et al. Sex differences in neuropsychological performance as an effect of human immunodeficiency virus infection: a pilot study in Zambia, Africa. J Nerv Ment Dis. 2012;200:336–42.
21. Hulgan T, Samuels DC, Bush W, Ellis RJ, Letendre SL, Heaton RK, CHARTER Group, et al. Mitochondrial DNA haplogroups and neurocognitive impairment during HIV infection. Clin Infect Dis. 2015;61:1476–84.
22. Marquine MJ, Sakamoto M, Dufour C, Rooney A, Fazeli P, Umlauf A, et al. HNRP Group. The impact of ethnicity/race on the association between the Veterans Aging Cohort Study (VACS) index and neurocognitive function among HIV-infected persons. J Neurovirol. 2016;22:442–54.
23. Mindt MR, Miranda C, Arentoft A, Byrd D, Monzones J, Fuentes A, et al. Aging and HIV/AIDS: neurocognitive implications for older HIV-positive Latina/o adults. Behav Med. 2014;40:116–23.
24. Duck KA, Connor JR. Iron uptake and transport across physiological barriers. Biometals. 2016;29:573–91.
25. Hadzhieva M, Kirches E, Mawrin C. Review: iron metabolism and the role of iron in neurodegenerative disorders. Neuropathol Appl Neurobiol. 2014;40:240–57.
26. Galbiati A, Marelli S, Giora E, Zucconi M, Oldani A, Ferini-Strambi L. Neurocognitive function in patients with idiopathic restless legs syndrome before and after treatment with dopamine-agonist. Int J Psychophysiol. 2015;95:304–9.
27. Pichler I, Del Greco MF, Gögele M, Lill CM, Bertram L, Do CB, et al. Serum iron levels and the risk of Parkinson disease: a Mendelian randomization study. PLoS Med. 2013;10:e1001462.
28. Crespo ÂC, Silva B, Marques L, Marcelino E, Maruta C, Costa S, et al. Genetic and biochemical markers in patients with Alzheimer's disease support a concerted systemic iron homeostasis dysregulation. Neurobiol Aging. 2014;35:777–85.
29. Bandyopadhyay S, Rogers JT. Alzheimer's disease therapeutics targeted to the control of amyloid precursor protein translation: maintenance of brain iron homeostasis. Biochem Pharmacol. 2014;88:486–94.
30. Ayton S, Faux NG, Bush AI. Alzheimer's disease neuroimaging initiative ferritin levels in the cerebrospinal fluid predict Alzheimer's disease outcomes and are regulated by *APOE*. Nat Commun. 2015;6:6760.
31. Scott SP, Murray-Kolb LE. Iron status Is associated with performance on executive functioning tasks in nonanemic young women. J Nutr. 2016;146:30–7.
32. Lozoff B, Smith JB, Kaciroti N, Clark KM, Guevara S, Jimenez E. Functional significance of early-life iron deficiency: outcomes at 25 years. J Pediatr. 2013;163:1260–6.
33. Berglund SK, Westrup B, Hägglöf B, Hernell O, Domellöf M. Effects of iron supplementation of LBW infants on cognition and behavior at 3 years. Pediatrics. 2013;131:47–55.
34. Khalil M, Riedlbauer B, Langkammer C, Enzinger C, Ropele S, Stojakovic T, et al. Cerebrospinal fluid transferrin levels are reduced in patients with early multiple sclerosis. Mult Scler J. 2014;20(12):1569–77.
35. Mitchell RM, Simmons Z, Beard JL, Stephens HE, Connor JR. Plasma biomarkers associated with ALS and their relationship to iron homeostasis. Muscle Nerve. 2010;42:95–103.
36. Mizuno S, Mihara T, Miyaoka T, Inagaki T, Horiguchi J. CSF iron, ferritin and transferrin levels in restless legs syndrome. J Sleep Res. 2005;14:43–7.
37. Earley CJ, Connor JR, Beard JL, Malecki EA, Epstein DK, Allen RP. Abnormalities in CSF concentrations of ferritin and transferrin in restless legs syndrome. Neurology. 2000;54:1698–700.
38. LeVine SM, Lynch SG, Ou CN, Wulser MJ, Tam E, Boo N. Ferritin, transferrin and iron concentrations in the cerebrospinal fluid of multiple sclerosis patients. Brain Res. 1999;821:511–5.
39. Simpson IA, Ponnuru P, Klinger ME, Myers RL, Devraj K, Coe CL, et al. A novel model for brain iron uptake: introducing the concept of regulation. J Cereb Blood Flow Metab. 2015;35:48–57.
40. Granziera C, Daducci A, Simioni S, Cavassini M, Roche A, Meskaldji D, et al. Micro-structural brain alterations in aviremic HIV+ patients with minor neurocognitive disorders: a multi-contrast study at high field. PLoS ONE. 2013;8:e72547.
41. Gkouvatsos K, Papanikolaou G, Pantopoulos K. Regulation of iron transport and the role of transferrin. Biochim Biophys Acta. 1820;2012:188–202.
42. Leitner DF, Connor JR. Functional roles of transferrin in the brain. Biochim Biophys Acta. 2012;1820:393–402.
43. Arosio P, Ingrassia R, Cavadini P. Ferritins: a family of molecules for iron storage, antioxidation and more. Biochim Biophys Acta. 2009;1790:589–99.
44. Feelders RA, Vreugdenhil G, Eggermont AM, Kuiper-Kramer PA, van Eijk HG, Swaak AJ. Regulation of iron metabolism in the acute-phase response: interferon gamma and tumour necrosis factor alpha induce hypoferraemia, ferritin production and a decrease in circulating transferrin receptors in cancer patients. Eur J Clin Invest. 1998;28:520–7.
45. Todorich B, Zhang X, Slagle-Webb B, Seaman WE, Connor JR. Tim-2 is the receptor for H-ferritin on oligodendrocytes. J Neurochem. 2008;107:1495–505.
46. Todorich B, Zhang X, Connor JR. H-ferritin is the major source of iron for oligodendrocytes. Glia. 2011;59:927–35.
47. Fisher J, Devraj K, Ingram J, Slagle-Webb B, Madhankumar AB, Liu X, Klinger M, Simpson IA, Connor JR. Ferritin: a novel mechanism for delivery of iron to the brain and other organs. Am J Physiol Cell Physiol. 2007;293:C641–9.
48. Ritchie RF, Palomaki GE, Neveux LM, Navolotskaia O. Reference distributions for the negative acute-phase proteins, albumin, transferrin, and transthyretin: a comparison of a large cohort to the world's literature. J Clin Lab Anal. 1999;13:280–6.
49. Kushner I. The phenomenon of the acute phase response. Ann NY Acad Sci. 1982;389:39–48.
50. Singh N, Haldar S, Tripathi AK, Horback K, Wong J, Sharma D, et al. Brain iron homeostasis: from molecular mechanisms to clinical significance and therapeutic opportunities. Antioxid Redox Signal. 2014;20:1324–63.
51. Fuchs D, Zangerle R, Artner-Dworzak E, Weiss G, Fritsch P, Tilz GP, et al. Association between immune activation, changes of iron metabolism and anaemia in patients with HIV infection. Eur J Haematol. 1993;50:90–4.
52. Pugliese A, Gennero L, Pescarmona GP, Beccattini M, Morra E, Orofino G, et al. Serum citrate levels, haptoglobin haplotypes and transferrin receptor (CD71) in patients with HIV-1 infection. Infection. 2002;30:86–9.
53. Salomé MA, Grotto HZ. Human immunodeficiency virus-related anemia of chronic disease: relationship to hematologic, immune, and iron metabolism parameters, and lack of association with serum interferon-gamma levels. AIDS Patient Care STDS. 2002;16:361–5.

54. Armitage AE, Stacey AR, Giannoulatou E, Marshall E, Sturges P, Chatha K, et al. Distinct patterns of hepcidin and iron regulation during HIV-1, HBV, and HCV infections. Proc Natl Acad Sci USA. 2014;111:12187–92.
55. Perrella O, Finelli L, Munno I, Perrella A, Soscia E, Carrieri PB. Cerebrospinal fluid ferritin in human immunodeficiency virus infection: a marker of neurologic involvement? J Infect Dis. 1993;168:1079–80.
56. Deisenhammer F, Miller RF, Brink NS, Harrison MJ, Thompson EJ. Cerebrospinal fluid ferritin in HIV infected patients with acute neurological episodes. Genitourin Med. 1997;73:181–3.
57. Lleó A, Cavedo E, Parnetti L, Vanderstichele H, Herukka SK, Andreasen N, et al. Cerebrospinal fluid biomarkers in trials for Alzheimer and Parkinson diseases. Nat Rev Neurol. 2015;11:41–55.
58. Dickens AM, Anthony DC, Deutsch R, Mielke MM, Claridge TD, Grant I, et al. Cerebrospinal fluid metabolomics implicate bioenergetic adaptation as a neural mechanism regulating shifts in cognitive states of HIV-infected patients. AIDS. 2015;29:559–69.
59. Tarawneh R, Head D, Allison S, Buckles V, Fagan AM, Ladenson JH, et al. Cerebrospinal fluid markers of neurodegeneration and rates of brain atrophy in early Alzheimer disease. JAMA Neurol. 2015;72:656–65.
60. Patton SM, Coe CL, Lubach GR, Connor JR. Quantitative proteomic analyses of cerebrospinal fluid using iTRAQ in a primate model of iron deficiency anemia. Dev Neurosci. 2012;34:354–65.
61. Hyacinthe C, De Deurwaerdere P, Thiollier T, Li Q, Bezard E, Ghorayeb I. Blood withdrawal affects iron store dynamics in primates with consequences on monoaminergic system function. Neuroscience. 2015;290:621–35.
62. Clendenen TV, Koenig KL, Arslan AA, Lukanova A, Berrino F, Gu Y, et al. Factors associated with inflammation markers, a cross-sectional analysis. Cytokine. 2011;56:769–78.
63. Antinori A, Arendt G, Becker JT, Brew BJ, Byrd DA, Cherner M, et al. Updated research nosology for HIV-associated neurocognitive disorders. Neurology. 2007;69:1789–99.
64. Burtis C, Ashwood E, Bruns D, editors. Tietz textbook of clinical chemistry and molecular diagnostics. Elsevier Saunders: St. Louis; 2012.
65. de Almeida SM, Rotta I, Ribeiro CE, Smith D, Wang R, Iudicello J, Potter M, Vaida F, Letendre S, Ellis RJ, HNRC Group. Blood–CSF barrier and compartmentalization of CNS cellular immune response in HIV infection. J Neuroimmunol. 2016;301:41–8.
66. Gichohi-Wainaina WN, Tanaka T, Towers GW, Verhoef H, Veenemans J, Talsma EF, et al. Associations between common variants in iron-related genes with haematological traits in populations of African Ancestry. PLoS ONE. 2016;11:e0157996.
67. Hozumi I, Hasegawa T, Honda A, Ozawa K, Hayashi Y, Hashimoto K, et al. Patterns of levels of biological metals in CSF differ among neurodegenerative diseases. J Neurol Sci. 2011;303:95–9.
68. Clardy SL, Earley CJ, Allen RP, Beard JL, Connor JR. Ferritin subunits in CSF are decreased in restless legs syndrome. J Lab Clin Med. 2006;147:67–73.
69. Clardy SL, Wang X, Boyer PJ, Earley CJ, Allen RP, Connor JR. Is ferroportin-hepcidin signaling altered in restless legs syndrome? J Neurol Sci. 2006;247:173–9.
70. Earley CJ, Connor JR, Beard JL, Clardy SL, Allen RP. Ferritin levels in the cerebrospinal fluid and restless legs syndrome: effects of different clinical phenotypes. Sleep. 2005;28:1069–75.
71. Congdon EL, Westerlund A, Algarin CR, Peirano PD, Gregas M, Lozoff B, et al. Iron deficiency in infancy is associated with altered neural correlates of recognition memory at 10 years. J Pediatr. 2012;160:1027–33.
72. Doom JR, Georgieff MK. Striking while the iron is hot: understanding the biological and neurodevelopmental effects of iron deficiency to optimize intervention in early childhood. Curr Pediatr Rep. 2014;2:291–8.
73. Lozoff B, Beard J, Connor J, Barbara F, Georgieff M, Schallert T. Long-lasting neural and behavioral effects of iron deficiency in infancy. Nutr Rev. 2006;64(Suppl (5 Pt 2)):34–43.
74. Minchella PA, Armitage AE, Darboe B, Jallow MW, Drakesmith H, Jaye A, et al. Elevated hepcidin is part of a complex relation that links mortality with iron homeostasis and anemia in men and women with HIV infection. J Nutr. 2015;145:1194–201.
75. Chang HC, Bayeva M, Taiwo B, Palella FJ Jr, Hope TJ, Ardehali H. Short communication: high cellular iron levels are associated with increased HIV infection and replication. AIDS Res Hum Retroviruses. 2015;31:305–12.
76. Drakesmith H, Chen N, Ledermann H, Screaton G, Townsend A, Xu XN. HIV-1 Nef down-regulates the hemochromatosis protein HFE, manipulating cellular iron homeostasis. Proc Natl Acad Sci USA. 2005;102:11017–22.
77. Skjørringe T, Møller LB, Moos T. Impairment of interrelated iron- and copper homeostatic mechanisms in brain contributes to the pathogenesis of neurodegenerative disorders. Front Pharmacol. 2012;3:169.
78. Speeckaert MM, Speeckaert R, Delanghe JR. Biological and clinical aspects of soluble transferrin receptor. Crit Rev Clin Lab Sci. 2010;47(5–6):213–28.
79. Flax VL, Adair LS, Allen LH, Shahab-Ferdows S, Hampel D, Chasela CS, Teqha G, Daza EJ, Corbett A, Davis NL, Kamwendo D, Kourtis AP, van der Horst CM, Jamieson DM, Bengley ME, BAN Study Team. Plasma micronutrient concentrations are altered by antiretroviral therapy and lipid-based nutrient supplements in lactating HIV-infected Malawian women. J Nutr. 2015;145:1950–7.
80. Ganz T, Nemeth E. Iron balance and the role of hepcidin in chronic kidney disease. Semin Nephrol. 2016;36:87–93.
81. Happe S, Kundmüller L, Reichelt D, Husstedt IW, Evers S. Comorbidity of restless legs syndrome and HIV infection. J Neurol. 2007;254:1401–6.
82. Provini F, Chiaro G. Neuroimaging in restless legs syndrome. Sleep Med Clin. 2015;10:215–26.
83. Meyers DG. The iron hypothesis—does iron cause atherosclerosis? Clin Cardiol. 1996;19:925–9.
84. Gill AJ, Kovacsics CE, Vance PJ, Collman RG, Kolson DL. Induction of heme oxygenase-1 deficiency and associated glutamate-mediated neurotoxicity is a highly conserved HIV phenotype of chronic macrophage infection that is resistant to antiretroviral therapy. J Virol. 2015;89:10656–67.
85. Cheng HT, Yen CJ, Chang CC, Huang KT, Chen KH, Zhang RY, Lee PY, Miaw SC, Huang JW, Chiang CK, Wu KD, Hung KY. Ferritin heavy chain mediates the protective effect of heme oxygenase-1 against oxidative stress. Biochim Biophys Acta. 2015;1850:2506–17.
86. Earley CJ, Connor J, Garcia-Borreguero D, Jenner P, Winkelman J, Zee PC, et al. Altered brain iron homeostasis and dopaminergic function in restless legs syndrome (Willis–Ekbom disease). Sleep Med. 2014;15:1288–301.
87. Kim J, Wessling-Resnick M. Iron and mechanisms of emotional behavior. J Nutr Biochem. 2014;25:1101–7.
88. Ortancil O, Sanli A, Eryuksel R, Basaran A, Ankarali H. Association between serum ferritin level and fibromyalgia syndrome. Eur J Clin Nutr. 2010;64(308–12):78.
89. Fennema-Notestine C, Ellis RJ, Archibald SL, Jernigan TL, Letendre SL, Notestine RJ, CHARTER Group, et al. Increases in brain white matter abnormalities and subcortical gray matter are linked to CD4 recovery in HIV infection. J Neurovirol. 2013;19:393–401.
90. Li J, Wu G, Wen Z, Zhang J, Lei H, Gui X, et al. White Matter Development is Potentially Influenced in Adolescents with Vertically Transmitted HIV Infections: a Tract-Based Spatial Statistics Study. AJNR Am J Neuroradiol. 2015;36:2163–9.
91. Hoare J, Fouche JP, Spottiswoode B, Donald K, Philipps N, Bezuidenhout H, et al. A diffusion tensor imaging and neurocognitive study of HIV-positive children who are HAART-naive "slow progressors". J Neurovirol. 2012;18:205–12.
92. Clifford DB. HIV-associated neurocognitive disorder. Curr Opin Infect Dis. 2017;30:117–22.
93. Campbell GR, Rawat P, Bruckman RS, Spector SA. Human Immunodeficiency Virus type 1 Nef inhibits autophagy through transcription factor EB sequestration. PLoS Pathog. 2015;11:e1005018.
94. Biasiotto G, Di Lorenzo D, Archetti S, Zanella I. Iron and neurodegeneration: is ferritinophagy the link? Mol Neurobiol. 2016;53:5542–74.
95. Wang W, Knovich MA, Coffman LG, Torti FM, Torti SV. Serum ferritin: past, present and future. Biochim Biophys Acta. 2010;1800:760–9.

16

Magnesium sulfate treatment for juvenile ferrets following induction of hydrocephalus with kaolin

Domenico L. Di Curzio[1,2], Emily Turner-Brannen[2], Xiaoyan Mao[2] and Marc R. Del Bigio[2,3*]

Abstract

Background: Previous work with 3-week hydrocephalic rats showed that white matter damage could be reduced by the calcium channel antagonist magnesium sulfate ($MgSO_4$). We hypothesized that $MgSO_4$ therapy would improve outcomes in ferrets with hydrocephalus induced with kaolin at 15 days.

Methods: MRI was performed at 29 days to assess ventricle size and stratify ferrets to treatment conditions. Beginning at 31 days age, they were treated daily for 14 days with $MgSO_4$ (9 mM/kg/day) or sham saline therapy, and then imaged again before sacrifice. Behavior was examined thrice weekly. Histological and biochemical ELISA and myelin enzyme activity assays were performed at 46 days age.

Results: Hydrocephalic ferrets exhibited some differences in weight and behavior between treatment groups. Those receiving $MgSO_4$ weighed less, were more lethargic, and displayed reduced activity compared to those receiving saline injections. Hydrocephalic ferrets developed ventriculomegaly, which was not modified by $MgSO_4$ treatment. Histological examination showed destruction of periventricular white matter. Glial fibrillary acidic protein content, myelin basic protein content, and myelin enzyme activity did not differ significantly between treatment groups.

Conclusion: The hydrocephalus-associated disturbances in juvenile ferret brains are not ameliorated by $MgSO_4$ treatment, and lethargy is a significant side effect.

Keywords: Hydrocephalus, Ferret, Kaolin, Magnesium sulfate, Brain

Background

Hydrocephalus is a common neurological condition where cerebrospinal fluid (CSF) flow dynamics are altered, leading to enlargement of ventricular cavities in the brain. The histopathologic consequences of hydrocephalus depend on the age of onset, rate of ventricular enlargement, and the etiology [1]. The brain damage induced by hydrocephalus is multifactorial with mechanical factors leading to primary destruction of periventricular axons due to gradual physical stretching and compression, accumulation of metabolic waste products in the CSF, and ischemic changes causing decreased white matter blood flow that contributes to axonal and oligodendroglial damage [2, 3]. Elevated calcium (Ca^{2+}) coincides with increased white matter content of calpain I, along with heightened immunoreactivity in periventricular axons exhibited by young hydrocephalic rats with appreciable axonal damage, which suggest that calcium-mediated proteolysis may be associated with axonal cytoskeletal damage found in hydrocephalus [4].

Magnesium (Mg^{2+}) is a calcium channel antagonist; extracellular Mg^{2+} antagonizes Ca^{2+} influx by blocking voltage and receptor-mediated calcium channels along with NMDA channel receptors in a voltage-dependent manner [5, 6]. Intracellular Mg^{2+} is regulated by at least five distinct transporters [7]. Peripherally administered Mg^{2+} enters brain tissue of rabbits and cats, albeit to a lesser magnitude than muscle [8]. Magnesium sulfate ($MgSO_4$) administration by bolus or short-term infusion (e.g. 3 days) has shown short-term (hours to <7 days)

*Correspondence: marc.delbigio@umanitoba.ca
[3] Department of Pathology, University of Manitoba Brodie 401-727 McDermot Avenue, Winnipeg, MB R3E 3P5, Canada

outcome improvements in animal models of experimental spinal cord injury [9], reversible focal cerebral ischemia [10], kainate induced neuron degeneration [11], hypoxic-ischemic brain damage [12, 13], and traumatic brain injury [14–16]. Few experiments have looked at longer-term benefits of magnesium. A bolus of magnesium chloride after fluid percussion brain injury in adult rats was associated with improved motor outcome at 4 weeks [17].

Clinically, $MgSO_4$ has been used to suppress uterine contractions during premature labor and to reduce convulsions in pregnant women with preeclampsia [18]. In these circumstances, there is an association between maternal receipt of $MgSO_4$ and reduced risk of cerebral palsy in the offspring; this suggests that it could be neuroprotective in preterm birth although the benefit in term birth is much less clear [19, 20]. In infants with hypoxic-ischemic encephalopathy, the composite results of five clinical trials indicate a significant reduction in the unfavorable short-term outcome but a trend to increased mortality overall [21]. If effective, its protective mechanism remains unclear. $MgSO_4$ is a vasodilator that might improve cerebral circulation [22]. It can also reduce monocyte-mediated proinflammatory cytokine production and increase intracellular magnesium levels, which may be beneficial in decreasing inflammation [23].

Pharmacologic intervention might be a useful supplement to surgical shunts for the management of hydrocephalus [24]. We previously showed that $MgSO_4$ was beneficial in hydrocephalic rats [25]. Three-week old rats received kaolin injections into the cisterna magna to induce hydrocephalus; after 2 weeks, they were treated with parenteral administration of $MgSO_4$ for 2 more weeks. There was reduced reactive astrogliosis in the frontal cerebrum and improved gait performance on an accelerating rotating cylinder task. Despite these benefits, research with rodents is limiting because they have a small volume of white matter, which is the main region of damage in human brains. Moreover, stroke research has provided a valuable lesson in the major setbacks that can occur when basing clinical treatment on the success of pharmacological studies with rodents; this has prompted the necessity of preclinical treatment efficacy in gyrencephalic brains before proceeding to human trials [26]. Thus, we developed a model of hydrocephalus in 2-week old ferrets using injection of kaolin (aluminum silicate) into the cisterna magna, and we showed similarities to other animal models and the human condition [27]. Ferrets are born with relatively immature brains which develop a complex gyrencephalic morphology that has been studied extensively [28, 29]; consequently they are useful for modeling the neurologic disorders of human fetuses and infants [30]. Our overall goal is to develop a pharmacologic intervention that could be used to mitigate brain damage in the period prior to definitive shunt therapy. We hypothesized that $MgSO_4$ treatment would lead to behavioral, structural, and/or biochemical improvements in juvenile ferrets with experimental kaolin-induced hydrocephalus.

Methods

Animals

Twenty pigmented sable ferret kits (n = 13 males and n = 7 females) were obtained from Marshall Farms (North Rose, NY) at postnatal day 7 (P7) in 4 l along with their mothers (jills). The kits stayed with their mothers in enclosed cages until P46. The cages were located in a room kept on a 12:12 h (6 a.m.–6 p.m.) light–dark cycle, and the room temperature and relative humidity were 21–22 °C and ~35–45 %, respectively. Food and water were provided ad libitum; the kits started eating solid food around P30. For identification, tattoos were imprinted on their paws. All animals were treated humanely according to the guidelines set forth by the Canadian Council on Animal Care. The institutional animal ethics committee approved the experimental protocols (protocol #11-012). All efforts were made to minimize the number of animals used and ensure the least amount of suffering experienced.

Hydrocephalus induction

Hydrocephalus was induced using kaolin (aluminum silicate; Sigma, St. Louis MO) as described previously [27]. Briefly, kaolin injections were performed on all 4 litters at P15 (5 per litter—total n = 20; weight 69–93 g). They were anesthetized using 2.5 % isoflurane in oxygen, and the dorsum of their necks were shaved and cleansed. Using a 27-gauge needle, 0.2 mL of 20 % sterile kaolin suspension (250 mg/mL in 0.9 % saline) was injected percutaneously into the cisterna magna under aseptic conditions. Animals were monitored during recovery and observed for signs of discomfort and/or neurological impairment and then were otherwise returned to their mothers. Subcutaneous (sc) injections of buprenorphine (0.03 mg/kg) and sterile 0.45 % saline were given every 12 h for 2 days to decrease potential pain and possible dehydration, respectively. They were weighed daily, and those experiencing severe neurologic impairment or weight loss were sacrificed to cease further suffering.

Magnetic resonance imaging and assignment to treatment groups

The T2-weighted MR images of the brain were obtained using with a 7 Tesla Bruker Biospec/3 MR scanner (Karlsruhe, Germany) as previously described [27]. The first images were attained 2 days post kaolin injections at

P17 to confirm successful hydrocephalus induction with kaolin, and then 14 days post kaolin at P29 to examine ventricle size and stratify treatment groups. The areas of the lateral ventricles to cerebrum brain area, third ventricle width to cerebrum width, cerebral aqueduct area to midbrain area, and fourth ventricle area to hindbrain area ratios were measured as previously described [27]. Ferrets were stratified based on ventricle size and assigned listwise to saline (0.9 % NaCl) and $MgSO_4$ treatment groups. A third set of MR images was taken after the 14-day drug treatment period at P45, no more than 24 h before euthanasia, to assess ventricle size again.

Drug preparation and administration

The $MgSO_4$ and/or NaCl treatments were administered starting 16 days post-kaolin at P31 (n = 8 for $MgSO_4$ and n = 8 for NaCl). All animals were weighed daily, and their weights were used to calculate treatment volumes. Stock solutions of 1.0 M $MgSO_4$ and 0.9 M NaCl were prepared in distilled H_2O at room temperature and stored at 4 °C; the solutions were labeled A and B, and treatments were given blindly based upon a volume drug to body weight formula. They received either a ~9 mM/kg/day dosage of $MgSO_4$ or NaCl daily for 14 days, which were administered by sc injections given 3 times per day on weekdays (~3 mM/kg/dose) and 2 times per day on weekends (~4.5 mM/kg/dose) to ensure that all animals received the entire dosage. This calculated dosage was derived from testing different $MgSO_4$ concentrations with rodents in a previous study, where 8.2 mM/kg/day was found to be protective [25]. The ferrets received their first injection in the morning before behavioral testing. Their second daily injection was given in the late afternoon, and the third injection was administered near midnight to maintain trough levels. Because of the expense, we could not conduct a dose-escalation study.

Behavioral testing

Previous work with kaolin-induced hydrocephalic ferrets [27] showed that they differed from controls in a limited number of the behavioral tests previously studied [31]; these were chosen for the current study. Behavioral testing commenced at P10-11 and continued 3 times weekly until P43-44 for all kits (n = 16). Behavior tests were conducted prior to the daily drug administration to minimize the effect of lethargy in the $MgSO_4$ recipients. The kits were not exposed to the test situations prior to testing. Open field behavior was assessed using two apparatuses. The first chamber was an enclosed square (44 × 43 × 29 cm) with 15 light beam sensors on each axis to quantitate ambulatory, vertical, and total movements (Opto-Varimex 3; Columbus Instruments International Corp., Columbus, OH, USA). Animals were observed individually for 3 min and tested once per session. The second chamber was a 75 × 75 × 45 cm transparent plastic square, where the kits were videotaped, and motor performance was analyzed for 3 min using HVS Image 2100 Plus Tracking System software (HVS Image Ltd, Twickenham, Middlesex, UK). Quantitative measures were performed after dividing the chamber into 100 (7.5 × 7.5 cm) squares and included the length of path traversed and the number and percent of squares entered. Qualitative observations were also recorded in the second chamber for pivoting, crawling, walking, running, and rearing.

Sacrifice and brain dissection

Ferrets were euthanized within 24 h of final MRI using isoflurane anesthesia (5 %) followed by carbon dioxide (CO_2) narcosis and exsanguination by transcardiac perfusion at ~P46 or when humane endpoints were met as described previously [27]. Ferret brains were rapidly removed, photographed, and then split in the parasagittal plane 1 mm from the midline. The right hemisphere was dissected into anterior frontal lobe, dorsal frontal cerebrum, and dorsal parietal cerebrum, which were frozen in liquid nitrogen (N_2) and stored at −70 °C. The left hemisphere was immersion fixed in cold 3 % buffered paraformaldehyde for several days; then it was sliced in the coronal plane, dehydrated, and embedded in paraffin wax.

Histology and immunohistochemistry

All paraffin blocks were sectioned coronally (6 μm thickness) and stained with hematoxylin and eosin (H and E). The cerebrum at the level of the anterior horn of the lateral ventricles was stained with solochrome cyanine and counterstained with eosin for visualization of myelin. Sections were immunostained with rabbit polyclonal anti-glial fibrillary acidic protein (GFAP; 1:10,000 dilution; DAKO Z0334; Glostrup, Denmark) to label astrocytes and reactive astrocytes. The primary antibody underwent 1.5 h incubation at room temperature. This was followed by incubation with appropriate biotinylated secondary antibody, followed by reaction with streptavidin-peroxidase, detection with diaminobenzidine (DAB, Sigma D5905), and finally counterstaining with hematoxylin. Negative controls were treated without the primary antibody. Corpus callosum thickness was measured using 100× ocular magnification at the sagittal midline and above the lateral angle of the anterior horn of the lateral ventricle. The second site was chosen because fragmentation of the midline region in some hydrocephalic brains preventing proper measurement of corpus callosum thickness. For comparative purposes, non-hydrocephalic ferrets from our previous experiment [27] were also examined.

Myelin enzymes and enzyme-linked immunosorbent assays

Frozen dorsal frontal and parietal cerebrum samples were homogenized using a radio immunoprecipitation assay (RIPA) buffer including protease inhibitors phenylmethylsulfonyl fluoride (PMSF) and aprotinin, which likely explain the lower myelin enzyme activities than were obtained previously [27]. Total protein quantification was determined with the Micro BCA (Pierce) Protein Assay kit (Thermo Scientific, Rockford, Illinois, USA). Dorsal frontal cerebrum homogenates were used to quantify myelin basic protein (MBP) and GFAP content by using ELISAs, as previously described in detail [27]. Colorimetric assays were performed in triplicate, and results are shown in μg of MBP or GFAP per gram of protein and averaged per sample. Dorsal parietal cerebrum samples were used to quantify the enzyme activity of UDP-galactose:ceramide galactosyltransferase (CGalT) and glycerylphosphorylcholine phosphocholine phosphodiesterase (GPC-PP) using the artificial substrate p-nitrophenylphosphorylcholine (pNPP). Both are enzymes that are enriched in myelin. They were quantified in triplicate as described previously [32, 33].

Atomic absorption spectroscopy

Flame atomic absorption spectroscopy (FAAS) was performed to determine Mg levels in anterior forebrain samples as indicated previously [34] except for the following differences. Ferrets were given their last dose of $MgSO_4$ or NaCl 35–152 min (mean 68.88 ± 13.46) before sacrifice. Forebrain samples were thawed and weighed then dissolved in 18 M sulfuric acid and 16 M nitric acid over gentle heat. Standards were prepared from a 1000 μg mL^{-1} Mg standard solution (Alfa Aesar 88077) at concentrations of 0.50, 0.40, and 0.20 μg mL^{-1}, along with a 1 % nitric acid blank. Mg content was measured using Atomic Absorption Spectrometer AAnalyst 400 with a PerkinElmer Lamp (Intensitron) using a wavelength of 285.21 nm. Measurements were performed in triplicate and averaged to obtain concentrations (μg Mg^{2+} per gram brain tissue).

Statistical analysis

All data are presented as mean ± SEM, unless otherwise indicated. Quantitative data were analyzed to confirm a normal distribution, and p values ≤ 0.05 were considered statistically significant. Statistical analyses for the behavioral tasks, MRI, and all biochemical analyses were conducted with the juvenile ferrets (n = 15). Data were assessed using ANOVA and two-tailed t-tests for behavioral testing, ventricle size, histological data, and biochemical assays to compare $MgSO_4$ and NaCl hydrocephalic treatment groups. Qualitative assessments for motor and behavioral development were analyzed separately from quantitative measures. Statistical analyses were conducted using the SPSS 19.0 software program.

Results

Mortality

Of the 20 kaolin-injected juvenile ferrets, three were euthanized due to severe neurological deficits within the first 2 days post-injection (P16), one was euthanized on P22 due to severe weight loss and neurological impairment, and one was euthanized on P43 due to persistently low weight and neurological impairment despite only slight ventricle enlargement (this animal was initially assigned to receive $MgSO_4$). Two of the remaining ferrets were nonhydrocephalic; these were used for comparative purposes only. The focus of the results is on the hydrocephalic ferrets (n = 13; 8 males and 5 females) that survived the 14-day drug therapy period. All were euthanized within 24 h of the final MRI between postnatal days P45–P46.

Ventricle size on magnetic resonance imaging

Ventricular expansion was noticeable 2 days after kaolin injections, where the lateral ventricles were already significantly larger compared to the nonhydrocephalic animals ($p < 0.010$, t test). From this time onward, the hydrocephalic ferrets displayed enhanced signal in the periventricular white matter on the T2-weighted MR images indicating elevated water content. At 14 days post-kaolin injections (P29), MR images showed a range of ventriculomegaly in the hydrocephalic ferrets (Fig. 1). This was particularly evident in the lateral and third ventricles, which were significantly enlarged (both $p < 0.05$, t tests). Ferrets were stratified according to ventricle size and alternately assigned to $MgSO_4$ or NaCl treatment groups to ensure that there was no significant difference between hydrocephalic groups before therapy. Both hydrocephalic groups displayed further expansion of the ventricles during the therapeutic period, exhibiting significant progressive enlargement of the lateral (Fig. 2; Table 1) and third ventricles (all $p < 0.05$, t tests). Comparison of the NaCl- and $MgSO_4$-treated ferrets showed no significant differences for any of the ventricle regions (all $p > 0.05$, t tests; Table 1).

Body weight and behavioral assessments

Behavioral testing began at P10–11 to determine baseline performance before kaolin injection was performed at P15. Successful induction of hydrocephalus was

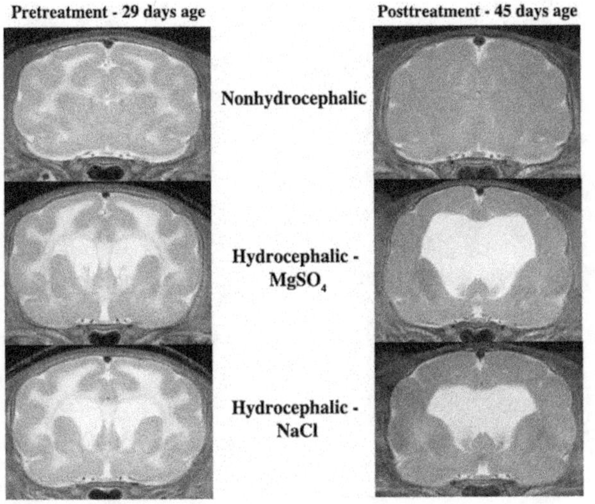

Fig. 1 T2-weighted magnetic resonance images showing frontal coronal slices of brains of ferrets without hydrocephalus as well as ferrets that were treated with $MgSO_4$ or NaCl between 29 and 45 days age. Progressive ventriculomegaly is evident in these examples of both treatments

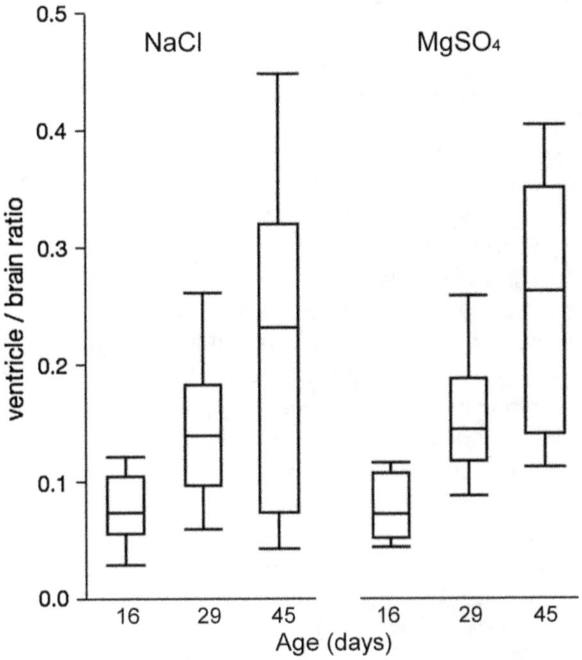

Fig. 2 *Box plots* (mean ± standard error of mean) showing cross sectional ratio of the lateral ventricle frontal horn areas to the cerebrum on the magnetic resonance images. The 16-day images were obtained 2 days after kaolin injection, the 29-day images were 14 days after kaolin injection and immediately prior to onset of drug treatment, and the 45-day images were obtained at the end of the treatment period shortly prior to termination (n = 7 for NaCl and n = 6 for $MgSO_4$ each at all time points). In comparison to non-hydrocephalic controls (not shown) and previous time points the ventricles enlarged progressively at successive time points ($p < 0.05$). There were no significant differences between the $MgSO_4$ and NaCl treatment groups

typically associated with weight loss for several days following injection. Overall, the hydrocephalic ferrets weighed 39 % less than nonhydrocephalic ferrets at P21 ($p < 0.001$, *t* test) and 25 % less at P28 ($p = 0.009$, *t* test). After the 14-day treatment period, the $MgSO_4$-treated hydrocephalic ferrets weighed significantly less than the NaCl hydrocephalic group during and after treatment (all $p < 0.05$, ANOVA; Table 1).

By the end of the pretreatment period (P28–P30), all the ferrets were crawling, similar to previously assessed motor development [27]. Walking commenced on P34–37, with no appreciable differences between hydrocephalic groups. Qualitatively, both groups reached motor and behavioral developmental milestones at the same time, although several of the $MgSO_4$-treated hydrocephalic ferrets (n = 5) were more unsteady and engaged in less exploratory behavior. Unlike our previous finding [27], the hydrocephalic ferrets did not become hyperactive or wander in circles within the enclosure. $MgSO_4$-treated ferrets were more lethargic than NaCl-treated animals. Quantitative activity measurements showed that the hydrocephalic $MgSO_4$ group displayed significantly less ambulatory movement, fewer cell entries, less distance traveled overall, and less supported rearing, compared to the NaCl group during the first week of treatment (all $p < 0.05$, ANOVA; data not shown). These between-group discrepancies were evident primarily during transition to walking phase of development but dissipated by the last behavioral time point measured and were not significantly different post-treatment (Table 1).

Structural and biochemical changes in brain

Macrophages that had engulfed kaolin and associated collagen deposition were microscopically identified throughout the basal subarachnoid space, having spread from the cisterna magna injection site; only rare macrophages were present in the fourth ventricle. Ventriculomegaly was accompanied by cerebral thinning surrounding the lateral ventricles and decreased depth of cerebral sulci. Intact white matter structures such as the internal capsule showed equivalent myelin staining in hydrocephalic and non-hydrocephalic ferrets. There was thinning and fraying of the periventricular white matter in all hydrocephalic ferrets; these damaged regions had no myelin staining. The corpus callosum thickness did not differ between the $MgSO_4$ and NaCl treatment groups (Fig. 3; Table 1). In comparison to non-hydrocephalic ferrets, there was a slight but not statistically significant reduction of cerebral MBP content in the hydrocephalic ferrets; however, there was no difference between treatment groups (Table 1). To determine if the severity of ventriculomegaly had any

Table 1 Results of magnesium sulfate treatment on hydrocephalic ferrets

	Non-hydrocephalic controls	NaCl-treated hydrocephalus	$MgSO_4$-treated hydrocephalus
Sample size	2	7	6
Lateral ventricle area index (P29/pre-treat)	0.012 ± 0.002	0.147 ± 0.024*	0.155 ± 0.023*
Lateral ventricle area index (P45/post-treat)	0.006 ± 0.0005	0.219 ± 0.053*#	0.254 ± 0.046*#
Percent enlargement ventricles during treatment	–	48.9 ± 23.1	63.9 ± 24.4
Body weight (g) (P29/pre-treat)	148.0 ± 8.0	114.3 ± 4.8*	106.8 ± 9.1*
Body weight (g) (P45/post-treat)	264.5 ± 34.5#	288.3 ± 12.8#	170.0 ± 31.0*@#
Rearing activity (beam breaks per 3 min) (P43/post-treat)	71 ± 16	57 ± 15	22 ± 20*
Ambulatory activity (beam breaks per 3 min) (P43/post-treat)	541 ± 21	460 ± 44	321 ± 71*
Total activity (beam breaks per 3 min) (P43/post-treat)	684 ± 20	584 ± 54	443 ± 89*
Number cells entered—open field (per 3 min) (P43/post-treat)	88 ± 7	115 ± 12	111 ± 15
Distance traveled—open field (m per 3 min) (P43/post-treat)	5.64 ± 0.39	7.58 ± 0.95	7.11 ± 1.08
Medial corpus callosum thickness (μm)	965 ± 95	410 ± 71*	315 ± 97*
Lateral corpus callosum thickness (μm)	665 ± 45	330 ± 50*	245 ± 59*
MBP content frontal cerebrum (μg MBP/g protein)	72.19 ± 12.75	64.25 ± 19.66	56.07 ± 14.15
CGalT activity parietal cerebrum (nM/mg protein/h)	0.029 ± 0.008	0.075 ± 0.024	0.051 ± 0.014
GPC-PP activity parietal cerebrum (nM/mg protein/h)	15.25 ± 1.83	14.42 ± 0.90	11.64 ± 1.20
GFAP content frontal cerebrum (μg GFAP/g protein)	0.64 ± 0.02	0.90 ± 0.13	0.70 ± 0.12
Frontal cerebrum magnesium (μg Mg^{2+}/g brain tissue)	133.64 ± 4.97	135.59 ± 10.37	150.89 ± 5.23

All data are presented as mean ± SEM. Behavior and ventricle size are specified at by postnatal day (P) age. All brain structural and biochemical data are at P46

CGalT ceramide galactosyltransferase

GFAP glial fibrillary acidic protein

GPC-PP glycerylphosphorylcholine phosphocholine phosphodiesterase

MBP myelin basic protein

* $p < 0.05$ control vs. hydrocephalic, *t* tests or ANOVA

@ $p < 0.05$ NaCl vs. $MgSO_4$-treated ferrets, *t* tests or ANOVA

\# $p < 0.05$ P29 (pre-treat) vs. P45 (post-treat), *t* tests

impact on the MBP content, both treatment groups were subdivided into moderate and severe hydrocephalus. Subgroup analyses of the 4 most severely affected ferrets in each group showed no significant differences between groups (data not shown). It should be noted that the MBP content at P46 is just beginning the rapid accumulation phase [27]; this is comparable to human brain shortly after full term gestation.

In periventricular and perivascular foci of the white matter adjacent to the frontal horns of the lateral ventricles, NaCl and $MgSO_4$-treated hydrocephalic ferrets displayed similar GFAP immunostaining of hypertrophic astrocytes (Fig. 3). ELISA analysis of GFAP content was 27 % lower in the $MgSO_4$ hydrocephalic group compared to NaCl group, but the difference was not statistically significant ($p = 0.375$, ANOVA; Table 1). Subgroup analysis of the most severely affected ferrets also did not reveal significant differences in GFAP content between treatment groups (data not shown).

Myelin enzyme activity was measured in hydrocephalic ferret brains. CGalT is active in oligodendrocytes during myelin production [35]; we previously showed highest activity from P35–P56 [27]. There were no significant differences between hydrocephalic treatment groups (Table 1). GPC-PP is abundant in mature myelin [36]; we previously showed that the activity began to increase at P35 [27]. Compared to the untreated hydrocephalic ferrets, the $MgSO_4$ group tended to show lower GPC-PP activity than the NaCl group ($p = 0.056$) (Table 1), but subgroup analysis still did not reach significance (data not shown).

Mg^{2+} in anterior forebrain samples was slightly, but not significantly, higher in the $MgSO_4$ group compared to the NaCl-treated group ($p = 0.38$, *t* test) (Table 1).

Discussion

Mg^{2+} was shown to have mild protective benefits in rats with experimental hydrocephalus treated from 5 to 7 weeks age but not in rats treated from 1 to 3 weeks age [25, 34]. We had hoped that $MgSO_4$ treatment would also yield therapeutic benefits in young hydrocephalic ferrets. As has been recommended for preclinical stroke and brain trauma studies [26, 37], the experimental design included randomization, blinding, and multiple

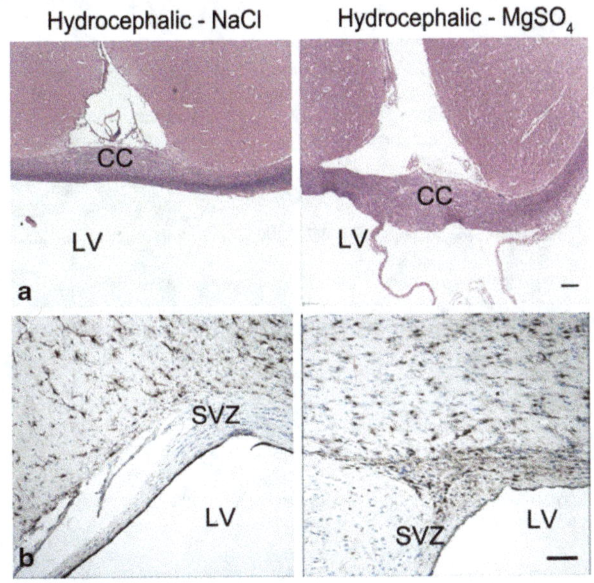

Fig. 3 Photomicrographs showing white matter above the frontal horn of the lateral ventricle in 46-day-old hydrocephalic ferret brains, after a 14-day treatment period with $MgSO_4$ or NaCl. **a** (*upper pair*)—corpus callosum *CC* thinning is evident in both animals (solochrome cyanine stains myelin *blue*, with *pink* eosin counterstain). **b** (*lower pair*)—GFAP immunolabeling (*brown*) showing hypertrophic reactive astrocytes in periventricular white matter near the lateral angle of the frontal horn. There is no obvious difference between the two groups of hydrocephalic ferrets. Objective magnification: **a**-40x, **b**-100x; *Scale bar* = 100 μm. Lateral ventricles *LV*, Subventricular zone SVZ

outcome measures. However, in comparison to NaCl-treated hydrocephalic ferrets, we did not find any behavioral, histological, or biochemical evidence to support the hypothesis that $MgSO_4$ therapy, at the same dose that was effective in rats, benefits hydrocephalic ferrets. Treated ferrets had transient sedation, which is well-documented [38], impaired weight gain, and tendency to greater progression of ventriculomegaly. Despite more severely enlarged ventricles, $MgSO_4$ treatment was associated with reduced GFAP accumulation in ferrets albeit not significantly; this finding is similar to that seen in hydrocephalic rats treated from 5 to 7 weeks age [25]. Reduced astroglial reaction has also been reported in kaolin-induced and congenitally hydrocephalic H-Tx rats treated with minocycline or decorin [39–41]. Although reduced GFAP accumulation is often considered an indicator of benefit, another possibility is that Mg^{2+}, which blocks signaling between astrocytes [42], simply masks the astrocytic response to brain damage.

Why was $MgSO_4$ therapy unsuccessful in hydrocephalic ferrets? Rationale for the experiment was based upon a previously-demonstrated neuroprotective effect in juvenile hydrocephalic rats and a range of experimental data from other neurological disorders. Technical and design aspects must be considered. It remains unclear whether entry of Mg^{2+} into brain is via the choroid plexus and CSF or through the blood brain barrier [43, 44], although the observed side effect of sedation indicates entry into the brain [8, 45, 46]. Lethargy is a potential confounder in the behavioral assessments, and it prevented complete blinding of the investigators. More importantly, weight gain was retarded in the $MgSO_4$ treated ferrets, possibly because lethargy impaired feeding or because of the effect of Mg^{2+} on intestinal smooth muscle [7]. Undernutrition might have had a negative effect on the outcome. This might be overcome experimentally by using a matched feeding strategy. Unfortunately, ferrets are obligate carnivores with short intestinal tracts; they can require special diets when they are ill [47], and therefore might not be the ideal animal for studies where feeding is compromised. Periodic subcutaneous injections would result in troughs and peaks; in rats Mg^{2+} levels peak at approximately 2 h and return to normal levels within 4 h after injection [25]. We had considered using osmotic minipumps, but none would accommodate sufficiently large volumes for the treatment period nor could they adjust for the increasing weight of the maturing ferrets. Furthermore, based on discussions with the veterinarians, the potential complications (maternal biting of the surgical site and sloughing of the skin over the minipumps) outweighed the potential benefits. During the treatment period, we did observe that the $MgSO_4$-treated ferrets experienced some skin irritation at the injection sites; rotating the locations of the injections minimized this. Oral administration potentially provides longer periods of exposure; however, peak levels are not as high as those that follow parenteral administration [48]. We also observed that some $MgSO_4$-treated ferrets began gagging and/or vomiting immediately after injections, which would have made repeated gavage difficult. In a clinical situation, tube feeding would negate this confounder. Perhaps the intervention was timed incorrectly. If the ventricular enlargement is too mild a therapeutic benefit might be difficult to detect or if the intervention is too late, no benefit might be possible. However, subgroup analysis of the 4 most severely affected ferrets in each group as well as the least severely affected still showed no significant differences between treatment groups.

We must also consider that the rodent experimental studies considered in the Introduction do not translate to larger animals. The majority documented only short-term benefit. In short term studies of brain hypoxic-ischemic damage in immature rat, sheep, and pig models, $MgSO_4$ has had inconsistent outcomes and results have been confounded by mild hypothermia; for this condition reviewers concluded "peripherally administered $MgSO_4$ is unlikely to be neuroprotective" [49]. A meta-analysis of

8 randomized controlled trials with a total of 786 head-injured patients indicates that $MgSO_4$ has no significant improvement for mortality, but there is borderline improvement in the glasgow outcome scale [50].

Conclusion

Young hydrocephalic ferrets at the age during which cerebral myelin production is just beginning did not exhibit behavioral benefits or white matter protection from $MgSO_4$ therapy. Although $MgSO_4$ seems to be safe in other situations, it was associated with severe sedation, which can compromise feeding. Considering the experimental and epidemiologic evidence that Mg^{2+} might protect the developing brain in other diseases, this negative result should not completely exclude its possible benefits in hydrocephalus. However, preclinical testing might have to be done in a larger animal model wherein continuous delivery is possible or more control can be achieved over feeding. We will continue to explore other pharmacological agents that can be used as a supplement to shunt treatment of hydrocephalus in gyrencephalic animal models.

Authors' contributions

DDC carried out the drug administration, behavioral work, dissections and histology, ELISAs, myelin enzyme activity assays, statistical analyses, and drafted the manuscript. DDC also assisted in the induction of hydrocephalus, MR imaging, and atomic absorption spectroscopy. ETB assisted in the induction of hydrocephalus, drug administration, behavioral work, MR imaging, and dissections. XM assisted with the MR imaging, behavioral tasks, ELISAs, myelin enzyme activity assays, and data collection. MDB conceived the study including its design and coordination, carried out the hydrocephalus induction, and guided writing of the manuscript. All authors read and approved the final manuscript.

Author details

[1] Department of Human Anatomy & Cell Science, University of Manitoba, Winnipeg, MB, Canada. [2] Children's Hospital Research Institute of Manitoba, Winnipeg, MB, Canada. [3] Department of Pathology, University of Manitoba Brodie 401-727 McDermot Avenue, Winnipeg, MB R3E 3P5, Canada.

Acknowledgements

The authors thank Dr. Richard Buist for performing MR imaging and Dr. Douglas Goltz for supervising the magnesium ion assay.
This work was funded by Grants from the Canadian Institutes of Health Research (Grant # 109756) and from Research Manitoba to Dr. Del Bigio. Dr. Del Bigio holds the Canada Research Chair in Developmental Neuropathology. Domenico Di Curzio had a Graduate Studentship from Research Manitoba.

Competing interests

The authors declare that they have no competing interests.

References

1. Del Bigio MR. Pathophysiologic consequences of hydrocephalus. Neurosurg Clin N Am. 2001;12:639–49.
2. Del Bigio MR. Neuropathological changes caused by hydrocephalus. Acta Neuropathol (Berl). 1993;85:573–85.
3. Del Bigio MR. Neuropathology and structural changes in hydrocephalus. Dev Disabil Res Rev. 2010;16:16–22.
4. Del Bigio MR. Calcium-mediated proteolytic damage in white matter of hydrocephalic rats? J Neuropathol Exp Neurol. 2000;59:946–54.
5. Simpson JI, Eide TR, Schiff GA, Clagnaz JF, Hossain I, Tverskoy A, Koski G. Intrathecal magnesium sulfate protects the spinal cord from ischemic injury during thoracic aortic cross-clamping. Anesthesiology. 1994;81:1493–9.
6. Fawcett WJ, Haxby EJ, Male DA. Magnesium: physiology and pharmacology. Br J Anaesth. 1999;83:302–20.
7. de Baaij JH, Hoenderop JG, Bindels RJ. Magnesium in man: implications for health and disease. Physiol Rev. 2015;95:1–46.
8. Hilmy MI, Somjen GG. Distribution and tissue uptake of magnesium related to its pharmacological effects. Am J Physiol. 1968;214:406–13.
9. Suzer T, Coskun E, Islekel H, Tahta K. Neuroprotective effect of magnesium on lipid peroxidation and axonal function after experimental spinal cord injury. Spinal Cord. 1999;37:480–4.
10. Marinov MB, Harbaugh KS, Hoopes PJ, Pikus HJ, Harbaugh RE. Neuroprotective effects of preischemia intraarterial magnesium sulfate in reversible focal cerebral ischemia. J Neurosurg. 1996;85:117–24.
11. Wolf G, Fischer S, Hass P, Abicht K, Kelhoff G. Magnesium sulphate subcutaneously injected protects against kainate-induced convulsions and neurodegeneration: in vivo study on the rat hippocampus. Neuroscience. 1991;43:31–4.
12. Goni-de-Cerio F, Alvarez A, Lara-Celador I, Alvarez FJ, Alonso-Alconada D, Hilario E. Magnesium sulfate treatment decreases the initial brain damage alterations produced after perinatal asphyxia in fetal lambs. J Neurosci Res. 2012;90(10):1932–40.
13. Sameshima H, Ikenoue T. Long-term magnesium sulfate treatment as protection against hypoxic-ischemic brain injury in seven-day-old rats. Am J Obstet Gynecol. 2001;184:185–90.
14. Esen F, Erdem T, Aktan D, Kalayci R, Cakar N, Kaya M, Telci L. Effects of magnesium administration on brain edema and blood-brain barrier breakdown after experimental traumatic brain injury in rats. J Neurosurg Anesthesiol. 2003;15:119–25.
15. Hoane MR. Assessment of cognitive function following magnesium therapy in the traumatically injured brain. Magnes Res. 2007;20:229–36.
16. Saatman KE, Bareyre FM, Grady MS, McIntosh TK. Acute cytoskeletal alterations and cell death induced by experimental brain injury are attenuated by magnesium treatment and exacerbated by magnesium deficiency. J Neuropathol Exp Neurol. 2001;60:183–94.
17. McIntosh TK, Vink R, Yamakami I, Faden AI. Magnesium protects against neurological deficit after brain injury. Brain Res. 1989;482:252–60.
18. Duley L, Gulmezoglu AM, Henderson-Smart DJ, Chou D. Magnesium sulphate and other anticonvulsants for women with pre-eclampsia. Cochrane Database Syst Rev. 2010;(11):CD000025. doi:10.1002/14651858.CD000025.pub2.
19. Doyle LW, Crowther CA, Middleton P, Marret S. Antenatal magnesium sulfate and neurologic outcome in preterm infants: a systematic review. Obstet Gynecol. 2009;113:1327–33.
20. Nguyen TM, Crowther CA, Wilkinson D, Bain E. Magnesium sulphate for women at term for neuroprotection of the fetus. Cochrane Database Syst Rev. 2013;2:CD009395.
21. Tagin M, Shah PS, Lee KS. Magnesium for newborns with hypoxic-ischemic encephalopathy: a systematic review and meta-analysis. J Perinatol. 2013;33:663–9.
22. Brewer RP, Parra A, Lynch J, Chilukuri V, Borel CO. Cerebral blood flow velocity response to magnesium sulfate in patients after subarachnoid hemorrhage. J Neurosurg Anesthesiol. 2001;13:202–6.
23. Sugimoto J, Romani AM, Valentin-Torres AM, Luciano AA, Kitchen CMR, Funderburg N, Mesiano S, Bernstein HB. Magnesium decreases inflammatory cytokine production: a novel innate immunomodulatory mechanism. J Immunol. 2012;188(12):6338–46.
24. Del Bigio MR, Di Curzio DL. Nonsurgical therapy for hydrocephalus: a comprehensive and critical review. Fluids Barriers CNS. 2016;13:3.
25. Khan OH, Enno T, Del Bigio MR. Magnesium sulfate therapy is of mild benefit to young rats with kaolin-induced hydrocephalus. Pediatr Res. 2003;53:970–6.
26. Fisher M, Feuerstein G, Howells DW, Hurn PD, Kent TA, Savitz SI, Lo EH. Update of the stroke therapy academic industry roundtable preclinical recommendations. Stroke. 2009;40:2244–50.

27. Di Curzio DL, Buist RJ, Del Bigio MR. Reduced subventricular zone proliferation and white matter damage in juvenile ferrets with kaolin-induced hydrocephalus. Exp Neurol. 2013;248:112–28.
28. Lockard BI. The forebrain of the ferret. Lab Anim Sci. 1985;35:216–28.
29. Hayes SG, Murray KD, Jones EG. Two epochs in the development of gamma-aminobutyric acidergic neurons in the ferret thalamus. J Comp Neurol. 2003;463:45–65.
30. Empie K, Rangarajan V, Juul SE. Is the ferret a suitable species for studying perinatal brain injury? Int J Dev Neurosci. 2015;45:2–10.
31. Christensson M, Garwicz M. Time course of postnatal motor development in ferrets: ontogenetic and comparative perspectives. Behav Brain Res. 2005;158:231–42.
32. Del Bigio MR, Kanfer JN, Zhang YW. Myelination delay in the cerebral white matter of immature rats with kaolin-induced hydrocephalus is reversible. J Neuropathol Exp Neurol. 1997;56:1053–66.
33. Kanfer JN, McCartney D. An unusual phosphodiesterase activity towards p-nitrophenylphosphorylcholine present in rat brain membranes. Neurochem Res. 1990;15:987–92.
34. Khan OH, McPhee LC, Moddemann LN, Del Bigio MR. Calcium antagonism in neonatal rats with kaolin-induced hydrocephalus. J Child Neurol. 2007;22:1161–6.
35. Koul O, Jungalwala FB. UDP-galactose: ceramide galactosyltransferase of rat central nervous system myelin during development. Neurochem Res. 1986;11:231–9.
36. Sok DE, Kim MR. Brain myelin-bound Zn(2+)-glycerophosphocholine cholinephosphodiesterase is a glycosylphosphatidylinositol-anchored enzyme of two different molecular forms. Neurochem Res. 1994;19:97–103.
37. Diaz-Arrastia R, Kochanek PM, Bergold P, Kenney K, Marx CE, Grimes CJ, Loh LT, Adam LT, Oskvig D, Curley KC, Salzer W. Pharmacotherapy of traumatic brain injury: state of the science and the road forward: report of the Department of Defense Neurotrauma Pharmacology Workgroup. J Neurotrauma. 2014;31:135–58.
38. Rude RK, Singer FR. Magnesium deficiency and excess. Annu Rev Med. 1981;32:245–59.
39. McAllister JP 2nd, Miller JM. Minocycline inhibits glial proliferation in the H-Tx rat model of congenital hydrocephalus. Cerebrospinal Fluid Res. 2010;7:7.
40. Xu H, Tan G, Zhang S, Zhu H, Liu F, Huang C, Zhang F, Wang Z. Minocycline reduces reactive gliosis in the rat model of hydrocephalus. BMC Neurosci. 2012;13:148.
41. Botfield H, Gonzalez AM, Abdullah O, Skjolding AD, Berry M, McAllister JP 2nd, Logan A. Decorin prevents the development of juvenile communicating hydrocephalus. Brain. 2013;136:2842–58.
42. Stout C, Charles A. Modulation of intercellular calcium signaling in astrocytes by extracellular calcium and magnesium. Glia. 2003;43:265–73.
43. Oppelt WW, MacIntyre I, Rall DP. Magnesium exchange between blood and cerebrospinal fluid. Am J Physiol. 1963;205:959–62.
44. Chutkow JG. Uptake of magnesium into the brain of the rat. Exp Neurol. 1978;60:592–602.
45. Hallak M, Berman RF, Irtenkauf SM, Evans MI, Cotton DB. Peripheral magnesium sulfate enters the brain and increases the threshold for hippocampal seizures in rats. Am J Obstet Gynecol. 1992;167:1605–10.
46. Hallak M. Effect of parenteral magnesium sulfate administration on excitatory amino acid receptors in the rat brain. Magnes Res. 1998;11:117–31.
47. Orosz SE. Critical care nutrition for exotic animals. J Exotic Pet Med. 2013;22:163–77.
48. Turner PV, Brabb T, Pekow C, Vasbinder MA. Administration of substances to laboratory animals: routes of administration and factors to consider. J Am Assoc Lab Anim Sci. 2011;50:600–13.
49. Galinsky R, Bennet L, Groenendaal F, Lear CA, Tan S, van Bel F, Juul SE, Robertson NJ, Mallard C, Gunn AJ. Magnesium is not consistently neuroprotective for perinatal hypoxia-ischemia in term-equivalent models in preclinical studies: a systematic review. Dev Neurosci. 2014;36:73–82.
50. Li W, Bai YA, Li YJ, Liu KG, Wang MD, Xu GZ, Shang HL, Li YF. Magnesium sulfate for acute traumatic brain injury. J Craniofac Surg. 2015;26:393–8.

17

Role of cationic drug-sensitive transport systems at the blood-cerebrospinal fluid barrier in *para*-tyramine elimination from rat brain

Shin-ichi Akanuma†, Yuhei Yamazaki†, Yoshiyuki Kubo and Ken-ichi Hosoya*

Abstract

Background: *para*-Tyramine (*p*-TA) is a biogenic amine which is involved in multiple neuronal signal transductions. Since the concentration of *p*-TA in dog cerebrospinal fluid (CSF) has been reported to be greater than that in plasma, it is proposed that clearance of cerebral *p*-TA is important for normal function. The purpose of this study was to examine the role of the blood–brain barrier and blood-cerebrospinal fluid barrier (BCSFB) in *p*-TA clearance from the brain.

Methods: In vivo [^{3}H]*p*-TA elimination from rat cerebral cortex and from CSF was examined after intracerebral and intracerebroventricular administration, respectively. To evaluate BCSFB-mediated *p*-TA transport, [^{3}H]*p*-TA uptake by isolated rat choroid plexus and conditionally immortalized rat choroid plexus epithelial cells, TR-CSFB3 cells, was performed.

Results: The half-life of [^{3}H]*p*-TA elimination from rat CSF was found to be 2.9 min, which is 62-fold faster than that from rat cerebral cortex. In addition, this [^{3}H]*p*-TA elimination from the CSF was significantly inhibited by co-injection of excess unlabeled *p*-TA. Thus, carrier-mediated *p*-TA transport process(es) are assumed to take part in *p*-TA elimination from the CSF. Since it is known that transporters at the BCSFB participate in compound elimination from the CSF, [^{3}H]*p*-TA transport in ex vivo and in vitro models of rat BCSFB was examined. The [^{3}H]*p*-TA uptake by isolated rat choroid plexus and TR-CSFB3 cells was time-dependent and was inhibited by unlabeled *p*-TA, indicating carrier-mediated *p*-TA transport at the BCSFB. The *p*-TA uptake by isolated choroid plexus and TR-CSFB3 cells was not reduced in the absence of extracellular Na^+ and Cl^-, and in the presence of substrates of typical organic cation transporters. However, this *p*-TA uptake was significantly inhibited by cationic drugs such as propranolol, imipramine, amantadine, verapamil, and pyrilamine. Moreover, *p*-TA uptake by TR-CSFB3 cells took place in an oppositely-directed H^+ gradient manner. Therefore, this suggested that *p*-TA transport at the BCSFB involves cationic drug-sensitive transport systems which are distinct from typical plasma membrane organic cation transporters.

Conclusion: Our study indicates that *p*-TA elimination from the CSF is greater than that from the cerebral cortex. Moreover, it is suggested that cationic drug-sensitive transport systems in the BCSFB participate in this *p*-TA elimination from the CSF.

Keywords: Biogenic amine, Blood-cerebrospinal fluid barrier, Blood–brain barrier, Choroid plexus, Clearance, Transporter, *para*-tyramine, *p*-TA

Background

para-Tyramine (*p*-TA) is one of the trace amines derived from tyrosine and present in fermented foods such as cheese [1, 2]. In the brain, *p*-TA acts as a neuromodulator, which supports neuronal actions by several neurotransmitters such as L-glutamate and norepinephrine [3, 4]. In addition, *p*-TA binds to trace amine-associated receptor 1, which is a G protein-coupled receptor and is a therapeutic target for schizophrenia [5]. It has been reported that, after activating the receptor, serotonergic and dopaminergic neuronal actions via serotonin receptor 1A and presynaptic

*Correspondence: hosoyak@pha.u-toyama.ac.jp
†Shin-ichi Akanuma and Yuhei Yamazaki contributed equally to this work
Department of Pharmaceutics, Graduate School of Medicine and Pharmaceutical Sciences, University of Toyama, 2630 Sugitani, Toyama 930-0194, Japan

dopamine D2 receptor, respectively, are reduced [6–10]. Since *p*-TA has a variety of roles in neuronal signal transduction, it is important to understand the homeostatic systems governing the *p*-TA concentration in the brain.

It is considered that the neural concentration of *p*-TA is maintained by a balance between production and clearance and there are reports that the activity of in vivo blood-to-brain transport of *p*-TA is low [11, 12]. In addition, Faraj et al. [13] have shown that the *p*-TA concentration in the cerebrospinal fluid (CSF) of dogs is approximately 2.6-fold lower than that in plasma although *p*-TA is produced in the brain. Therefore, it is conceivable that the *p*-TA clearance from the brain is relatively greater compared with that of *p*-TA production. Regarding the metabolic pathway of *p*-TA, it is known to be metabolized to octopamine and *p*-hydroxyphenylacetate via dopamine β-hydroxylase and monoamine oxidase, respectively [14]. Brain barriers are involved in the clearance of several neural compounds: the blood-brain barrier (BBB), which is formed by brain capillary endothelial cells, directly separates the brain from the circulating blood [15]. In addition, the cerebrospinal fluid (CSF) is separated from the circulating blood by the blood-CSF barrier (BCSFB) composed of choroid plexus epithelial cells [15]. Recent reports have shown that these barriers play a role in brain-to-blood transport of endogenous anionic and cationic compounds such as homovanillic acid and histamine [16, 17]. Therefore, there is a possibility that the BBB and/or BCSFB transport *p*-TA from the brain to the circulating blood and play a role in the *p*-TA clearance system in the brain.

These cells express a variety of plasma membrane transporters which contribute to compound transport across the BBB and BCSFB. In rat brain capillary endothelial cells, mRNAs of serotonin transporter [SERT/solute carrier (Slc) 6a4], organic cation transporter 1–3 (OCT1–3/Slc22a1–3), multidrug and toxin extrusion 1–2 (MATE1–2/Slc47a1–2), organic cation/carnitine transporter 1–2 (OCTN1–2/Slc22a4–5), and plasma membrane monoamine transporter (PMAT/Slc29a4) have been reported to be expressed [18, 19]. Among these transporters, it has been demonstrated that PMAT is involved in 1-methyl-4-phenylpyridinium (MPP^+) efflux transport at the BBB, at least in part [18]. Regarding the BCSFB, the mRNA expression of these transporters has also been reported [18]. In addition, our previous studies have shown that PMAT and OCT3 are involved in the elimination of histamine and creatinine, respectively, from rat CSF [16, 20]. Taking these reports into consideration, it is possible that several cationic transporters at these brain barriers take part in the clearance of cationic compounds from the brain. It is known that *p*-TA is a substrate of plasma membrane transporters, such as SERT, OCT3, PMAT, and dopamine transporter (DAT/Slc6a3) [21–24] and, thus, it is hypothesized that *p*-TA in the brain is eliminated via these plasma membrane transporters at the brain barriers.

To increase our knowledge of the homeostatic mechanism(s) governing the cerebral *p*-TA concentration, the purpose of this study was to examine the role of the brain barriers in *p*-TA clearance from the brain. To examine *p*-TA elimination across the BBB, we used an intracerebral microinjection technique. To evaluate BCSFB-mediated *p*-TA efflux transport, in vivo intracerebroventricular administration and ex vivo transport studies using isolated choroid plexus were performed. In addition, the properties of *p*-TA uptake were examined using an in vitro model of rat BCSFB, conditionally immortalized rat choroid plexus epithelial cells (TR-CSFB3 cells).

Methods

Reagents

Butanol, *n* [1-^{14}C] ([^{14}C]*n*-butanol, 2 mCi/mmol), mannitol, D-[1-^{14}C] ([^{14}C]D-mannitol, 55 mCi/mmol), and tyramine hydrochloride, [ring-3,5-^{3}H]-([^{3}H]*p*-TA, 50 Ci/mmol) were obtained from American Radiolabeled Chemicals (St. Louis, MO, USA). All other reagents were commercially available.

Animals

Wistar rats (male, 6-week-old, ~ 160 g) were purchased from Japan SLC (Hamamatsu, Japan) and maintained in a controlled environment.

In vivo technique for evaluating *p*-TA elimination across the BBB [25]

Anesthetized rats, obtained by intraperitoneally injecting pentobarbital sodium solution (50 mg/kg), were fixed in a stereotaxic apparatus (SR-5R; Narishige, Tokyo, Japan). Physiological buffer A (0.5 μL; 122 mM NaCl, 25 mM $NaHCO_3$, 10 mM D-glucose, and 10 mM 2-[4-(2-hydroxyethyl)-1-piperazinyl]ethansulfonic acid (HEPES)-NaOH, 3 mM KCl, 1.4 mM $CaCl_2$, 1.2 mM $MgSO_4$, 0.4 mM K_2HPO_4, pH 7.4) containing [^{3}H]*p*-TA (120 nCi/0.5 μL, 2.0 μM) and [^{14}C]D-mannitol (6.0 nCi/0.5 μL, 220 μM) was injected into the parietal cortex area two region of the brain over a period of 1 min. [^{14}C]D-Mannitol, a BBB-impermeable marker, was used to normalize the actual injection volume. At a designated time, each rat was decapitated, and the ipsilateral cerebrum was removed. During the procedure, the behavior of rats and abnormal morphology of the brain was monitored, and there was no apparent change in the anesthetized conditions and brain structure. The tissue was dissolved in 2 N NaOH (2 mL) at 55 °C for 3 h and then mixed with 10 mL Hionic-Fluor (PerkinElmer, Boston, MA, USA). The radioactivity was measured in a liquid scintillation counter equipped with an appropriate crossover correction for ^3H and ^{14}C (LSC-6101; Hitachi-Aloka Medical, Tokyo, Japan). The percentage of [^3H]*p*-TA remaining in the ipsilateral cerebrum (%) was obtained from Eq. 1.

$$\left[^3\mathrm{H}\right]p\text{-TA remaining in the ipsilateral cerebrum (\%)} = \frac{\left[^3\mathrm{H}\right]p\text{-TA}/\left[^{14}\mathrm{C}\right]D\text{-mannitol in the cerebrum}}{\left[^3\mathrm{H}\right]p\text{-TA}/\left[^{14}\mathrm{C}\right]D\text{-mannitol in the injectate}} \times 100 \quad (1)$$

Lateral ventricular micro-administration [26]

Rats were anesthetized by intraperitoneally injecting pentobarbital solution (50 mg/kg), and the head was fixed in the SR-5R (Narishige). A hole was drilled in the skull, 1.5 mm to the left and 0.5 mm posterior to the bregma, into which a needle was fixed as a cannula for injection. Then, 10 μL buffer A containing [^3H]*p*-TA (400 nCi) and [^{14}C]D-mannitol (5 nCi), with or without unlabeled 75 mM *p*-TA, was injected into the left lateral ventricle over a period of 20 s. At designated times, CSF (50 μL) was withdrawn by cisternal puncture and the levels of ^3H and ^{14}C in the CSF and injectate were measured in a liquid scintillation counter (LSC-6101; Hitachi-Aloka Medical). The rats exhibited no abnormal behavior during this technique.

The kinetic parameters of this study were obtained using a one-compartmental model (Eq. 2), where $C_{CSF}(t)$, $k_{e,CSF}$, and $V_{d,CSF}$ are the concentration in CSF at time t, the elimination rate constant from the CSF, and the distribution volume in the CSF, respectively, of either [^3H]*p*-TA or [^{14}C]D-mannitol.

$$C_{CSF}(t) = \frac{\text{Dose}}{V_{d,CSF}} \times \exp\left(-k_{e,CSF} \times t\right) \quad (2)$$

In addition, "$C_{CSF}(t)$/dose × 100" is the percentage of the residual concentration of the compound in the CSF normalized by the amount of injectate (% of dose/mL CSF). By multiplying k_e by $V_{d,CSF}$, the apparent elimination clearance from the CSF (CL_{CSF}) was obtained.

Transport study using choroid plexus [27]

Rats were decapitated and the choroid plexus in the lateral ventricles was isolated. After preincubation of the choroid plexus in buffer A for 1 min at 37 °C, a transport reaction was initiated by applying buffer A containing 1.0 μCi [^3H]*p*-TA and 0.05 μCi [^{14}C]*n*-butanol, a marker of water space in the choroid plexus [28], in the absence or presence of unlabeled compounds. Na^+-free or Cl^--free buffer was prepared by equimolar replacement of NaCl and $NaHCO_3$ with lithium chloride and potassium bicarbonate or that of NaCl, KCl, and $CaCl_2$ with sodium gluconate, potassium gluconate, and calcium gluconate, respectively. At designated times, the uptake buffer was removed, and the choroid plexus was solubilized by adding 3 N KOH. A liquid scintillation cocktail (Hionic-Fluor; PerkinElmer) was added to the sample, and ^3H- and ^{14}C-radioactivities were measured using an LSC-6101 (Hitachi-Aloka Medical).

Uptake by conditionally immortalized rat choroid plexus epithelial cells [29]

TR-CSFB3 cells were cultured at 33 °C as described previously. Kitazawa et al. have determined the apical localization of Na^+, K^+-ATPase from an immunocytochemical study using TR-CSFB3 cells cultured onto a glass slide [29]. It has also been demonstrated that the apical-to-cell uptake capacity of [^3H]L-proline in TR-CSFB3 cells seeded onto a Transwell® was similar to the uptake value of [^3H]L-proline in TR-CSFB3 cells seeded onto a culture plate [29]. The cells were plated onto collagen I-coated 24-well culture plates (BD-Biosciences, Franklin Lakes, NJ, USA) at a density of 1.0×10^5 cells/well and cultured for 2 days at 33 °C. At 37 °C, the cells were washed three times with buffer A and 200 μL [^3H]*p*-TA-containing buffer A (0.75 μCi/mL) was applied. Na^+- or Cl^--free buffer A was prepared as described in the previous section. To stop the uptake reaction, cells were rinsed three times with 4 °C buffer A. The cells were subsequently solubilized with 1 N NaOH solution and incubated at room temperature for 12 h. After neutralization with 1 N HCl, the cellular protein and [^3H]*p*-TA-derived radioactivity were determined using a detergent-compatible protein assay kit (BIO-RAD, Hercules, CA, USA) and liquid scintillation counting, respectively.

Data analyses

The distribution volume of [^3H]*p*-TA in isolated rat choroid plexus and TR-CSFB3 cells, namely the tissue/medium ratio and cell/medium ratio, respectively, was obtained from the following equations (Eqs. 3, 4).

$$\text{Tissue/medium ratio } (\mu\text{L}/\mu\text{L ChP}) = \frac{\left[^3\mathrm{H}\right]p\text{-TA in the choroid plexus (dpm/ChP)}/\left[^3\mathrm{H}\right]p\text{-TA concentration in buffer (dpm/}\mu\text{L)}}{\left[^{14}\mathrm{C}\right]n\text{-Butanol in the choroid plexus (dpm/ChP)}/\left[^{14}\mathrm{C}\right]n\text{-Butanol concentration in buffer (dpm/}\mu\text{L)}} \quad (3)$$

$$\text{Cell/medium ratio } (\mu\text{L/mg protein}) = \frac{\text{Intracellular } [^3\text{H}]p\text{-TA per cellular protein amount (dpm/mg protein)}}{[^3\text{H}]p\text{-TA concentration in buffer (dpm/}\mu\text{L)}} \quad (4)$$

The initial uptake clearance of [^{3}H]p-TA by isolated rat choroid plexus and TR-CSFB3 cells was calculated using Eqs. 5 and 6, respectively.

$$\begin{aligned}&\text{Tissue/medium ratio } (\mu\text{L}/\mu\text{L ChP})\\&\quad = \text{Initial uptake clearance } (\mu\text{L}/(\text{min } \mu\text{L ChP}))\\&\quad\times \text{Time (min)} + \text{Initial distribution volume}\\&\quad(\mu\text{L}/\mu\text{L ChP})\end{aligned} \quad (5)$$

$$\begin{aligned}&\text{Cell/medium ratio}(\mu\text{L/mg protein})\\&\quad = \text{Initial uptake clearance}\\&\quad(\mu\text{L}/(\text{min mg protein})) \times \text{Time (min)}\\&\quad + \text{Initial distribution volume}\\&\quad(\mu\text{L/mg protein})\end{aligned} \quad (6)$$

The equation was fitted using the nonlinear least-squares regression analysis program, MULTI [30]. To examine the initial uptake process, a linear correlation analysis was performed. The coefficient of determination (r^2) of [^{3}H]p-TA uptake by isolated rat choroid plexus from 0.25 min to 1.0 min was found to be 0.981, which was greater than that from 0.25 min to 2.0 min ($r^2 = 0.822$). This suggested that the initial [^{3}H]p-TA uptake by isolated rat choroid plexus is reflected in the data up to 1 min. Regarding the uptake of [^{3}H]p-TA by TR-CSFB3 cells, the r^2 of the [^{3}H]p-TA uptake from 0.25 min to 2.0 min was calculated as 0.989, which is similar to that of [^{3}H]p-TA uptake by isolated rat choroid plexus from 0.25 min to 1.0 min and is close to 1. This result suggests that the cell/medium ratio at all time points reflects the initial [^{3}H]p-TA uptake process.

The kinetic parameters for p-TA uptake by TR-CSFB3 cells were obtained from Eq. 7:

$$V = (V_{\max} \times [\text{S}])/(K_{\text{m}} + [\text{S}]) + K_{\text{d}} \times [\text{S}] \quad (7)$$

where V is the uptake rate of p-TA, [S] is the p-TA concentration in buffer, K_m is the Michaelis–Menten constant, and K_d is the non-saturable transport clearance. The equation was fitted using the MULTI program [30]. The kinetic parameters are presented as the mean ± standard deviation (S.D.). Other data represent the mean ± standard error of the mean (S.E.M.). The statistical significance of differences between the means was determined using the unpaired Student's t test for two groups and one-way analysis of variance followed by Dunnett's test for more than three groups.

Results

Evaluation of p-TA elimination from rat cerebral cortex

The time-course of the percentage [^{3}H]p-TA remaining in rat ipsilateral cerebrum at 5, 10, 20, and 40 min after microadministration into the parietal cortex area 2 is shown in Fig. 1a. There was no significant difference between the values at 5, 10, 20, and 40 min ($p = 0.143$), although a tendency for a time-dependent decrease was observed. As a reference value, the half-life ($t_{1/2}$) of the percentage of cerebral [^{3}H]p-TA remaining after microinjection into the cerebral cortex was calculated to be 178 ± 68 min.

In vivo p-TA elimination from rat CSF

Figure 1b shows the time profile of "C_{CSF}(t)/dose × 100" values of [^{3}H]p-TA and [^{14}C]D-mannitol after intracerebroventricular injection. The residual concentration in CSF of [^{3}H]p-TA at 1.0, 1.5, and 2.0 min was significantly lower than that of [^{14}C]D-mannitol. [^{3}H]p-TA was eliminated from the CSF with a $t_{1/2}$ of 2.85 ± 0.83 min, which is 3.0-fold faster than the $t_{1/2}$ of [^{14}C]D-mannitol. From the $V_{d,CSF}$ and $k_{e,CSF}$ values of [^{3}H]p-TA ($V_{d,CSF}$, 159 ± 16 μL/rat; $k_{e,CSF}$, $2.43 \times 10^{-1} \pm 0.72 \times 10^{-1}$ min^{-1}), the CL_{CSF} of [^{3}H]p-TA was found to be 38.6 ± 12.0 μL/rat. The kinetic parameters for [^{14}C]D-mannitol, $V_{d,CSF}$, $k_{e,CSF}$, and CL_{CSF}, were calculated to be 135 ± 11 μL/rat, $8.07 \times 10^{-2} \pm 6.09 \times 10^{-2}$ min^{-1}, and 10.9 ± 8.3 μL/rat, respectively. To examine the possible contribution of carrier-mediated p-TA elimination system(s) from the CSF, the effect of unlabeled excess p-TA on the concentration ratio of [^{3}H]p-TA and [^{14}C]D-mannitol was examined. The [^{3}H]p-TA/[^{14}C]D-mannitol residual concentration ratio at 2 min was significantly (1.1-fold) increased by co-administration of 75 mM unlabeled p-TA into the rat cerebroventricle compared with that in the control (Fig. 1c), indicating that [^{3}H]p-TA elimination from rat CSF was inhibited by excess unlabeled p-TA.

[^{3}H]p-TA uptake by isolated rat choroid plexus

In order to examine whether p-TA was eliminated from the CSF across the BCSFB, a [^{3}H]p-TA transport study using isolated rat choroid plexus was performed. [^{3}H]p-TA was time-dependently taken up into the isolated rat choroid plexus with an initial uptake rate and an initial distribution volume of 1.19 ± 0.31 μL/(min μL

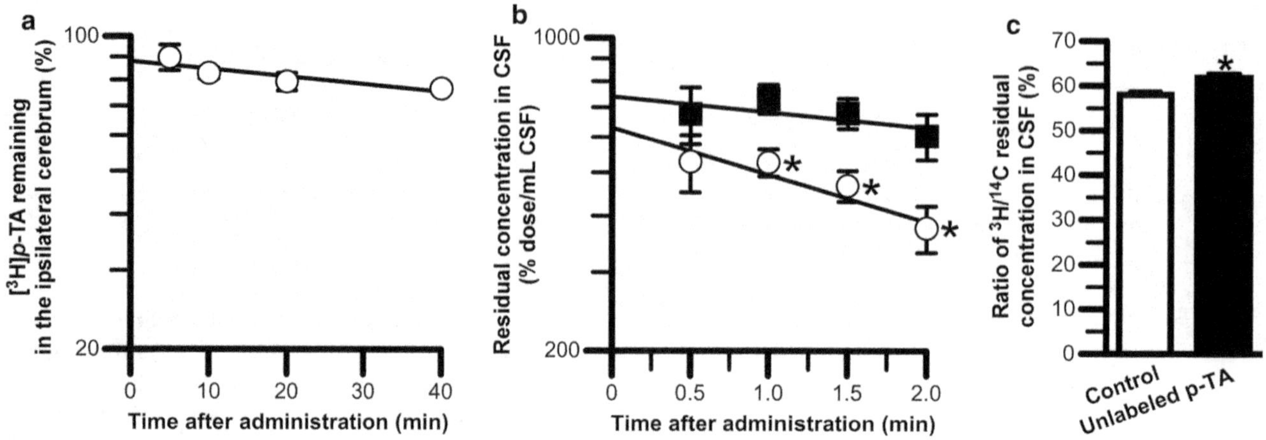

Fig. 1 In vivo analyses of *p*-TA elimination from rat brain or cerebrospinal fluid. **a** Time profile of [^{3}H]*p*-TA remaining in the ipsilateral cerebrum after injection into rat cerebral cortex. A mixture of [^{3}H]*p*-TA (120 nCi) and [^{14}C]D-mannitol (6 nCi) dissolved in 0.5 μL buffer A was injected. The solid line was obtained by MULTI analysis. Each point represents the mean ± S.E.M. ($n = 3$). **b** Time profile of the residual CSF concentration (% dose × 100) of [^{3}H]*p*-TA (open circles) and [^{14}C]D-mannitol (closed squares) after administration into rat lateral ventricles and sampled from the cisterna magna. Buffer A containing [^{3}H]*p*-TA (400 nCi/10 μL) and [^{14}C]D-mannitol (5 nCi/10 μL) was injected into rat lateral ventricles. The solid line was obtained by MULTI analysis. Each point represents the mean ± S.E.M. ($n = 3$–4). *$p < 0.05$, significantly different from the value for [^{14}C]D-mannitol. **c** Increase in the residual CSF concentration of [^{3}H]*p*-TA at 2 min normalized to that of [^{14}C]D-mannitol by simultaneous administration of unlabeled 75 mM *p*-TA. Each column represents the mean ± S.E.M. ($n = 3$–5). *$p < 0.05$, significantly different from the control

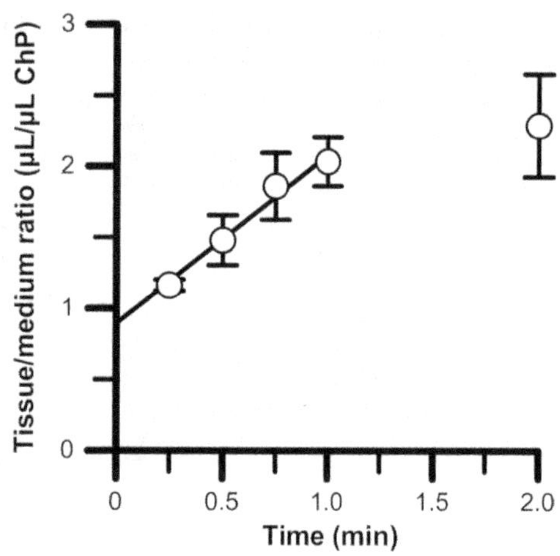

Fig. 2 Time-dependent uptake of [^{3}H]*p*-TA by isolated rat choroid plexus. The choroid plexus was incubated with [^{3}H]*p*-TA (1 μCi/sample, 1 μM) and [^{14}C]*n*-butanol (0.05 μCi/sample, 250 nM) at 37 °C. The solid line was obtained by MULTI analysis. Each point represents the mean ± S.E.M. ($n = 3$–6)

ChP) and 0.895 ± 0.223 μL/μL ChP, respectively (Fig. 2). As shown in Table 1, 10 mM unlabeled *p*-TA significantly inhibited this [^{3}H]*p*-TA uptake by 34%. The absence of extracellular Na^+ or Cl^- did not significantly affect the [^{3}H]*p*-TA uptake by isolated rat choroid plexus (Table 1), indicating that Na^+ and/or Cl^--cotransport systems are not involved in *p*-TA uptake by the rat choroid plexus. To examine *p*-TA transport mechanism(s) on the choroid plexus, the compound/drug-sensitivities to [^{3}H]*p*-TA uptake were examined (Table 1). Several cationic drugs, such as propranolol, pyrilamine, amantadine, imipramine, and verapamil, significantly inhibited [^{3}H]*p*-TA uptake by the isolated rat choroid plexus by more than 29%. Among typical SLC transporter substrates/inhibitors, choline exhibited 28% inhibition of [^{3}H]*p*-TA uptake. However, [^{3}H]*p*-TA uptake by the isolated rat choroid plexus was not significantly altered in the presence of serotonin (a substrate of SERT), MPP^+ (a typical substrate of OCT and PMAT), tetraethylammonium (TEA; a typical substrate of OCT, OCTN, and MATE), and *p*-aminohippurate (PAH; a typical substrate of organic anion transporter, OAT).

Characteristics of [^{3}H]*p*-TA uptake by TR-CSFB3 cells

To clarify the characteristics of *p*-TA transport at the BCSFB, a [^{3}H]*p*-TA transport study using an in vitro model of rat BCSFB, TR-CSFB3 cells, was performed. TR-CSFB3 cells exhibited time-dependent [^{3}H]*p*-TA uptake with an initial uptake rate and an initial distribution volume of 2.93 ± 0.32 μL/(min mg protein) and 2.25 ± 0.24 μL/mg protein (Fig. 3a, open circles). At 2 min, [^{3}H]*p*-TA uptake by TR-CSFB3 cells at 4 °C was significantly reduced by 86% (Fig. 3a, closed square). In addition, concentration-dependent *p*-TA uptake by TR-CSFB3 cells consisted of saturable and non-saturable components with apparent K_m, V_{max} and K_d values of 3.48 ± 0.83 mM, 7.26 ± 1.61 nmol/(min mg protein), and $9.78 \times 10^{-1} \pm 0.66 \times 10^{-1}$ μL/(min mg protein), respectively (Fig. 3b). Moreover, 10 mM *p*-TA significantly

Table 1 Effect of Na^+- or Cl^--replacement, and co-presence of compounds on [^{3}H]*p*-TA uptake by isolated rat choroid plexus

Compounds	Concentration (mM)	Percentage of control
Na^+/Cl^--replacement		
Control		100 ± 5
Na^+-free		93.6 ± 3.9
Cl^--free		98.4 ± 5.8
Co-presence of compounds		
Control		100 ± 9
p-TA	10	65.9 ± 4.6**
Propranolol	10	61.0 ± 5.4**
Pyrilamine	10	61.2 ± 0.8**
Amantadine	10	61.4 ± 0.6**
Imipramine	1	67.4 ± 1.1*
Verapamil	1	70.8 ± 1.1*
Choline	10	72.3 ± 4.6*
Serotonin	10	79.6 ± 2.2
MPP^+	10	84.7 ± 6.3
TEA	10	93.0 ± 3.1
PAH	10	95.4 ± 5.1

[^{3}H]*p*-TA uptake by isolated rat choroid plexus (1 μCi/sample) was performed at 37 °C for 45 s in the absence (control) or presence of Na^+ and Cl^- without (control) or with unlabeled compounds. Each value represents the mean ± S.E.M. ($n = 3$–8)

MPP^+ 1-methyl-4-phenylpyridinium, *PAH* *p*-aminohippurate, *TEA* tetraethylammonium, *p-TA para*-tyramine

*$p < 0.05$ and **$p < 0.01$, significantly different from control

inhibited the [^{3}H]*p*-TA uptake by 48% (Table 2). [^{3}H]*p*-TA uptake by TR-CSFB3 cells was significantly inhibited by more than 30% in the presence of several kinds of cationic drugs/compounds, such as propranolol, imipramine, amantadine, nicotine, desipramine, pyrilamine, and verapamil. In contrast, this [^{3}H]*p*-TA uptake was not significantly altered by L-carnitine (a typical substrate of OCTN), pyrimethamine (a substrate of MATE), norepinephrine (a substrate of norepinephrine transporter), PAH, serotonin, and cimetidine (a substrate of OCT and MATE). In addition, the [^{3}H]*p*-TA uptake by TR-CSFB3 cells was significantly increased, but not decreased, by the co-presence of tyrosine (a precursor of *p*-TA), choline (a substrate of OCT), MPP^+, and TEA (Table 2).

The extracellular inorganic anion sensitivity of [^{3}H]*p*-TA uptake by TR-CSFB3 cells was examined and was found not to be altered in the absence of extracellular Cl^-, whereas it was significantly increased, but not decreased, in the absence of extracellular Na^+ (Table 2). This result indicates that Na^+- and Cl^--cotransporters are not involved in *p*-TA transport into the choroid plexus. The [^{3}H]*p*-TA uptake by TR-CSFB3 cells was significantly reduced by 50% at an extracellular pH of 6.0 (Fig. 4a, closed column), and increased 1.8-fold at an extracellular pH of 8.4 (Fig. 4a, hatched column). In order to examine the intracellular pH effect, TR-CSFB3 cells were treated with ammonium chloride, since the intracellular pH is increased by treatment with ammonium

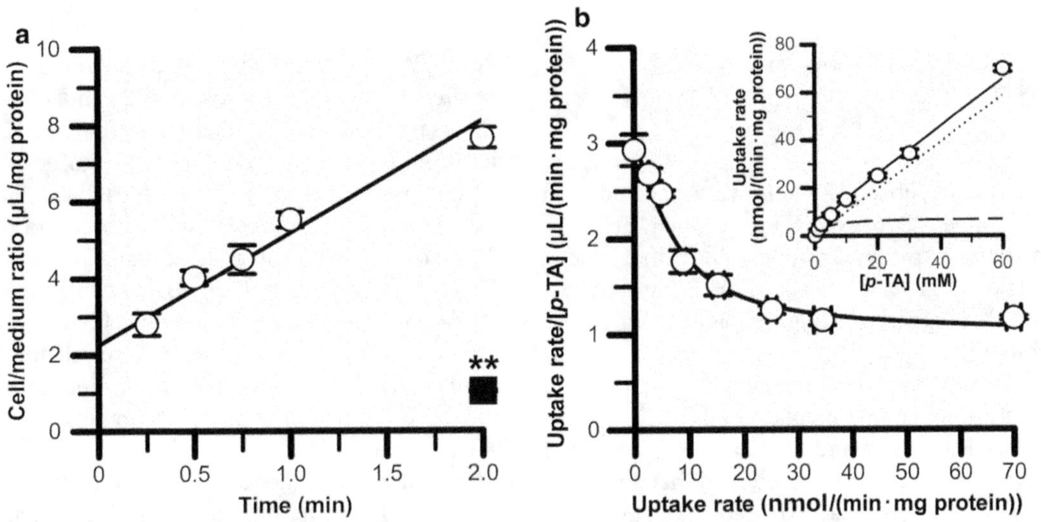

Fig. 3 Time-, temperature-, and concentration-dependence of [^{3}H]*p*-TA uptake by TR-CSFB3 cells. **a** [^{3}H]*p*-TA uptake (0.15 μCi/well, 19 nM) was measured at 37 °C (open circles) and 4 °C (closed square) for indicated times. The solid line was obtained by MULTI analysis. Each point represents the mean ± S.E.M. ($n = 3$). **$p < 0.01$, significantly different from [^{3}H]*p*-TA uptake at 37 °C for 2 min. **b** *p*-TA uptake, over the concentration range 20 nM–60 mM, was measured at 37 °C for 2 min. The data were subjected to Eadie–Scatchard analysis in addition to Michaelis–Menten kinetics (inset). The solid, dashed, and dotted lines, which were fitted by the MULTI program, represent overall, saturable, and non-saturable transport, respectively. Each point represents the mean ± S.E.M. ($n = 3$)

Table 2 Effect of Na^+- or Cl^--replacement, and co-presence of compounds on [^{3}H]*p*-TA uptake by TR-CSFB3 cells

Compounds	Concentration (mM)	Percentage of control
Na^+/Cl^--replacement		
Control		100 ± 3
Na^+-free		153 ± 8**
Cl^--free		103 ± 4
Co-presence of compounds		
Control		100 ± 1
p-TA	10	51.8 ± 3.7**
Propranolol	10	29.0 ± 4.2**
Imipramine	10	31.5 ± 2.9**
Amantadine	10	45.3 ± 2.4**
Nicotine	10	52.2 ± 3.8**
Desipramine	10	63.4 ± 1.9**
Pyrilamine	10	65.4 ± 10.8**
Verapamil	3.0	69.6 ± 6.7*
L-Carnitine	10	75.0 ± 5.7
Norepinephrine	10	96.1 ± 7.3
PAH	10	110 ± 6
Serotonin	10	114 ± 5
Cimetidine	10	115 ± 2
Tyrosine	10	140 ± 17**
Choline	10	150 ± 6**
MPP^+	10	155 ± 19**
TEA	10	168 ± 13**
Control (1% DMSO)		100 ± 5
Pyrimethamine (1% DMSO)	0.2	91.0 ± 7.3

[^{3}H]*p*-TA uptake by TR-CSFB3 cells (0.15 μCi/well) was performed at 37 °C for 2 min in the absence (control) or presence of Na^+ and Cl^- without (control) or with unlabeled compounds. Each value represents the mean ± S.E.M. ($n = 3$)

DMSO dimethyl sulfoxide, *MPP^+* 1-methyl-4-phenylpyridinium, *PAH* p-aminohippurate, *TEA* tetraethylammonium, *p-TA para*-tyramine

*$p < 0.05$ and **$p < 0.01$, significantly different from control

chloride (acute), and subsequent removal of ammonium chloride (pretreated) reduces the intracellular pH [31]. An increase in the intracellular pH significantly reduced [^{3}H]*p*-TA uptake by TR-CSFB3 cells at pH 7.4 and pH 8.4 by 37% and 42%, respectively (Fig. 4b, acute and closed column), compared with respective untreated conditions (Fig. 4b, untreated and open column). In contrast, a reduction in intracellular pH increased [^{3}H]*p*-TA uptake by TR-CSFB3 cells to 126% and 191% at pH 7.4 and pH 8.4, respectively (Fig. 4b, pretreated and hatched column), relative to the respective untreated conditions.

Discussion

In this study, *p*-TA elimination from the brain and CSF was investigated in rats (Fig. 1). To clarify the involvement of the BCSFB in *p*-TA elimination from the CSF, a *p*-TA transport study using isolated rat choroid plexus, which forms the BCSFB, was carried out (Fig. 2 and Table 1). Since carrier-mediated transport properties were observed in this study using rat choroid plexus, *p*-TA transport characteristics were examined in in vitro rat BCSFB model cells (Figs. 3, 4, and Table 2).

The percentage of [^{3}H]*p*-TA remaining in the ipsilateral cerebrum tended to be reduced in a time-dependent manner (Fig. 1a), although there was no significant difference between the values at examined time points. It is known that *p*-TA is converted via enzymes in neural cells to several metabolites, such as octopamine [14]. Thus, it is suggested that *p*-TA and its metabolites are eliminated to a degree from the brain across the BBB. However, this $t_{1/2}$, as a reference record (178 min), was 62-fold longer than that of the residual concentration of [^{3}H]*p*-TA in the CSF (Fig. 1b). These results show that *p*-TA elimination from the CSF makes a major contribution to cerebral *p*-TA clearance relative to that from the brain parenchyma or interstitial fluid. In addition, the CL_{CSF} for [^{3}H]*p*-TA was 3.5-fold higher than that of [^{14}C]D-mannitol, a marker compound for bulk flow of CSF [26, 32]. Taking the inhibitory effect of *p*-TA elimination from the CSF by excess unlabeled *p*-TA (Fig. 1c) into consideration, this suggests that carrier-mediated transport system(s), which are distinct from CSF bulk flow, are involved in *p*-TA elimination from the CSF.

After intracerebroventricular administration, it is possible that [^{3}H]*p*-TA is distributed to the brain parenchyma and/or taken up into ependymal cells and choroid plexus epithelial cells [33]. It is known that transporters at the BCSFB participate in the elimination of several compounds from the CSF [15]. We have shown that [^{3}H]*p*-TA was time-dependently taken up into ex vivo isolated rat choroid plexus (Fig. 2) and in vitro choroid plexus epithelial cells, which form the BCSFB (Fig. 3). In addition, this [^{3}H]*p*-TA uptake was significantly inhibited by unlabeled 10 mM *p*-TA (Tables 1, 2). Since the initial distribution volume of *p*-TA was found to be 159 μL (Fig. 1b), the concentration in rat CSF of unlabeled *p*-TA after a 10 μL intracerebroventricular microinjection of 75 mM unlabeled *p*-TA was calculated to be 4.7 mM, which is similar to that in the in vitro self-inhibition studies. Therefore, it is suggested that some transport systems at the BCSFB take part in carrier-mediated elimination of *p*-TA from the CSF.

Since the apical membrane of the choroid plexus faces the [^{3}H]*p*-TA-containing buffer in the uptake study using isolated choroid plexus, it appears that the characteristics of [^{3}H]*p*-TA uptake by rat choroid plexus reflects the CSF-to-cell transport direction at the BCSFB. In this study, the choroid plexus from the lateral ventricle was used in the *p*-TA transport study. Although there are

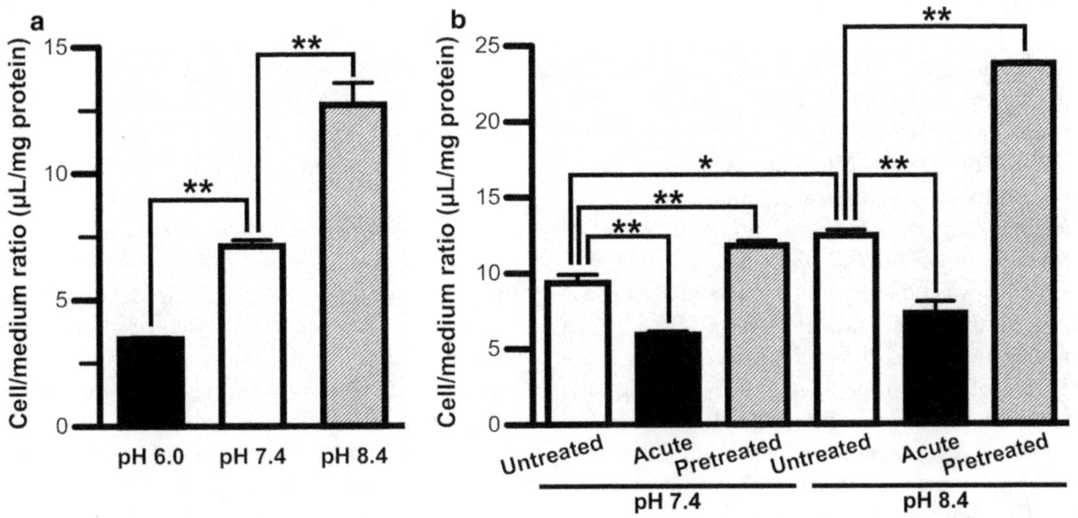

Fig. 4 Extra- and intra-cellular pH dependence of [^{3}H]*p*-TA uptake by TR-CSFB3 cells. **a** [^{3}H]*p*-TA uptake (0.15 μCi/well) at pH 6.0, pH 7.4, and pH 8.4 was tested at 37 °C for 2 min. Each column represents the mean ± S.E.M. ($n = 3$). **$p < 0.01$, significant difference between the groups. **b** TR-CSFB3 cells were preincubated with buffer A at pH 7.4 or pH 8.4 in the absence (untreated and acute) or presence (pretreated) of 30 mM ammonium chloride for 20 min. After removal of the buffer, the cells were incubated with [^{3}H]*p*-TA (0.15 μCi/well) at pH 7.4 or pH 8.4 in the absence (untreated and pretreated) or presence (acute) of 30 mM ammonium chloride at 37 °C for 2 min. Each column represents the mean ± SEM ($n = 3$–6). *$p < 0.05$ and **$p < 0.01$, significant difference between the groups

known regional differences in physiological and transport functions between the choroid plexuses from the lateral, third, and fourth ventricles [34, 35], Ogawa et al. [26] have reported that the in vivo uptake rate which is extrapolated from in vitro benzylpenicillin transport in rat choroid plexus from the lateral ventricle, is in good agreement with that of saturable in vivo elimination of benzylpenicillin from the CSF. *p*-TA transport across the apical membrane of the isolated rat choroid plexus was found to be 7.14 μL/(min rat) since the total volume of rat choroid plexus has been reported to be 6 μL (7.14 μL/(min rat) = 1.19 μL/μL ChP × 6 μL/rat) [26]. Regarding the polarity of TR-CSFB3 cells after seeding onto a culture plate and glass slide, it has been reported that membrane protein localization onto the plasma membrane of choroid plexus epithelial cells is mostly retained [29]. As the surface area of TR-CSFB3 cells and rat lateral ventricle choroid plexus epithelium has been reported to be 20 cm^2/mg protein [18] and 75 cm^2/rat [36], respectively, the initial *p*-TA uptake clearance estimated from the uptake study using TR-CSFB3 cells was calculated to be 11.0 μL/(min rat) (= 2.93 μL/(min mg protein) ÷ 20 cm^2/mg protein × 75 cm^2/rat). This estimated initial *p*-TA uptake clearance from the transport study using TR-CSFB3 cells is consistent with that using isolated rat choroid plexus. Taking these findings into consideration, there is a high possibility that the characteristics of *p*-TA uptake by TR-CSFB3 cells reflect the *p*-TA transport properties of the apical membrane of the BCSFB.

These BCSFB-mediated [^{3}H]*p*-TA uptake clearance values obtained from the uptake studies of isolated rat choroid plexus (7.14 μL/(min rat) and TR-CSFB3 cells (11.0 μL/(min rat)) were 18.5 and 28.5% of the in vivo total [^{3}H]*p*-TA elimination clearance from rat CSF (38.6 μL/(min rat), Fig. 1b). As the elimination clearance of [^{14}C]D-mannitol from rat CSF was found to be 10.9 μL (Fig. 1b), 28.2% of the total [^{3}H]*p*-TA clearance would reflect the CSF bulk flow and diffusion to the brain parenchyma. As the other pathways for *p*-TA elimination from the CSF, the remainder of which corresponds to (43.3–53.5%), the incorporation of *p*-TA into the neural cells facing the cerebroventricles, including the ependymal cells, is a possibility. Further analysis to check the radioactivities in choroid plexus and neural cells surrounding the cerebroventricle could help these cells contribute to *p*-TA elimination from the CSF. Nevertheless, it is considered that the BCSFB is involved in the carrier-mediated *p*-TA elimination from the CSF, at least in part, since an inhibitory effect of unlabeled excess *p*-TA on [^{3}H]*p*-TA uptake by isolated rat choroid plexus (Table 1) and TR-CSFB3 cells (Table 2) was observed.

p-TA uptake by TR-CSFB3 cells exhibited saturable and non-saturable kinetics (Fig. 3b). The clearance of the saturable process of *p*-TA transport (V_{max}/K_m) was found to be 2.09 μL/(min mg protein), which is 2.1-fold higher than that of the non-saturable process [K_d, 0.978 μL/(min mg protein)]. This result indicates that the transporter-mediated process makes a major contribution to apical p-TA transport at the BCSFB. It has been reported that human OCT3 and PMAT accept p-TA as a substrate with a K_m of 0.281 and 283 μM, respectively [21, 22]. However, the K_m value of p-TA uptake by TR-CSFB3 cells (3.48 mM) was inconsistent with these values. mRNA expression of OCT1–2, OCTN1–2, and MATE in addition to OCT3 and PMAT as typical organic cation transporters has been reported [18] but no attenuation of [^{3}H]p-TA transport into TR-CSFB3 cells and/or isolated rat choroid plexus was observed in the presence of these transporter inhibitors, such as MPP^+, TEA, L-carnitine, pyrimethamine, and cimetidine (Tables 1, 2). In summary, these lines of evidence suggest that typical organic cation transporters which are expressed in the BCSFB are not involved in p-TA transport across the BCSFB. Other plasma membrane transporters for p-TA are known: i.e. several Na^+-, Cl^--dependent Slc molecules, such as DAT and SERT. However, in the uptake study using isolated rat choroid plexus and TR-CSFB3 cells, [^{3}H]p-TA uptake was not attenuated in the absence of extracellular Na^+ and Cl^- (Tables 1, 2). The K_m value of human DAT- and SERT-mediated p-TA transport has been reported to be 1.7 and 52.7 μM, respectively [23, 24], which is different from the K_m value obtained for p-TA uptake by TR-CSFB3 cells. In addition, [^{3}H]p-TA uptake by both isolated rat choroid plexus and TR-CSFB3 cells was not significantly changed in the presence of serotonin, a substrate of SERT (Tables 1, 2). Consequently, we conclude that typical organic cation transporters and the Na^+- and Cl^--dependent Slc family do not play a role in apical p-TA transport at the BCSFB.

We showed that p-TA transport into TR-CSFB3 cells exhibited an oppositely-directed H^+-gradient (Fig. 4). Cationic drug transport system(s) in several tissues and blood-central nervous system barriers have been proposed [37–43]. It has been reported that human intestinal epithelial cells transport several cationic drugs, such as bisoprolol and metoprolol, in an extracellular pH-dependent manner [37, 38]. Our previous reports have shown that nicotine is taken up into rat hepatocytes and lung via unidentified transport system(s) which recognize several cationic drugs and exhibit a H^+/substrate antiport behavior [39, 40]. Moreover, it has been shown that H^+/substrate antiport system(s) involve blood-to-brain transport across the BBB of cationic compounds and drugs, such as pyrilamine, oxycodone, and nicotine, although the molecular identification of the system(s) has not been reported [41–43]. p-TA uptake by isolated rat choroid plexus (Table 1) and TR-CSFB3 cells (Table 2) was significantly inhibited by cationic drugs which also inhibited the uptake of pyrilamine, oxycodone, and nicotine by an in vitro BBB model cell line [41, 42]. Thus, it is suggested that cationic drug-sensitive transport system(s), similar to the systems in the BBB, are present on the apical membrane of the BCSFB and are involved in p-TA elimination across the BCSFB from the CSF.

In patients with Parkinson's disease and depression, monoamine oxidase inhibitors, such as selegiline, are regularly prescribed. It is widely known that patients who take p-TA-enriched foods exhibit neural side-effects such as migraine when receiving pharmacotherapy with monoamine oxidase inhibitors [44, 45]. As one reason for the above side-effects, the activation of noradrenergic signal transduction has been proposed by monoamine oxidase inhibition and, thus, an increase in the neural p-TA concentration. Many monoamine oxidase inhibitors, including selegiline, are cationic and lipophilic drugs. This study has demonstrated that p-TA elimination across the BCSFB from the CSF is inhibited by cationic and lipophilic compounds (Tables 1, 2). Thus, it is possible that the administration of cationic drugs causes an increase in p-TA in the brain via the inhibition of BCSFB-mediated p-TA elimination and exacerbates neuronal actions induced by excess p-TA. Further studies on the identification of p-TA transport molecule(s) which also recognize cationic drugs are needed, since this could help improve the pharmacotherapy of these patients in addition to increasing our understanding of the role of the BCSFB in homeostasis of p-TA levels in the brain. Moreover, it is considered that our findings about the in vitro characteristics of tyramine transport at the BCSFB (Tables 1, 2), such as inhibition by cationic drugs and promotion by the presence of several compounds (i.e., tyrosine, choline, MPP^+, and TEA), are helpful for identifying the responsible molecule(s) for tyramine transport at the BCSFB.

Conclusion

Our study demonstrates the greater contribution of p-TA elimination from the CSF to the clearance of p-TA from the brain parenchyma in vivo. From the transport studies using isolated choroid plexus and TR-CSFB3 cells, p-TA efflux transport at the BCSFB was shown to involve cationic drug-sensitive transport systems. These are distinct from typical plasma membrane organic cation transporters in the BCSFB. This study provides a new view of the role of the BCSFB in homeostasis of trace amines in the brain, including p-TA.

Abbreviations

BBB: blood–brain barrier; BCSFB: blood-cerebrospinal fluid barrier; $C_{CSF}(t)$: concentration in CSF at time t; CSF: cerebrospinal fluid; DAT: dopamine transporter; DMSO: dimethyl sulfoxide; HEPES: 2-[4-(2-hydroxyethyl)-1-piperazinyl] ethansulfonic acid; $k_{e,CSF}$: elimination rate constant from the CSF; K_d: clearance of non-saturable transport; K_m: Michaelis–Menten constant; MATE: multidrug and toxin extrusion; MPP^+: 1-phenyl-4-phenylpyridinium; OCT: organic cation transporter; OCTN: organic cation/carnitine transporter; PMAT: plasma membrane monoamine transporter; p-TA: *para*-tyramine; [S]: the p-TA concentration in buffer; S.D.: standard deviation; S.E.M.: standard error of the mean; SERT:

serotonin transporter; Slc: solute carrier; TR-CSFB: conditionally immortalized rat choroid plexus epithelial cells; *V*: uptake rate; $V_{d,CSF}$: distribution volume in the CSF.

Authors' contributions
SA contributed to the design of this study, carried out the in vivo experiments, performed data collection and analysis, and drafted the manuscript. YY carried out most of the experiments. YK participated in the coordination of the study. KH took part in writing the manuscript. All authors read and approved the final manuscript.

Acknowledgements
The authors thank Dr. Tetsuya Terasaki (Tohoku University, Sendai, Japan) for kindly supplying TR-CSFB3 cells and Mr. Hirokazu Shimada (University of Toyama, Toyama, Japan) for help with the in vitro methods used in this study.

Competing interests
The authors declare that they have no competing interests.

Funding
This research was supported by the Japan Society for the Promotion of Science (JSPS) KAKENHI [Grant Numbers JP16H05110 and JP16K08365] and the Research Grant from the Smoking Research Foundation.

References
1. Borkum JM. Migraine triggers and oxidative stress: a narrative review and synthesis. Headache. 2016;56:12–35.
2. Ledonne A, Berretta N, Davoli A, Rizzo GR, Bernardi G, Mercuri NB. Electrophysiological effects of trace amines on mesencephalic dopaminergic neurons. Front Syst Neurosci. 2011;5:56.
3. Youdim MB, Weinstock M. Therapeutic applications of selective and non-selective inhibitors of monoamine oxidase A and B that do not cause significant tyramine potentiation. Neurotoxicology. 2004;25:243–50.
4. Revel FG, Moreau JL, Gainetdinov RR, Bradaia A, Sotnikova TD, Mory R, et al. TAAR1 activation modulates monoaminergic neurotransmission, preventing hyperdopaminergic and hypoglutamatergic activity. Proc Natl Acad Sci USA. 2011;108:8485–90.
5. Revel FG, Moreau JL, Pouzet B, Mory R, Bradaia A, Buchy D, et al. A new perspective for schizophrenia: TAAR1 agonists reveal antipsychotic- and antidepressant-like activity, improve cognition and control body weight. Mol Psychiatry. 2013;18:543–56.
6. Wolinsky TD, Swanson CJ, Smith KE, Zhong H, Borowsky B, Seeman P, et al. The Trace Amine 1 receptor knockout mouse: an animal model with relevance to schizophrenia. Genes Brain Behav. 2007;6:628–39.
7. Lindemann L, Meyer CA, Jeanneau K, Bradaia A, Ozmen L, Bluethmann H, et al. Trace amine-associated receptor 1 modulates dopaminergic activity. J Pharmacol Exp Ther. 2008;324:948–56.
8. Xie Z, Miller GM. Beta-phenylethylamine alters monoamine transporter function via trace amine-associated receptor 1: implication for modulatory roles of trace amines in brain. J Pharmacol Exp Ther. 2008;325:617–28.
9. Bradaia A, Trube G, Stalder H, Norcross RD, Ozmen L, Wettstein JG, et al. The selective antagonist EPPTB reveals TAAR1-mediated regulatory mechanisms in dopaminergic neurons of the mesolimbic system. Proc Natl Acad Sci USA. 2009;106:20081–6.
10. Leo D, Mus L, Espinoza S, Hoener MC, Sotnikova TD, Gainetdinov RR. Taar1-mediated modulation of presynaptic dopaminergic neurotransmission: role of D2 dopamine autoreceptors. Neuropharmacology. 2014;81:283–91.
11. Oldendorf WH. Brain uptake of radiolabeled amino acids, amines, and hexoses after arterial injection. Am J Physiol. 1971;221:1629–39.
12. James JH, Escourrou J, Fischer JE. Blood-brain neutral amino acid transport activity is increased after portacaval anastomosis. Science. 1978;200:1395–7.
13. Faraj BA, Camp VM, Ansley JD, Scott J, Ali FM, Malveaux EJ. Evidence for central hypertyraminemia in hepatic encephalopathy. J Clin Invest. 1981;67:395–402.
14. Berry MD. Mammalian central nervous system trace amines. Pharmacologic amphetamines, physiologic neuromodulators. J Neurochem. 2004;90:257–71.
15. Ohtsuki S, Terasaki T. Contribution of carrier-mediated transport systems to the blood–brain barrier as a supporting and protecting interface for the brain; importance for CNS drug discovery and development. Pharm Res. 2007;24:1745–58.
16. Usui T, Nakazawa A, Okura T, Deguchi Y, Akanuma SI, Kubo Y, et al. Histamine elimination from the cerebrospinal fluid across the blood-cerebrospinal fluid barrier: involvement of plasma membrane monoamine transporter (PMAT/SLC29A4). J Neurochem. 2016;139:408–18.
17. Mori S, Takanaga H, Ohtsuki S, Deguchi T, Kang YS, Hosoya K, et al. Rat organic anion transporter 3 (rOAT3) is responsible for brain-to-blood efflux of homovanillic acid at the abluminal membrane of brain capillary endothelial cells. J Cereb Blood Flow Metab. 2003;23:432–40.
18. Okura T, Kato S, Takano Y, Sato T, Yamashita A, Morimoto R, et al. Functional characterization of rat plasma membrane monoamine transporter in the blood–brain and blood-cerebrospinal fluid barriers. J Pharm Sci. 2011;100:3924–38.
19. Wakayama K, Ohtsuki S, Takanaga H, Hosoya K, Terasaki T. Localization of norepinephrine and serotonin transporter in mouse brain capillary endothelial cells. Neurosci Res. 2002;44:173–80.
20. Tachikawa M, Kasai Y, Takahashi M, Fujinawa J, Kitaichi K, Terasaki T, et al. The blood-cerebrospinal fluid barrier is a major pathway of cerebral creatinine clearance: involvement of transporter-mediated process. J Neurochem. 2008;107:432–42.
21. Chen L, Pawlikowski B, Schlessinger A, More SS, Stryke D, Johns SJ, et al. Role of organic cation transporter 3 (SLC22A3) and its missense variants in the pharmacologic action of metformin. Pharmacogenet Genom. 2010;20:687–99.
22. Engel K, Wang J. Interaction of organic cations with a newly identified plasma membrane monoamine transporter. Mol Pharmacol. 2005;68:1397–407.
23. Hilber B, Scholze P, Dorostkar MM, Sandtner W, Holy M, Boehm S, et al. Serotonin-transporter mediated efflux: a pharmacological analysis of amphetamines and non-amphetamines. Neuropharmacology. 2005;49:811–9.
24. Sitte HH, Huck S, Reither H, Boehm S, Singer EA, Pifl C. Carrier-mediated release, transport rates, and charge transfer induced by amphetamine, tyramine, and dopamine in mammalian cells transfected with the human dopamine transporter. J Neurochem. 1998;71:1289–97.
25. Kakee A, Terasaki T, Sugiyama Y. Brain efflux index as a novel method of analyzing efflux transport at the blood–brain barrier. J Pharmacol Exp Ther. 1996;277:1550–9.
26. Ogawa M, Suzuki H, Sawada Y, Hanano M, Sugiyama Y. Kinetics of active efflux via choroid plexus of beta-lactam antibiotics from the CSF into the circulation. Am J Physiol. 1994;266:R392–9.
27. Suzuki H, Sawada Y, Sugiyama Y, Iga T, Hanano M. Transport of benzylpenicillin by the rat choroid plexus in vitro. J Pharmacol Exp Ther. 1987;242:660–5.
28. Suzuki H, Sawada Y, Sugiyama Y, Iga T, Hanano M. Transport of cimetidine by the rat choroid plexus in vitro. J Pharmacol Exp Ther. 1986;239:927–35.
29. Kitazawa T, Hosoya K, Watanabe M, Takashima T, Ohtsuki S, Takanaga H, et al. Characterization of the amino acid transport of new immortalized choroid plexus epithelial cell lines: a novel in vitro system for investigating transport functions at the blood-cerebrospinal fluid barrier. Pharm Res. 2001;18:16–22.
30. Yamaoka K, Tanigawara Y, Nakagawa T, Uno T. A pharmacokinetic analysis program (multi) for microcomputer. J Pharmacobiodyn. 1981;4:879–85.
31. Ohta KY, Inoue K, Hayashi Y, Yuasa H. Molecular identification and functional characterization of rat multidrug and toxin extrusion type transporter 1 as an organic cation/H^+ antiporter in the kidney. Drug Metab Dispos. 2006;34:1868–74.
32. Suzuki H, Sawada Y, Sugiyama Y, Iga T, Hanano M. Saturable transport of cimetidine from cerebrospinal fluid to blood in rats. J Pharmacobiodyn. 1985;8:73–6.
33. Akanuma S, Sakurai T, Tachikawa M, Kubo Y, Hosoya K. Transporter-mediated L-glutamate elimination from cerebrospinal fluid: possible involve-

ment of excitatory amino acid transporters expressed in ependymal cells and choroid plexus epithelial cells. Fluids Barriers CNS. 2015;12:11.
34. Quay WB. Regional differences in metabolism and composition of choroid plexuses. Brain Res. 1966;2:378–89.
35. Krunic N, Adamson SL, Coceani F. Differential uptake and catabolism of prostaglandin (PG)E(2) versus PGF(2alpha) in the sheep choroid plexus during development. Brain Res Dev Brain Res. 2000;119:11–9.
36. Keep RF, Jones HC. A morphometric study on the development of the lateral ventricle choroid plexus, choroid plexus capillaries and ventricular ependyma in the rat. Brain Res Dev Brain Res. 1990;56:47–53.
37. Fukao M, Ishida K, Horie A, Taguchi M, Nozawa T, Inoue H, et al. Variability of bioavailability and intestinal absorption mechanisms of metoprolol. Drug Metab Pharmacokinet. 2014;29:162–7.
38. Ishida K, Horie A, Nishimura M, Taguchi M, Fujii N, Nozawa T, et al. Variability of bioavailability and intestinal absorption characteristics of bisoprolol. Drug Metab Pharmacokinet. 2013;28:491–6.
39. Tega Y, Akanuma S, Kubo Y, Hosoya K. Involvement of the H^+/organic cation antiporter in nicotine transport in rat liver. Drug Metab Dispos. 2015;43:89–92.
40. Tega Y, Yuzurihara C, Kubo Y, Akanuma SI, Ehrhardt C, Hosoya KI. Functional expression of nicotine influx transporter in A549 human alveolar epithelial cells. Drug Metab Pharmacokinet. 2016;31:99–101.
41. Tega Y, Akanuma S, Kubo Y, Terasaki T, Hosoya K. Blood-to-brain influx transport of nicotine at the rat blood–brain barrier: involvement of a pyrilamine-sensitive organic cation transport process. Neurochem Int. 2013;62:173–81.
42. Okura T, Hattori A, Takano Y, Sato T, Hammarlund-Udenaes M, Terasaki T, et al. Involvement of the pyrilamine transporter, a putative organic cation transporter, in blood–brain barrier transport of oxycodone. Drug Metab Dispos. 2008;36:2005–13.
43. Yamazaki M, Fukuoka H, Nagata O, Kato H, Ito Y, Terasaki T, et al. Transport mechanism of an H1-antagonist at the blood–brain barrier: transport mechanism of mepyramine using the carotid injection technique. Biol Pharm Bull. 1994;17:676–9.
44. Youdim MB, Bakhle YS. Monoamine oxidase: isoforms and inhibitors in Parkinson's disease and depressive illness. Br J Pharmacol. 2006;147(Suppl 1):S287–96.
45. Sathyanarayana Rao TS, Yeragani VK. Hypertensive crisis and cheese. Indian J Psychiatry. 2009;51:65–6.

18

Fluid outflow in the rat spinal cord: the role of perivascular and paravascular pathways

Shinuo Liu[1*], Magdalena A. Lam[1], Alisha Sial[1], Sarah J. Hemley[1], Lynne E. Bilston[2] and Marcus A. Stoodley[1]

Abstract

Background: Cerebrospinal fluid (CSF) is thought to flow into the brain via perivascular spaces around arteries, where it mixes with interstitial fluid. The precise details concerning fluid outflow remain controversial. Although fluid dynamics have been studied in the brain, little is known about spinal cord fluid inflow and outflow. Understanding the normal fluid physiology of the spinal cord may give insight into the pathogenesis of spinal cord oedema and CSF disorders such as syringomyelia. We therefore aimed to determine the fluid outflow pathways in the rat spinal cord.

Methods: A fluorescent tracer, Alexa-Fluor®-647 Ovalbumin, was injected into the extracellular space of either the cervicothoracic lateral white matter or the grey matter in twenty-two Sprague–Dawley rats over 250 s. The rats were sacrificed at 20 or 60 min post injection. Spinal cord segments were sectioned and labelled with vascular antibodies for immunohistochemistry.

Results: Fluorescent tracer was distributed over two to three spinal levels adjacent to the injection site. In grey matter injections, tracer spread radially into the white matter. In white matter injections, tracer was confined to and redistributed along the longitudinal axonal fibres. Tracer was conducted towards the pial and ependymal surfaces along vascular structures. There was accumulation of tracer around the adventitia of the intramedullary arteries, veins and capillaries, as well as the extramedullary vessels. A distinct layer of tracer was deposited in the internal basement membrane of the tunica media of arteries. In half the grey matter injections, tracer was detected in the central canal.

Conclusions: These results suggest that in the spinal cord interstitial fluid movement is modulated by tissue diffusivity of grey and white matter. The central canal, and the compartments around or within blood vessels appear to be dominant pathways for fluid drainage in these experiments. There may be regional variations in fluid outflow capacity due to vascular and other anatomical differences between the grey and white matter.

Keywords: Cerebrospinal fluid, Outflow, Spinal cord, Syringomyelia, Perivascular, Interstitial fluid

Background

Details of the circulation of cerebrospinal fluid (CSF) and interstitial fluid (ISF) of the central nervous system remain controversial [1, 2]. In recent decades, the concept of CSF circulating through the brain parenchyma, as a mechanism for metabolite transport and clearance [1–4], has gained momentum. ISF consists of water and solutes that are the by-products of cellular metabolism and synaptic transmission in the extracellular space. There may even be a component of ISF that passes across the brain capillary endothelium (although compelling in vivo evidence is contentious) [4–8]. Perivascular spaces have received renewed interest as a crucial facilitator of fluid inflow in neural tissue [9–13]. If CSF can enter brain parenchyma, there must also be efflux pathways [3]. The assumption is that ISF must be cleared, probably into the subarachnoid space [14, 15], but the precise mechanism is unclear.

The "glymphatic" theory of fluid homeostasis posits that fluid flow into and out of the parenchyma is via arterial and venular pathways respectively [10, 16, 17]. Studies to date have largely focused on the brain, with few investigations of spinal cord. Although there is some

*Correspondence: shinuo.liu@hdr.mq.edu.au
[1] Department of Clinical Medicine, Faculty of Medicine and Health Sciences, Macquarie University, Suite 407, Clinic Building, 2 Technology Place, Sydney, NSW 2109, Australia

evidence of similar mechanisms governing fluid ingress [18–20], how fluid egresses from the cord is almost unknown [21, 22]. Compared to the brain the spinal cord is not only much smaller, but the arrangement of the grey and white matter is reversed. Furthermore, spinal cord axonal tracts are oriented parallel to its long axis. These fundamental anatomical differences mean diffusion and transport of fluid in grey and white matter are likely to be different [3, 14, 23].

Syringomyelia is a puzzling condition where fluid filled cysts develop in the spinal cord, usually secondary to another pathology, such as trauma, that results in CSF obstruction in the subarachnoid space. There is emerging evidence that its pathogenesis is a dynamic process involving imbalances in fluid inflow and outflow. The important contribution of perivascular spaces to mechanisms of fluid entry into syrinxes has been characterised in previous animal experiments [19, 24, 25]. Recent work [26] on fluid outflow pathways in an ovine model of post-traumatic syringomyelia indicated diffuse fluid movement away from the syrinx cavity and towards the central canal and perivascular spaces. However, the precise pathways of fluid drainage in the spinal cord under normal physiological conditions, and whether perivascular spaces play a crucial role in this context are unknown. A more complete understanding of the mechanisms governing spinal cord fluid homeostasis may lead to new insights into the pathogenesis of syringomyelia.

In this study, we aimed to determine the fluid outflow pathways in the rat spinal cord. We injected a fluorescent tracer of the extracellular space, ovalbumin conjugated to the fluorophore Alexa-Fluor®-647 (AFO-647), into the spinal grey and white matter of Sprague–Dawley rats. Our hypotheses were: (1) fluid outflow from the spinal cord is via the perivenular spaces; and (2) the pattern of fluid flow in the white matter is different from that of grey matter.

Methods

Ethics approval was obtained from Macquarie University Animal Ethics Committee (ARA 2016/032–5). Outflow from the grey and white matter was separately investigated at two time points in 22 male Sprague–Dawley rats, weighing from 155–345 g. Ten animals were used in the white matter injection studies, while 12 were used in the grey matter injection studies.

Surgical procedure

After induction of general anaesthesia with 4% isoflurane in oxygen, the animal was positioned prone in a stereotactic frame, and maintained under anaesthesia with 2.5% isoflurane (adjusted as necessary) in 0.2 L/min of oxygen. Heart rate, oxygen saturation, respiratory rate and rectal temperature were continuously recorded.

Under an operating microscope, a dorsal midline occipitocervical incision was made followed by subperiosteal muscle dissection. Segmental laminectomies at C7/T1 or T1/T2 were performed with fine rongeurs. A window of thecal sac, eccentric to the right, was exposed. A 34G Nanofil needle, loaded onto a glass syringe (World Precision Instruments, Florida, USA), punctured the dura in a single pass. For grey matter studies, the entry point of the needle was 0.5 mm right of the midline at the C7/T1 interspace. For white matter studies the entry was at least 1 mm right of the midline at the T1/T2 interspace, where the grey matter is less prominent. The needle passed into the parenchyma to a depth of 1 mm targeting either the junction of the ventral and dorsal horns (for grey matter injections), or the lateral white matter funiculus. An Ultramicro pump (World Precision Instruments, Florida, USA) was used to deliver 500 nL of Ovalbumin Alexa-Fluor®-647 conjugate (Life Technologies, Victoria, Australia) with 10% fluorescent microspheres (v/v %) (Thermo Fisher Scientific, Massachusetts) at a rate of 2 nL/s. The needle was left in situ for either 20 or 60 min from the start of the injection. By either the 20 or 60 min time point, the animal underwent transcardiac perfusion with heparinised 0.1 M phosphate buffered saline (PBS) followed by 4% paraformaldehyde (PFA) (Lancaster Synthesis, Pelham, New Hampshire).

Tissue processing

The spinal cord and brain were harvested en bloc for macroscopic fluorescent imaging. After post fixation in 4% PFA overnight, the specimen was stored in 30% sucrose for cryoprotection. The spinal cord was segmented from C2 to T4. Each segment was snap frozen, and 40 μm axial sections were taken on a cryostat and mounted onto glass slides.

Immunohistochemistry

The glass slides were washed twice for 10 min in tris–phosphate buffered saline, and then in 50% ethanol for cellular permeabilization. After application of 15% normal donkey serum (NDS) blocking solution, the slides were incubated overnight with 1:100 Rat Endothelial Cell Antibody (RECA-1, Abcam, Cambridge, United Kingdom) in 4% NDS. The secondary antibody, 1:400 anti-mouse IgG Alexa-Fluor®-488 (Molecular Probes, Life Technologies, New York, USA) was then applied. This was followed by anti-actin α-smooth muscle antibody at 1:400 dilution (SMA-Cy3, Sigma-Aldrich, St. Louis, Montana). Primary and secondary controls were established to exclude autofluorescence. The slides were cover-slipped with fluorescent mounting medium (DAKO, NSW, Australia).

Image acquisition

After post fixation, macroscopic white-light and single channel fluorescent images were captured with the in-vivo MS FX PRO (Bruker, Billerica, MA). The fluorescence camera was set at excitation and emission wavelengths of 630 and 700 nm respectively, with an exposure time of 4 s.

Spinal cord axial sections from C2 to T4 were imaged with a Zeiss Axio Imager Z1 fluorescence microscope (Carl Zeiss Microimaging GmbH, Germany) for qualitative and quantitative analysis. The fluorescent microspheres, which have a diameter of 1 μm, were used to verify the location of the injection site as their size prevents significant displacement. SMA- and RECA-1-positive vessels were identified as arterioles. SMA-negative, RECA-1-positive vessels were designated venules or capillaries. Those with largest diameter ≥ 6.5 μm were considered venules, and those < 6.5 μm capillaries. Further delineation of vascular and anatomical structures was undertaken with confocal microscopy (LSM 880, Carl Zeiss Microimaging GmbH, Germany).

Image analysis

Quantitative analysis of fluorescent signal intensity was performed using Image J, version 1.46r [27]. Subtraction of background fluorescence was performed in all measurements. In macroscopic fluorescent acquisitions, the spinal segment levels were identified by counting nerve roots on the white light images (Fig. 1a). These were then overlaid onto the fluorescence images. Mean pixel densities were measured in each spinal segment from C2 to T4 to yield fluorescence intensities.

In fluorescent photomicrographs of axial sections, the integrated density of the tracer (mean pixel density multiplied by area) was calculated. The mean pixel densities of the white and grey matter were measured separately. At least three sections were analysed per spinal level from C2 to T4, and then averaged to give a mean integrated density.

Statistical analysis

Grey matter and white matter integrated densities were compared using two-way analysis of variance (ANOVA) and adjusted for multiple comparison using Bonferroni's post hoc tests (GraphPad Prism v7.02, GraphPad Software Inc, California). A p value < 0.05 was considered statistically significant. All values were expressed as mean ± standard error of the mean (SEM).

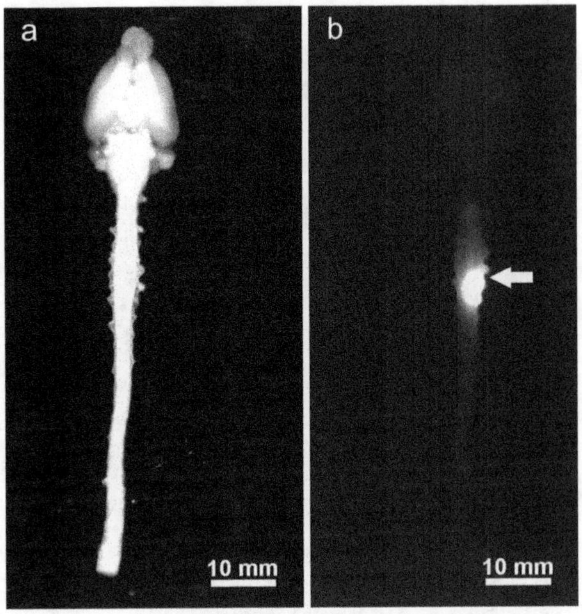

Fig. 1 White light and single fluorescence channel acquisition of harvested brain and spinal cord with the in-vivo MS FX PRO Multispectral Imager System. Brightness and contrast have been uniformly adjusted for optimal visualisation. **a** White light enabled spinal level localisation. **b** Macroscopic appearance of tracer distribution. There is a sharp drop off in fluorescence intensity within 1–2 spinal levels rostral and caudal to injection site at C7/8 (arrow)

Results

Rostral–caudal tracer distribution

In macroscopic fluorescent imaging, tracer was observed to be localised to the injection site in all experiments (Fig. 1b). The macroscopic mean fluorescence intensity was determined for each spinal cord level. A sharp drop-off in intensity within two levels rostral and caudal to the injection site was observed (Fig. 2). At the 60 min time point, but not at the 20 min time point, the cord had significantly higher mean fluorescence intensities after white matter injections (WMi) compared to grey matter injections (GMi) (two way ANOVA, p = 0.0026). On post hoc analysis, significance was reached one and two levels rostral to the injection point (p = 0.045 and 0.026 respectively) (Fig. 2b). Post hoc analysis also demonstrated a significant difference between white and grey matter injections at the 20 min time point one level caudal to the injection site (p = 0.034) (Fig. 2a).

Axial tracer distribution

Quantification of AFO-647 intensity from microscopic analysis of axial sections is summarised in Fig. 3a–d. The fluorescence intensity within the grey and white

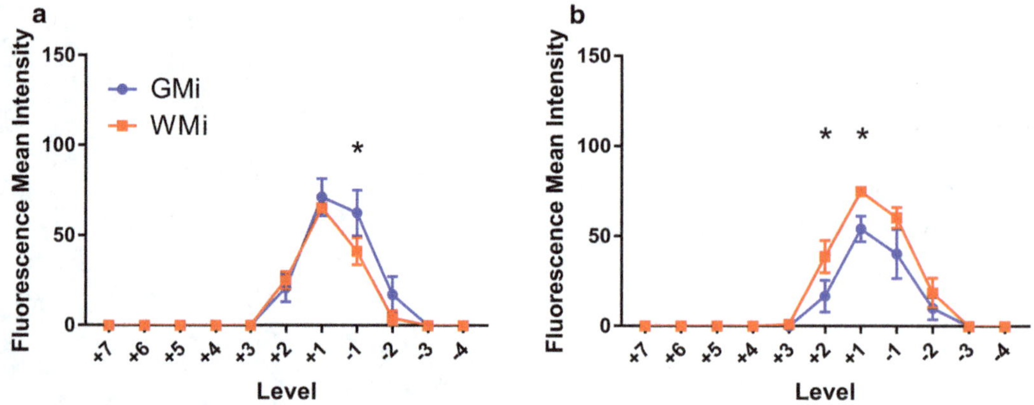

Fig. 2 Quantification of rostral–caudal tracer fluorescence (mean fluorescence intensity) per spinal level after grey (n = 10) and white (n = 10) matter injections at 20 min (**a**, left panel) and at 60 min (**b**, right panel). Each spinal cord level ("Level") is expressed as the number of levels rostral (positive integers) or caudal (negative integers) to injection site. All error bars are expressed as ± SEM. In both white and grey matter injections at both time points, there was a sharp drop off of tracer fluorescence within 2 levels rostral and caudad to the injection. At the 20 min time point **a**, there was no difference in fluorescence intensity between white and grey matter injections, but on post hoc analysis a significant difference was reached at − 1 level caudal to the injection site (*p = 0.0341). At the 60 min time point **b**, fluorescence intensity was significantly higher in the white matter injections compared to the grey matter injections (p = 0.0026). On post hoc analysis significant differences were observed at + 1 and + 2 levels rostral to the injection point (*p = 0.0448 and 0.0259 respectively)

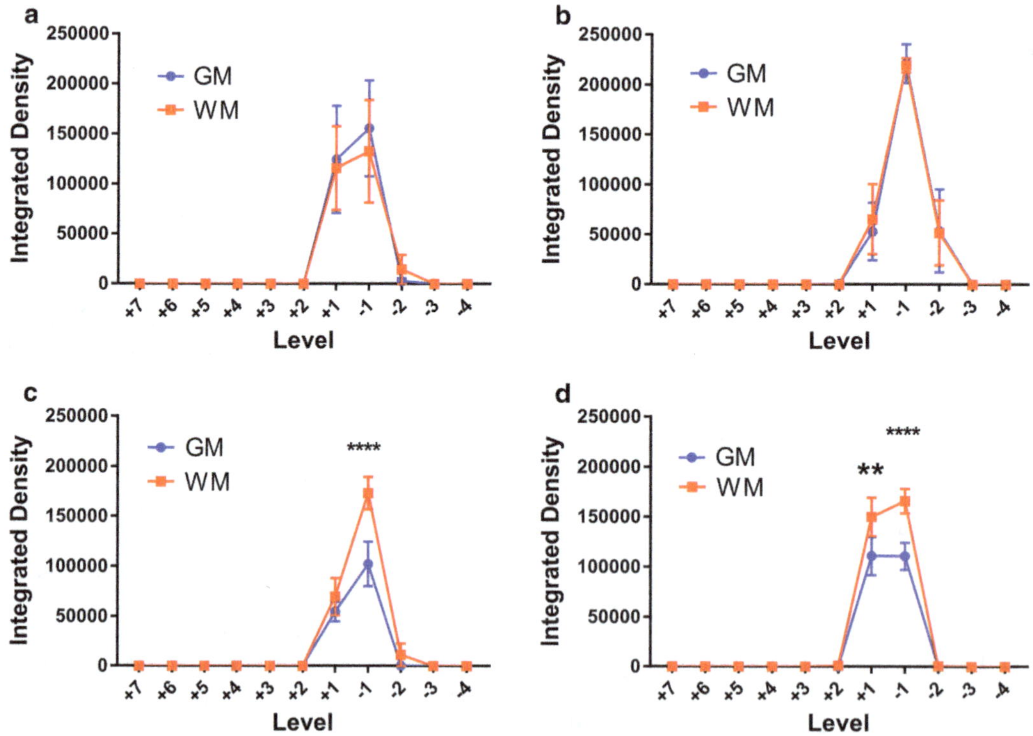

Fig. 3 Quantification of microscopic axial section tracer fluorescence (integrated density) per spinal level after grey and white matter injections. Each spinal cord level ("Level") is expressed as the number of levels rostral (positive integers) or caudal (negative integers) to injection site. All error bars are expressed as ± SEM. **a** After grey matter injections at 20 min (n = 5) there was no statistical difference between grey and white matter fluorescence. **b** This was also observed in grey matter injections after 60 min (n = 5). However, after white matter injections at **c** 20 min (n = 5) and at **d** 60 min (n = 5), there was significantly greater tracer fluorescence in the white matter compared to the grey matter (p = 0.0094 and 0.0041 for 20 and 60 min respectively). On post hoc analysis, a statistically significant difference was observed at one level caudal to the injection site (***p < 0.0001) at 20 min (**c**), and one level rostral and caudal at 60 min (**d**) (**p = 0.0017, ****p < 0.0001)

matter, expressed as integrated density, is represented in relation to spinal level at the 20 and 60 min time points separately. After white matter injections, at both 20 and 60 min, fluorescence was significantly greater in the white matter compared to grey matter ($p=0.0094$ and 0.0041 for 20 and 60 min respectively) (Fig. 3c, d). On post hoc analysis, at the 20 min time point, a significant difference was observed at one level caudal to the injection site ($p<0.0001$). At 60 min, white matter fluorescence was found to be significantly greater one level rostrally ($p=0.0017$) and caudally ($p<0.0001$). Following grey matter injections, however, tracer fluorescence was not significantly different between grey and white matter, at either time point (Fig. 3a, b).

Pattern of tracer distribution: grey matter injections

In six of 12 animals, in which grey matter injections were performed, tracer was delivered to the junction of the ventral and dorsal horns. There was a continuous radial decrease in fluorescence intensity in all directions away from the injection site. Tracer signal was detected in the white matter surrounding the grey matter at the injection level (Fig. 4e). In rostral and caudal axial sections, tracer was detected predominantly in the grey matter.

In the other six animals, in which grey matter injections were performed, tracer was delivered into either the middle of the ventral or dorsal horn. Although the highest fluorescence intensity was found within the grey matter, there was substantial tracer signal in the adjacent white matter. In rostral and caudal sections there was prominent tracer signal in the white matter (Fig. 4f). In all but one animal, tracer was detected in the contralateral grey matter.

Pattern of tracer distribution: white matter injections

In eight of 10 animals the distribution of AFO-647 conformed to the shape of the lateral funiculus, staying primarily in the white matter (Fig. 4g). A radial reduction in tracer fluorescence was also observed. A small amount of tracer entered the lateral horn of the grey matter. Rostrocaudally, ovalbumin was almost exclusively found in the white matter (Fig. 4h). Within this subgroup of animals, no tracer was detected in the contralateral grey matter except in one animal.

In two of 10 animals, there was a similar pattern of tracer spread in the white matter but considerable ovalbumin also redistributed into the grey matter. Rostrocaudally, however, tracer was confined to the white matter.

Tracer in relation to vascular structures

In all animals fluorescent tracer accumulated around or within the walls of arterioles, venules and capillaries in both the grey and white matter (Figs. 5, 6g). Arterioles were more numerous in the grey matter than the white matter (Fig. 4d). Selective tracer labelling of vascular structures was particularly evident in areas of low background tracer concentration (Fig. 5a, d). In the white matter, tracer concentrated along arterioles and venules that extended from the grey matter to the pia (Fig. 5d).

Tracer co-localised with arterioles and venules of the ventral median fissure in all but one animal (a white matter injection, sacrificed at 20 min) (Fig. 5d, f, h). Tracer was present in the wall of the anterior spinal artery (ASA) and its central branch in 10 animals (Fig. 5d), of which nine were grey matter injections. Fluorescence was further present in the walls of the arterial vasocorona in 13 animals (Fig. 6d–f), of which 10 were white matter injections. Confocal microscopy demonstrated tracer deposition external to the smooth muscle layer of the ASA. Additionally, there was a distinct layer of tracer between the endothelial and smooth muscle layers (Fig. 5e). This pattern of tracer distribution was also observed in parenchymal arterioles and other extramedullary arteries, such as the central branch of the ASA and the arterial vasocorona. AFO-647 was discretely deposited external to the endothelial layer of capillaries and venules of the cord parenchyma (Figs. 5h, i, 6g).

In at least six animals (two from white matter injections), tracer deposited prominently around "remote" arterioles (Fig. 5f, g). These labelled vessels were far removed from the bulk of the contiguous tracer at the injection site. Tracer labelling of the pia and subpial space was generally limited or absent as fluorescence intensity decreased from the site of injection towards the cord surface. Instead, ovalbumin concentrated around vessels that traversed the cord parenchyma towards the pial surface. Tracer appeared to be transported from the injection site to the extramedullary vasculature (Fig. 6i), along these conduit-like arterioles and venules.

Central canal

Fluorescent tracer was detected in the central canal ependymal cell layer in 6 of 12 grey matter injections. In three animals, central canal tracer fluorescence was present in at least eight contiguous spinal levels, rostral to the injection site. Furthermore, tracer was observed within the lumen of the canal, confirmed by confocal microscopy. The bordering layer of ependymal cells was heterogeneously delineated by fluorescence. Nuclear labelling by tracer was absent. The apical ends displayed greater tracer intensity compared to the basal surface (Fig. 6a–c). In two animals, central canal ependymal tracer was detected rostrally over only 2 spinal levels. In one animal, tracer extended caudally only from T1 to T4. No tracer was found in the central canal in any of the white matter injection animals.

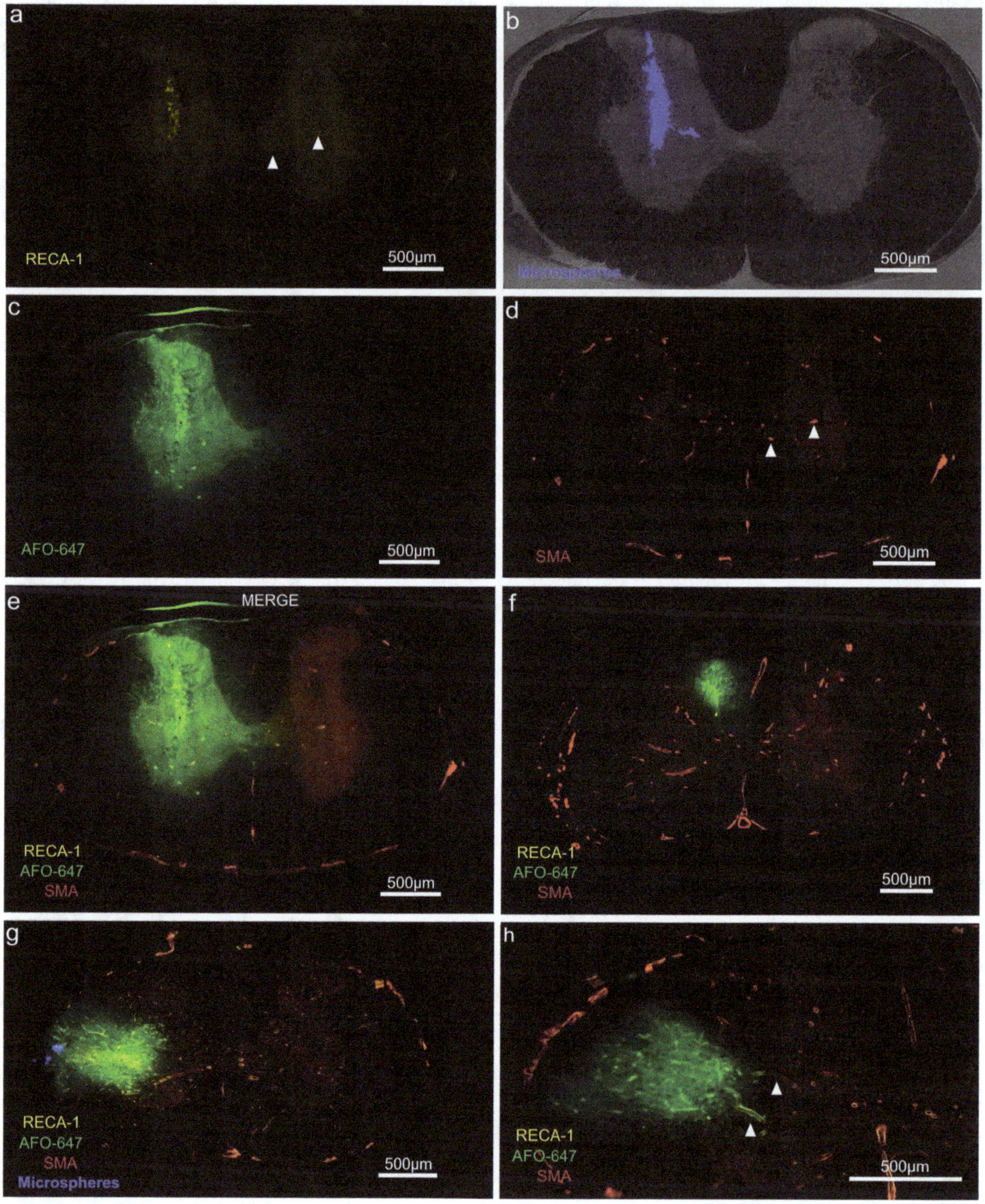

Fig. 4 Typical axial sections at the cervicothoracic junction after injection of fluorescent tracer into the spinal grey and white matter. **a**–**e** Grey matter injection. **a** RECA-1 and **d** SMA immunofluorescent staining of arterioles. Examples of grey matter arterioles are marked by arrow heads in **a**, **d**. Arterioles were present in greater numbers in the grey matter compared to white matter. **b** Fluorescent microspheres confirmed the Nanofil needle had traversed the grey matter. **c**, **e** Radial redistribution of tracer from the middle of the grey matter in all directions. **f** Axial section rostral to a grey matter injection site where a significant amount of tracer had spread into dorsal column. Note tracer fluorescence was mainly confined to the dorsal white matter column at this level. **g** After delivery into the white matter, AFO-647 tracer conformed to the shape of the lateral funiculus with limited spread into the grey matter. **h** In rostral sections in the same animal, tracer was confined to the white matter. Arrow heads demonstrating selective tracer deposition around arterioles. All fluorescent photomicrographs were taken at ×20 magnification

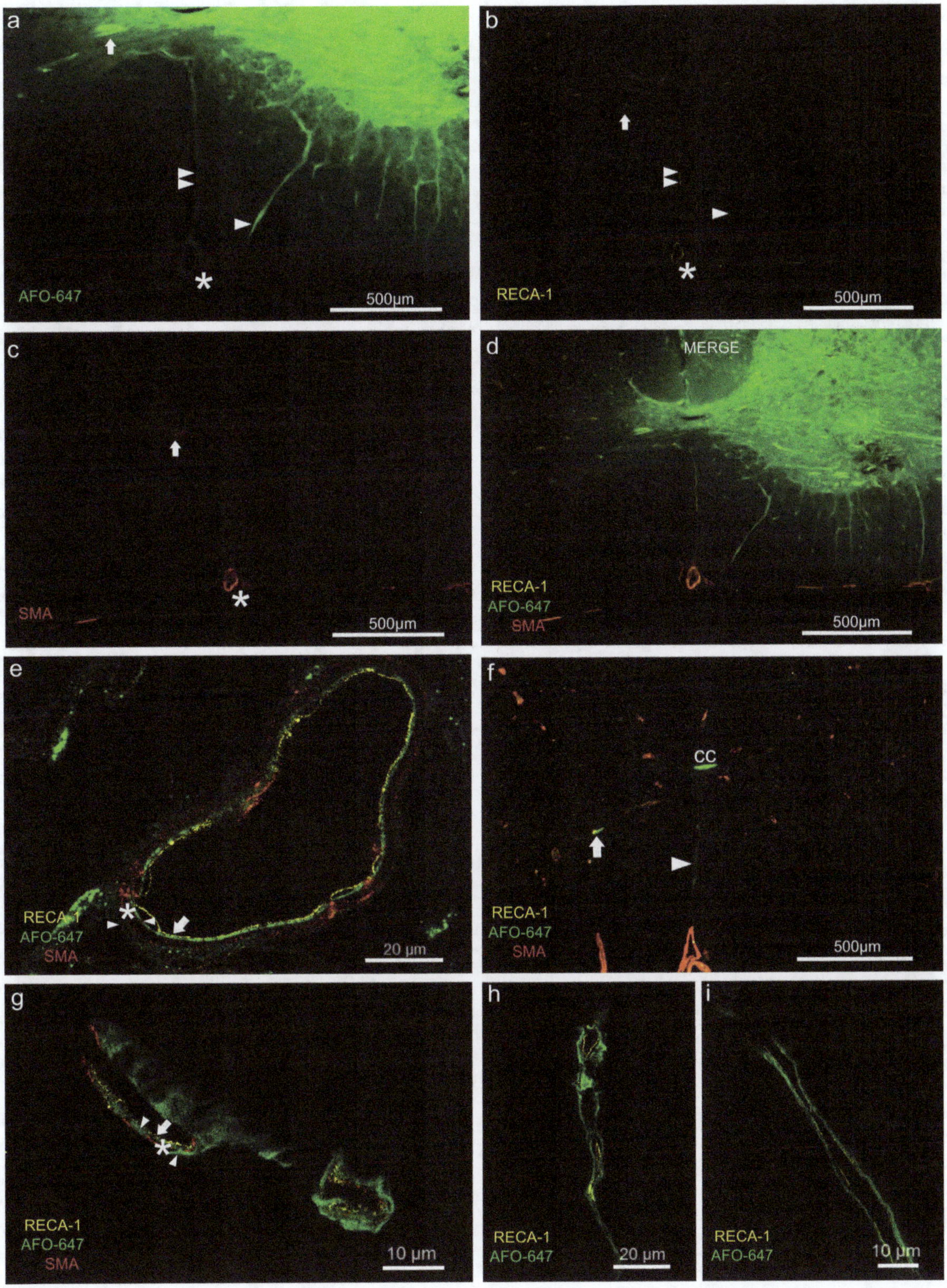
a
AFO-647
500µm
b
RECA-1
500µm
c
SMA
500µm
d
MERGE
RECA-1
AFO-647
SMA
500µm
e
RECA-1
AFO-647
SMA
20 µm
f
cc
RECA-1
AFO-647
SMA
500µm
g
RECA-1
AFO-647
SMA
10 µm
h
RECA-1
AFO-647
20 µm
i
RECA-1
AFO-647
10 µm

(See figure on previous page.)

Fig. 5 Relationship of injected tracer to vascular structures. **a–d** Fluorescent microscopy of grey matter injection. Tracer co-localised with the wall of the anterior spinal artery (asterisk). A radially directed venule (single arrow head) and veins (note RECA-1 positive and SMA negative) in the ventral median sulcus (double arrow heads) appeared to conduct ovalbumin away from the injection site towards the pial surface. Prominent accumulation of tracer around an arteriole (marked by arrow) against a relatively low background fluorescence suggests it is a pathway for fluid outflow. **e** Confocal photomicrograph of the anterior spinal artery found in **d**. A layer of AFO-647 tracer (indicated by right pointing arrow head) was detected external to the tunica media (SMA positive, indicated by asterisk). Another distinct layer of fluorescent tracer was also found internal to the tunica media layer (left pointing arrow head), separate from the endothelial layer (RECA-1, marked by arrow). **f** Pronounced tracer deposition around a "remote" arteriole (arrow) and vein in the ventral median sulcus (arrow head). These vessels were one level rostral to the grey matter injection site, and therefore tracer accumulation around these structures could not be explained by contiguous tracer spread. It is likely ovalbumin was transported over a distance in the spaces around these vessels. Note tracer labelling of the central canal (indicated by "cc"). **g** "Peri- and para-arterial" pattern of tracer deposition in specific compartments external and internal to the tunica media of parenchymal arterioles (arrow heads, arrow and asterisk denote the same anatomical layers as in **e**). **h** Tracer accumulation between the adventitia and the glia limitans of veins in the ventral median sulcus (found in **f**). **i** The same "para-venular" pattern demonstrated in a radially directed parenchymal venule, found in **d**. All fluorescent and confocal photomicrographs were taken at ×20 and ×63 magnification respectively

Effect of time

Figure 7a–d compares tracer fluorescence intensity in both the white and grey matter at the 20 min time point to that of the 60 min group. The same data derived from the quantification of axial tracer fluorescence was used to assess the effect of time on tracer distribution. There was no statistically significant difference in the grey matter fluorescence intensities between the two time points after either grey or white matter injection (Fig. 7a, b). However, on post hoc analysis significantly greater grey matter fluorescence was observed at one spinal level rostral to the white matter injection site after 60 min compared to 20 min ($p < 0.0001$). There was no overall significant difference in the white matter fluorescence intensities between the two time points after either grey or white matter injections. Post hoc analyses demonstrated significantly higher white matter fluorescence at 60 min compared to 20 min at one level caudal ($p = 0.009$) and one level rostral ($p < 0.0001$) to the injection site following grey matter and white matter injections respectively (Fig. 7c, d). At the longer time point, it appeared that after white matter injections there was greater redistribution of tracer from the white matter into the grey matter, and also along white matter tracts rostrally. After grey matter injections, there also appeared to be greater tracer spread into the lateral white matter caudally with time.

Discussion

In this study, the distribution of fluorescent tracer up to 60 min after injection into the spinal cord interstitium was limited to the adjacent two to three spinal cord levels. Tracer was distributed in a radial pattern after delivery into the grey matter, with dissemination into white matter. The absence of statistically significant differences between tracer fluorescence intensities of the grey and white matter after grey matter injections (Fig. 3a, b) is consistent with this observation. However, there was limited redistribution of tracer from white into grey matter after white matter injections. The statistically significant differences between grey and white matter tracer fluorescence intensities after white matter injections support this observation. There was some evidence these patterns were amplified over time. Greater spread of tracer along white matter tracts longitudinally was also observed. There was prominent labelling of all vascular structures by AFO-647. Tracer appeared to be conducted away from the injection site towards the pial surface by depositing around radially projecting arterioles and venules. Support for this inference was provided by the detection of tracer fluorescence around extramedullary vessels. This finding was unlikely to have been secondary to diffusion (or other means of contiguous solute transport such as bulk flow) of tracer because of the general absence of subpial fluorescence (Fig. 6e, i), particularly after grey matter injections. Further microscopic analysis revealed accumulation of ovalbumin both in the perivascular and paravascular spaces of arterial vessels, which will be discussed below.

Although it was not possible in this study to conclude whether diffusion or bulk flow governed interstitial tracer movement, our findings are in concordance with theoretical and animal models of spinal ISF movement from other groups. Confinement of tracer to white matter tracts is characteristic of anisotropic diffusion, well described in the literature on CNS diffusion tensor imaging [23], and has been confirmed in the developing rat spinal cord in ex vivo experiments [28, 29]. Here, fluid diffuses along, and is constrained by, myelinated white matter fibres that run parallel to its long axis. The unmyelinated grey matter, however, is the site of penetrating arteries and its extracellular space (ECS) is rich with somas and neurites that have no preferential orientation. Diffusion here is isotropic which may explain why in our experiments tracer in the grey matter was able to redistribute in all directions. Convection enhanced delivery (CED) studies in animal spinal cord have yielded similar

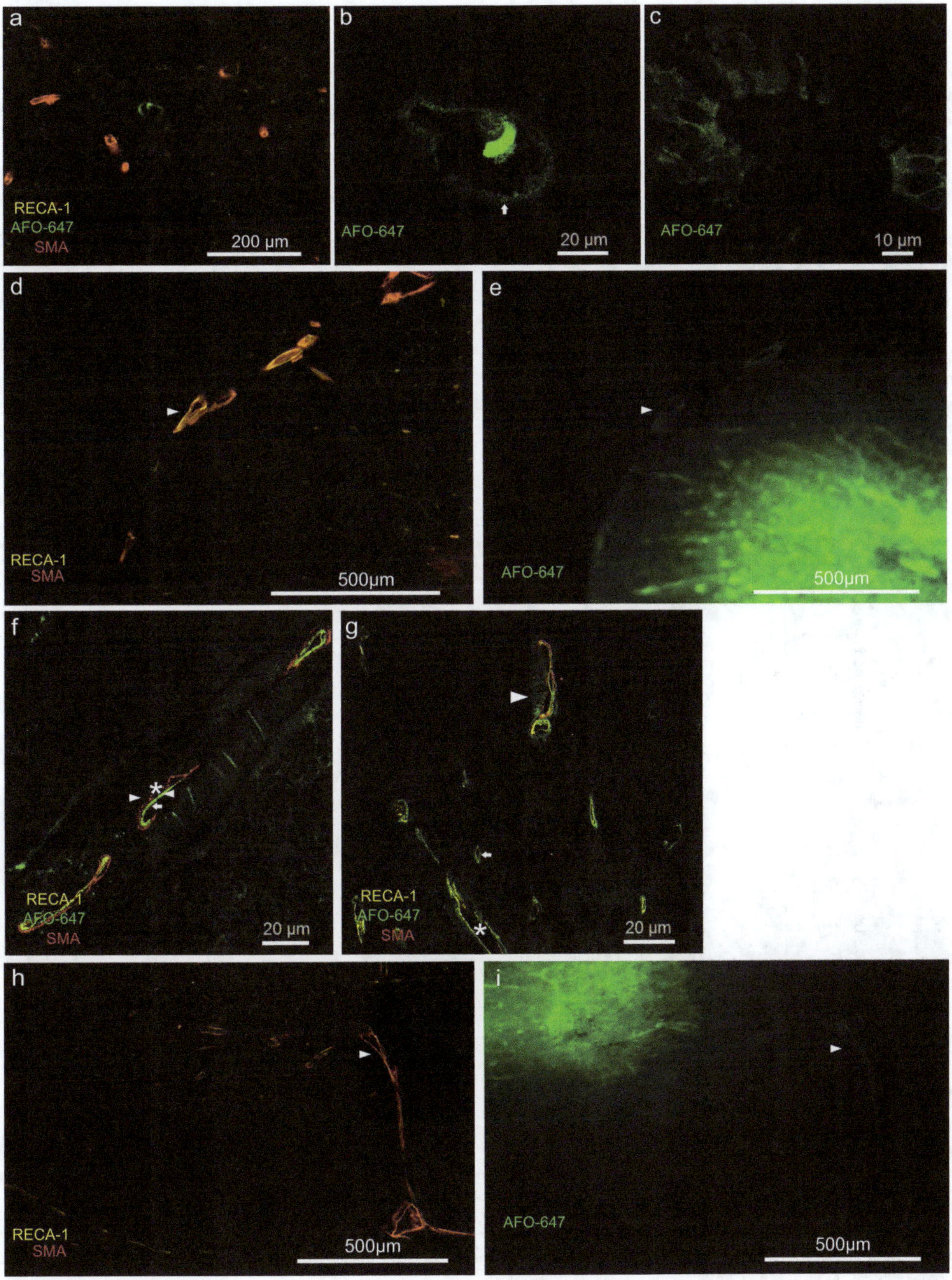
a
RECA-1
AFO-647
SMA
200 μm
b
AFO-647
20 μm
c
AFO-647
10 μm
d
RECA-1
SMA
500μm
e
AFO-647
500μm
f
RECA-1
AFO-647
SMA
20 μm
g
RECA-1
AFO-647
SMA
20 μm
h
RECA-1
SMA
500μm
i
AFO-647
500μm

(See figure on previous page.)

Fig. 6 Tracer delivered into the spinal cord parenchyma accumulated around ependymal and extramedullary structures. Fluorescent (**a**) and confocal (**b**) micrographs demonstrating tracer accumulation in the central canal. Note the presence of tracer within the lumen in **b** (12 o'clock position). **c** Confocal microscopy of central canal in another experiment. The ependymal cells were heterogeneously delineated by fluorescence, with the noted absence of nuclear tracer signal. In both **b** and **c**, the apical ends displayed greater tracer intensity compared to the basal surface. **d, e** Tracer deposition around the arterial vasocorona (arrow heads, note RECA-1 and SMA positivity) of the dorsal spinal cord surface. **f** Confocal microscopy view of the same arterial vasocorona demonstrating the characteristic "peri-arterial" and "para-arterial" distribution of the tracer (arrow heads) with respect to the tunica media (asterisk) and endothelium (arrow). The absence of subpial tracer signal excludes the possibility of contiguous tracer spread from injection site to artery. The arterial vasocorona could be the dominant pathway for fluid outflow from the white matter. **g** Fluid outflow appeared to involve all vascular structures. Confocal microscopy of grey matter showing arteriolar (arrow head), venular (asterisk) and capillary (arrow) labelling by tracer. Note the "paravascular" location of tracer in venules and capillaries. **h, i** Fluorescent microscopy of grey matter injection demonstrating conduction of tracer along the central branch of the anterior spinal artery towards the ventral median fissure. This suggests drainage of interstitial fluid towards the pial surface via vascular structures. All fluorescent and confocal photomicrographs were taken at ×20 and ×63 magnification respectively

findings of anisotropic movement of ligands through the white matter tracts [30, 31]. Endo et al. [21], employing Evan's blue tracer, observed comparable results to ours but described almost no tracer penetration into grey matter after white matter injections. Moreover, Evan's blue tracer was redistributed further rostrocaudally from the injection site in the white matter compared to the grey matter. These differences could be secondary to the larger delivered volume of tracer (2 μL) in their experiments, and the smaller molecular size of Evan's blue compared

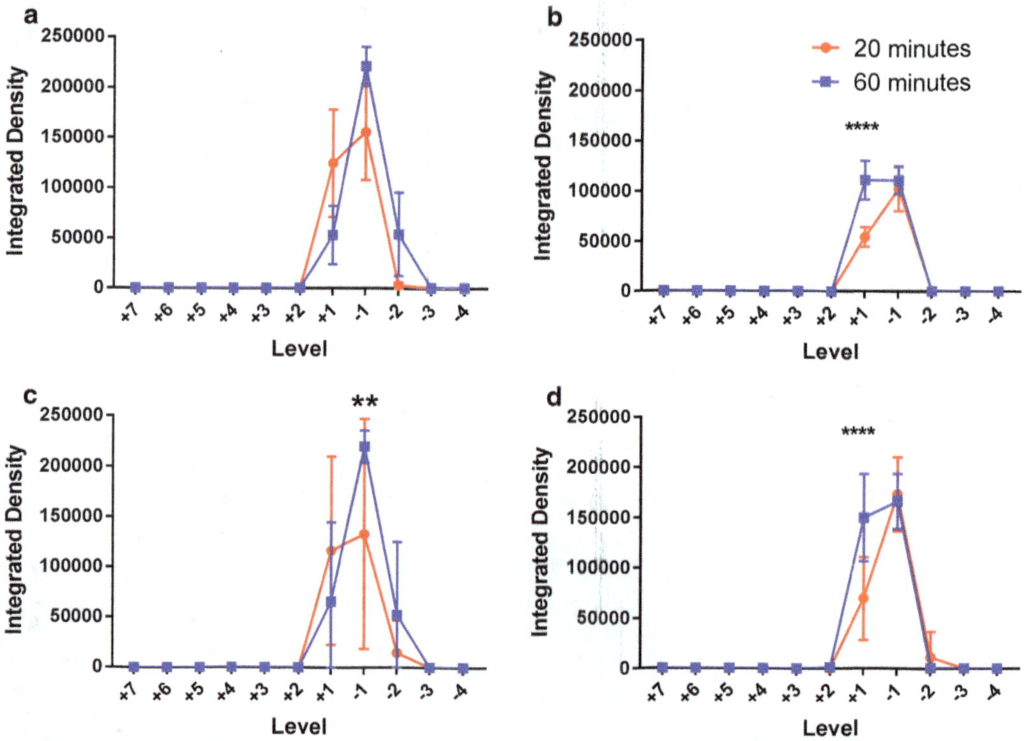

Fig. 7 Comparison of tracer fluorescence (integrated density) in axial sections at the 20 and 60 min time points per spinal level to assess the effect of time on tracer distribution. Each spinal cord level ("Level") is expressed as the number of levels rostral (positive integers) or caudal (negative integers) to injection site. All error bars are expressed as SEM. **a** After grey matter injections, no statistical significant difference between the time points was observed in the fluorescence intensity in the grey matter. **b** Following injection of tracer in the white matter, no statistically significant difference was observed between the 20 and 60 min groups in the grey matter. However, on post hoc analysis there was significantly greater fluorescence at +1 level rostral to the injection site after 60 min (****$p < 0.0001$). Similarly, after both **c** grey matter injections and **d** white matter injections, there was no overall statistical significant difference between the 20 and 60 min groups in the white matter. However, post hoc analysis demonstrated greater integrated densities at 60 min (compared to 20 min) −1 level caudal (**$p = 0.009$) and +1 level rostral (****$p < 0.0001$) to the injection site in **c** grey matter and **d** white matter injections respectively

to ovalbumin. Like other CED models and earlier ex vivo work on spinal cord ISF movement [14, 28, 30–34], in Endo's study a large durotomy was performed, resulting in substantial CSF leak and altered hydraulic integrity of the subarachnoid space and perivascular spaces, which may in turn alter fluid inflow dynamics. Computational simulation of the rat spinal cord by Sarntinoranont et al. [35] yielded a lower hydraulic conductivity in the grey matter and thus increased tissue resistance. They showed that diffusion of macromolecules *through* ECS is limited by tortuosity (higher in grey matter) and efficacy of diffusion diminishes as the square of distance. Diffusion *along* ECS is unaffected by these factors [1, 36]. This would account for the greater penetration of tracer from grey to white matter (compared to white to grey matter) in this study, and the higher fluorescence signal rostral to the injection site observed at 60 min in white matter injections (Fig. 2b). It may also explain the apparent increase in white matter fluorescence after white matter injections at 60 min compared to 20 min, and the absence of this in the grey matter after delivery of tracer into the grey matter (Fig. 7a, d).

Perivascular clearance

Various authors have used the terms "Virchow-Robin space", "perivascular space" and "paravascular space" interchangeably, but also at times to refer to discrete anatomical compartments. A comprehensive review of the ultrastructure of the "perivascular" space is beyond the scope of this article, but readers are referred to excellent treatises by Bakker et al. [37] and others [3, 38–40]. For our purposes, we distinguish the "peri-arterial space", which consists of multiple compartments within the pial sheath that accompanies the arteriole/artery as it enters the CNS parenchyma, from the "para-arterial space". The latter is the space formed by the glia limitans and the pial sheath of the penetrating artery. The "para-venular space" is formed by the venular adventitia and the glia limitans. Collectively the "para-arterial" and para-venular" spaces form the paravascular compartment. Henceforth, "perivascular space" loosely refers to all the compartments between vessel and glia limitans. These descriptions have been derived from brain studies [2, 3, 37, 38]. Ultrastructural studies of the rat spinal perivascular space suggest similar anatomy [41].

There is compelling evidence from our study supporting the importance of the vascular basement membrane in fluid outflow in the spinal cord. Controversy still surrounds the relationship of CSF, ISF and perivascular flow in the brain. There are two prominent contemporary theories of brain perivascular flow—the "glymphatic" system [10, 42] and a vascular basement membrane model [11]. The former was borne out of experiments on transgenic mice where intraventricular, intracerebral, and intracisternal injections of CSF tracers established CSF inflow into brain via a "para-arterial" route, bulk interstitial flow, and "para-venous" outflow. Other groups later raised concerns regarding the methodology and interpretation of observations [2–4, 8, 43–46]. The Carare–Weller group has long promulgated that fluid influx is via the para-arterial space and clearance of solutes and ISF occurs via the "peri-arterial" vascular basement membrane found within the tunica media. Their model has been backed by experiments from their own laboratory [11, 38, 47, 48] and from other groups employing intravital multiphoton microscopy [49]. They also assert that at the level of the capillaries, there is adjacent bidirectional flow of fluid, with inflow occurring adjacent to the glia limitans, and outflow of ISF occurring next to the endothelium. Notably, there is no venular involvement in fluid transport. The major points of dissent are: (1) the types of vascular structure(s) that are involved in ISF and solute egress; and (2) the precise relationship of the outflowing fluid to the various compartments surrounding these vessels. In this study, confocal microscopy demonstrated the presence of tracer not only in the "para-arterial" and "para-venular" spaces, but also in the "peri-arterial" compartment. It appeared that arterioles, venules and even capillaries are implicated in fluid outflow, and hence elements of both dominant theories (that are based on brain studies) have relevance in the spinal cord. Moreover, the vascular basement membrane (as proposed by Carare–Weller) has been shown here to play an important role in solute clearance in the spinal cord, which in turn suggests ISF outflow occurs both within and outside the wall of the arteriole. While injection pump pressure could confound our interpretation of interstitial perivascular tracer deposition, it is unlikely to explain tracer accumulation around only some extramedullary vessels and "remote" arterioles that are far removed from the bulk of the tracer. Moreover, our infusion rate of 0.12 μL/min is lower than that employed by other groups [3, 50], and thus is unlikely to alter the physiological drainage pathways. Uniform perivascular distribution of tracer around the spinal pial surface, which has been previously observed following cisterna magna injections [20, 41], was not detected in our experiments. Therefore, accidental delivery into, or recirculation of tracer from the cord back into the subarachnoid space are highly improbable.

Our findings raise the possibility of a model of spinal perivascular fluid dynamics characterised by rapid bidirectional movement. Some authors have suggested that there is little or no directed net fluid displacement in the perivascular space, a concept that aligns with earlier experimental data [2, 51]. A recent mathematical modelling study proposed that although there might be fast water movement to-and-fro in the perivascular space, solute transfer is facilitated by advection or dispersion [43]. Dispersion is in turn driven by arterial pulsations, which authors of disparate theories can all agree underlie the mechanism of perivascular flow [11, 16, 18, 52]. Additionally, solutes may freely communicate between the "para-arterial space" and the "peri-arterial" space through porous barriers that have been confirmed in ultrastructural studies of the spinal cord [2, 39, 41]. If this "convection" [3] theory of bidirectional fluid displacement also applies to the "para-venous" space, then tracer molecules injected into the cord parenchyma would disperse along both arteriolar and venular pathways by way of the capillaries [11]. Initially, there is "peri-arterial" drainage of solutes via the vascular basement membrane, but tracer is then able to infiltrate the "para-arterial" space. As pulsations are much stronger in arteries, tracer is propelled further along arterioles (towards the extramedullary arteries) compared to venules. This is reflected in the preponderance of tracer around extramedullary arteries and "remote" arterioles. However, we would also expect greater "para-venular" tracer deposition at 60 min compared to 20 min. This was, however, not observed, challenging this conjecture on perivascular fluid outflow. Future studies would mandate longer time points to investigate para-venular tracer distribution.

Central canal

Central canal labelling by tracer was detected in 50% of grey matter injection experiments, with a predilection for rostral migration. This corresponds to the earlier observation by Milhorat [22] of cephalad flow within the central canal, which gave rise to the theory that it acts as a "sink" for excess solutes and fluid from the cord interstitium. Previous work by our group and others has indicated that the central canal is a route of clearance in normal and injured rat and ovine cords [18–20, 24–26, 53, 54]. Bedussi et al. have suggested that in the brain, ISF drains preferentially towards the ependymal surface. However, this was only true in close proximity to the ependymal lining and the effect decreased away from the ventricles [15]. In the spinal cord the distance between the ependymal and pial surfaces is much smaller, so the relevance of this hypothesis is unclear. A more likely explanation for the disparate central canal labelling between grey and white matter injected animals is that diffusivity differences (which in turn are dependent on factors such as tortuosity and distance) at the grey/white matter junction result in the central canal playing a critical role in fluid outflow from the grey matter. It was not possible to clarify, based on confocal micrographs, whether tracer migration into the central canal was transcellular, paracellular or both. Further ultrastructural studies may address this.

Clinical relevance

Findings from these experiments may contribute to a clearer understanding of various spinal cord pathologies. Although outflow pathways have been shown here to involve all vascular structures, there may be regional variations. In the spinal grey matter, there is prominent drainage of solutes and ISF via the numerous ramifying arteries from the ventral median sulcus, as well as into the central canal. In the white matter, outflow efficiency may differ as there are fewer arterioles, and greater reliance on the smaller arterial vasocorona. Extrapolating further, extra-canalicular syringomyelia (a consequence of spinal cord injuries) may be partly precipitated by pathological processes disproportionately compromising ISF drainage via white matter perivascular spaces. Outflow is unable to keep up with fluid influx, ultimately leading to fluid accumulation. Similarly, this may partially explain why spinal cord oedema preferentially follows white matter tracts, as in the grey matter there may be more robust drainage pathways.

Limitations

As some authors have emphasized [10] that for maintenance of perivascular bulk flow the hydraulic parameters of the subarachnoid and perivascular spaces cannot be compromised. Although CSF losses were not observed during injections in this study, small leaks cannot be ruled out and may account for the relatively limited longitudinal displacement of ovalbumin, and the absence of statistical significance in tracer redistribution between 20 and 60 min. The apparent lack of tracer displacement between the two time points could also be explained by the possibility that these experiments were, at least partially, an investigation of spinal convection enhanced delivery. Other groups have noted that in CED studies, spinal cord injury results in migration of tracer across the grey–white border [31]. We used the smallest calibre needle possible, but there was still some evidence of local parenchymal trauma due to the cyclical movements of respiration. Unlike in Endo's study where Evan's blue did not cross the grey/white junction after white matter injections, tracer in this study was not completely contained within white matter at the level of injection. As with other tracer studies, labelling of the "pial glial" layer and the smooth muscle basement membrane may be explained by selective binding of tracer or by a sieving effect [8]. Fluid passage within the dorsal white columns was not directly investigated. As this area is isolated from the rest of the white matter the pattern of fluid outflow could theoretically be different. In future investigations of spinal cord fluid outflow, longer experimental time points are recommended. This would validate some of the observed differences between grey and white matter tracer distribution patterns. It may also provide insight into whether spinal CED was actually investigated in these experiments, as well as the role arterial pulsations might play in driving tracer outflow—para-venular tracer deposition may increase with time (see above). It was not possible to quantify the amount of tracer outflow via the various pathways due to the semi-quantitative nature of our results. Finally, these findings were obtained in anaesthetised prone small animals and extrapolation of these findings to upright large mammals should proceed cautiously as volatile anaesthetics are known to alter cardiovascular parameters and CSF production, which in turn affects CSF hydrodynamics [8].

Conclusions

This study investigated the pattern and pathways of fluid outflow in the rat spinal cord. Our results suggest interstitial fluid is transported radially in the grey matter, and along the parallel axonal fibres in the white matter. Fluid outflow appears to be limited predominantly to a few spinal segments after 60 min. Paravascular and perivascular pathways, including both arterial and venous routes, likely play important roles in fluid efflux. The precise mechanisms by which the vascular basement membrane of arteries act as a conduit for fluid and solute drainage from the spinal cord warrants further investigation. There may be regional variations in fluid outflow pattern within the spinal cord due to the presence of the central canal and differences between grey and white matter in vascular anatomy. These results suggest interstitial fluid dynamics are more complicated than that described by the glymphatic model.

Abbreviations

AFO-647: Alexa Fluor Ovalbumin 647; ASA: anterior spinal artery; CED: convection enhanced delivery; CFD: computational fluid dynamics; CNS: central nervous system; CSF: cerebrospinal fluid; ECS: extracellular space; GM: grey matter; GMi: grey matter injection; ISF: interstitial fluid; MRI: magnetic resonance imaging; NDS: normal donkey serum; PBS: phosphate buffered solution; PFA: paraformaldehyde; RECA-1: rat endothelial cell antigen-1; SAS: subarachnoid space; SEM: standard error of mean; SMA: smooth muscle antibody; WM: white matter; WMi: white matter injection.

Authors' contributions

MAS and LEB conceived the original idea; MAS, LEB, SL and MAL experimental design; MAL, SL, SJH, AS, conducted the experiments at Macquarie University. SL analysed the data. SL interpreted the results of the data analysis. SL drafted the manuscript; all authors reviewed the manuscript. All authors read and approved the final manuscript.

Author details

[1] Department of Clinical Medicine, Faculty of Medicine and Health Sciences, Macquarie University, Suite 407, Clinic Building, 2 Technology Place, Sydney, NSW 2109, Australia. [2] Neuroscience Research Australia, Prince of Wales Clinical School, University of New South Wales, Margarete Ainsworth Building, Barker Street, Randwick, Sydney, NSW 2031, Australia.

Competing interests

The authors declare that they have no competing interests.

Datasets

The datasets used and/or analysed during the current study are available from the corresponding author on reasonable request.

Funding

This work was supported by the Column of Hope Research Foundation and the National Health and Medical Research Council.

References

1. Coles JA, Myburgh E, Brewer JM, McMenamin PG. Where are we? The anatomy of the murine cortical meninges revisited for intravital imaging, immunology, and clearance of waste from the brain. Prog Neurobiol. 2017;156:107–48.
2. Brinker T, Stopa E, Morrison J, Klinge P. A new look at cerebrospinal fluid circulation. Fluids Barriers CNS. 2014;11:10.
3. Hladky SB, Barrand MA. Mechanisms of fluid movement into, through and out of the brain: evaluation of the evidence. Fluids Barriers CNS. 2014;11:26.
4. Spector R, Keep RF, Robert Snodgrass S, Smith QR, Johanson CE. A balanced view of choroid plexus structure and function: focus on adult humans. Exp Neurol. 2015;267:78–86.
5. Abbott NJ. Evidence for bulk flow of brain interstitial fluid: significance for physiology and pathology. Neurochem Int. 2004;45:545–52.
6. Hladky SB, Barrand MA. Fluid and ion transfer across the blood–brain and blood–cerebrospinal fluid barriers; a comparative account of mechanisms and roles. Fluids Barriers CNS. 2016;13:19.
7. Mokgokong R, Wang S, Taylor CJ, Barrand MA, Hladky SB. Ion transporters in brain endothelial cells that contribute to formation of brain interstitial fluid. Pflugers Arch. 2014;466:887–901.
8. Spector R, Robert Snodgrass S, Johanson CE. A balanced view of the cerebrospinal fluid composition and functions: focus on adult humans. Exp Neurol. 2015;273:57–68.
9. Rennels ML, Gregory TF, Blaumanis OR, Fujimoto K, Grady PA. Evidence for a 'paravascular' fluid circulation in the mammalian central nervous system, provided by the rapid distribution of tracer protein throughout the brain from the subarachnoid space. Brain Res. 1985;326:47–63.
10. Iliff JJ, Wang M, Liao Y, Plogg BA, Peng W, Gundersen GA, Benveniste H, Vates GE, Deane R, Goldman SA, et al. A paravascular pathway facilitates CSF flow through the brain parenchyma and the clearance of interstitial solutes, including amyloid β. Sci Transl Med. 2012;4:147ra111.
11. Carare RO, Bernardes-Silva M, Newman TA, Page AM, Nicoll JA, Perry VH, Weller RO. Solutes, but not cells, drain from the brain parenchyma along basement membranes of capillaries and arteries: significance for cerebral amyloid angiopathy and neuroimmunology. Neuropathol Appl Neurobiol. 2008;34:131–44.
12. Bilston LE, Fletcher DF, Brodbelt AR, Stoodley MA. Arterial pulsation-driven cerebrospinal fluid flow in the perivascular space: a computational model. Comput Methods Biomech Biomed Eng. 2003;6:235–41.
13. Cserr HF, Cooper DN, Milhorat TH. Flow of cerebral interstitial fluid as indicated by the removal of extracellular markers from rat caudate nucleus. Exp Eye Res. 1977;25(Suppl):461–73.
14. Sykova E, Nicholson C. Diffusion in brain extracellular space. Physiol Rev. 2008;88:1277–340.
15. Bedussi B, van Lier MG, Bartstra JW, de Vos J, Siebes M, VanBavel E, Bakker EN. Clearance from the mouse brain by convection of interstitial fluid towards the ventricular system. Fluids Barriers CNS. 2015;12:23.
16. Iliff JJ, Wang M, Zeppenfeld DM, Venkataraman A, Plog BA, Liao Y, Deane R, Nedergaard M. Cerebral arterial pulsation drives paravascular CSF-interstitial fluid exchange in the murine brain. J Neurosci. 2013;33:18190–9.
17. Jessen NA, Munk AS, Lundgaard I, Nedergaard M. The glymphatic system: a Beginner's guide. Neurochem Res. 2015;40:2583–99.

18. Stoodley MA, Brown SA, Brown CJ, Jones NR. Arterial pulsation-dependent perivascular cerebrospinal fluid flow into the central canal in the sheep spinal cord. J Neurosurg. 1997;86:686–93.
19. Stoodley MA, Jones NR, Brown CJ. Evidence for rapid fluid flow from the subarachnoid space into the spinal cord central canal in the rat. Brain Res. 1996;707:155–64.
20. Wei F, Zhang C, Xue R, Shan L, Gong S, Wang G, Tao J, Xu G, Zhang G, Wang L. The pathway of subarachnoid CSF moving into the spinal parenchyma and the role of astrocytic aquaporin-4 in this process. Life Sci. 2017;182:29–40.
21. Endo T, Fujii Y, Sugiyama SI, Zhang R, Ogita S, Funamoto K, Saito R, Tominaga T. Properties of convective delivery in spinal cord gray matter: laboratory investigation and computational simulations. J Neurosurg Spine. 2016;24:359–66.
22. Milhorat THNS, Heger I, Nobandegani F, Murray S. Ultrastructural evidence of sink function of central canal of spinal cord as demonstrated by clearance of horseradish peroxidase. Proc Electron Microsc Soc Am. 1992;50:700–1.
23. Rossi C, Boss A, Steidle G, Martirosian P, Klose U, Capuani S, Maraviglia B, Claussen CD, Schick F. Water diffusion anisotropy in white and gray matter of the human spinal cord. J Magn Reson Imaging. 2008;27:476–82.
24. Brodbelt AR, Stoodley MA, Watling AM, Tu J, Jones NR. Fluid flow in an animal model of post-traumatic syringomyelia. Eur Spine J. 2003;12:300–6.
25. Stoodley MA, Gutschmidt B, Jones NR. Cerebrospinal fluid flow in an animal model of noncommunicating syringomyelia. Neurosurgery. 1999;44:1065–76.
26. Wong J, Hemley S, Jones N, Cheng S, Bilston L, Stoodley M. Fluid outflow in a large-animal model of posttraumatic syringomyelia. Neurosurgery. 2012;71:474–80.
27. Schneider CA, Rasband WS, Eliceiri KW. NIH Image to ImageJ: 25 years of image analysis. Nat Methods. 2012;9:671–5.
28. Prokopova S, Vargova L, Sykova E. Heterogeneous and anisotropic diffusion in the developing rat spinal cord. NeuroReport. 1997;8:3527–32.
29. Ellingson BM, Ulmer JL, Kurpad SN, Schmit BD. Diffusion tensor MR imaging in chronic spinal cord injury. AJNR Am J Neuroradiol. 2008;29:1976–82.
30. Lonser RR, Gogate N, Morrison PF, Wood JD, Oldfield EH. Direct convective delivery of macromolecules to the spinal cord. J Neurosurg. 1998;89:616–22.
31. Wood JD, Lonser RR, Gogate N, Morrison PF, Oldfield EH. Convective delivery of macromolecules into the naive and traumatized spinal cords of rats. J Neurosurg. 1999;90:115–20.
32. Simonova Z, Svoboda J, Orkand P, Bernard CC, Lassmann H, Sykova E. Changes of extracellular space volume and tortuosity in the spinal cord of Lewis rats with experimental autoimmune encephalomyelitis. Physiol Res. 1996;45:11–22.
33. Svoboda J, Sykova E. Extracellular space volume changes in the rat spinal cord produced by nerve stimulation and peripheral injury. Brain Res. 1991;560:216–24.
34. Sykova E, Vargova L, Prokopova S, Simonova Z. Glial swelling and astrogliosis produce diffusion barriers in the rat spinal cord. Glia. 1999;25:56–70.
35. Sarntinoranont M, Chen X, Zhao J, Mareci TH. Computational model of interstitial transport in the spinal cord using diffusion tensor imaging. Ann Biomed Eng. 2006;34:1304–21.
36. Nicholson C, Chen KC, Hrabetova S, Tao L. Diffusion of molecules in brain extracellular space: theory and experiment. Prog Brain Res. 2000;125:129–54.
37. Bakker EN, Bacskai BJ, Arbel-Ornath M, Aldea R, Bedussi B, Morris AW, Weller RO, Carare RO. Lymphatic clearance of the brain: perivascular, paravascular and significance for neurodegenerative diseases. Cell Mol Neurobiol. 2016;36:181–94.
38. Morris AW, Sharp MM, Albargothy NJ, Fernandes R, Hawkes CA, Verma A, Weller RO, Carare RO. Vascular basement membranes as pathways for the passage of fluid into and out of the brain. Acta Neuropathol. 2016;131:725–36.
39. Woollam DH, Millen JW. The perivascular spaces of the mammalian central nervous system and their relation to the perineuronal and subarachnoid spaces. J Anat. 1955;89:193–200.
40. Weller RO, Sharp MM, Christodoulides M, Carare RO, Mollgard K. The meninges as barriers and facilitators for the movement of fluid, cells and pathogens related to the rodent and human CNS. Acta Neuropathol. 2018;135:363–85.
41. Lam MA, Hemley SJ, Najafi E, Vella NGF, Bilston LE, Stoodley MA. The ultrastructure of spinal cord perivascular spaces: implications for the circulation of cerebrospinal fluid. Sci Rep. 2017;7:12924.
42. Simon MJ, Iliff JJ. Regulation of cerebrospinal fluid (CSF) flow in neurodegenerative, neurovascular and neuroinflammatory disease. Biochim Biophys Acta. 2016;1862:442–51.
43. Asgari M, de Zélicourt D, Kurtcuoglu V. Glymphatic solute transport does not require bulk flow. Sci Rep. 2016;6:38635.
44. Jin BJ, Smith AJ, Verkman AS. Spatial model of convective solute transport in brain extracellular space does not support a "glymphatic" mechanism. J Gen Physiol. 2016;148:489–501.
45. Smith AJ, Yao X, Dix JA, Jin BJ, Verkman AS. Test of the 'glymphatic' hypothesis demonstrates diffusive and aquaporin-4-independent solute transport in rodent brain parenchyma. Elife. 2017. https://doi.org/10.7554/eLife.27679.
46. Abbott NJ, Pizzo ME, Preston JE, Janigro D, Thorne RG. The role of brain barriers in fluid movement in the CNS: is there a 'glymphatic' system? Acta Neuropathol. 2018;135:387–407.
47. Hawkes CA, Jayakody N, Johnston DA, Bechmann I, Carare RO. Failure of perivascular drainage of beta-amyloid in cerebral amyloid angiopathy. Brain Pathol. 2014;24:396–403.
48. Weller RO, Djuanda E, Yow HY, Carare RO. Lymphatic drainage of the brain and the pathophysiology of neurological disease. Acta Neuropathol. 2009;117:1–14.
49. Arbel-Ornath M, Hudry E, Eikermann-Haerter K, Hou S, Gregory JL, Zhao L, Betensky RA, Frosch MP, Greenberg SM, Bacskai BJ. Interstitial fluid drainage is impaired in ischemic stroke and Alzheimer's disease mouse models. Acta Neuropathol. 2013;126:353–64.
50. Morrison PF, Laske DW, Bobo H, Oldfield EH, Dedrick RL. High-flow microinfusion: tissue penetration and pharmacodynamics. Am J Physiol. 1994;266:R292–305.
51. Ichimura T, Fraser PA, Cserr HF. Distribution of extracellular tracers in perivascular spaces of the rat brain. Brain Res. 1991;545:103–13.
52. Schley D, Carare-Nnadi R, Please CP, Perry VH, Weller RO. Mechanisms to explain the reverse perivascular transport of solutes out of the brain. J Theor Biol. 2006;238:962–74.
53. Stoodley MA, Jones NR, Yang L, Brown CJ. Mechanisms underlying the formation and enlargement of noncommunicating syringomyelia: experimental studies. Neurosurg Focus. 2000;8:1–7.
54. Murtha LA, Yang Q, Parsons MW, Levi CR, Beard DJ, Spratt NJ, McLeod DD. Cerebrospinal fluid is drained primarily via the spinal canal and olfactory route in young and aged spontaneously hypertensive rats. Fluids Barriers CNS. 2014;11:12.

19

Functional brain-specific microvessels from iPSC-derived human brain microvascular endothelial cells: the role of matrix composition on monolayer formation

Moriah E. Katt[1,2*], Raleigh M. Linville[1,3], Lakyn N. Mayo[1,2], Zinnia S. Xu[1,3] and Peter C. Searson[1,2]

Abstract

Background: Transwell-based models of the blood–brain barrier (BBB) incorporating monolayers of human brain microvascular endothelial cells (dhBMECs) derived from induced pluripotent stem cells show many of the key features of the BBB, including expression of transporters and efflux pumps, expression of tight junction proteins, and physiological values of transendothelial electrical resistance. The fabrication of 3D BBB models using dhBMECs has so far been unsuccessful due to the poor adhesion and survival of these cells on matrix materials commonly used in tissue engineering.

Methods: To address this issue, we systematically screened a wide range of matrix materials (collagen I, hyaluronic acid, and fibrin), compositions (laminin/entactin), protein coatings (fibronectin, laminin, collagen IV, perlecan, and agrin), and soluble factors (ROCK inhibitor and cyclic adenosine monophosphate) in 2D culture to assess cell adhesion, spreading, and barrier function.

Results: Cell coverage increased with stiffness of collagen I gels coated with collagen IV and fibronectin. On 7 mg mL^{-1} collagen I gels coated with basement membrane proteins (fibronectin, collagen IV, and laminin), cell coverage was high but did not reliably reach confluence. The transendothelial electrical resistance (TEER) on collagen I gels coated with basement membrane proteins was lower than on coated transwell membranes. Agrin, a heparin sulfate proteoglycan found in basement membranes of the brain, promoted monolayer formation but resulted in a significant decrease in transendothelial electrical resistance (TEER). However, the addition of ROCK inhibitor, cAMP, or cross-linking the gels to increase stiffness, resulted in a significant improvement of TEER values and enabled the formation of confluent monolayers.

Conclusions: Having identified matrix compositions that promote monolayer formation and barrier function, we successfully fabricated dhBMEC microvessels in cross-linked collagen I gels coated with fibronectin and collagen IV, and treated with ROCK inhibitor and cAMP. We measured apparent permeability values for Lucifer yellow, comparable to values obtained in the transwell assay. During these experiments we observed no focal leaks, suggesting the formation of tight junctions that effectively block paracellular transport.

Keywords: Brain microvascular endothelial cells, Stem cells, Transendothelial electrical resistance, Microvessels, Tissue-engineering

*Correspondence: mknigh14@jhu.edu
[1] Institute for Nanobiotechnology, Johns Hopkins University, Baltimore, MD, USA
Full list of author information is available at the end of the article

Background

Brain microvascular endothelial cells (BMECs) are highly specialized with tight junctions that effectively eliminate paracellular transport, transporters to deliver essential nutrients to the brain, and efflux pumps to transport unwanted substrates back into circulation [1, 2]. The lack of physiologically relevant BMEC lines has been a major roadblock to blood–brain barrier (BBB) research [3], however, stem cell technology has provided a potential solution to this problem [4].

Human induced pluripotent stem cells (hiPSC) have been used extensively to study cells with neuronal lineages in both health and disease [5–7]. More recently iPSCs have been differentiated into brain microvascular endothelial cells (dhBMECs) from a number of iPSC lines including: BC1 [8], IMR90-4 [4, 9–11], ARiPS [11], DF6-9-9T [12], DF19-9-11T [12], H9 embryonic stem cells, as well as patient lines from Huntington's disease [13]. All of these iPSC lines produce dhBMECs with characteristics of the BBB, including high transendothelial electrical resistance (TEER), greater than 1000 Ω cm^2 for cells from healthy individuals, claudin-5- and occludin-positive tight junctions, polarized P-gp efflux, $\geq$ 90% endothelial purity, and many other important characteristics of the BBB [4, 8–15]. Therefore, differentiated iPSCs play an important role in BBB research since they provide a renewable and reproducible source of human BMECs.

Accumulating evidence suggests that in addition to their barrier function, human brain microvascular endothelial cells exhibit other unique characteristics that contribute to their phenotype. For example, in cell culture hBMECs and dhBMECs do not undergo a transition from cobblestone to spindle morphology under shear flow [16, 17]. Similarly hBMECs and dhBMECs do not elongate and align in response to the high curvature of capillary dimensions [8, 18].

While 2D transwell models provide an important tool in BBB research [1, 19], recent attention has focused on the fabrication of 3D models that recapitulate the cylindrical microvessel geometry and shear flow. Advances in tissue engineering have enabled fabrication of functional endothelial microvessels in a gel matrix [20–25], however, attempts to recapitulate the key characteristics of the BBB using primary or immortalized BMECs have had limited success [26–28]. Stem-cell derived hBMECs provide a potential solution to this problem, although incorporation of dhBMECs into tissue-engineered BBB models has been challenging since dhBMECs are less adherent and proliferative than other endothelial cells.

The objective of this work was to identify matrix compositions for the formation of confluent dhBMEC monolayers and maintenance of barrier function. We first screened adhesion and spreading of dhBMECs on 2D collagen I gels as a function of gel stiffness, composition (collagen I and collagen I + laminin/entactin), surface modification (fibronectin, laminin, collagen IV, perlecan, and agrin), and the addition of soluble factors [ROCK inhibitor Y-27632 and cyclic adenosine monophosphate (cAMP)]. We then assessed barrier function of dhBMEC monolayers on porous supports with different coatings or bulk hydrogels. Finally, having identified conditions that promote formation of confluent monolayers with physiological barrier properties in 2D, we then demonstrated the formation of perfusable brain-specific microvessels with confluent monolayers of dhBMECs in a genipin—crosslinked collagen I matrix coated with fibronectin and collagen IV with the addition of the ROCK inhibitor Y-27632 and cAMP in the perfusion media during seeding.

Methods

Cell culture and differentiation

BC1 GFP iPSCs were cultured and differentiated as previously reported [8]. Briefly, iPSCs were cultured on matrigel-coated tissue culture flasks (Corning, Corning, New York, USA) in TeSR-E8™ medium (StemCell Technologies, Vancouver, BC, Canada) to 50% confluence. Then the media was switched to unconditioned media without basic fibroblast growth factor [DMEM/F12 supplemented with 80% KOSR, 1% non-essential amino acids, 0.5% glutaMAX, and 0.836 μM beta-mercaptoethanol (Life Technologies, Carlsbad, California, USA)] for 7 days, then transferred to endothelial cell medium [endothelial cell serum free medium, 1% human platelet poor-derived serum, 20 ng mL^{-1} bFGF (R&D Systems, Minneapolis, Minnesota, USA), 10 μM retinoic acid (Sigma, St. Louis, Missouri, USA)]. Cells were then sub-cultured on collagen IV and fibronectin coated plates for 1 h before being subsequently passaged onto the experimental substrate at a density of 1×10^6, or 5×10^6 cells mL^{-1} on transwells. In previous work we have shown that confluent monolayers are formed on collagen IV and fibronectin-coated glass and transwell supports at this density [8]. The medium was changed 24 h following subculture and every 48 h after that. Where indicated cells were treated with 10 μM ROCK inhibitor (Y-27632) (ATCC, Manassas, Virginia, USA) for the first 24 h and 100 μM dibutyryl cyclic AMP (Sigma) throughout culture following subculture.

Matrix formation

Unless otherwise stated, gels were fabricated from collagen I (Corning) ranging from 4 to 7 mg mL^{-1} neutralized with sodium hydroxide. Laminin/entactin (Corning) was added to collagen I gels at densities of 0.25–1 mg mL^{-1}.

Collagen I gels were formed at 37 °C for 30 min and then coated with 50 μg mL^{-1} of proteins and heparan sulfate proteoglycans at 37 °C overnight. The thickness of the gels was 300–500 μm. Where indicated, the gels were cross-linked with 20 mM genipin (Sigma) for 2 h and washed with PBS for 24–48 h at room temperature before coating. Genipin is a low molecular weight cross-linker that has been used previously to enhance vascular stability and increases the stiffness of collagen fivefold [29]. Collagen I gels were coated with collagen IV (Sigma), fibronectin (Life Technologies), laminin (Sigma), agrin (R&D Systems), and/or perlecan (R&D Systems).

Immunofluorescence

To image monolayers, the gels were fixed and stained, then inverted on a glass slide. Four days after seeding, gels were washed with PBS then fixed in 3.7% paraformaldehyde for 10 min. Cells were then permeablized for 1 h in 0.1% Triton-X100 and blocked for 1 h in 10% donkey serum in PBS. Primary antibodies were incubated overnight at 4 °C in 10% donkey serum followed by 1 h incubation with secondary antibodies in 10% donkey serum. Cells were stained for ZO-1 (Life Technologies), claudin-5 (Life Technologies), and DAPI as described previously [8]. Imaging was performed on a Nikon TiE confocal microscope using 40× objective and NIS Advanced Research software (Nikon, Minato, Tokyo, Japan). The images are maximum intensity projections of confocal z-stacks with a z spacing of 0.4 μm.

Transendothelial electrical resistance

Transendothelial electrical resistance (TEER) was measured daily for 1 week after seeding on polyester 12-well transwell membranes with a 0.4 μm pore size (Corning), as previously described [8]. TEER measurements were recorded using a STX2 probe with EVOM2 (World Precision Instruments, Sarasota, Florida, USA). Peak TEER values on coated transwells were typically recorded between days 2 and 4 and were used for comparison to experiments where monolayers were formed on bulk gels (300–500 μm thick) in the transwell inserts, as described above. Note that TEER values on 12-well transwell inserts are typically 2.5-fold higher than the values of around 2000 Ω cm^2 reported on 24-well inserts [8, 10]. All TEER experiments were performed in triplicate (3 wells) for each of three distinct differentiations.

Cell coverage and junctional analysis

The endothelial cell coverage on different substrates was measured from phase contrast images of cells on coated gels daily for 3 days. Images were taken following a wash and media exchange step to ensure only adherent cells were considered in analysis. Images were taken in three randomly selected areas of the plate for three separate differentiations, resulting in at least nine images per condition. Images were then analyzed using Image J to determine the percent coverage. Cell area was calculated from maximum intensity ZO-1 projection images manually using ImageJ on at least 75 cells per condition. Measurements of cell–cell junction width were obtained from claudin-5 confocal z-stack images with a slice height of 0.4 μm from at least 150 junctions. Slices where the claudin-5 junctions were clear and in focus, which ranged from 3 to 10 slices, were stacked and the width of the junction in the collective images were measured in NIS Advanced Research software (Additional file 1: Figure S1).

Statistical analysis

Statistical differences in coverage and TEER were determined using one-way ANOVA, with Tukey's multiple comparisons test. P values of less than 0.05 were considered statistically significant (*), with $P \leq 0.01$ represented with **, and $P \leq 0.001$ represented with ***.

Microvessel fabrication and characterization

Microvessels were fabricated as previously reported [22]. Briefly, neutralized 7 mg mL^{-1} collagen I was injected into a polydimethylsiloxane and glass enclosure around a 150 μm diameter Nitinol template rod and allowed to gel at 37 °C. 2% agarose was injected at the ends of the collagen I to prevent delamination. After template rod removal, channels were cross-linked with 20 mM genipin for 2 h and washed with PBS for 24–48 h. The platform was then treated overnight with endothelial cell medium containing 50 μg mL^{-1} fibronectin and 100 μg mL^{-1} collagen IV at 37 °C. Endothelial cell media was supplemented with 10 μM retinoic acid, 400 μM dibutyryl cyclic AMP, 20 μM phosphodiesterase inhibitor Ro-20-1724 (Sigma), and 3% 70 kDa dextran (Sigma) to promote vascular stability [29–31]. dhBMECs were introduced into the channel at a density of 6×10^7 cells mL^{-1} under low flow and allowed to settle and adhere for 1 h. Low shear flow (~ 0.1 dyn cm^{-1}) was applied for the first 24 h; during this time the media was additionally supplemented with 10 μM ROCK inhibitor. Flow was increased after 24 h to 1.0 dyn cm^{-1}.

Three days after seeding, the permeability of the microvessels to Lucifer yellow was measured using methods reported previously [22, 32]. 100 μM Lucifer yellow (Sigma) was perfused through microvessels for 45 min, and fluorescence images recorded every 5 min. Images were analyzed using ImageJ, and apparent permeability was calculated from $P_{app} = (d/4)(1/\Delta I)(dI/dt)$ where d is the vessel diameter, ΔI is the initial increase in fluorescence intensity due to perfusion in the lumen, and (dI/dt) is the rate of increase in fluorescence intensity. Imaging was performed on a Nikon TiE microscope using 10× objective and NIS Advanced Research software. Permeability was measured in microvessels seeded from three distinct differentiations.

Results

Extracellular matrix (ECM)

To assess cell adhesion and spreading, dhBMECs were seeded onto gels with different composition, stiffness, and coatings. To compare adhesion across different conditions we measured the coverage of the dhBMECs over the first 72 h of culture. In general, cells either adhered to the matrix and formed monolayers, or showed poor adhesion and formed small mounds that eventually detached from the matrix (Additional file 1: Figure S2).

ECM composition and concentration

To assess the role of ECM stiffness on monolayer formation, dhBMECs were seeded onto collagen I gels coated with fibronectin and collagen IV. The fractional coverage of dhBMECs was strongly dependent on ECM stiffness, with coverages ranging from 7 ± 1% on 4 mg mL^{-1} gels to 72 ± 7% on 7 mg mL^{-1} gels 72 h after seeding (Fig. 1a). For the lowest collagen concentrations (4 and 5 mg mL^{-1}), the cell coverage decreased with time as mounds of cells coalesced on the surface. In contrast to the dhBMECs, other widely used human- and animal-derived ECs form confluent monolayers when seeded onto collagen I gels in this concentration range [22–24, 33, 34]. For the highest collagen concentrations (6 and 7 mg mL^{-1}), the cell coverage increased with time due to spreading and proliferation.

We assessed monolayer formation on 7 mg mL^{-1} collagen I gels with the addition of 0.25, 0.5, 0.75, and 1 mg mL^{-1} laminin/entactin and coated with collagen IV and fibronectin (Fig. 1b). The laminin concentrations were based on previous studies of neuronal outgrowth and cerebral organoid development [35, 36]. The addition of laminin/entactin did not change the cell coverage, even at the highest concentration (Fig. 1b). In each case the coverage increased with time, up to around 70% after 72 h, similar to the control with no laminin/entactin.

Basement membrane components: fibronectin, laminin, collagen IV, perlecan, and agrin

To assess the role of basement membrane proteins on adhesion and spreading in more detail, 7 mg mL^{-1} collagen gels were coated with combinations of basement membrane proteins. Monolayers formed on collagen I gels coated with combinations of basement membrane proteins were not fully confluent, leaving large openings in the monolayer that did not close following 3 days of culture. However, in all cases, coating with basement membrane proteins resulted in higher cell coverage compared to the control with no coating (Fig. 1c). There was no statistical difference in the area covered by the cells between coating with one, two, or three components.

Coating collagen I gels with heparan sulfate proteoglycans resulted in a highly variable propensity for monolayer formation (Fig. 1d). On gels coated with perlecan or a combination of perlecan, fibronectin, and collagen IV, dhBMECs showed poor adhesion, similar to the uncoated control. In contrast, on gels with agrin or a combination of agrin, fibronectin, and collagen IV, complete monolayers were formed. Monolayer formation was also observed on gels coated with agrin and perlecan or a combination of agrin, perlecan, fibronectin, and collagen IV. These results suggest that agrin is important in promoting adhesion of dhBMECs.

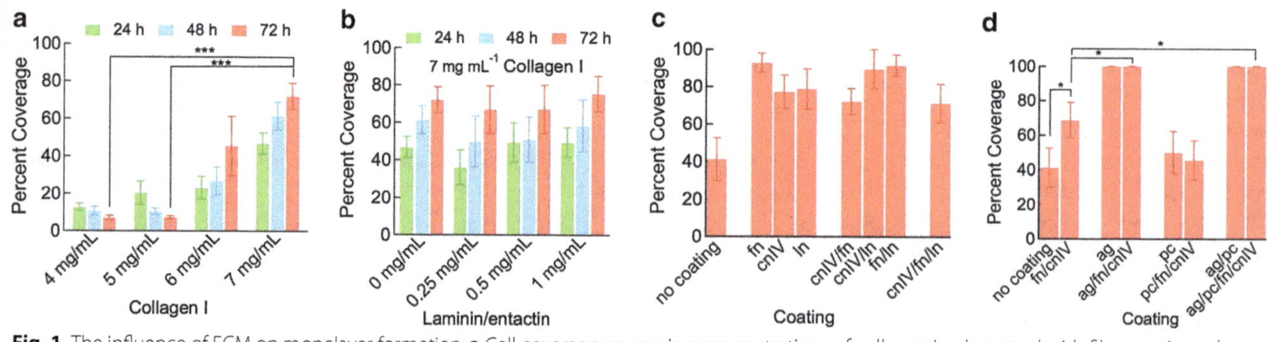

Fig. 1 The influence of ECM on monolayer formation. **a** Cell coverage on varying concentrations of collagen I gels coated with fibronectin and collagen IV at 24, 48, and 72 h following seeding. **b** Cell coverage on 7 mg mL^{-1} collagen I gels supplemented with laminin/entactin and coated with fibronectin and collagen IV. **c** Coverage on 7 mg mL^{-1} collagen I gel coated with the proteins indicated fn—fibronectin, cnIV—collagen IV, ln—laminin. All coatings result in significantly higher coverage compared to uncoated collagen I gels ($P < 0.05$), with no difference between different coatings ($P > 0.05$). **d** Coverage on 7 mg mL^{-1} collagen I gel coated with selected proteins (fn—fibronectin, cnIV—collagen IV) and selected heparan sulfate proteoglycans (ag—agrin, pc—perlecan). Bars represent mean ± standard error, * represents $p < 0.05$, *** represents $p < 0.001$

Barrier function

Cell adhesion and spreading is important for monolayer formation, but does not necessarily confirm barrier function. The formation of tight junctions minimizes paracellular transport, a key feature of the BBB. To assess barrier function we measured the transendothelial electrical resistance (TEER) of dhBMEC monolayers on transwell membranes and on transwell membranes modified with bulk collagen I gels (Fig. 2a).

Barrier function of monolayers on transwell membranes coated with basement membrane components

TEER values for dhBMEC monolayers on transwell membranes coated with fibronectin and collagen IV were around 4400 Ω cm^2 48 h after seeding, and were used as the control. To avoid the influence of the different coatings on dhBMEC purification/selection, cells were sub-cultured in tissue culture flasks coated with collagen IV and fibronectin for 1 h before seeding on the coated transwell membranes. After the subculture step, TEER values of dhBMEC monolayers on membranes coated with fibronectin and collagen IV were around 5700 cm^2. hBMEC monolayers on membranes coated with fibronectin, fibronectin and collagen IV, or collagen IV and laminin showed similarly high TEER values (Fig. 2b). In contrast, the TEER of dhBMECs on agrin-coated membranes was 5 Ω cm^2, significantly lower than the control. These results show that the formation of a confluent monolayer is not sufficient to confirm barrier formation since agrin promotes monolayer formation (Fig. 1d), but these monolayers failed to develop barrier properties, as indicated by the low TEER values. However, monolayers on membranes coated with agrin and fibronectin show similar TEER to fibronectin-coated membranes and the control.

Barrier function of monolayers on collagen I gels

To assess barrier function of monolayers under conditions relevant for 3D, we measured TEER values of monolayers on collagen I gels on the transwell membranes (Fig. 2c, Additional file 1: Figure S3). Cell monolayers on fibronectin-coated gels showed TEER values of 840 Ω cm^2, significantly lower than on the transwell membranes. Similar TEER values were obtained for gels coated with fibronectin, collagen IV, and laminin. Monolayers on gels coated with agrin, exhibited TEER values about 100 Ω cm^2. Monolayers on gels coated with agrin and other basement membrane components exhibited TEER values from 80 to 400 Ω cm^2.

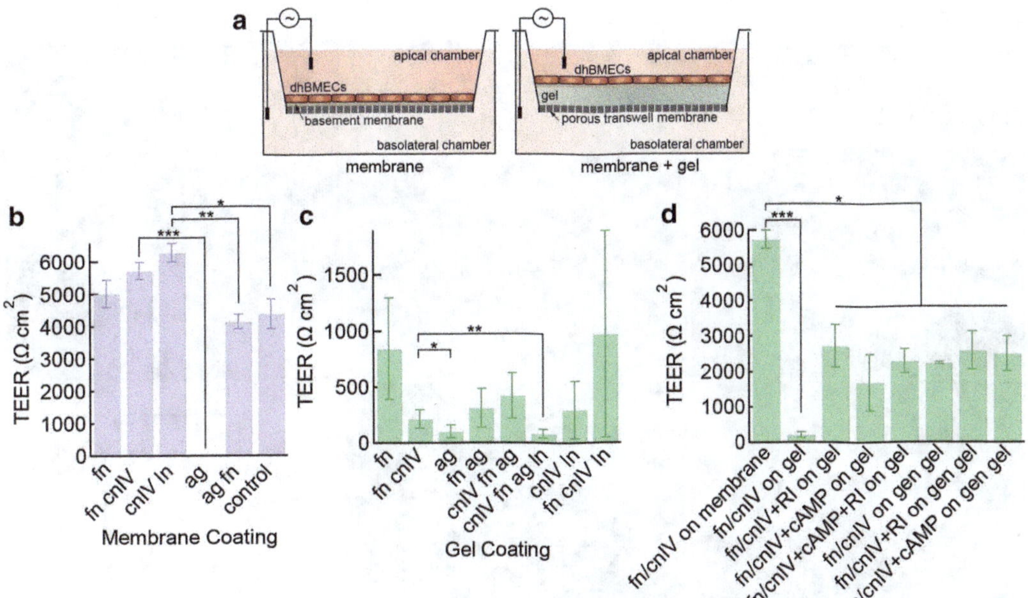

Fig. 2 Barrier function of dhBMEC monolayers. **a** Schematic illustration of transwell assay for TEER measurements for dhBMEC monolayers on coated membranes or collagen I gels and membrane coatings. **b** Peak TEER on membranes coated with basement membrane proteins and heparan sulfate proteoglycans that resulted in monolayer formation coverage where the control is cells directly subcultured onto fn + cnIV coated membranes, compared to cells subcultured on plastic tissue culture plates coated with collagen IV and fibronectin before plating onto coated transwells. **c** Peak TEER taken on membranes coated with collagen gels and basement membrane coating mixtures. **d** Peak TEER on transwells with collagen gels coated with fibronectin and collagen IV, and different combinations of ROCK inhibitor Y27632, cAMP, and genipin treatment. Bars represent mean ± standard error, * represents $p < 0.05$, ** represents $p < 0.01$, *** represents $p < 0.001$

Effects of soluble factors on the barrier properties of the monolayers

Based on the results from screening matrix materials and coatings, collagen I gels (7 mg mL^{-1}) coated with fibronectin and collagen IV show a good combination of monolayer formation and barrier function, although the TEER values were about fivefold lower than on fibronectin-coated transwell membranes. Soluble factors can also modulate adhesion, spreading, and barrier function, and hence we assessed two molecules: the ROCK inhibitor Y-27632 (RI) and cyclic adenosine monophosphate (cAMP). RI did not significantly increase adhesion to the collagen I gels (results not shown), but increased the TEER of monolayers on collagen I gels coated with fibronectin and collagen IV from 215 to 2700 Ω cm^2 (Fig. 2d, Additional file 1: Figure S2). cAMP had no effect on monolayer formation (data not shown), but also showed a significant increase in TEER, from 215 to 1700 Ω cm^2 (Fig. 2d), similar to the increase seen with the addition of RI. The combination of cAMP and RI did not result in a further increase in TEER (Fig. 2d).

Cross-linking

As shown above (Fig. 1a), the coverage of dhBMECs on uncoated collagen I gels increased with increasing stiffness, but did not result in the formation of confluent monolayers even at a concentration 7 mg mL^{-1}. While confluent monolayers were formed on 7 mg mL^{-1} gels coated with fibronectin and collagen IV, TEER values were about fivefold lower than on transwell membranes with no gel. To assess whether some of the loss of TEER on gels could be recovered, we used a small molecular cross-linker to increase the gel stiffness. Based on previous work, we estimate that cross-linking results in a fivefold increase in stiffness [29]. Cross-linking did not influence the rate of monolayer formation on 7 mg mL^{-1} gels coated with fibronectin and collagen IV (data not shown), but the TEER increased significantly to 2200 Ω cm^2. The addition of RI and cAMP did not further increase the TEER.

Formation of cell–cell junctions

To confirm the formation of cell–cell junctions on gels that promote monolayer formation, we performed immunofluorescence imaging of zona-occludens 1 (ZO-1) (Additional file 1: Figure S4) and claudin-5 (Fig. 3a). Monolayers formed on gels are similar to monolayers formed on glass but show larger cell areas, consistent with the decrease in adhesion, where fewer cells adhere and hence need to spread out to form junctions with neighboring cells (Additional file 1: Figure S4). Claudin-5-positive junctions were observed on collagen I gels coated with agrin, agrin and fibronectin, and fibronectin and collagen IV, although all conditions show significant

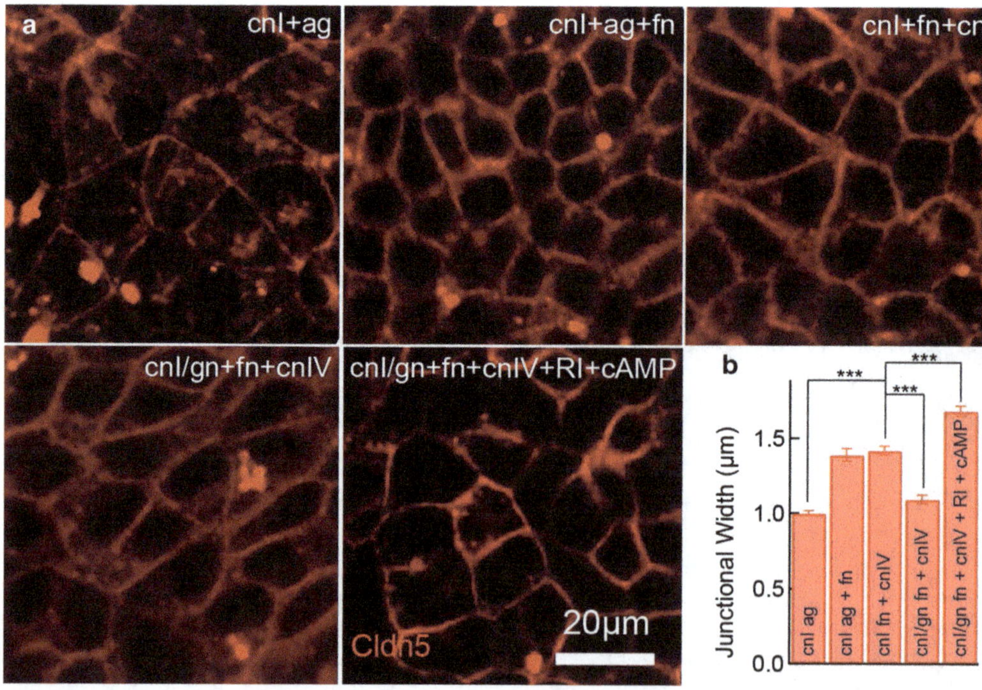

Fig. 3 Tight junction formation of dhBMEC monolayers. **a** Maximum intensity projection of claudin-5 confocal z-stack of dhBMECs monolayers on coated collagen I (cnI) and genipin cross-linked collagen I gels. **b** Width of claudin-5 junctions. Bars represent mean ± standard error, *** represents $p < 0.001$

intracellular staining. The most distinct claudin-5 networks with the lowest level of intracellular expression were obtained for genipin-treated collagen I gels coated with fibronectin and collagen IV, and with ROCK inhibitor and cAMP added to the media. To gain insight into the degree of cell–cell overlap and the strength of the junction, we used confocal microscopy to determine the width of the claudin-5 junctional stain. Agrin-coated collagen I gels have the narrowest junction width, whereas gels with fibronectin and collagen IV showed significantly wider junctions (Fig. 3b). Although genipin cross-linked gels show low junction width, the incorporation of ROCK inhibitor and cAMP resulted in a significant increase.

Fabrication of perfusable brain-specific dhBMEC microvessels

The ability to derive hBMECs with BBB phenotype from iPSCs provides the opportunity to develop a new generation of tissue-engineered BBB models. dhBMECs form monolayers with expression of tight junction markers and very high TEER on glass and transwell membranes [8]. However, compared to other ECs commonly used in tissue engineering, formation of dhBMEC monolayers is much more difficult on ECM materials, representing a major barrier to the integration of these cells in 3D BBB models. Having screened gel concentrations, coatings, and soluble factors, we next used these results to form dhBMEC microvessels (Fig. 4a).

We first seeded GFP-labeled dhBMECs in cylindrical channels within a 7 mg mL^{-1} collagen I matrix coated with collagen IV and fibronectin. Cells seeded under these conditions resulted in poor adhesion and death of the majority of cells over the first 24 h, as evidenced by blebbing and loss of intracellular fluorescence (data not shown). Using fibronectin and/or agrin to coat the vessels did not significantly increase coverage or cell viability. To overcome the low density of adherent cells, sequential seeding, with cells seeded every 3 days, resulted in higher cell densities in the microvessel, although not sufficient for microvessel formation.

The addition of ROCK inhibitor to the media reduced the large amount of cell death in the first 24 h of culture following seeding in channels. In conjunction with sequential seeding, the addition of ROCK inhibitor resulted in nearly confluent microvessels. The inclusion of cAMP had a similar result, but by different means. Rather than inhibiting cell death, cAMP increased the rate of adhesion and spreading, as reported elsewhere [37]. Combining ROCK inhibitor and cAMP into the media made moderate improvements, with the number

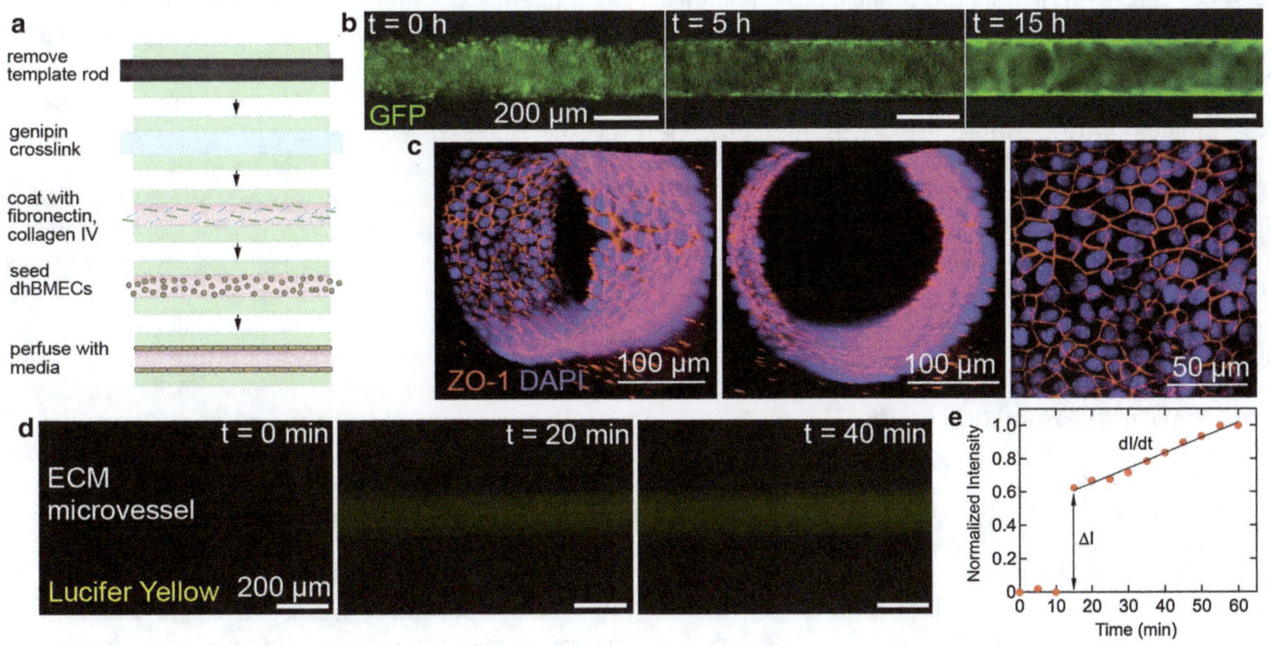

Fig. 4 Functional microvessels formed from dhBMECs. **a** Schematic of microvessel construction. **b** BC1 GFP—dhBMEC (GFP) growth in genipin cross-linked 7 mg mL^{-1} collagen gel, coated with collagen IV and fibronectin, with RI, cAMP, Ro-20-1724, and 70 kDa dextran. **c** Confocal image of a dhBMEC microvessel, cross section, and projected image at the bottom of the microvessel. ZO-1 (red), DAPI (blue). **d** Sequence of fluorescence images during a Lucifer yellow permeability experiment. **e** Normalized fluorescence intensity versus time following Lucifer yellow introduction into the microvessel

of cells adhering to the collagen increasing, but still unable to form confluent microvessels (data not shown).

Cross-linking the collagen I gel proved essential for microvessel formation. Following cross-linking with genipin, fully confluent microvessels were formed within 24 h (Fig. 4b). Functional dhBMEC microvessels were formed in genipin cross-linked gels coated with collagen IV and fibronectin, and with RI and cAMP in the culture media. Phosphodiesterase inhibitor Ro-20-1724 and 70 kDa dextran were also incorporated into the culture medium to promote long term vessel stability, as adhesion and survival were no longer the primary concern [30]. Using these conditions functional microvessels were maintained for more than 1 week with a single seeding.

Confocal images of the dhBMEC microvessels show a network of well-defined cell–cell junctions (Fig. 4c). The cells do not elongate and align under flow, as we have shown previously [38].

To assess barrier function we measured the permeability of Lucifer yellow, a small anionic salt (Fig. 4d) [39]. The flow rate was about 200 μL h^{-1} corresponding to a shear stress of about 1 dyn cm^{-2}, typical of post-capillary venules [1]. The permeability was calculated from the fluorescence intensity using standard methods developed for microvessels (Fig. 4e) [32]. The Lucifer yellow permeability in the dhBMEC microvessels was $0.70 \pm 0.21 \times 10^{-6}$ cm s^{-1}, similar to the value of $0.37 \pm 0.11 \times 10^{-6}$ cm s^{-1} obtained for dhBMEC monolayers using the transwell assay [8]. This permeability value is much lower than that reported in other brain microvessel models with permeability values over an order of magnitude higher using larger molecular probes [27] and in HUVEC microvessels [22]. In addition to showing very low permeability, the microvessels also showed no detectable focal leaks. Focal leaks are characterized by localized plumes of increased fluorescence, and were not observed with the 5 min imaging frequency. Focal leaks of much larger fluorescently-labeled probes have been observed in microvessels formed from HUVECs and HMVECs at this imaging frequency [22, 33]. The fact that we observe no characteristic focal leaks with a small molecule further supports the formation of physiological tight junctions.

Discussion

Cell adhesion

The interstitial space in the brain includes a complex ECM composed of hyaluronic acid, laminin, proteoglycans, and tenascins [40–43]. In vitro models of the BBB need to take into account the brain ECM, but also must meet additional requirements; an ECM material must provide structural support and chemical cues to maintain barrier function. We considered hyaluronic acid (HA), fibrin, and collagen I, three structural materials commonly used in tissue engineering. In preliminary work we showed that dhBMECs exhibit very poor adhesion on HA and hence this matrix material was not considered further. Fibrin, another common structural hydrogel used in microvessel models [44], is rapidly digested by BMECs and hence was not a candidate matrix material. Therefore, we selected collagen I as the structural matrix for our BBB model. Collagen I is the most prevalent structural protein in the body, and is widely used in in vitro models [22, 25, 45], but is not present in the brain [43]. However, collagen I provides a stable, structural matrix that can be modified to promote adhesion, spreading of dhBMECs and promote barrier function. In previous work we have also shown that gels based on collagen I can recapitulate the morphology and low levels of GFAP expression associated with quiescent astrocytes in the human brain [40], providing a structural support that mimics the stiffness of the brain.

Matrix stiffness is known to play an important role in promoting adhesion and spreading of endothelial cells and other cell types [46–50]. Here we show that dhBMECs form mounds on softer collagen I gels, but spread and form confluent regions on 6 and 7 mg mL^{-1} collagen I gels. The collagen I concentrations correspond to a stiffness of 189 ± 4, 1840 ± 76, and 3800 ± 162 Pa for 4, 6, and 8 mg mL^{-1} respectively, based on AFM measurements reported previously [40], and in agreement with previous reports in the literature [51]. The bulk shear modulus for the human, rat, and pig brain is around 200–300 Pa [35, 52], corresponding to around 4 mg mL^{-1} collagen. The monotonic increase in dhBMEC coverage with stiffness suggests that other factors are important in establishing the endothelium in vivo, compared to the relative importance of bulk stiffness in vitro.

Brain capillaries and microvessels are surrounded by a basement membrane, which is composed of laminin, fibronectin, collagen IV, and heparan sulfate proteoglycans agrin, perlecan, and collagen XVIII [53–55]. The makeup of the BMEC basement membrane is unique and critical for BMEC barrier formation [56–60]. Here we investigated the role of fibronectin, laminin, collagen IV, perlecan, and agrin as surface coatings to mimic components of the basement membrane in the brain. The addition of basement membrane proteins fibronectin, collagen IV, and laminin promoted adhesion and spreading. This result is consistent with similar experiments using primary porcine cerebral endothelial cells [53]. The addition of agrin and perlecan, two heparin sulfate proteoglycans present in the basement membrane in the BBB, resulted in very different responses. While perlecan had no apparent influence on adhesion and spreading, agrin had the largest effect in promoting adhesion and spreading. Agrin loss has been associated with BBB dysfunction and breakdown, and agrin coating has been reported to decrease permeability, proliferation, and increase junctional staining of murine bEnd5 cells [61]. Although agrin promoted adhesion, monolayers showed weak claudin-5 junctional staining and agrin abolished barrier function.

Cell–cell overlap may be important for BMECs as it likely enhances the formation of stable tight junctions that keep the brain isolated from circulation. Evidence of large cell–cell overlap has been inferred from 2D shear stress experiments, where the cells do not migrate far from their starting position when compared to HUVECs [17]. We hypothesize that larger cell–cell overlap helps to increase and maintain barrier function. In our indirect measurement of cell–cell overlap we found that cells plated on 7 mg mL^{-1} collagen I gels crosslinked with genipin, coated with collagen IV and fibronectin, and cultured with ROCK inhibitor and cAMP, show evidence of significantly more cell–cell overlap. Laminin/entactin was selected as an additional ECM component as it is present in the developing brain and has been shown to be an important additive to ECM to support the maintenance of endothelial cells [40, 54]. No change in adhesion was observed with the addition of laminin/entactin into the ECM.

Barrier function

TEER values for dhBMEC monolayers decreased from 5500 Ω cm^2 on transwell membranes coated with fibronectin and collagen IV, to 215 Ω cm^2 on 7 mg mL^{-1} collagen gels coated with fibronectin and collagen IV, highlighting the important role of substrate stiffness on adhesion and barrier function. This high TEER value is consistent with recent publications using derived hBMECs in monoculture [14, 62], and is approaching the calculated electrical resistance of brain microvessels of around 8000 Ω cm^2 [63], and significantly higher than other hBMEC cell lines, which are typically $\leq$ 200 Ω cm^{-2} [64–66]. The addition of agrin promoted monolayer formation (Fig. 1d), but down-regulated barrier function (Fig. 2c), illustrating that improved adhesion and spreading does not necessarily predict improved barrier function. However, the addition of fibronectin restored barrier function. The origin of this effect is beyond the scope of this study, however, we speculate that agrin promotes the formation of focal adhesions to the detriment of cell–cell junctions.

Treatment with ROCK inhibitor, cAMP, or cross-linking with genipin resulted in recovery of the TEER on bulk gels to about 2500 Ω cm^2, about half of the value on transwell membranes (no gel). Combinations of treatment with ROCK inhibitor, cAMP, or cross-linking also resulted in TEER values of around 2500 Ω cm^2 for all dhBMEC monolayers. ROCK inhibitor is commonly used to prevent apoptosis in embryonic and induced pluripotent stem cell cultures [67] and has been shown to play a role in the adhesion of cancer cells [68]. In addition, ROCK inhibitor has been shown to enhance survival, adhesion, and TEER following cryopreservation of dhBMECs, possibly by decreasing cellular stress as measured by actin stress fiber formation [69]. cAMP is well known to contribute to barrier function in the BBB [70, 71], and improve barrier function in monolayers and in vitro microvessel models [23, 37].

We speculate that the maximum TEER values for monolayers on gels (around 2500 Ω cm^2) are lower than for dhBMECs on transwell inserts (around 5500 Ω cm^2) due to the relatively rough surface morphology of the gels and the resulting difficulty in forming a good seal with the sidewalls at the perimeter. Claudin-5 positive tight junctional networks were formed using a number of the gel conditions, including genipin cross-linked collagen I gels with ROCK inhibitor and cAMP. In summary, these results show that monolayer formation, barrier function, and tight junction formation can be achieved in cross-linked collagen I gels coated with fibronectin and collagen IV, and treated with ROCK inhibitor and cAMP. These results provide key insight into strategies for tissue engineering perfusable dhBMEC microvessels. ROCK inhibitor does not increase the number of cells that adhere to the matrix, but rather the number of cells that survive the first 24 h and thus remain adhered. On collagen I gels, cell adhesion and spreading typically takes 24–48 h [72]. ROCK inhibitor may allow the cells more time to form these junctions before initiating apoptosis, just as it does in iPSC cultures, and allow the cells more time to form cadherin junctions with neighboring cells [67].

dhBMEC microvessels

Having identified matrix compositions and coatings that promote adhesion, spreading, and barrier function, we have successfully applied these conditions to the formation of functional brain-specific microvessels. Tissue-engineered models of the BBB have been reported using primary rat [26], immortalized human [28], and primary human [27] brain microvascular endothelial cells. All of these models show apparent permeabilities on the order of 10^{-6} cm s^{-1} for large molecular weight (3–40 kDa) dextran. In one study, the addition of astrocytes in the surrounding matrix resulted in a permeability of 0.6×10^{-6} cm s^{-1} for 4 kDa dextran [28]. Permeability to high molecular weight dextrans is typical for tumor vasculature, but is not physiological in the BBB. Here we show an apparent permeability of 0.7×10^{-6} cm s^{-1} for Lucifer yellow (MW 442), similar to values obtained in the transwell assay. Furthermore, in contrast to microvessels using other endothelial cell types, we detect no transient focal leaks. These results suggest that microvessels formed from dhBMECs can mimic the barrier function of the BBB.

Conclusions

To assess the parameters that control adhesion, spreading, and survival of dhBMECs, we systematically screened matrix stiffness (collagen I, crosslinking with genipin), compositions (laminin/entactin), protein coatings (fibronectin, laminin, collagen IV, perlecan, and agrin), and soluble factors in the culture medium (ROCK inhibitor and cyclic adenosine monophosphate). Increasing matrix stiffness increased adhesion but did not result in monolayer formation. Coating 7 mg mL^{-1} collagen I gels with fibronectin, collagen IV, and laminin resulted in high coverage but unreliable monolayer formation. However, coating collagen I gels with agrin, with or without fibronectin and collagen IV, resulted in monolayer formation. The addition of ROCK inhibitor or cAMP to the culture medium, or gel cross-linking, resulted in a significant increase in TEER to around 2500 Ω cm^2. Based on these results, we successfully fabricated dhBMEC microvessels in cross-linked collagen I gels coated with fibronectin and collagen IV, and treated with ROCK inhibitor and cAMP. We measured apparent permeability values for Lucifer yellow, comparable to values obtained in the transwell assay. During these experiments we observed no focal leaks, suggesting the formation of tight junctions that effectively block paracellular transport.

Abbreviations

AFM: atomic force microscopy; ag: agrin; BBB: blood–brain barrier; BMEC: brain microvascular endothelial cell; cAMP: cyclic adenosine monophosphate; cnI: collagen I; cnI/gn: genipin treated collagen I; cnIV: collagen IV; dhBMEC: derived human brain microvascular endothelial cell; EC: endothelial cell; ECM: extracellular matrix; fn: fibronectin; HA: hyaluronic acid; hBMEC: human brain microvascular endothelial cell; hiPSC: human induced pluripotent stem cell; HMVEC: human microvascular endothelial cells; HUVEC: human umbilical vein endothelial cells; iPSC: induced pluripotent stem cell; KOSR: knockout serum replacement; ln: laminin; PBS: phosphate buffered saline; pc: perlecan; RI: rho-associate kinase inhibitor; ROCK: rho-associated kinase; TEER: transendothelial electrical resistance; ZO-1: zona occludin 1.

Authors' contributions

MK, RL and LM performed the experiments. MK, RL, LM, ZX, and PS analyzed the data. MK, and PS wrote the manuscript. All authors read and approved the final manuscript.

Author details

[1] Institute for Nanobiotechnology, Johns Hopkins University, Baltimore, MD, USA. [2] Department of Materials Science and Engineering, Johns Hopkins University, Baltimore, MD, USA. [3] Department of Biomedical Engineering, Johns Hopkins University, Baltimore, MD, USA.

Competing interests

The authors declare that they have no competing interests.

Funding

The authors gratefully acknowledge support from DTRA (HDTRA1-15-1-0046).

References

1. Wong A, Ye M, Levy A, Rothstein J, Bergles D, Searson PC. The blood–brain barrier: an engineering perspective. Front in Neuroeng. 2013;6:7.
2. Abbott NJ, Rönnbäck L, Hansson E. Astrocyte–endothelial interactions at the blood–brain barrier. Nat Rev Neurosci. 2006;7:41–53.
3. Neuwelt EA, Bauer B, Fahlke C, Fricker G, Iadecola C, Janigro D, Leybaert L, Molnár Z, O'donnell ME, Povlishock JT. Engaging neuroscience to advance translational research in brain barrier biology. Nat Rev Neurosci. 2011;12:169–82.
4. Lippmann ES, Al-Ahmad A, Azarin SM, Palecek SP, Shusta EV. A retinoic acid-enhanced, multicellular human blood–brain barrier model derived from stem cell sources. Sci Rep. 2014;4:4160.
5. Mahairaki V, Ryu J, Peters A, Chang Q, Li T, Park TS, Burridge PW, Talbot CC Jr, Asnaghi L, Martin LJ. Induced pluripotent stem cells from familial Alzheimer's disease patients differentiate into mature neurons with amyloidogenic properties. Stem cells Dev. 2014;23:2996–3010.
6. Jung YW, Hysolli E, Kim KY, Tanaka Y, Park IH. Human induced pluripotent stem cells and neurodegenerative disease: prospects for novel therapies. Curr Opin Neurol. 2012;25:125.
7. Heman-Ackah SM, Bassett AR, Wood MJA. Precision modulation of neurodegenerative disease-related gene expression in human iPSC-derived neurons. Sci Rep. 2016;6:28420.
8. Katt ME, Xu ZS, Gerecht S, Searson PC. Human brain microvascular endothelial cells derived from the BC1 iPS cell line exhibit a blood–brain barrier phenotype. PLoS ONE. 2016;11:e0152105.
9. Kokubu Y, Yamaguchi T, Kawabata K. In vitro model of cerebral ischemia by using brain microvascular endothelial cells derived from human induced pluripotent stem cells. Biochem Biophys Res Commun. 2017;486:577–83.
10. Mantle JL, Min L, Lee KH. Minimum transendothelial electrical resistance thresholds for the study of small and large molecule drug transport in a human in vitro blood–brain barrier model. Mol Pharm. 2016;13:4191–8.
11. Appelt-Menzel A, Cubukova A, Günther K, Edenhofer F, Piontek J, Krause G, Stüber T, Walles H, Neuhaus W, Metzger M. Establishment of a human blood–brain barrier co-culture model mimicking the neurovascular unit using induced pluri-and multipotent stem cells. Stem cell Rep. 2017;8:894–906.
12. Lippmann ES, Azarin SM, Kay JE, Nessler RA, Wilson HK, Al-Ahmad A, Palecek SP, Shusta EV. Derivation of blood–brain barrier endothelial cells from human pluripotent stem cells. Nat Biotechnol. 2012;30:783–91.
13. Lim RG, Quan C, Reyes-Ortiz AM, Lutz SE, Kedaigle AJ, Gipson TA, Wu J, Vatine GD, Stocksdale J, Casale MS. Huntington's disease iPSC-derived brain microvascular endothelial cells reveal WNT-mediated angiogenic and blood–brain barrier deficits. Cell Rep. 2017;19:1365–77.
14. Hollmann EK, Bailey AK, Potharazu AV, Neely MD, Bowman AB, Lippmann ES. Accelerated differentiation of human induced pluripotent stem cells to blood–brain barrier endothelial cells. Fluids Barriers CNS. 2017;14:9.
15. Wilson HK, Canfield SG, Hjortness MK, Palecek SP, Shusta EV. Exploring the effects of cell seeding density on the differentiation of human pluripotent stem cells to brain microvascular endothelial cells. Fluids Barriers CNS. 2015;12:13.
16. Reinitz A, DeStefano J, Ye M, Wong AD, Searson PC. Human brain microvascular endothelial cells resist elongation due to shear stress. Microvasc Res. 2015;99:8–18.
17. DeStefano JG, Xu ZS, Williams AJ, Yimam N, Searson PC. Effect of shear stress on iPSC-derived human brain microvascular endothelial cells (dhBMECs). Fluids Barriers CNS. 2017;14:20.
18. Ye M, Sanchez HM, Hultz M, Yang Z, Bogorad M, Wong AD, Searson PC. Brain microvascular endothelial cells resist elongation due to curvature and shear stress. Sci Rep. 2014;4:4681.

19. Cecchelli R, Berezowski V, Lundquist S, Culot M, Renftel M, Dehouck MP, Fenart L. Modelling of the blood–brain barrier in drug discovery and development. Nat Rev Drug Discov. 2007;6:650–61.
20. Bogorad MI, DeStefano J, Wong AD, Searson PC. Tissue-engineered 3D microvessel and capillary network models for the study of vascular phenomena. Microcirculation. 2017. https://doi.org/10.1111/micc.12360.
21. Bogorad MI, DeStefano J, Karlsson J, Wong AD, Gerecht S, Searson PC. Review: in vitro microvessel models. Lab Chip. 2015;15:4242–55.
22. Wong AD, Searson PC. Live-cell imaging of invasion and intravasation in an artificial microvessel platform. Can Res. 2014;74:4937–45.
23. Chrobak KM, Potter DR, Tien J. Formation of perfused, functional microvascular tubes in vitro. Microvasc Res. 2006;71:185–96.
24. Song JW, Munn LL. Fluid forces control endothelial sprouting. Proc Natl Acad Sci. 2011;108:15342–7.
25. Lee VK, Lanzi AM, Ngo H, Yoo SS, Vincent PA, Dai G. Generation of multiscale vascular network system within 3D hydrogel using 3D bio-printing technology. Cell Mol Bioeng. 2014;7:460–72.
26. Deosarkar SP, Prabhakarpandian B, Wang B, Sheffield JB, Krynska B, Kiani MF. A novel dynamic neonatal blood–brain barrier on a chip. PLoS ONE. 2015;10:e0142725.
27. Herland A, van der Meer AD, FitzGerald EA, Park TE, Sleeboom JJ, Ingber DE. Distinct contributions of astrocytes and pericytes to neuroinflammation identified in a 3D human blood–brain barrier on a chip. PLoS ONE. 2016;11:e0150360.
28. Partyka PP, Godsey GA, Galie JR, Kosciuk MC, Acharya NK, Nagele RG, Galie PA. Mechanical stress regulates transport in a compliant 3D model of the blood–brain barrier. Biomaterials. 2017;115:30–9.
29. Chan KL, Khankhel AH, Thompson RL, Coisman BJ, Wong KH, Truslow JG, Tien J. Crosslinking of collagen scaffolds promotes blood and lymphatic vascular stability. J Biomed Mater Res Part A. 2014;102:3186–95.
30. Linville RM, Boland NF, Covarrubias G, Price GM, Tien J. Physical and chemical signals that promote vascularization of capillary-scale channels. Cell Mol Bioeng. 2016;9:73–84.
31. Wong KH, Truslow JG, Tien J. The role of cyclic AMP in normalizing the function of engineered human blood microvessels in microfluidic collagen gels. Biomaterials. 2010;31:4706–14.
32. Bogorad MI, Searson PC. Real-time imaging and quantitative analysis of doxorubicin transport in a perfusable microvessel platform. Integr Biol. 2016;8:976–84.
33. Price GM, Wong KH, Truslow JG, Leung AD, Acharya C, Tien J. Effect of mechanical factors on the function of engineered human blood microvessels in microfluidic collagen gels. Biomaterials. 2010;31:6182–9.
34. Zheng Y, Chen J, Craven M, Choi NW, Totorica S, Diaz-Santana A, Kermani P, Hempstead B, Fischbach-Teschl C, López JA. In vitro microvessels for the study of angiogenesis and thrombosis. Proc Natl Acad Sci. 2012;109:9342–7.
35. Prang P, Muller R, Eljaouhari A, Heckmann K, Kunz W, Weber T, Faber C, Vroemen M, Bogdahn U, Weidner N. The promotion of oriented axonal regrowth in the injured spinal cord by alginate-based anisotropic capillary hydrogels. Biomaterials. 2006;27:3560–9.
36. Lancaster MA, Renner M, Martin C-A, Wenzel D, Bicknell LS, Hurles ME, Homfray T, Penninger JM, Jackson AP, Knoblich JA. Cerebral organoids model human brain development and microcephaly. Nature. 2013;501:373–9.
37. Morandini R, Ghanem G, Portier-Lemarie A, Robaye B, Renaud A, Boeynaems JM. Action of cAMP on expression and release of adhesion molecules in human endothelial cells. Am J PhysiologyHeart Circ Physiol. 1996;270:H807–16.
38. DeStefano JG, Williams A, Wnorowski A, Yimam N, Searson PC, Wong AD. Real-time quantification of endothelial response to shear stress and vascular modulators. Integr Biol (Camb). 2017;9:362–74.
39. Irvine JD, Takahashi L, Lockhart K, Cheong J, Tolan JW, Selick H, Grove JR. MDCK (Madin–Darby canine kidney) cells: a tool for membrane permeability screening. J Pharm Sci. 1999;88:28–33.
40. Placone AL, McGuiggan PM, Bergles DE, Guerrero-Cazares H, Quiñones-Hinojosa A, Searson PC. Human astrocytes develop physiological morphology and remain quiescent in a novel 3D matrix. Biomaterials. 2015;42:134–43.
41. Johansson S, Svineng G, Wennerberg K, Armulik A, Lohikangas L. Fibronectin-integrin interactions. Front Biosci. 1997;2:d126–46.
42. Zimmermann DR, Dours-Zimmermann MT. Extracellular matrix of the central nervous system: from neglect to challenge. Histochem Cell Biol. 2008;130:635–53.
43. Yamaguchi Y. Lecticans: organizers of the brain extracellular matrix. Cell Mol Life Sci CMLS. 2000;57:276–89.
44. Nakatsu MN, Sainson RC, Aoto JN, Taylor KL, Aitkenhead M, Pérez-del-Pulgar S, Carpenter PM, Hughes CC. Angiogenic sprouting and capillary lumen formation modeled by human umbilical vein endothelial cells (HUVEC) in fibrin gels: the role of fibroblasts and Angiopoietin-1☆. Microvasc Res. 2003;66:102–12.
45. Yeon JH, Ryu HR, Chung M, Hu QP, Jeon NL. In vitro formation and characterization of a perfusable three-dimensional tubular capillary network in microfluidic devices. Lab Chip. 2012;12:2815–22.
46. Buxboim A, Ivanovska IL, Discher DE. Matrix elasticity, cytoskeletal forces and physics of the nucleus: how deeply do cells 'feel' outside and in? J Cell Sci. 2010;123:297–308.
47. Yeung T, Georges PC, Flanagan LA, Marg B, Ortiz M, Funaki M, Zahir N, Ming W, Weaver V, Janmey PA. Effects of substrate stiffness on cell morphology, cytoskeletal structure, and adhesion. Cell Motil Cytoskeleton. 2005;60:24–34.
48. Yeung T, Georges PC, Flanagan LA, Marg B, Ortiz M, Funaki M, Zahir N, Ming W, Weaver V, Janmey PA. Effects of substrate stiffness on cell morphology, cytoskeletal structure, and adhesion. Cell Motil Cytoskelet. 2005;60:24–34.
49. Discher DE, Janmey P, Wang Y. Tissue cells feel and respond to the stiffness of their substrate. Science. 2005;310:1139–43.
50. Ruoslahti E, Pierschbacher MD. New perspectives in cell adhesion: RGD and integrins. Science. 1987;238:491–7.
51. Raub CB, Unruh J, Suresh V, Krasieva T, Lindmo T, Gratton E, Tromberg BJ, George SC. Image correlation spectroscopy of multiphoton images correlates with collagen mechanical properties. Biophys J. 2008;94:2361–73.
52. Georges PC, Miller WJ, Meaney DF, Sawyer ES, Janmey PA. Matrices with compliance comparable to that of brain tissue select neuronal over glial growth in mixed cortical cultures. Biophys J. 2006;90:3012–8.
53. Tilling T, Engelbertz C, Decker S, Korte D, Hüwel S, Galla HJ. Expression and adhesive properties of basement membrane proteins in cerebral capillary endothelial cell cultures. Cell Tissue Res. 2002;310:19–29.
54. Ruoslahti E. Brain extracellular matrix. Glycobiology. 1996;6:489–92.
55. Knox S, Whitelock J. Perlecan: how does one molecule do so many things? Cell Mol Life Sci CMLS. 2006;63:2435–45.
56. Thomsen MS, Birkelund S, Burkhart A, Stensballe A, Moos T. Synthesis and deposition of basement membrane proteins by primary brain capillary endothelial cells in a murine model of the blood–brain barrier. J Neurochem. 2017;140:741–54.
57. Thomsen MS, Routhe LJ, Moos T. The vascular basement membrane in the healthy and pathological brain. J Cereb Blood Flow Metab. 2017;37:3300–17.
58. Osada T, Gu Y-H, Kanazawa M, Tsubota Y, Hawkins BT, Spatz M, Milner R, Del Zoppo GJ. Interendothelial claudin-5 expression depends on cerebral endothelial cell–matrix adhesion by β1-integrins. J Cereb Blood Flow Metab. 2011;31:1972–85.
59. Tilling T, Korte D, Hoheisel D, Galla HJ. Basement membrane proteins influence brain capillary endothelial barrier function in vitro. J Neurochem. 1998;71:1151–7.
60. Savettieri G, Di Liegro I, Catania C, Licata L, Pitarresi GL, D'Agostino S, Schiera G, De Caro V, Giandalia G, Giannola LI. Neurons and ECM regulate occludin localization in brain endothelial cells. NeuroReport. 2000;11:1081–4.
61. Steiner E, Enzmann GU, Lyck R, Lin S, Rüegg MA, Kröger S, Engelhardt B. The heparan sulfate proteoglycan agrin contributes to barrier properties of mouse brain endothelial cells by stabilizing adherens junctions. Cell Tissue Res. 2014;358:465–79.
62. Qian T, Maguire SE, Canfield SG, Bao X, Olson WR, Shusta EV, Palecek SP. Directed differentiation of human pluripotent stem cells to blood–brain barrier endothelial cells. Sci Adv. 2017;3:e1701679.
63. Smith QR, Rapoport SI. Cerebrovascular permeability coefficients to sodium, potassium, and chloride. J Neurochem. 1986;46:1732–42.
64. Eigenmann DE, Xue G, Kim KS, Moses AV, Hamburger M, Oufir M. Comparative study of four immortalized human brain capillary endothelial cell lines, hCMEC/D3, hBMEC, TY10, and BB19, and optimization of culture

conditions, for an in vitro blood–brain barrier model for drug permeability studies. Fluids Barriers CNS. 2013;10:33.

65. Daniels BP, Cruz-Orengo L, Pasieka TJ, Couraud PO, Romero IA, Weksler B, Cooper JA, Doering TL, Klein RS. Immortalized human cerebral microvascular endothelial cells maintain the properties of primary cells in an in vitro model of immune migration across the blood brain barrier. J Neurosci Methods. 2013;212:173–9.
66. Khan NA. Novel in vitro and in vivo models to study central nervous system infections due to *Acanthamoeba* spp. Exp Parasitol. 2010;126:69–72.
67. Watanabe K, Ueno M, Kamiya D, Nishiyama A, Matsumura M, Wataya T, Takahashi JB, Nishikawa S, Nishikawa SI, Muguruma K. A ROCK inhibitor permits survival of dissociated human embryonic stem cells. Nat Biotechnol. 2007;25:681–6.
68. Wang L, Xue L, Yan H, Li J, Lu Y. Effects of ROCK inhibitor, Y-27632, on adhesion and mobility in esophageal squamous cell cancer cells. Mol Biol Rep. 2010;37:1971–7.
69. Wilson HK, Faubion MG, Hjortness MK, Palecek SP, Shusta EV. Cryopreservation of brain endothelial cells derived from human induced pluripotent stem cells is enhanced by rho-associated coiled coil-containing kinase inhibition. Tissue Eng Part C Methods. 2016;22:1085–94.
70. Deli MA, Ábrahám CS, Kataoka Y, Niwa M. Permeability studies on in vitro blood–brain barrier models: physiology, pathology, and pharmacology. Cell Mol Neurobiol. 2005;25:59–127.
71. Tóth A, Veszelka S, Nakagawa S, Niwa M, A Deli M. Patented in vitro blood–brain barrier models in CNS drug discovery. Recent Pat CNS Drug Discov. 2011;6:107–18.
72. Gumbiner BM. Cell adhesion: the molecular basis of tissue architecture and morphogenesis. Cell. 1996;84:345–57.

20

Monoclonal antibody exposure in rat and cynomolgus monkey cerebrospinal fluid following systemic administration

Qin Wang[1*], Luisette Delva[1], Paul H. Weinreb[1], Robert B. Pepinsky[1], Danielle Graham[1], Elvana Veizaj[1], Anne E. Cheung[1,2], Weiping Chen[1], Ivan Nestorov[1], Ellen Rohde[1,3], Robin Caputo[1,4], Geoffrey M. Kuesters[1,5], Tonika Bohnert[1] and Liang-Shang Gan[1,6]

Abstract

Background: Many studies have focused on the challenges of small molecule uptake across the blood–brain barrier, whereas few in-depth studies have assessed the challenges with the uptake of antibodies into the central nervous system (CNS). In drug development, cerebrospinal fluid (CSF) sampling is routinely used as a surrogate for assessing CNS drug exposure and biomarker levels. In this report, we have studied the kinetic correlation between CSF and serum drug concentration–time profiles for five humanized monoclonal antibodies in rats and cynomolgus monkeys and analyzed factors that affect their CSF exposure.

Results: Upon intravenous (IV) bolus injection, antibodies entered the CNS slowly and reached maximum CSF concentration (${}^{CSF}T_{max}$) in one to several days in both rats and monkeys. Antibody serum and CSF concentration–time curves converged until they became parallel after ${}^{CSF}T_{max}$ was reached. Antibody half-lives in CSF (${}^{CSF}t_{½}$) approximated their serum half-lives (${}^{serum}t_{½}$). Although the intended targets of these antibodies were different, the steady-state CSF to serum concentration ratios were similar at 0.1–0.2% in both species. Independent of antibody target and serum concentration, CSF-to-serum concentration ratios for individual monkeys ranged by up to tenfold from 0.03 to 0.3%.

Conclusion: Upon systemic administration, average antibodies CSF-to-serum concentration ratios in rats and monkeys were 0.1–0.2%. The ${}^{CSF}t_{½}$ of the antibodies was largely determined by their long systemic $t_{½}$ (${}^{systemic}t_{½}$).

Introduction

The blood brain barrier (BBB) is the single most significant obstacle that impedes the delivery of therapeutics to targets in the central nervous system (CNS). For medications that interact with targets in the CNS, it is essential for therapeutic and/or safety reasons to obtain accurate kinetic relationships between CNS and systemic circulation levels. It is also important to understand the factors that affect this relationship in order to project CNS drug levels based on their systemic concentration–time profiles. In practice, cerebrospinal fluid (CSF) is the most accessible and widely used sampling matrix for measuring drug and biomarker levels in the CNS. CSF sampling is inconvenient, and therefore requires rigorous study design to minimize the number of time points that need to be collected. Several excellent reviews highlight the scientific rationale and utility of using CSF as a surrogate for assessing CNS drug exposure levels [1–5]. Although there are numerous studies examining the rates of small molecule drug penetration across the blood brain barrier (BBB) and blood CSF barrier (BCSFB), there are few in-depth studies looking at the kinetics of antibody transmission into and out of CSF, especially with respect to the key factors that govern CSF antibody exposure. Considerations include the time needed for an antibody to reach maximum CSF drug concentration (${}^{CSF}T_{max}$), antibody CSF half-life (${}^{CSF}t_{½}$) and the length of time required for achieving steady-state antibody levels

*Correspondence: qin.wang@biogen.com
[1] Biogen, Inc., 250 Binney Street, Cambridge, MA 02142, USA

between CSF and systemic circulation. In this study, we report the kinetic relationships of CSF versus serum concentration–time profiles of five humanized monoclonal antibodies in rats and cynomolgus monkeys following systemic administration and factors that affect their CSF antibody exposures. These findings have important implications for assessing CNS antibody drug kinetics in humans.

Materials and methods

Materials

In this study, we tested five human monoclonal antibodies (mAb). All five antibodies are highly selective and have subnanomolar affinities for their respective targets. Antibody A (BIIB054) preferentially binds to aggregated forms of α-synuclein and binds human, non-human primate (NHP), and rat α-synuclein with similar affinity. Antibody B (399 H0/L0) recognizes JC virus, which is found in humans [6], but is not present in NHP or rats. Antibody C (BIIB076) and antibody D (40E8) bind to the microtubule-binding protein tau. Antibody C recognizes a linear sequence within tau and binds to human and NHP, but not rat tau. Antibody D is specific for phosphorylated tau and recognizes phosphorylated human, NHP, and rat tau. Antibody E (BIIB033, opicinumab) binds LRR- and Ig-domain-containing Nogo receptor interacting protein 1 (LINGO-1) and exhibits similar affinity for human, NHP, and rat LINGO-1. Antibodies A, C, D, and E are fully human antibodies, and antibody B is a humanized rabbit antibody. Antibodies, A, B, C, and D contain a wildtype human IgG1 Fc, while antibody E contains an aglycosylated human IgG1-Fc designed to reduce effector function [7]. Antibody A (BIIB054), antibody C (BIIB076), and antibody E (BIIB033) are currently being assessed in clinical trials.

Methods

Rat PK studies. Adult male Sprague–Dawley rats (250–300 g) (Charles-River Laboratory, Wilmington, MA) were housed at constant temperature (22 ± 2 °C) and relative humidity (50–70%) under a regular light/dark schedule (light, 7:00 A.M. to 7:00 P.M.). Food and water were freely available. The dose administration route was either by tail vein (mAbs A, B, C and D) or intraperitoneal injection (mAb E). At various time points after dose administration, the animals were euthanized by CO_2 asphyxiation and immediately followed by CSF collection via cisterna magna puncture and blood collection via cardiac puncture. The rats used to evaluate antibody E were adult male Brown Norway rats (average weight 150–200 g). The procedures were essentially the same. For brain and spinal cord collection, perfusion was performed promptly following CSF/blood collection with 15 mL of saline via a peristaltic pump inserted into the left ventricle. Whole blood samples were left on the bench for about 15–30 min and spun at 3000 rpm (approximately 1000×*g*) for 10 min to isolate serum. All samples were stored at − 80 °C until analysis. All experimental procedures were approved and monitored by Biogen's Institutional Animal Care and Use Committee (IACUC).

Studies in NHP were carried out at SNBL (Everett, WA) with approved IACUC accreditation. Briefly, young adult cynomolgus monkeys (2.5–4 kg), were individually housed in cages that complied with the Animal Welfare Act, corresponding guidelines and standard operating procedures (SOPs) of SNBL. Approximately 1 week prior to dose administration, a single lumbar intrathecal catheter (advanced cranially into the thoracic region) was surgically implanted to allow repeated CSF sampling. Prior to dose administration, CSF was collected from the catheter for baseline measurements. The intravenous (IV) dose was administered via primed butterfly infusion lines over 1–2 min. At pre-selected sampling time points, blood (1 mL) and CSF (0.5 mL) were collected from restrained, conscious animals. Serum and CSF samples were prepared as described above for rat studies. CSF samples were visually examined for blood contamination and contaminated samples were excluded.

The concentrations of antibodies A–E in serum and CNS specimens were measured using enzyme-linked immunosorbent assays (ELISAs). A generic sandwich ELISA format similar to the one described [8] was optimized for testing of each antibody. Because the capture and detection reagents are human IgG specific rather than target specific, the assays could be used to quantify human or humanized IgG molecules in non-human biological matrices including NHP and rat samples with minor modifications [8, 9]. The assays measured total mAb concentrations that included both unbound and soluble ligand-bound antibody. Capture and detection reagents were purchased from Southern Biotech (http://www.southernbiotech.com). Briefly, for the analysis of antibody A–D samples, 96-well ELISA plates were coated with the capture antibody, monkey-adsorbed goat anti-human IgG, at 1 μg/mL. The plates were blocked and washed, and standards (STDs), quality controls (QCs), or study samples containing test articles were added to the plate. The plates were again washed, and a 1:7500 dilution (50 ng/mL) of enzyme conjugated detection antibody (goat anti-human IgG-HRP), was added to the wells. After washing, the HRP substrate tetramethylbenzidine (TMB) was added. The HRP reaction was stopped following the addition of 1 N H_2SO_4 and the absorbance at 450 nm was measured on a microplate reader. Standard calibration curves were generated and the concentrations of the controls and samples were interpolated from their respective standard curves. On average, the quantitation ranges of the ELISAs were between 16 and 4400 ng/mL. Lower limits of quantitation were generally 16 ng/mL for CSF and 50 ng/mL for serum samples. Antibody E samples were quantified as previously described [10]. Pharmacokinetic modeling was carried out using Phoenix 6.4.0 software (http://www.certara.com).

Results

The pharmacokinetic properties of five human antibodies in serum and CSF were evaluated in rats and NHPs. A two-compartment first order pharmacokinetic model fit the concentration–time curves for all five antibodies well. Serum and CSF concentration–time profiles for antibodies A (10 mg/kg), B (10 mg/kg), C (20 mg/kg) and D (20 mg/kg) in rats following IV administration are shown in Fig. 1. Serum concentration profiles showed a multi-exponential decrease. All 4 antibodies appeared in the CSF slowly, with ${}^{CSF}T_{max}$ ranging between 6 and 48 h. Serum and CSF concentration–time curves became parallel after ${}^{CSF}T_{max}$. CSF antibody concentrations were approximately 1000-fold lower than serum concentrations. Since antibody E was dosed by intraperitoneal (IP) injection in Brown-Norway rats, the serum and CNS tissue concentration–time profiles for CSF, brain, and spinal cord are plotted separately in Fig. 2. Following IP administration (30 mg/kg), ${}^{serum}T_{max}$ was observed 6–24 h after dosing. The ${}^{CSF}T_{max}$, ${}^{brain}T_{max}$ and ${}^{Spinal\_cord}T_{max}$ were achieved 1–2 days following ${}^{serum}T_{max}$. Like the data shown in Fig. 1 for IV dosing, serum and CSF concentration–time curves following IP administration also became parallel after ${}^{CSF}T_{max}$. Concentration–time curves in brain (for antibodies A and E) and spinal cord (for antibody E) paralleled those in CSF, although the antibody concentrations in these CNS tissues were slightly higher than in CSF (Figs. 1, 2). No evidence for target-mediated clearance was observed, which is consistent with either the lack of cross-reactivity of the antibodies to rodent targets (antibodies B and C) or the low level of target in the periphery (antibodies A, D, and E).

Antibodies A, C and D were also evaluated in cynomolgus monkeys. The serum and CSF concentration–time profiles are plotted in Figs. 3, 4 and 5. As observed in rats, serum concentration profiles for each antibody in NHP

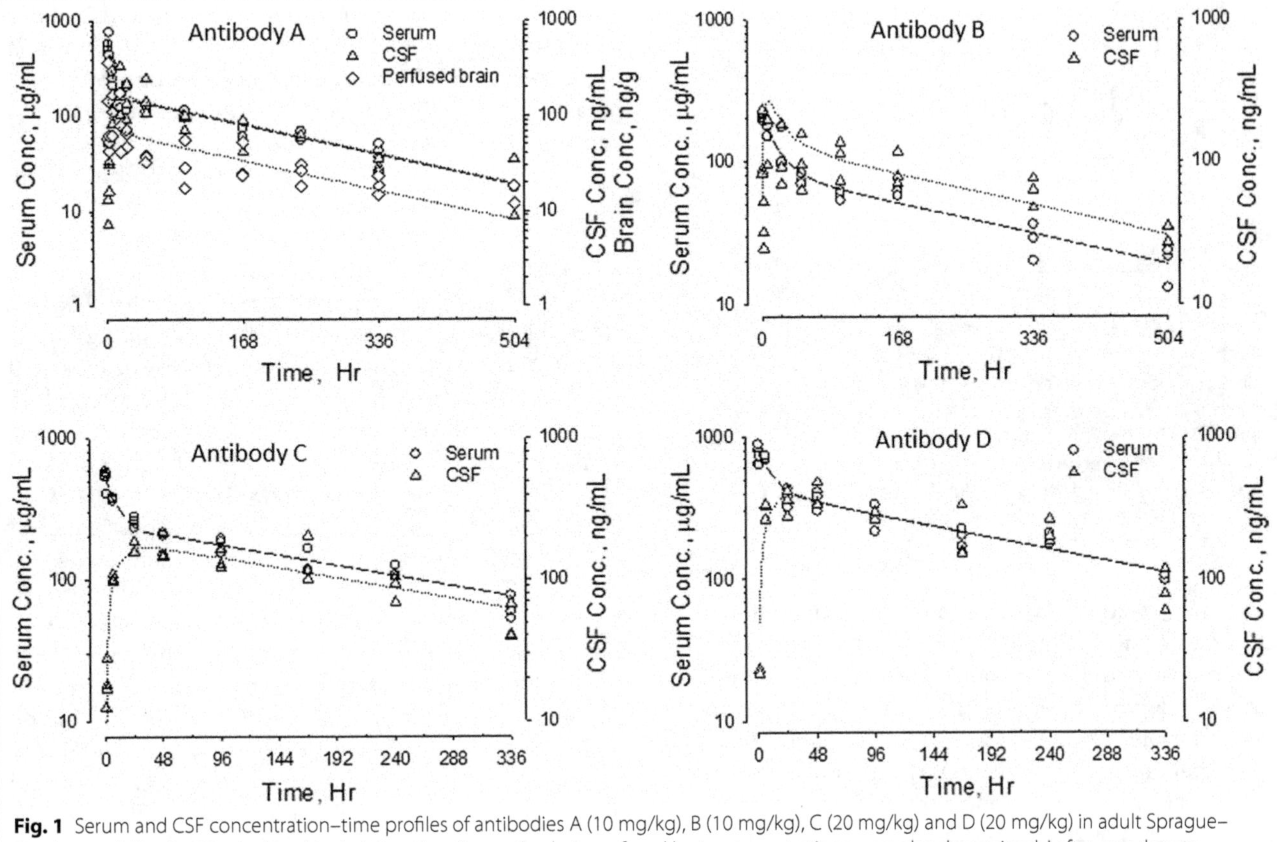

Fig. 1 Serum and CSF concentration–time profiles of antibodies A (10 mg/kg), B (10 mg/kg), C (20 mg/kg) and D (20 mg/kg) in adult Sprague–Dawley rats following single dose IV administration. For antibody A, perfused brain concentrations were also determined. Left *y-axes* denote antibody serum concentration in μg/mL (open circle). Right *y-axes* denote antibody CSF or brain concentrations in ng/mL (open triangle). Data for each individual animal are plotted separately

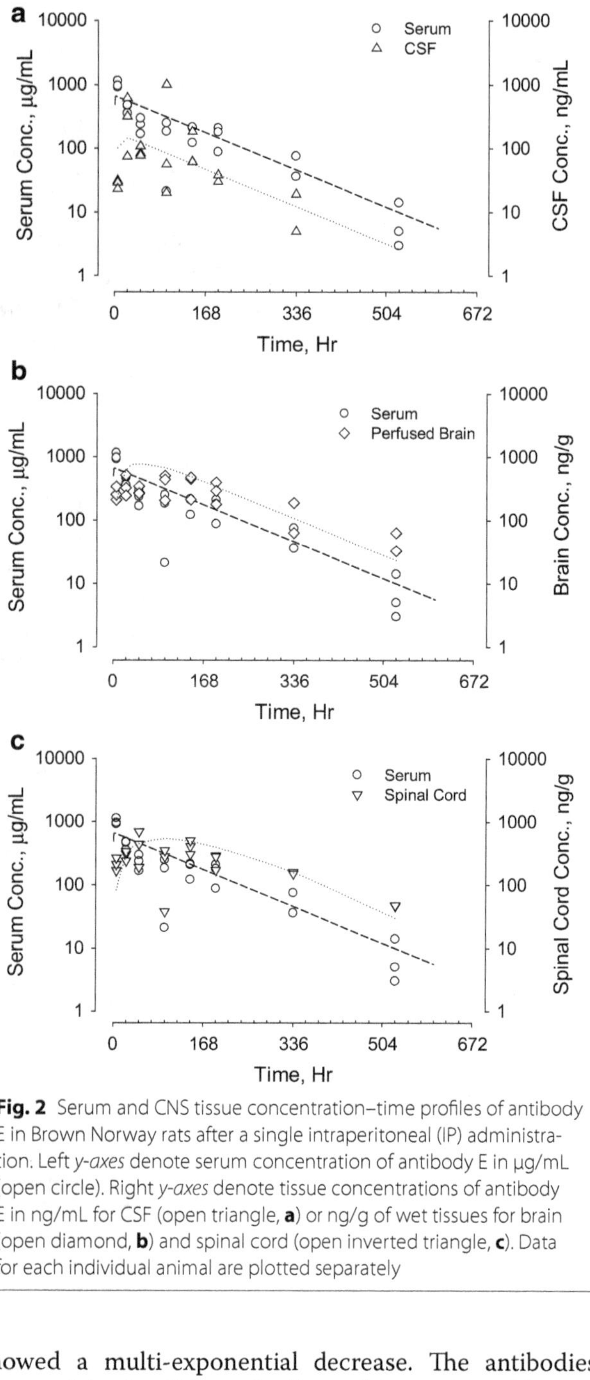

Fig. 2 Serum and CNS tissue concentration–time profiles of antibody E in Brown Norway rats after a single intraperitoneal (IP) administration. Left *y-axes* denote serum concentration of antibody E in µg/mL (open circle). Right *y-axes* denote tissue concentrations of antibody E in ng/mL for CSF (open triangle, **a**) or ng/g of wet tissues for brain (open diamond, **b**) and spinal cord (open inverted triangle, **c**). Data for each individual animal are plotted separately

showed a multi-exponential decrease. The antibodies appeared in the CSF gradually, peaking at 24–96 h after IV administration. Serum and CSF concentration–time curves became parallel after ${}^{CSF}T_{max}$, and CSF antibody concentrations on average were approximately 1000-fold lower than serum concentrations. Figure 3 shows antibody A serum and CSF concentration time curves after single IV doses of 20 and 100 mg/kg. The serum concentrations were proportional to antibody dose and the CSF concentrations were proportional to the antibody serum concentrations. Figure 4 shows serum and CSF concentration time curves following IV dosing of antibody C at 30 and 100 mg/kg (panel a) and antibody D at 30 mg/kg (panel b). The pharmacokinetic profiles of antibodies A, C and D were similar. Although the inter-subject variations in serum concentration–time profiles for all three antibodies were relatively small, there was an approximately tenfold variation in CSF-to-serum concentration ratios. To better understand the variability seen in the CSF measurements, we analyzed serum and CSF concentration–time curves of individual animals from the three NHP studies. Representative results from four animals are shown in Fig. 5. For the individual animals, ${}^{CSF}t_{½}$ and ${}^{serum}t_{½}$ were similar, but the CSF-to-serum concentration ratios varied from 0.03 to 0.32%. The variation in CSF-to-serum ratios was random and occurred in all studies irrespective of intended target and dose strength.

Results of non-compartmental analysis (NCA) of the pharmacokinetic parameters for the five antibodies characterized in Figs. 1, 2, 3 and 4 are summarized in Table 1. All five antibodies exhibited high serum exposures (${}^{serum}AUC$), and long half-lives ($t_{½}$) in both serum and CNS tissues. Following IV administration, antibodies appeared in the CSF gradually, reaching maximum CSF concentration (${}^{CSF}C_{max}$) between 16 and 48 h in rats and 2–3 days in cynomolgus monkeys (${}^{CSF}T_{max}$). For all five antibodies, serum and CSF concentration–time curves became parallel 2–3 days after dose administration, with CSF concentrations roughly one thousand times lower than the corresponding serum concentrations and independent of dose. For example, antibody A had a ${}^{CSF}AUC\text{-to-}{}^{serum}AUC$ ratio of 0.15 ± 0.07% at 20 mg/kg (N = 4) and 0.16 ± 0.08% at 100 mg/kg (N = 11). Antibody C had an average ${}^{CSF}AUC\text{-to-}{}^{serum}AUC$ ratio of 0.09 ± 0.06% at 30 mg/kg (N = 12) and 0.10 ± 0.05% at 100 mg/kg (N = 6). Taking into consideration low and high dose groups, antibody A had relatively long ${}^{serum}t_{½}$ of 18 ± 3 days and ${}^{CSF}t_{½}$ of 21 ± 6 days in monkeys (N = 15). On the other hand, antibody C had a relatively short ${}^{serum}t_{½}$ of 6 ± 2 days and ${}^{CSF}t_{½}$ of 8 ± 3 days in monkeys (N = 18).

Upon entering the CNS, there are four possible clearance mechanisms: (1) movement back across the BBB and/or BCSFB via a first order non-specific process; (2) active/facilitated transport out of the CNS by efflux transporters located at the membrane sites of the BBB and/or BCSFB, an energy-requiring process against the antibody concentration gradient; (3) biotransformation/metabolism, and (4) convection carried by brain ISF/CSF flow and drainage. For mass balance at steady-state, solute concentration in the CNS is determined by the rate entering the CNS divided by the sum of the four possible clearance mechanisms out of the same compartment. To simplify the analysis, we treated the brain tissue and CSF

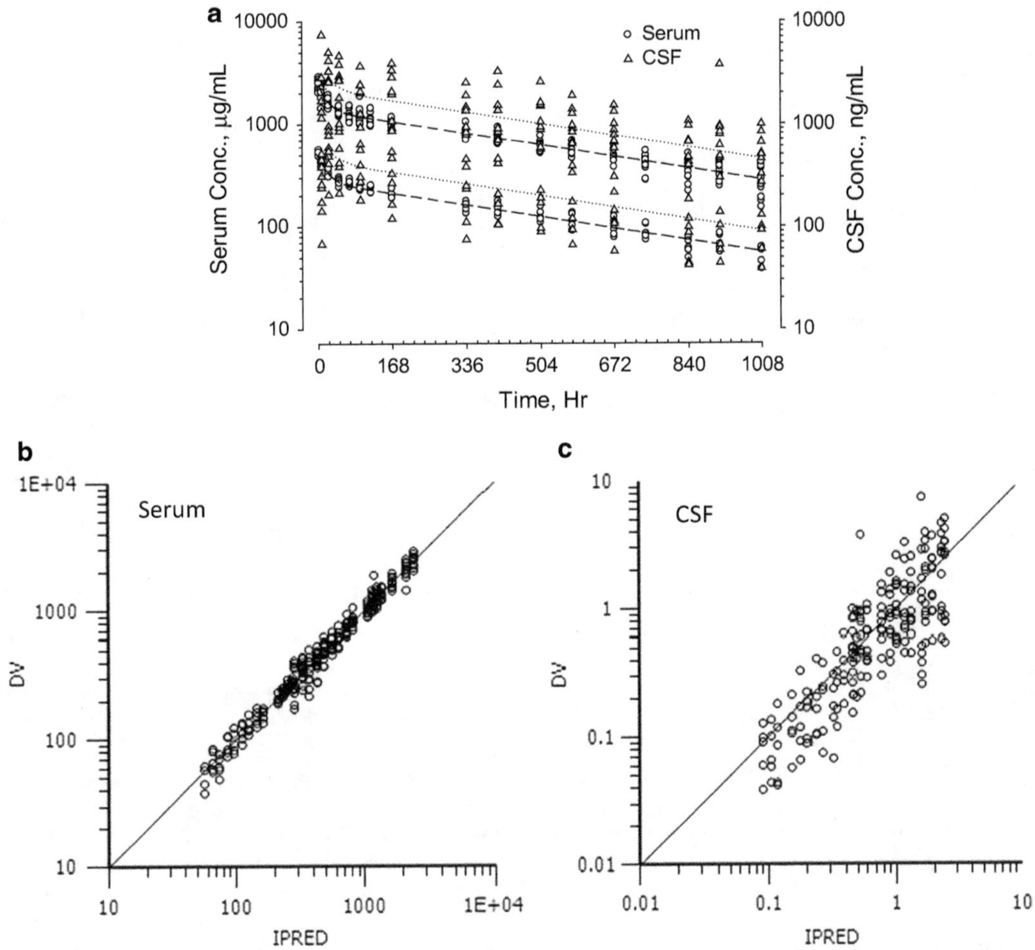

Fig. 3 Serum and CSF concentration–time profiles of antibody A in adult male cynomolgus monkeys (**a**) after a single IV administration of 20 mg/kg (N=4) or 100 mg/kg (N=11). Left *y-axes* denote serum concentrations in µg/mL (open circle). Right *y-axes* denote CSF concentrations in ng/mL (open triangle). Data for each individual animal are plotted separately. Plots for observed (*y-axis*) versus predicted (*x-axis*) antibody A concentrations in serum (**b**) and CSF (**c**) are on log scales

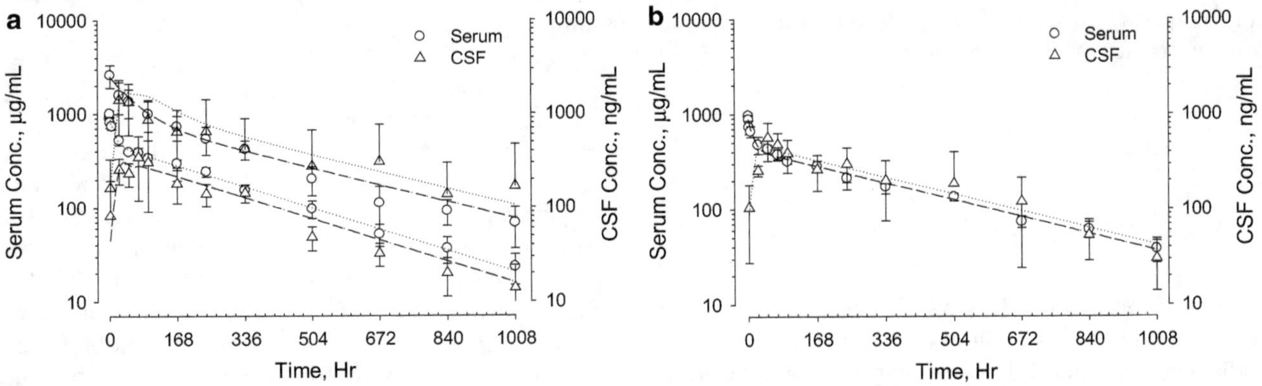

Fig. 4 Mean serum and CSF concentration–time profiles in adult male cynomolgus monkeys following single IV dose administration of antibody C (**a**) at 30 mg/kg (N=6) or 100 mg/kg (N=12) and following a single IV administration of antibody D (**b**) at 30 mg/kg. Left *y-axes* denote serum concentrations in µg/mL (open circle). Right *y-axes* denote CSF concentration in ng/mL (open triangle)

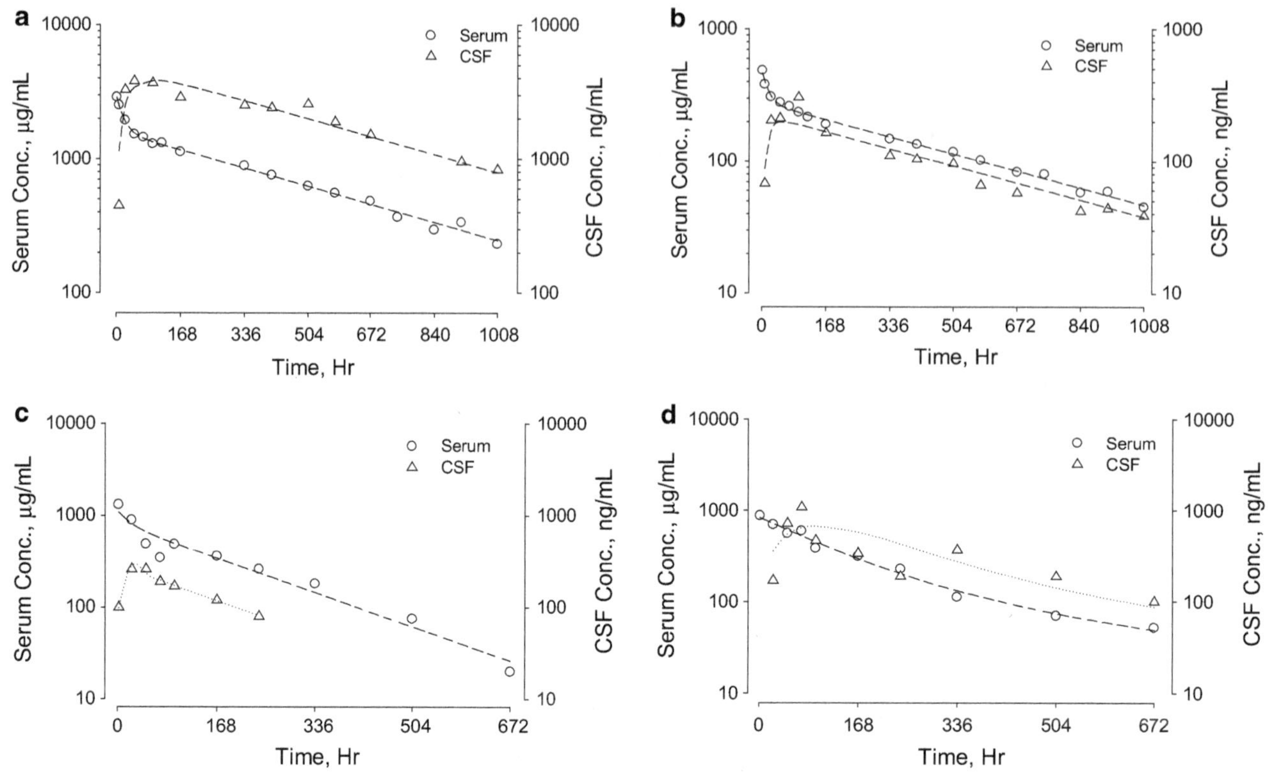

Fig. 5 Representative serum and CSF concentration–time profiles of antibodies A and C from individual cynomolgus monkeys. **a** Represents antibody A at 100 mg/kg, **b** represents antibody A at 20 mg/kg, and **c**, **d** represent antibody C at 30 mg/kg in selective animals. Left *y-axes* denote serum concentrations in µg/mL (open circle). Right *y-axes* denote CSF concentration in ng/mL (open triangle)

as one fast equilibrium homogeneous compartment as shown in Eq. 1: where R_{in} is the rate of passage into the CNS in amount per time; CL_{out} is the total clearance out of the CNS in volume per time; ${}^{CSF}C$ and ${}^{serum}C$ denote the steady-state drug concentrations in CSF and systemic circulation, respectively; $PS_{A\ to\ B}$ and $PS_{B\ to\ A}$ represent directional first order kinetics across BBB from apical to basolateral and from basolateral to aoical, respectively; and Cl_{efflux}, $Cl_{metabolism}$ and $Q_{convection}$ represent the individual clearance mechanisms indicated.

$$
\begin{aligned}
{}^{CSF}C &= \frac{R_{in}}{CL_{out}} \\
&= \frac{PS_{A\ to\ B} \times {}^{serum}C}{PS_{B\ to\ A} + CL_{Efflux} + CL_{metabolism} + Q_{convection}}
\end{aligned}
\tag{1}
$$

Without consumption of energy, passive diffusion or facilitated transcytosis requires a favorable concentration gradient and occurs only from high to low concentrations. Therefore, passive diffusion out of the CNS is not a feasible clearance mechanism for antibodies. Thus far, there has been no reported evidence for a high efficiency efflux pump or massive brain specific catabolism for antibodies or human IgGs. Unlike the other clearance mechanisms described above, convection by ISF/CSF flow does not require a favorable concentration gradient, specific transporter, or energy and is not structurally restricted by stoichiometry. If one assumes that convection is the most plausible and efficient mechanism for CNS removal of antibodies, Eq. 1 can be re-arranged and simplified to Eq. 2.

$$
\frac{{}^{CSF}C_{ss}}{{}^{serum}C_{ss}} \approx \frac{PS_{A\ to\ B}}{Q_{convection}} \approx 0.1\% \tag{2}
$$

In this model, the major factors that determine CNS exposures of therapeutic antibodies are two independent processes: an antibody's ability to cross the BBB, and clearance dominated by the mechanism of convection, which is closely associated with the brain's ISF/CSF production rate. Assuming rapid equilibrium across the various CNS compartments and CSF antibody concentration as a surrogate for CNS drug levels, the pharmacokinetic modeling of CNS antibody concentration can be simplified to Eq. 3, where ${}^{CNS}V$ is the apparent volume of distribution for CNS, ${}^{CSF}C$ and ${}^{serum}C$ denote

Table 1 Pharmacokinetic parameters of antibodies A, B, C, D and E in rodents and non-human primates

Test article	Animal info	Dose	Serum PK parameters[a]				CSF PK parameters[a]				$^{CSF}AUC/^{Serum}AUC$ ratio (%)
			$^{serum}C^{c}_{max}$	$^{serum}T^{c}$	$^{serum}AUC_{INF}$	$^{serum}t_{1/2}$	$^{CSF}C^{c}_{max}$	$^{CSF}T^{c}_{max}$	$^{CSF}AUC_{INF}$	$^{CSF}t_{1/2}$	
		mg/kg	µg/mL	H	µg*h/mL	H	ng/mL	H	ng*h/mL	H	
A	Rat[b]	10 (IV)	560		40,400	155	200	16	38,000	185	0.09
B	Rat[b]	10 (IV)	208		31,700	234	110	24	48,400	245	0.15
C	Rat[b]	20 (IV)	778		108,500	169	380	48	94,000	136	0.09
D	Rat[b]	20 (IV)	559		67,100	173	170	24	48,000	143	0.07
E	Rat[b,d]	30 (IP)	1000	6	71,000	80	340	24	54,000	44	0.075
A	NHP (N=4)	20 (IV)	520±35		171,400±23,100	402±39	590±270	42±36	258,000±124,600	423±44	0.15±0.07
	NHP (N=11)	100 (IV)	2270±650		854,700±266,500	456±87	2670±2060	43±30	1,441,200±798,100	531±152	0.16±0.08
C	NHP (N=11)	30 (IV)	1220±390		163,200±36,000	156±34	680±710	48±29	140,300±73,300	201±71	0.09±0.06
	NHP (N=6)	100 (IV)	4210±790		467,300±76,500	126±31	2210±810	64±29	538,300±231,300	181±39	0.10±0.05
D	NHP (N=4)	30 (IV)	980±70		179,700±22,400	290±35	580±240	60±24	194,400±106,800	257±44	0.10±0.04

[a] Pharmacokinetic calculation was based on linear-log noncompartmental analysis for both CSF and serum profiles

[b] Rat PK parameters were based on mean data

[c] Maximum serum and CSF levels were based on the highest observed serum and CSF concentration, respectively

[d] Pharmacokinetic parameters from Ref. [7]

the antibody concentrations in CSF and serum, respectively, and $PS_{product}$ and $Q_{convection}$ are independent parameters that govern entering and exiting the CNS. Entering CNS ($PS_{product}$) requires overcoming the BBB/BCSFB, whereas exiting CNS ($Q_{convection}$) to a large extent does not. Both processes are independent of systemic clearance mechanisms.

$$\frac{{}^{CNS}Vd\,{}^{CSF}C}{dt} = PS_{product} \times {}^{serum}C - Q_{convection} \times {}^{CSF}C \tag{3}$$

The apparent linearity of the predicted vs. experimentally measured serum and CSF data for antibody A in Fig. 3b, c confirm that the model has little bias over a wide range of antibody concentrations. Although the variation in serum pharmacokinetic profiles are small (Fig. 3b), the differences in CSF to serum ratios are relatively large (Fig. 3c). Similar variations were observed for antibody C (Fig. 4a). For the 12 monkeys that received 30 mg/kg of antibody C, ${}^{CSF}AUC\text{-}to\text{-}{}^{serum}AUC$ ratios ranged from 0.03 to 0.23%.

Discussion

The CSF-to-serum ratio of 0.1–0.2% that we measured for five independent antibodies in rats and NHPs agrees well with published results for other antibodies. CSF-to-total serum IgG ratios of 0.1–0.2% in healthy humans have been reported by several groups [11–13]. Similarly, for therapeutic antibodies in humans, there are many reports from sparse CSF sampling that was used to estimate CSF-to-serum ratios. For example, in patients treated with rituximab for neurological autoimmune diseases, the (lumbar) CSF to serum antibody ratios were approximately 0.1–0.2% [14]. Trastuzumab had a CSF-to-serum ratio of 0.3% in a 62-year-old patient with meningeal carcinomatosis treated by weekly IV administration [15]. MGAWN1, an antibody against West Nile virus, had a CSF-to-serum ratio of 0.25% in healthy volunteers [16]. CSF to serum ratios for anti-LINGO-1 mAb BIIB033 measured 2 weeks post dose are 0.032–0.079% in healthy volunteers and 0.03–0.13% in individuals with multiple sclerosis [17]. Finally, a murine analog of anti-amyloid beta mAb solanezumab had a CSF to plasma ratio in rats of approximately 0.1% [18]. Of special note, the CSF to serum ratios of 0.032–0.079% for BIIB033 (antibody E) observed in healthy volunteers, matches well with the 0.075% value we report here in rats for the same antibody.

There are many studies exploring the mechanisms by which antibodies cross the BBB [19]. Garg and Balthasar studied antibody distribution in neonatal Fc receptor (FcRn) deficient mice. Although the plasma AUC of ^{125}I-labeled antibody was significantly reduced in FcRn−/− mice, the brain-to-plasma exposures remained unchanged at 0.22% in wildtype and FcRn−/− mice. Similar to what we observed in rats and NHP, the brain concentration–time profiles paralleled the plasma profiles in wildtype and FcRn−/− mice (i.e., ${}^{brain}t_{½}$ was equal to ${}^{plasma}t_{½}$) [20]. Other proposed mechanisms include a low-rate nonspecific adsorptive mechanism involving transcytosis, endocytosis, or macropinocytosis [20–23]. Unlike with small molecules, it is challenging to accurately measure antibody concentrations in brain tissues. With CNS-to-serum concentration ratios for antibodies of only 0.1–0.2%, it is critical to prepare brain tissues that are free of residual blood. Brain ISF levels can be determined by microdialysis, but this is a technically challenging method for antibodies due to their large size. Thus, brain tissue data provides a rough estimate of CNS drug levels but must be interpreted with caution. In both preclinical and clinical settings, CSF has been widely accepted as a surrogate for assessing CNS drug levels [2, 5, 24]. In investigating CNS exposure levels in animals, euthanasia followed by perfusion and collection of brain and CSF samples could impact the data. Further work is needed to understand potential differences that might arise due to sample handling.

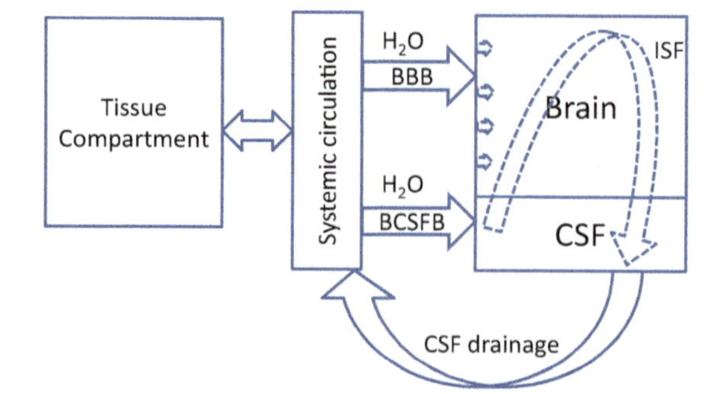

Fig. 6 Diagram for water flow into and out of the CNS

Although CSF is largely produced at the choroid plexus (CP) and secreted into the four ventricles of the brain, recent studies indicate there are other sources of CSF [24–27]. As illustrated in Fig. 6, water is secreted into the CNS by endothelial cells of the BBB, forming brain ISF, and by choroid plexus (CP) into ventricles, forming CSF [25, 28]. CSF also enters the brain interstitial spaces via peri-capillary (Virchow–Robin) spaces [27, 28]. The junctures between brain parenchyma and CSF interfaces are relatively loose and allow exchange of solutes between brain ISF and CSF [24, 29, 30]. Moving away from BBB and BCSFB, ISF/CSF carries solutes and eventually drains into blood at multiple locations, including the dural sinus [27, 31, 32]. There has been no report that BBB and/or BCSFB are involved in CSF drainage/reabsorption.

For the factors that determine the CNS exposure of an antibody, $PS_{product}$ and $Q_{convection}$ are two independent processes that cannot be simplified by inter-compartmental clearance and are independent of systemic clearance mechanisms. Large inter-subject variations in CNS antibody exposures need to be taken into consideration even if there is little variation in a drug's serum concentration–time profile. Variation can be introduced at the CNS level by an individual's $PS_{product}/Q_{convection}$ ratio. From a pharmacokinetic modeling point of view, these two parameters are highly correlated and difficult to differentiate other than through a change in their ratio. That said, the $PS_{product}$ value of an antibody can be assessed using in vitro methods [23] and an individual's CSF production rate can be assessed by MRI [33]. On average, rats have 150 μL CSF by volume, which undergoes turnover 11 times per day. In contrast, healthy humans have an average CSF volume of 580 mL and a turnover rate of 4 times per day [1]. The CSF turnover rate sets the efficiency of convective clearance out of the CNS. It is well documented that CSF production rates vary under different conditions, including circadian rhythm [33–36], normal aging [36–39], concurrent medications such as the carbonic anhydrase inhibitor acetazolamide [40, 41] and the proton pump inhibitor omeprazole [42, 43], and in disease conditions such as hydrocephalus [26, 44] and Alzheimer's disease (AD) [45, 46]. Alterations in CSF production rates can have profound effects on CNS clearance of medications and waste products. In individuals with AD, reduced brain ISF/CSF turnover is probably caused by decreased brain ISF/CSF production and increased CSF volume [45, 46]. BAN2401, a monoclonal antibody targeting amyloid beta protein, has a CSF-to-serum ratio in AD patients of 0.04–0.08% at 24 h following dose administration, but increases to 0.29–0.81% after 10–14 days [47]. These data suggest that ${}^{CSF}T_{max}$ for BAN2401 is > 24 h and that ${}^{CSF}C$ levels have not yet peaked 24 h after dose administration. CSF-to-serum ratios of greater than 0.1–0.2% have also been reported for other antibody therapies in individuals with AD [13, 48, 49]. CSF-to-serum total albumin and IgG ratios are also elevated in AD patients [12, 13], consistent with AD patients has reduced CSF clearance rates [45, 46].

Linking CSF production rates with CNS clearance of antibodies potentially has broad applications, since it enables the estimation of antibody kinetics between the CSF and systemic circulation and would allow for rational design of CSF sampling schedules and projection of CNS drug exposures in selected patient groups. For example, for antibodies, delayed ${}^{CSF}T_{max}$ and steady-state CSF-to-serum concentration ratios are observed. These should be taken into consideration when designing CSF sampling schemes. In patients with reduced CSF production, either due to disease or concurrent medications, higher CSF drug exposures should be expected. Unfortunately, the factors that affect CSF production rates and, more importantly, the subsequent impact on their ability to clear CNS waste have not yet been fully investigated and/or appreciated.

In summary, from an extensive analysis of the pharmacokinetics of five human antibodies in rats and monkeys, we show that antibodies enter the CNS slowly, with ${}^{CSF}T_{max}$ around 24–72 h after IV administration, and that CSF and serum concentration–time curves become parallel after ${}^{CSF}T_{max}$, with average CSF-to-serum ratios of 0.1–0.2%. Prior to achieving ${}^{CSF}T_{max}$, CSF-to-serum ratios are not accurate indicators of CNS uptake or steady-state CSF-to-systemic concentration ratios. For antibodies with long systemic $t_{½}$s, ${}^{serum}t_{½}$ determines ${}^{CSF}t_{½}$. These studies should aid in the design of future studies to better understand factors that contribute to the elimination of antibodies from the CNS.

Abbreviations

BBB: blood–brain-barrier; CSF: cerebrospinal fluid; ISF: interstitial fluid; BCSFB: blood–CSF-barrier; mAb: monoclonal antibody.

Authors' contributions

The studies were conceived and designed by QW, PW and RP. The experiments were conducted by LD, EV, AC, WC, RC and GK. QW performed data analysis. QW, PW, DG, RP, IN, ER, TB and LG participated in the discussion and interpretation. The final manuscript was prepared by QW, LD, AC, PW and RP. The studies in their entirety were supervised by QW. All authors read and approved the final manuscript.

Author details

[1] Biogen, Inc., 250 Binney Street, Cambridge, MA 02142, USA. [2] Present Address: Ribon Therapeutic, 99 Hayden Ave #100, Lexington, MA 02421, USA. [3] Present Address: Intellia Therapeutics, 40 Erie St, Cambridge, MA 02139, USA. [4] Present Address: Thermo Fisher Scientific Inc, 790 Memorial Dr, Cambridge, MA 02139, USA. [5] Present Address: Merrimack pharmaceuticals, 1 Kendall Square, Cambridge, MA 02139, USA. [6] Present Address: Foresee pharmaceuticals, 1 Innovation Way, Suite 100, Newark, DE 19711, USA.

Competing interests

The authors declare that they have no competing interests.

Funding

This work was funded by Biogen, Inc. All authors and Biogen have approved the manuscript and this submission.

References

1. Hammarlund-Udenaes M, et al. On the rate and extent of drug delivery to the brain. Pharm Res. 2008;25(8):1737–50.

2. Lin JH. CSF as a surrogate for assessing CNS exposure: an industrial perspective. Curr Drug Metab. 2008;9(1):46–59.
3. Liu X, et al. Unbound drug concentration in brain homogenate and cerebral spinal fluid at steady state as a surrogate for unbound concentration in brain interstitial fluid. Drug Metab Dispos. 2009;37(4):787–93.
4. Badhan RK, Chenel M, Penny JI. Development of a physiologically-based pharmacokinetic model of the rat central nervous system. Pharmaceutics. 2014;6(1):97–136.
5. de Lange EC. Utility of CSF in translational neuroscience. J Pharmacokinet Pharmacodyn. 2013;40(3):315–26.
6. Plavina T, et al. Anti-JC virus antibody levels in serum or plasma further define risk of natalizumab-associated progressive multifocal leukoencephalopathy. Ann Neurol. 2014;76(6):802–12.
7. Pepinsky RB, et al. Structure of the LINGO-1-anti-LINGO-1 Li81 antibody complex provides insights into the biology of LINGO-1 and the mechanism of action of the antibody therapy. J Pharmacol Exp Ther. 2014;350(1):110–23.
8. Hall CM, et al. An extended range generic immunoassay for total human therapeutic antibodies in preclinical pharmacokinetic studies. J Immunol Methods. 2013;393(1–2):70–3.
9. Stubenrauch K, Wessels U, Lenz H. Evaluation of an immunoassay for human-specific quantitation of therapeutic antibodies in serum samples from non-human primates. J Pharm Biomed Anal. 2009;49(4):1003–8.
10. Pepinsky RB, et al. Exposure levels of anti-LINGO-1 Li81 antibody in the central nervous system and dose-efficacy relationships in rat spinal cord remyelination models after systemic administration. J Pharmacol Exp Ther. 2011;339(2):519–29.
11. Giasuddin AS, et al. Levels of serum immunoglobulin G, CSF IgG and IgG index in acute bacterial meningitis. Br J Biomed Sci. 1998;55(4):253–7.
12. Frolich L, et al. Integrity of the blood–CSF barrier in dementia of Alzheimer type: CSF/serum ratios of albumin and IgG. Eur Arch Psychiatry Clin Neurosci. 1991;240(6):363–6.
13. Leonardi A, et al. The integrity of the blood–brain barrier in Alzheimer's type and multi-infarct dementia evaluated by the study of albumin and IgG in serum and cerebrospinal fluid. J Neurol Sci. 1985;67(2):253–61.
14. Petereit HF, Rubbert-Roth A. Rituximab levels in cerebrospinal fluid of patients with neurological autoimmune disorders. Mult Scler. 2009;15(2):189–92.
15. Pestalozzi BC, Brignoli S. Trastuzumab in CSF. J Clin Oncol. 2000;18(11):2349–51.
16. Beigel JH, et al. Safety and pharmacokinetics of single intravenous dose of MGAWN1, a novel monoclonal antibody to West Nile virus. Antimicrob Agents Chemother. 2010;54(6):2431–6.
17. Tran JQ, et al. Randomized phase I trials of the safety/tolerability of anti-LINGO-1 monoclonal antibody BIIB033. Neurol Neuroimmunol Neuroinflamm. 2014;1(2):p.e18
18. Siemers ER, et al. Safety and changes in plasma and cerebrospinal fluid amyloid beta after a single administration of an amyloid beta monoclonal antibody in subjects with Alzheimer disease. Clin Neuropharmacol. 2010;33(2):67–73.
19. Greenwood J, et al. Current research into brain barriers and the delivery of therapeutics for neurological diseases: a report on CNS barrier congress London, UK, 2017. Fluids Barriers CNS. 2017;14(1):31.
20. Garg A, Balthasar JP. Investigation of the influence of FcRn on the distribution of IgG to the brain. AAPS J. 2009;11(3):553–7.
21. Haqqani AS, et al. Endosomal trafficking regulates receptor-mediated transcytosis of antibodies across the blood brain barrier. J Cereb Blood Flow Metab. 2017. https://doi.org/10.1177/0271678X17740031.
22. Mager I, et al. Targeting blood–brain-barrier transcytosis—perspectives for drug delivery. Neuropharmacology. 2017;120:4–7.
23. Stanimirovic DB, et al. Blood–brain barrier models: in vitro to in vivo translation in preclinical development of CNS-targeting biotherapeutics. Expert Opin Drug Discov. 2015;10(2):141–55.
24. Johanson CE, et al. Multiplicity of cerebrospinal fluid functions: new challenges in health and disease. Cerebrospinal Fluid Res. 2008;5:10.
25. Hladky SB, Barrand MA. Mechanisms of fluid movement into, through and out of the brain: evaluation of the evidence. Fluids Barriers CNS. 2014;11(1):26.
26. Oreskovic D, Klarica M. A new look at cerebrospinal fluid movement. Fluids Barriers CNS. 2014;11:16.
27. Brinker T, et al. A new look at cerebrospinal fluid circulation. Fluids Barriers CNS. 2014;11:10.
28. Hladky SB, Barrand MA. Fluid and ion transfer across the blood–brain and blood–cerebrospinal fluid barriers; a comparative account of mechanisms and roles. Fluids Barriers CNS. 2016;13(1):19.
29. Shen DD, Artru AA, Adkison KK. Principles and applicability of CSF sampling for the assessment of CNS drug delivery and pharmacodynamics. Adv Drug Deliv Rev. 2004;56(12):1825–57.
30. Benfenati V, Ferroni S. Water transport between CNS compartments: functional and molecular interactions between aquaporins and ion channels. Neuroscience. 2010;168(4):926–40.
31. Pollay M. The function and structure of the cerebrospinal fluid outflow system. Cerebrospinal Fluid Res. 2010;7:9.
32. Plog BA, Nedergaard M. The glymphatic system in central nervous system health and disease: past, present, and future. Annu Rev Pathol. 2017;13:379–94.
33. Battal B, et al. Cerebrospinal fluid flow imaging by using phase-contrast MR technique. Br J Radiol. 1004;2011(84):758–65.
34. Tan DX, Manchester LC, Reiter RJ. CSF generation by pineal gland results in a robust melatonin circadian rhythm in the third ventricle as an unique light/dark signal. Med Hypotheses. 2016;86:3–9.
35. Takahashi H, et al. Variation in supratentorial cerebrospinal fluid production rate in one day: measurement by nontriggered phase-contrast magnetic resonance imaging. Jpn J Radiol. 2011;29(2):110–5.
36. Nilsson C, et al. Circadian variation in human cerebrospinal fluid production measured by magnetic resonance imaging. Am J Physiol. 1992;262(1 Pt 2):R20–4.
37. May C, et al. Cerebrospinal fluid production is reduced in healthy aging. Neurology. 1990;40(3 Pt 1):500–3.
38. Gideon P, et al. Cerebrospinal fluid production and dynamics in normal aging: a MRI phase-mapping study. Acta Neurol Scand. 1994;89(5):362–6.
39. Kleine TO, et al. Transport and production of cerebrospinal fluid (CSF) change in aging humans under normal and diseased conditions. Zeitschrift fur Gerontol. 1993;26(4):251–5.
40. Jafarzadeh F, et al. Novel application of acetazolamide to reduce cerebrospinal fluid production in patients undergoing thoracoabdominal aortic surgery. Interact Cardiovasc Thorac Surg. 2014;18(1):21–6.
41. Del Bigio MR, Di Curzio DL. Nonsurgical therapy for hydrocephalus: a comprehensive and critical review. Fluids Barriers CNS. 2016;13:3.
42. Lindvall-Axelsson M, et al. Inhibition of cerebrospinal fluid formation by omeprazole. Exp Neurol. 1992;115(3):394–9.
43. Girod M, et al. Evaluation of the effect of oral omeprazole on canine cerebrospinal fluid production: a pilot study. Vet J. 2016;209:119–24.
44. Rutka JT. Cerebrospinal fluid production in patients with hydrocephalus. J Neurosurg. 2002;97(6):1269–70 **(discussion 1270)**.
45. Tarasoff-Conway JM, et al. Clearance systems in the brain-implications for Alzheimer disease. Nat Rev Neurol. 2015;11(8):457–70.
46. Suzuki Y, et al. Reduced CSF water influx in Alzheimer's disease supporting the beta-amyloid clearance hypothesis. PLoS ONE. 2015;10(5):e0123708.
47. Logovinsky V, et al. Safety and tolerability of BAN2401—a clinical study in Alzheimer's disease with a protofibril selective Abeta antibody. Alzheimers Res Ther. 2016;8(1):14.
48. Leyhe T, et al. Modulation of beta-amyloid by a single dose of GSK933776 in patients with mild Alzheimer's disease: a phase I study. Alzheimers Res Ther. 2014;6(2):19.
49. Miyoshi I, et al. Safety and pharmacokinetics of PF-04360365 following a single-dose intravenous infusion in Japanese subjects with mild-to-moderate Alzheimer's disease: a multicenter, randomized, double-blind, placebo-controlled, dose-escalation study. Int J Clin Pharmacol Ther. 2013;51(12):911–23.

Opportunities in posthemorrhagic hydrocephalus research: outcomes of the Hydrocephalus Association Posthemorrhagic Hydrocephalus Workshop

Jenna E. Koschnitzky[1*], Richard F. Keep[2], David D. Limbrick Jr.[3], James P. McAllister II[3], Jill A. Morris[4], Jennifer Strahle[3] and Yun C. Yung[5]

Abstract

The Hydrocephalus Association Posthemorrhagic Hydrocephalus Workshop was held on July 25 and 26, 2016 at the National Institutes of Health. The workshop brought together a diverse group of researchers including pediatric neurosurgeons, neurologists, and neuropsychologists with scientists in the fields of brain injury and development, cerebrospinal and interstitial fluid dynamics, and the blood–brain and blood–CSF barriers. The goals of the workshop were to identify areas of opportunity in posthemorrhagic hydrocephalus research and encourage scientific collaboration across a diverse set of fields. This report details the major themes discussed during the workshop and research opportunities identified for posthemorrhagic hydrocephalus. The primary areas include (1) preventing intraventricular hemorrhage, (2) stopping primary and secondary brain damage, (3) preventing hydrocephalus, (4) repairing brain damage, and (5) improving neurodevelopment outcomes in posthemorrhagic hydrocephalus.

Keywords: Hydrocephalus, Posthemorrhagic, Intraventricular hemorrhage, Germinal matrix hemorrhage, Blood brain barrier, Premature

Background

The Hydrocephalus Association hosted a workshop on July 25 and 26, 2016 at the National Institutes of Health, Neuroscience Center, to build research capacity and identify areas of opportunity for research around posthemorrhagic hydrocephalus (PHH). The Hydrocephalus Association was founded in 1983 by parents of children with hydrocephalus and developed a research program in 2009. Since then the Association has committed over $7 million to research, making it the largest non-profit, non-governmental funder of hydrocephalus research in the United States. The mission of the Hydrocephalus Association is to promote a cure for hydrocephalus and improve the lives of those affected by the condition. The Association strives to accomplish this mission by collaborating with patients, caregivers, researchers and industry, raising awareness, and funding innovative, high impact research to prevent, treat, and ultimately cure hydrocephalus.

The 2016 Hydrocephalus Association PHH Workshop was developed through the Hydrocephalus Association PHH Initiative, a multiyear initiative focused on increasing research efforts focused on PHH. The workshop agenda was developed by the workshop planning committee which was led by Hydrocephalus Association staff and included both an investigator in the Hydrocephalus Clinical Research Network (HCRN) and a family member of a person with hydrocephalus. The workshop brought together a diverse group of researchers including pediatric neurosurgeons, neurologists, and neuropsychologists

*Correspondence: jenna@hydroassoc.org
[1] Hydrocephalus Association, 4340 East West Highway, Bethesda, MD 20814, USA

together with scientists in the fields of brain injury and development, cerebrospinal and interstitial fluid dynamics, and the blood–brain and blood–CSF barriers. Workshop attendees also included Hydrocephalus Association staff and family members of people affected by hydrocephalus.

The primary focus of the workshop was on PHH of prematurity, although PHH can develop at any age, including in utero, after preterm birth, and in children and adults who have had a brain hemorrhage [1]. PHH develops after intraventricular extension of a hemorrhage [intraventricular hemorrhage, (IVH)] (Fig. 1). IVH grade (I–IV) is classified according to the extension (periventricular germinal tissue, ventricle, parenchyma) of hemorrhage and presence of ventricular dilation according to the Papile scale [2]. Both the source of the hemorrhage (e.g. periventricular vs. choroid plexus) and the degree of tissue injury related to the extension of the hemorrhage are linked to outcomes. Neonatal IVH occurs in up to 25% of preterm neonates [3–12] and results in hydrocephalus in 10% of these neonates, including 25% of neonates with grade III/IV IVH [13]. 38% of neonates with PHH require long term CSF diversion; the remaining either die or do not require a permanent shunt [13].

Advances in neonatology have improved survival rates for preterm neonates in recent decades [14]. In the early 1980 s, the rates of IVH decreased from 40–50 to 20% for premature neonates < 1500 g [15, 16]. However, for premature neonates 500–750 g, the rate of IVH remained high at 40–50% [15, 17, 18], and the trend in recent years shows a relative increase in IVH rates [13, 19, 20]. In the United States, the incidence of PHH of prematurity after IVH remained steady (8–10%) between 2000 and 2010; however, annual admissions for both IVH and PHH increased approximately 60% during the same time period [13]. The increase in IVH and PHH comes despite a recent decline in overall premature birth rate between 2007 and 2010 [13, 21].

PHH of prematurity is a common form of pediatric hydrocephalus, accounting for 20% of the shunted hydrocephalus cases in the United States [22] and is associated with significant morbidity and mortality [13]. This report details the major themes and the research opportunities discussed during the 2016 Hydrocephalus Association Posthemorrhagic Hydrocephalus Workshop. The views and recommendations in this report were developed by the listed authors and subsequently distributed to all workshop attendees for commentary. All feedback was then discussed and integrated into the report.

PHH of prematurity

PHH of prematurity is a common and particularly insidious form of pediatric hydrocephalus [22]. During the workshop, an overview of our current knowledge about PHH risks, pathophysiology, and treatments was presented.

Maternal and neonatal risk and protective factors

Many maternal factors can alter the risk of IVH in premature neonates. Some protective factors are related to health care including access to prenatal care, administration of antenatal corticosteroid regimens, and cesarean delivery [23]. Maternal health care disparities likely interact with other factors such as maternal race and

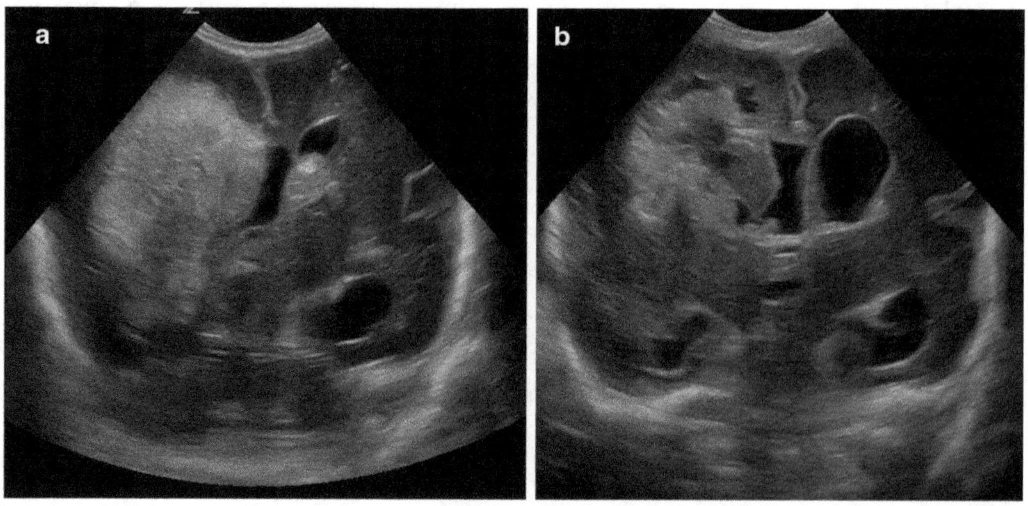

Fig. 1 Cranial Ultrasounds of Premature Infant after IVH. **a** Cranial ultrasound performed in a 5 day old 24 week gestation male showing grade IV intraventricular hemorrhage with intraventricular extension. **b** Cranial ultrasound performed in the same infant 12 days later showing interval development of hydrocephalus

education level which have also been associated with risk of IVH in preterm neonates. Unexpectedly, preeclampsia has been associated with a decreased risk of IVH [23–28].

Neonates born at term rarely develop IVH or PHH [29]. For premature neonates, the risk of IVH, and subsequently PHH, increases with decreased gestational age and weight [7, 13, 14]. Furthermore, the development of PHH is directly related to IVH grade, with over 75% of PHH patients having Grade III/IV IVH [13]. Male sex is also associated with an increased risk of PHH. Prenatal infection, specifically chorioamnionitis, can increase the risk of IVH and is related to gestational age [5, 23, 30–35]. Asian ethnicity seems to be protective [36].

Physiological risk factors

Premature neonates are especially vulnerable to IVH within the subependymal germinal matrix, a highly vascularized region consisting of neural and glial precursor cells [19, 30, 37, 38]. During early development, the germinal matrix undergoes rapid cellular proliferation and angiogenesis, but the thickness of the germinal matrix peaks and subsequently declines after 24 gestational weeks and is nearly absent by 36–37 gestational weeks [3, 19, 39–41]. This corresponds to the time-dependent risk of developing IVH and subsequent PHH. At developmental time points when premature birth is survivable, the germinal matrix is located along the walls of the lateral ventricles, primarily within the ganglionic eminence and over the developing caudate nucleus.

In preterm neonates, the germinal matrix is susceptible to hemorrhaging due to the immaturity of the vasculature, [3, 15, 19, 39, 42, 43] and sudden fluctuations in cerebral blood flow due to respiratory and hemodynamic instability [37, 38, 44]. The combination of immature vasculature and rapid changes in cerebral blood flow may lead to rupture of the germinal matrix vasculature and IVH [3, 19, 30].

Pathophysiology of PHH

Hydrocephalus represents an alteration in fluid balance within the brain and cranial cavity. It is traditionally held that under normal conditions cerebrospinal fluid (CSF) is primarily secreted into the cerebral ventricles by the choroid plexus (site of the blood–CSF barrier) and moves via bulk flow through the ventricular system and subarachnoid space before being absorbed at the arachnoid villi/granulations although it should be noted that these develop at about week 35 and 39, respectively [45]. In addition, some fluid secretion into brain parenchyma occurs across the cerebral microvasculature (site of the blood–brain barrier) and through Virchow-Robins spaces (also recently termed the "glymphatic" system) at the surface of the cerebral cortex in animal models [46–48]. Parenchymal interstitial fluid also enters the cerebral ventricles across the ependymal lining [49]. CSF can also be absorbed via cranial nerve lymphatics [50–52] and may pass retrogradely into cerebral microvessels [53–57]. An increase in CSF production or reduction in CSF absorption may result in ventriculomegaly if the system cannot compensate for the changes.

Secondary injury mechanisms occur following ventriculomegaly (reviewed in [58–60]). A detailed discussion of these secondary mechanisms is beyond the scope of this manuscript, but they include cerebral (mostly periventricular) edema, demyelination, axonal degeneration and impaired axoplasmic transport in periventricular white matter, cerebral hypoxia and ischemia, reduced metabolite levels, altered blood–brain and blood–CSF barriers, loss of cilia and junctional complexes on ependymal cells, ependymal denudation, changes in aquaporin channels, and altered neurodevelopmental trophic factors. These cytopathologies are found in most forms of congenital and acquired hydrocephalus and most likely overlap with the pathogenetic mechanisms involved in PHH.

As detailed above, the pathophysiology of hydrocephalus is multifactorial in nature, and the precise mechanisms underlying PHH of prematurity remain unclear [3]. PHH is traditionally thought to occur due to impediments in the CSF flow or absorption pathways. Acute, obstructive hydrocephalus can occur soon after IVH and may be due to blood physically blocking the most-narrow portions of the CSF spaces, i.e. the cerebral aqueduct, the foramina of Monro, the outlets of the fourth ventricle, or the subarachnoid spaces.

Multiple theories have been proposed to explain the development of "communicating" hydrocephalus after IVH including blockage of the arachnoid villi and arachnoid granulations due to microthrombi [61] or scarring [62]. Other theories include the CSF bulk flow hypothesis and the hydrodynamic theory. These theories are based on postulated changes in pressure gradients within the CSF or CSF and vascular systems, respectively [63, 64]. Few studies, however, have been conducted to test any of these theories.

Surprisingly, there have also been very few studies addressing the impact of IVH on the choroid plexus [65]. One recent study reports CSF hypersecretion occurs after IVH in a rodent model. This hypersecretion is caused by an upregulation in choroid plexus Na/K/Cl cotransporter activity associated with Toll-like receptor 4 activation [66].

In contrast, there is much evidence that IVH damages the ependymal cells that line the cerebral ventricles. Alterations in this CSF–brain interface may impact bulk fluid flow via ciliopathy and disrupt neurodevelopment by exposing the subventricular zone to CSF. An emerging mechanism appears to involve impaired junctional proteins, such as N-cadherin and connexin that not only provide structure for the ependymal lining of the ventricles but also influence progenitor cell proliferation, migration, and differentiation [67–70]. Recent evidence from preterm neonates with PHH also indicates that the neurogenic niche is compromised following IVH [71], and this primary effect could subsequently evolve into a type of hydrocephalus *ex vacuo,* in which the ventricles expand subsequent to impaired neurogenesis and neuronal differentiation [71].

Current treatments for PHH of prematurity

Treatments for PHH of prematurity fall into one of three categories: temporary non-surgical, temporary surgical, and permanent surgical. Temporary non-surgical treatments, including thrombolytic agents and diuretics, have been tested [72–77]; however, none of these interventions are currently recommended for use in neonates with PHH [78]. Temporary surgical treatments include ventricular access devices (VADs), external ventricular drains (EVDs), ventriculosubgaleal (VSG) shunts, and lumbar punctures. All four temporary surgical treatments are options in the management of PHH [79]; however, lumbar puncture is only recommended for immediate short-term removal of CSF [78]. Serial lumbar punctures are not recommended [78, 80].

Emerging treatments include endoscopic lavage with early removal of IVH. In one study, Schulz et al. reported a decrease in the rates of hydrocephalus and need for permanent shunt placement [81]. However, this treatment remains under investigation and long-term outcomes remain unclear.

If hydrocephalus persists despite temporary CSF diversion, placement of a ventriculoperitoneal (VP) shunt has been the treatment of choice. VP shunting has been the mainstay of long-term surgical management of hydrocephalus for over six decades. However, VP shunts frequently fail. In children, approximately 30-50% of shunts fail within the first 2 years [82–84] and 80% of shunt fail within 4 years [83], necessitating revision, externalization, or removal, all of which have associated costs and complications. Endoscopic third ventriculostomy (ETV), with or without choroid plexus cauterization (ETV-CPC), is an alternative treatment option and can obviate the need for a shunt. However, for treating PHH, the success rate in children less than 1 year of age is approximately 50% [85–90]. Evaluations of long-term neurological outcomes of ETV-CPC or ETV versus shunt are ongoing.

Review of clinical trials

Past clinical trials inform future clinical, translational, and basic science research. The workshop, reviewed clinical trials conducted in both premature neonates and adults with intracranial hemorrhage to identify areas of promise and obstacles that limit our ability to interpret and compare results.

Interventions that alter risk of IVH

Premature and/or (extremely) low birth weight neonates are vulnerable populations at risk for multiple co-morbidities such as IVH and neurological deficits. To improve survival rates and decrease such co-morbidities, interventions based on a variety of biological mechanisms have been tested and adopted by the medical community. These interventions can be broadly grouped into antenatal interventions, birth-related procedural interventions, and postnatal interventions (Table 1).

Antenatal interventions include administration of corticosteroids, phenobarbital, magnesium sulfate, and vitamin K. Antenatal corticosteroids administration is perhaps the most established intervention and has been shown to reduce severe grades of IVH as well as reduce mortality and respiratory distress syndrome [91, 92]. In extremely premature infants, improved outcomes in neonatal mortality and neurodevelopmental outcomes were dose dependent with an indication that these results were mediated by reduced rates of severe IVH [93]. Antenatal vitamin K administration also reduced IVH risk during the first 7 days of life in a small randomized trial [94]; however, an earlier meta-analysis concluded that antenatal vitamin K did not reduce risk of IVH or improve neurodevelopmental outcomes [95]. A recent meta-analysis indicated that, antenatal magnesium sulfate did not reduce the rates of IVH in preterm infants but may have beneficial effects on the rates of moderate to severe cerebral palsy [96]. In addition, antenatal phenobarbital had no effect on IVH risk in preterm infants (NCT00009620; [97, 98]).

Procedural interventions occurring at or close to the time of birth include mode of delivery and the timing of umbilical cord clamping. In many studies comparing vaginal and cesarean deliveries in preterm and very low birth weight infants, there did not appear to be IVH risk reduction associated with one form of delivery over the other [99–101]. By contrast, a study showed planned cesarean delivery is associated with a reduced risk of IVH in extremely preterm infants compared to vaginal delivery and emergency cesarean delivery [102]. A study comparing both antenatal corticosteroid administration and cesarean delivery reported that antenatal corticosteroid administration independently reduced IVH risk [103]. The choice of immediate/early vs. delayed cord clamping balances the desire to have neonatologists care for the preterm infant as soon as possible compared with the thought that additional blood flow from the placenta (placental transfusion) may minimize IVH and decrease the need for subsequent transfusions. An early study

Table 1 Summary of representative drug or physical intervention trials to reduce IVH or improve neurological outcomes in humans

Drug(s) or intervention	Dosage	Mechanism	Data class	Degree of IVH reduction	Neurological outcome improvement	References
Antenatal betamethasone	Single 2-dose (12 mg each); 24 mg	May reduce endothelial proliferation, vascular density, and increase pericyte vascular coverage [270]	Class 2, Class 2, Class 2, Class 2, Class 1, Class 2, Class 1	IVH reduction from 6 to 47 h, slowly increased 48 h ≥ 10 days); beneficial for women < 34 weeks GA; decreased IVH from 22–29 GA; decreased IVH even with incomplete course	Not significant, not examined in study; associated improved neurological outcome	[30, 91, 93, 114, 271–273]
Antenatal betamethasone/dexamethasone	Meta-study with unknown dosing	May reduce endothelial proliferation, vascular density, and increase pericyte vascular coverage	Class 2	Beneficial for women periviable ages 23–26 weeks GA	Not examined	[274]
Prophylactic indomethacin (oral or IV)	Oral 0.2 mg/kg daily for 3 days; 0.1 mg/kg IV for daily for 2 days	Inhibits cyclooxygenase-mediated production of prostaglandins, promotes germinal matrix vascular maturation	Class 2, Class 1, Class 1	50–80% reduction in IVH	Higher verbal scores in 3-8 yr old boys	[118, 275, 276]
Ibuprofen	Oral 5–10 mg/kg daily for 3 days	Inhibits cyclooxygenase-mediated production of prostaglandins	Class 2, Class 1	Mixed results: 0–80% reduction in IVH	Not examined	[118, 277]
Neonatal Ethamsylate	12.5 mg/kg daily for 4 days	Inhibits cyclooxygenase-mediated production of prostaglandins; possibly increases platelet aggregation	Class 1, Class 1, Class 1	Reduction in IVH	No decrease in mortality (possibly increased), no improvement in cognitive outcomes	[113, 278, 279]
Inhaled nitric oxide	Inhaled at 20 ppm	Mediates rapid vasodilation by stimulating guanylate cyclase, subsequent reduced phosphorylation of myosin, and relaxes smooth muscle cells	Class 1, Class 1	No reduction in IVH	No significant neurological improvement	[280, 281]
Phenobarbital	IV injections of 20–30 mg/kg loading dose, followed by 3–7 days of maintenance doses	Acts on GABA receptors and is thought to stabilize blood pressure and may protect against free radicals	Class 2, 3	Mixed results from 12 clinical trials; overall does not appear to reduce severe IVH or ventricular dilatation	Did not seem to attenuate neurological impairments	[282]
Prophylactic surfactant	Bolus or infusion delivery via endotracheal tube (e.g., 5 ml/kg)	Replenishes insufficient surfactant production in premature neonates in order to increase pulmonary compliance, increase alveolar gas exchange, and decrease hypoxia	Class 1, Class 1, Class 1	No reduction in IVH (though there was decrease in neonatal morbidity)	Not examined	[283–285]

Table 1 continued

Drug(s) or intervention	Dosage	Mechanism	Data class	Degree of IVH reduction	Neurological outcome improvement	References
Postnatal corticosteroids (typically dexamethasone)	0.12–0.5 mg/kg/day for several days	May reduce endothelial proliferation, vascular density, and increase pericyte vascular coverage	Class 1, Class 1	Possible trend towards reduction of neonatal IVH	Unclear neurological improvement	[286, 287]
Magnesium (magnesium sulfate)	4–6 g IV $MgSO_4$ loading dose, 2–4 g/h for 12–24 h	Tocolytic mechanisms include competition for calcium, prevent release of acetylcholine, and activation of myosin light chain kinase, which blocks myometrial contractions; neuroprotective effects may include stabilization of rapid blood pressure fluctuations, increased cerebral blood flow, and decreased neuroinflammation	Class 1, Class 1, Class 1, Class 2	No effect on IVH reduction	Possible neurological protection	[288–291]
Cesarean delivery	22–37 weeks gestational age planned delivery	Prevention of stresses associated with vaginal delivery	Class 2, Class 2	35% reduction in IVH in < 30 week preterm neonates	Not examined	[102, 292]
Delayed cord clamping	Delayed clamping usually performed 60–75 s (compared with 30–45 s)	Proposed mechanisms include cardiovascular transition with ventilation, establishment of red blood cell volume, decreased need for blood transfusion	Class 1, Class 1, Class 3, Class 3	Up to 50% reduction in preterm IVH; benefits unclear in term neonates	May improve fine motor and social domains at 4 years in low-risk children [293]	[288, 293–295]

and a meta-review appeared to show a reduction in IVH with delayed clamping [104, 105], although subsequent primary and meta-analysis studies showed no difference in the rate of IVH [106–108]. Encouraging, there may be some neurological and motor benefits to the infants when examined after 18 months [106].

Postnatal interventions that decrease the risk of IVH, but may not improve long-term neurological outcomes, include treatment with prophylactic indomethacin, ibuprofen, inositol, or ethamsylate [31, 109–114]. Early indomethacin or ibuprofen decreased IVH rates in preterm and very low birth weight infants [115–120]. In addition, indomethacin reduced the incidence of patent ductus arteriosus and the risk of severe periventricular and intraventricular hemorrhage, although rates of shunted hydrocephalus were not changed (NCT00009646; [120]). Inositol treatment reduced the risk of severe IVH as well as neonatal deaths, infant deaths, and retinopathy of prematurity [121–125]. In a systematic review of ethamsylate treatment in preterm and very low birth rate infants, Hunt and Hey found lower rates of IVH in treated infants who were born at less than 35 weeks gestation [113]. However, there were no differences in neonatal mortality or neurodevelopmental outcomes at 2 years.

Other postnatal interventions, such as inhaled nitrous oxide, phenobarbital, prophylactic surfactant, and corticosteroids, have had no effect on IVH rates [5, 126–129] but some were associated with other positive outcomes [5, 126, 128]. In contrast, multiple interventions for premature neonates increase the risk of IVH, which include red blood cell transfusions and rapid volume expansion [130–132]. Encouragingly, vitamin E supplementation in preterm infants reduces the risk of germinal matrix/intraventricular hemorrhage in a meta-analysis of 26 studies, though there was an associated higher risk of sepsis [133].

Neonatal interventions to stop development of progressive PHH

Pharmaceutical agents, drainage and irrigation of the ventricles, and temporizing devices have been tested to stop the development or progression of PHH after IVH. In these studies, the primary outcome is usually permanent shunt placement.

To date, pharmaceutical treatments have not been effective in stopping the development of PHH or its neurological disability [78, 134, 135]. These therapies include the use of diuretics to reduce CSF production [76, 77, 136] and fibrinolytic agents. The International Posthemorrhagic Ventricular Dilation (PHVD) Drug Trial Group tested acetazolamide plus furosemide treatment. In that trial, the combination resulted in higher rates of morbidity and did not decrease the need for a permanent shunt placement [76]. At the 1 year follow up, there was no difference in shunt placements but the group did report an increase in neurological morbidity [77]. A definitive Cochrane database review by Whitelaw et al. [43] and another study reported no difference in mortality or permanent shunt placement [78, 137]. Intraventricular thrombolytic agents, including recombinant tissue plasminogen activator (rtPA) [138], streptokinase [73, 75, 139], and urokinase [140], have been tested but are also not recommended for clinical use [78]. The two randomized studies testing streptokinase reported no difference in rates of shunt dependent hydrocephalus and also increased concerns about the development of meningitis and secondary IVH [75, 139].

Recently, a phase one clinical trial for the use of PNEUMOSTEM®, human umbilical cord blood derived mesenchymal stem cells, in preterm infants with grade III–IV IVH was completed. The primary outcome is unexpected death or anaphylactic shock and the secondary outcome is death or the development of shunt dependent hydrocephalus; results are pending (NCT02274428). The same group is now enrolling infants in a follow up study (NCT02673788). In related work, multiple clinical trials are underway or being analyzed to determine the effects of mesenchymal stem cells on the development of bronchopulmonary dysplasia in preterm infants (NCT01828957; NCT01897987; NCT02381366; NCT0244396).

In contrast to pharmaceutical treatments, trials that have attempted to physically wash out blood and other substances have shown more positive results [72, 141, 142]. Drainage and irrigation of the ventricles in the DRIFT (Drainage, Irrigation, and Fibrinolytic Therapy) randomized control trial did not decrease mortality or the need for permanent shunt insertion at 6 months, and the study was stopped early due to an increase the incidence of secondary intraventricular bleeding [72]. However, at 2 years, the DRIFT group had reduced rates of severe cognitive disability and death compared to the standard care group [141]. These results underscore the need for long term cognitive assessments in addition to near term outcomes such as shunt placement.

At this time, short-term temporizing procedures are often the first step in the clinical treatment of PHH, since the longevity of the condition may still be in question and, from a technical standpoint, the size of the neonate may preclude longer-term strategies such as permanent CSF shunting. Temporary surgical treatments include VADs, EVDs, VSG shunts, and lumbar punctures. Many studies have compared these treatment options but no clear results have emerged (reviewed in [78, 143, 144]). A recent prospective cohort study by the Hydrocephalus Clinical Research Network (HCRN) reported no difference in the rate of permanent shunt placement between EVDs or VSG shunts (SOPHH, NCT01480349) [145].

In future studies, morbidity, mortality, permanent shunt placement, and infection risk should all be considered as important factors. However, the timing of these interventions may have a greater impact on outcomes than the type of treatment. In one study, early treatment (based on ventricular index) with either reservoir placement or lumbar puncture was safe, effective, resulted in lower rates of permanent shunt placement, and reduced moderate-to-severe disability [146]. The results of a randomized control trial, the Early versus Late Ventricular Intervention Study (ELVIS, NCT00875758), are currently being analyzed.

Lessons from adult intracerebral and intraventricular hemorrhage clinical trials

In adults, IVH occurs as an extension of an initial intracerebral hemorrhage (ICH) with IVH occurring in about 40% of ICH cases [147, 148]. IVH size and degree of extension through the ventricular system predict poor outcomes and mortality [11, 149, 150]. Hydrocephalus develops in two-thirds of adult IVH cases and is an independent risk factor for poor neurological outcome [11, 12]. While both neonatal and adult IVH arise from parenchymal hemorrhage, the underlying causes differ between premature neonates (rupture of immature germinal matrix blood vessels) and adults (e.g., hypertension, amyloid angiopathy, anti-coagulant use; [151]). However, information from IVH in adults may inform neonatal studies.

In adults, ICH/IVH treatment has focused on three main approaches: limiting bleeding, clot removal, and reducing secondary brain injury. Hemostatic therapy (e.g., Factor VIIa, FAST trial NCT00127283; Tranexamic acid, TRAIGE trial, NCT02625948; platelet transfusion, PATCH trial, NCT02187120) and reducing blood pressure (e.g., ATACH, NCT01176565; INTERACT, NCT00716079) have undergone clinical trials to limit continued bleeding (clot expansion) in the early phase (< 24 h) after ICH. Although some of these studies have reported statistically significant effects on limiting bleeding, there has yet to be definitive evidence of improved outcomes [152–160].

The second therapeutic approach has centered on parenchymal or intraventricular clot removal. For ICH, standard surgical evacuation has not shown statistical benefit (e.g. STICH II trial, NCT01320423) and there is interest in using minimally invasive surgery (MIS) with or without tissue rtPA to lyse the clot (MISTIE II trial, NCT01827046; ICES trial, NCT00224770; ENRICH trial, NCT02880878) [161–163]. Evidence indicates that MIS is safe but whether it improves outcomes after ICH is still uncertain [162].

As in the premature population, a number of trials for adult ICH patients with IVH have combined EVD placement with administration of thrombolytic agents. A number of systematic meta-analyses have reported decreased mortality using this combination versus external ventricular drain (EVD) alone [164, 165]. Khan et al. [165] also reported a reduction in permanent shunt placement with the combination therapy while a non-significant reduction was reported by Gaberel et al. [164]. The recent large CLEAR III trial (NCT00784134) evaluated EVD with rtPA administration vs. EVD with saline in IVH patients. There was no significant improvement in the primary outcome measure (modified Rankin Score), but there was a significant reduction in mortality compared to EVD + saline [166]. There is debate about whether the particular thrombolytic (urokinase vs. rtPA) used to remove the clot is important [164, 165]. Two subsequent meta-analyses have been performed which include the results of the CLEAR trial [167, 168]. Wang et al. [88] reported that benefit of intraventricular thrombolysis (IVT) + EVD vs. EVD alone is limited to a reduction in mortality at the expense of an increased number of survivors with moderately-severe to severe disability; subgroup analyses did not suggest an advantage of urokinase over rtPA. In a recent meta-analysis and systematic review, Baker et al. [167] reported that intraventricular thrombolytic therapy for IVH resulted in reduced mortality and potentially better functional outcomes as measured by the modified Rankin Scale or Glasgow outcome scale.

Other newer minimally invasive approaches to adult IVH studied in small clinical trials include endoscopic surgery and controlled lumbar drainage for prevention of permanent shunt dependency. A randomized trial of combined IVT with lumbar drainage vs. IVT alone for prevention of permanent shunt dependency after ICH with severe IVH was stopped following interim analysis after 30 patients due to significant efficacy of the tested intervention [169]. A meta-analysis comparing neuroendoscopic surgery combined with EVD versus combination EVD plus IVT reported significant benefits in survival, functional outcomes, hematoma evacuation rates, and need for shunt placement in favor of endoscopic techniques [170]. These promising techniques will require large-scale validation with standardized protocols.

Compared to cerebral ischemia [171], there have been relatively few clinical trials of neuroprotectants to reduce ICH/IVH-induced secondary brain injury including hydrocephalus [151, 152]. As yet, those trials have not shown any statistical benefit. Iron, from hemoglobin, is one potential clot-derived neurotoxic factor [151]. Currently, there is a phase II clinical trial for deferoxamine, an iron chelator (iDEF; NCT02175225) and minocycline (MACH; NCT01805895, [172]), an anti-inflammatory agent that also chelates iron [173]. Additional promising therapies tested in small pilot clinical trials include fingolimod, which may reduce progression of perihematomal edema [174], and transcription factor peroxisome proliferator-activated receptor gamma (pioglitazone) which augments phagocytosis and modulates oxidative stress and inflammation (SHRINC; NCT00827892) [175].

With the exception of early clot expansion, where there is little data in the neonate, there are similarities in the approaches being examined in the adult and neonate. It is hoped that information from each age group may help in devising better ways for hematoma removal and reducing the impact of clot-induced, or derived, harmful factors.

Workshop recommendations: key areas for research and intervention

The development of PHH of prematurity involves a series of events resulting in multiple, simultaneous injury processes. Correctly predicting who is at risk, determining key time-points and targets for early interventions, and understanding the long-term effects of PHH are essential for preventing, minimizing, or reversing the development of hydrocephalus and improving long-term outcomes. During the workshop, key areas for research and interventions were identified and discussed (Fig. 2).

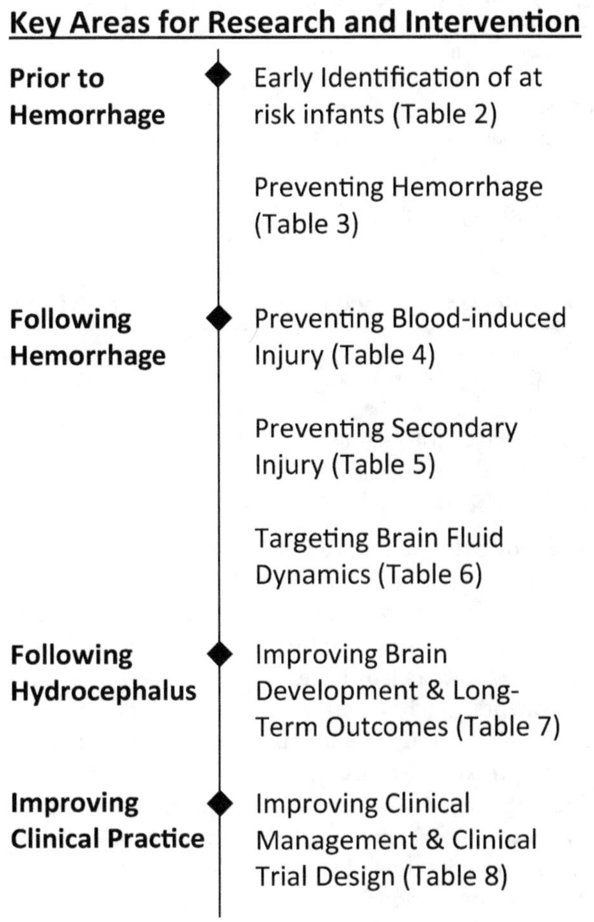

Fig. 2 Key areas for research and intervention. A schematic of the key areas for research and intervention identified during the workshop

Early identification

To optimize clinical management, it is essential to identify the premature neonates who are at highest risk of developing IVH and subsequently PHH. This is a key area for future research (Table 2). Many demographic and physiological factors are associated with IVH and PHH, but there are currently no established predictive models of PHH [176–180]. Predicting IVH and PHH with a high degree of sensitivity and specificity will improve clinical management and prognostication of high risk neonates and could be an essential component in the development and testing of new therapies. Identified biomarkers may provide insights to the pathophysiology of PHH and provide new therapeutic targets to prevent or minimize the condition. These tools could also be used as selection criteria for clinical trials testing the efficacy of new therapies.

Table 2 Early identification: research targets

Identifying genetic risk factors
Identifying susceptibility/risk factors of IVH and PHH
Identify diagnostic, prognostic, predictive, and monitoring biomarkers (e.g., molecular, cellular, imaging biomarkers)
Developing a prognostic scale

Prevention of hemorrhage

Premature neonates are uniquely susceptible to germinal matrix hemorrhage (GMH) and the germinal matrix vasculature is a major target for research (Table 3). Determining the tolerance of the germinal matrix to fluctuations in cerebral blood flow and the interplay between respiratory and cardiac instability and cerebral blood flow will help guide clinical management of premature neonates to reduce the risk of GMH. In addition, a more in depth understanding of germinal matrix development and physiology will provide new targets for prophylactic therapies aimed at strengthening or otherwise modifying the germinal matrix to make it less susceptible to hemorrhage. Determining how these therapies affect corticogenesis is a critical component and potential barrier to success.

Table 3 Preventing hemorrhage: research targets

Determining the tolerance of the germinal matrix to respiratory and cardiac instability
Understanding the development of the germinal matrix
Understanding the physiology of the blood/ventricular barrier of the germinal matrix
Determining how to modify the germinal matrix vasculature without altering corticogenesis

Table 4 Preventing blood-induced injury: research targets

Identifying mechanisms of toxicity
Elucidating the effects of IVH on ventricular ependymal and choroid plexus epithelium
Developing targeted therapeutics
Determining how to clear the blood clot rapidly and safely

Prevention of blood-induced injury

Once IVH occurs, blood and blood-derived products cause damage to the surrounding tissue. Developing methods to reduce such injury is a major research target (Table 4). Multiple labs have already identified key blood components, such as iron and lysophosphatidic acid (LPA), that can independently cause ventriculomegaly and progressive hydrocephalus [3, 67, 181–186]. Determining the mechanism(s) of action on both the ventricular ependyma and choroid plexus epithelia may allow the development of targeted therapies, such as iron chelation, LPA receptor antagonism, or reducing LPA production. Ependymal damage after IVH may be a cause of further injury by allowing blood and blood components direct access to underlying tissue and by affecting fluid flow within the brain [71]. As stated earlier, the choroid plexus is the site of the blood–CSF barrier and the primary site of CSF secretion. Alterations in either of these functions may exacerbate brain injury and alter fluid dynamics in the brain after IVH [66].

Careful time-series experimentation will be required to determine if there is a critical time window post-IVH in which these therapies are effective and if the timing can be achieved in a clinical setting. In addition, early blood evacuation with or without the use of thrombolytic agents may reduce damage and improve outcomes. Forthcoming results from the ELVIS trial should help clinical decision making. Active clearance of the blood clot remains a promising avenue for research. It may also be possible to speed up endogenous processes, such as macrophage clearance of the clot, that do not result in the release of additional blood products.

Prevention of secondary injury

Prevention or reduction of secondary injury processes and the damage caused by hydrocephalus are active areas of research, with multiple research targets (Table 5), and may have broad implications for preventing or minimizing the effects of hydrocephalus for many etiologies. Immediately after hemorrhage, blood coagulation begins through a cascade that activates thrombin [187, 188] and results in subarachnoid fibrosis and disruption of cerebrospinal fluid dynamics [58, 189–194]. Modulation of neuro-inflammatory pathways has thus been suggested as a strategy for mitigating the effects of IVH and potentially preventing the development of PHH. CSF levels of interleukin (IL)-1β, IL-6, IL-8, IL-18, transforming growth factor (TGF)-β1 and -β2, tumor necrosis factor (TNF)-α, and other cytokines and chemokines have all been implicated in PHH [194–200]. In a recent study by Habiyaremye et al. [201], XCL-1 was decreased in the CSF of neonates with PHH. Levels of CCL-19, IL-1α, IL-1β, IL-12, and CCL-3 were elevated but only absolute CCL-19 levels correlated with levels of CSF nucleated cells, neutrophils, and lymphocytes [201]. In addition, non-protein bound iron likely remains a source of injury well after the initial bleed [3, 182, 185, 202].

Table 5 Preventing secondary brain injury: research targets

Therapeutic modulation of neuroinflammation
Preventing fibrosis
Preventing ependymal damage
Minimizing edema

Recent studies have focused on reducing subarachnoid fibrosis and periventricular astrogliosis by targeting inflammatory and other signaling cascades and have had positive results in animal models [194, 203–205]. Other neuroprotective attempts to modulate calcium cytopathology have shown limited improvements [134, 206, 207]. As opposed to molecular targets, the results of the DRIFT trial suggest that ventricular drainage and irrigation to remove toxic substances, such as free iron and pro-inflammatory cytokines, provides long-term benefits [141]. To date, this is the only intervention that has improved outcomes in PHH in a randomized trial.

For treatment of both blood-induced injury and secondary injuries, the specificity of the compounds, mode of administration, dosing, toxicity, and proof of target engagement will become extremely important as therapies move toward first in human trials (see section: "Moving basic science discoveries into clinical practice"). The identification of potential therapeutic agents would be accelerated if appropriate in vitro preparations were developed that could be used for high-throughput screening of new or repurposed compounds.

Targeting brain fluid dynamics

IVH in premature neonates can result in altered brain fluid dynamics and hydrocephalus. Increased intracranial pressure (ICP) and hydrocephalus can cause additional damage through hypoxia, ischemia, and mechanical stress [58, 207–214]. This damage is especially apparent in white matter tracts [214–221]. Temporizing devices and permanent shunting can, at least partially, relieve these insults, but are only implemented after ventriculomegaly is apparent. Non-surgical methods that alter CSF dynamics could be used at earlier time points in isolation or later in conjunction with temporizing devices. Current targets for these interventions include pharmaceutical reduction of CSF production by the choroid plexus (reviewed in [134, 222]), increased CSF absorption (e.g., increase absorption through aquaporin channels [223–225], especially following IVH [226], as well as cranial nerve lymphatics [227]), and improved CSF flow (e.g., enhancement of natural processes that repair motile cilia). This list, however, also highlights the need for a better understanding of the choroid plexus response after IVH, alternative routes of CSF production and absorption, and the role of motile cilia in the development of hydrocephalus after hemorrhage. Strengthening cell–cell junctions between ependymal cells might also prevent or delay ventriculomegaly by maintaining ependymal integrity and increasing the total resistance of the ependymal layer [71, 228].

Although much research is still needed on CSF dynamics (Table 6), IVH and subsequent injury may also impact interstitial flow within the brain parenchyma. The recently proposed brain glymphatic system describes a pathway for fluid movement between CSF and brain parenchyma and within the parenchyma itself [229]. How IVH affects such movement is an important research question.

Understanding brain development and long-term outcomes after IVH

Premature neonates with Grade III or IV IVH are at a higher risk of poor neurodevelopmental and cognitive outcomes than preterm neonates without IVH or who have Grade I or II IVH [7, 230]. It is not clear if the development of progressive hydrocephalus significantly adds to this burden [30], but it is likely that the injury mechanisms involved in the development of PHH overlap with those related to neurodevelopmental and cognitive outcomes.

For the PHH population, improving long-term neurodevelopmental and cognitive outcomes is very important and should be a primary focus in clinical trials [231]. Understanding how blood products, destruction of the ependymal layer, and inflammatory processes alter brain maturation will be important for the development of rehabilitation strategies. Normalized brain development and function after therapeutic interventions could serve as additional markers of efficacy beyond the primary outcome measure of permanent shunt placement. For example, recent findings of altered CSF proteins [129–131, 152] and impaired adherens junctions in disrupted ventricular and subventricular zones [71] could be targeted and have long-lasting neurodevelopmental consequences. In the near term, ventricular drainage and irrigation may minimize the secondary damage that occurs soon after and in the months following a brain bleed, minimizing the need for additional therapies [141].

Improving functional outcomes is a priority for the hydrocephalus community and must become a priority in research [231]. Longitudinal clinical studies are needed to investigate the long-term neurobehavioral outcomes of PHH, ranging from the infant/toddler stage through adulthood. For patients with shunted hydrocephalus, it is important to study the longer term, cumulative effects of altered CSF dynamics along with periodic brain compression and increased ICP due to shunt malfunction on cognition and other measures of quality of life. Other areas of particular interest include the impact of non-surgical (e.g., occupational, speech, physical therapies) and surgical (CSF shunt management) treatments. For such long-term studies, the development of optimal psychometric and imaging-based instruments is a logical priority. Research priorities in relation to brain development and long-term outcomes after IVH are given in Table 7.

Table 6 Fluid dynamics: research targets

Understanding and targeting CSF fluid production
Understanding and targeting alternative routes for CSF absorption
Understanding and targeting CSF and brain interstitial fluid flow
Understanding changes in barrier function after IVH
Understanding and targeting ependymal cell–cell junctions

Improving clinical management and clinical trials

Focus on the clinical management of preterm neonates has intensified in recent years in parallel with advances in obstetrics and newborn medicine. Identifying and implementing best practices as well as testing the benefit, or lack thereof, of new techniques and therapies is an essential part of this process. However, in published work, substantial variability exists in the study populations as well as diagnosis and treatment thresholds, making comparisons between studies difficult.

Standardizing clinical protocols through quality improvement methodologies and/or clinical trials has become a priority for the field but more work needs to

Table 7 Brain development and long-term outcomes after IVH: research targets

Determining if PHH is associated with worse long-term neurodevelopmental, cognitive, and motor deficits compared to IVH and prematurity
Determining how damage to motile and primary cilia affects brain development
Understanding how cell proliferation from the ventricular and subventricular zones are altered after IVH
Identifying and targeting the mechanisms responsible for changes in cell proliferation
Linking neurodevelopmental and cognitive deficits to altered brain function
Developing targeted rehabilitation strategies for preterm neonates with IVH and PHH.
Determining mechanisms of tissue repair after PHH and how to enhance it
Determining the benefits of stem cell therapies on long-term outcomes
Determining impact of non-surgical interventions on long-term outcomes
Developing optimal psychometric and imaging-based instruments

be done. An early report from the HCRN demonstrated substantial variation in the treatment of PHH, even within this coordinated network [232]. In 2014, evidence-based guidelines for the management of PHH were published and provided specific recommendations while also identifying larger areas of uncertainty [78]. Wellons et al. [145] recently published the results of the HCRN's Shunting Outcomes in Post-Hemorrhagic Hydrocephalus (SOPHH), which compared two of the most common neurosurgical treatments for PHH, and, while no difference was found between the two treatments, SOPHH provides an excellent starting point for standardizing the diagnosis and treatment of PHH [145].

Study protocols also need to be standardized. Currently, research groups use different study populations and inclusion criteria (e.g., preterm vs. very preterm, low birth weight, very low birth weight, or IVH grade) as well as different diagnosis and treatment thresholds. As a first step, common classification data including gestational age at birth, weight at birth, and IVH grade should be collected in every study and, when possible, standard inclusion and exclusion criteria should be used.

Establishing standardized criteria for PHH diagnosis and treatment thresholds (e.g., physical criteria, ventricular size parameters, CSF and imaging biomarkers, etc.) will also help simplify the interpretation of comparative effectiveness research examining available treatments (e.g., CSF shunting versus ETV ± CPC) and studies testing emerging therapeutics. Outcome measures (e.g., ventriculomegaly, progressive hydrocephalus, symptomatic hydrocephalus, or permanent shunt placement) also need to be standardized and used consistently.

Table 8 Clinical management and clinical trials: targets

Developing standardized management and treatment protocols
Implementing standardized management and treatment protocols
Collecting common classification data (e.g., gestational age at birth, birth weight)
Using common study inclusion/exclusion criteria when possible
Developing standardized diagnosis criteria/definitions
Developing standardized treatment criteria/definitions
Developing standardized outcome measures/definitions

Standardizing clinical management and study protocols for preterm neonates is essential as new surgical and non-surgical strategies are developed. With powerful, multi-institutional and multi-dimensional clinical trial infrastructure, the collective efforts of committed investigators can be leveraged to address critical clinical questions relevant to the diagnosis and treatment of PHH over both the short- and long-term. Research priorities in relation to clinical management and clinical studies after IVH are given in Table 8.

Moving basic science discoveries into clinical practice

The workshop was designed to identify areas of opportunity and spur research efforts for PHH of prematurity, but the ultimate goal is to prevent IVH and PHH of prematurity or prevent associated brain injury. The process of moving basic science discoveries into clinical trials and then standard clinical practice, however, is slow and inefficient. During the workshop, participants identified multiple areas that could be improved and opportunities to speed up the transition from basic research to clinical trials.

Choosing the appropriate model

There is a wide range of animal models used for research in PHH of prematurity and germinal matrix hemorrhage (reviewed in [233, 234]), and no single animal model will be suitable for all biological questions. Most studies involve experimental induction of IVH in mice [67, 191, 235], rats [182, 185, 202, 236–243], rabbits [244–250], cats [251], dogs [252, 253], sheep [254], and pigs [255–258]. While the majority of these in vivo studies have employed intraventricular injection of whole blood or blood products, others have used alternative approaches [67, 247, 259–261]. In vitro models of IVH have also been used [262, 263]. Before studies begin, animal models should be reviewed to determine the model most suitable for the outcomes being measured, the clinical relevance of each model, and whether multiple animal models will be needed if the initial studies are positive [233, 234]. In addition, experimental parameters such as mode of IVH induction, intraventricular volume changes, and developmental age of animal models should be addressed when interpreting the results.

Streamlining preclinical research

There is a paucity of studies on non-surgical therapies in PHH and one goal is to increase this number and move these therapies into clinical trial. However, the literature is littered with clinical trials that proved to be costly failures. To avoid these mistakes, it is imperative that investigators conduct preclinical research at the highest standards of scientific rigor and demonstrate robust reproducibility. It is difficult for one lab or investigator to conduct all of the experiments necessary, but it is possible to streamline these efforts through the use of standardized protocols and active collaboration. In addition, publication of negative data would benefit the entire research community.

In addition to the success or failure of an experiment or series of experiments, there are other common stumbling blocks in the development of novel treatments. Many are related to the compound itself including its safety profile, metabolism, and tissue distribution. Mode of delivery can also prevent promising therapies from moving forward. On the business side, compound manufacturing, licensing, and commercialization are issues in which many investigators are not versed but can prevent a therapy from coming to market [264, 265]. Early identification of these issues can help investigators design meaningful translational studies.

Available resources for preclinical research

Private and public organizations provide useful resources to guide preclinical research. The Operation Brain Trauma Therapy (OBTT) consortium has published a framework for preclinical drug screening and could be a useful model for PHH research [266]. In addition, the National Institutes of Health (NIH) have developed general guidelines to improve scientific rigor and reproducibility (https://www.nih.gov/research-training/rigor-reproducibility/principles-guidelines-reporting-preclinical-research). The RIGOR guidelines and Stroke Therapy Academic Industry Roundtable (STAIR) recommendations have been developed for preclinical studies focused on stroke therapies [267–269]. These guidelines and recommendations are highly applicable to PHH research.

The National Institute of Neurological Disorders and Stroke (NINDS) has also developed programs to streamline preclinical therapeutic development (https://www.ninds.nih.gov/Current-Research/Research-Funded-NINDS/Translational-Research). For early-stage development, NINDS has created the IGNITE (Innovation Grants to Nurture Initial Translational Efforts) Program that include: (1) funding opportunities for assay development and screening potential therapeutic agents, (2) therapeutic agent characterization (pharmacokinetics, pharmacodynamics and in vivo efficacy studies for small molecules, biologics and biotechnology products and (3) the development and validation of animal models, model systems and/or pharmacodynamic markers. Additional information about this program can be found here: https://www.ninds.nih.gov/Current-Research/Research-Funded-NINDS/Translational-Research/Funding-Programs-Researchers/IGNITE.

For later-stage biologic and biotechnology products, NINDS has established the CREATE Bio (Cooperative Research to Enable and Advance Translational Enterprises for Biologics) program that includes an optimization track (agent optimizations) and a development track (IND enabling and optional small first in human Phase 1 clinical trials) funding opportunities (https://www.ninds.nih.gov/Current-Research/Research-Funded-NINDS/Translational-Research/CREATE-BIO). For later-stage drug development, NIH established the NIH Blueprint Neurotherapeutics Network (BPN) providing support for small molecule discovery and development (https://neuroscienceblueprint.nih.gov/bpdrugs/).

The Food and Drug Administration (FDA) also provides guidelines for good laboratory practices (GLP) which need to be followed for medical product development for preclinical trials (http://www.accessdata.fda.gov/scripts/cdrh/cfdocs/cfcfr/CFRSearch.cfm?CFRPart=58). Researchers should understand the guidelines and work with their institutions to establish GLP practices early in the drug development process. Resources are also available through the Alzheimer's Drug Discovery Foundation that cover topics from central nervous system drug discovery through commercialization (https://www.scienceexchange.com/group/addf-access/resources#catList).

Conducting clinical trials

Conducting clinical trials in PHH of prematurity present a number unique challenges. Extreme prematurity, very low birthweight, and medical comorbidities as well as often complex social issues all contribute to the vulnerability of this population. Thus, clinical studies must be held to the highest standards of good clinical practice (GCP), institutional human research protection offices, and federal agencies such as the NIH and FDA.

Despite its high prevalence within newborn medicine and hydrocephalus in general, PHH is relatively uncommon at any individual institution. Multi-institutional platforms are therefore critical to conducting meaningful human studies research in PHH. In addition to the

HA-supported HCRN, the NIH has worked to develop infrastructure for clinical studies for conditions like PHH. NINDS established the Network for Excellence in Neuroscience Clinical Trials (NeuroNext) that consists of one Clinical Coordinating Center (CCC), a Data Coordinating Center (DCC), and 25 Clinical Sites located throughout the United States (https://www.neuronext.org/). The standardized and accessible infrastructure of NeuroNext was designed to efficiently and rapidly conduct exploratory phase I and II clinical trials as well as biomarker validation studies.

Through the National Center for Advancing Translational Sciences (NCATS), the NIH also has important resources for early and late phase studies designed to repurpose drugs developed for other conditions (https://ncats.nih.gov/preclinical/repurpose). For example, the Molecular Libraries Small Molecule Repository (MLSMR) has over 350,000 compounds. Taking advantage of these resources can accelerate the process of therapy development.

Role of the Hydrocephalus Association

The HA can play a central role in accelerating hydrocephalus research by serving as a link between the two HA-supported clinical networks, the Hydrocephalus Clinical Research Network (HCRN.org) and Adult HCRN (AHCRN.org), the basic and translational researchers involved with the HA Network for Discovery Science (HANDS, HANDS.hydroassoc.org), and the patient community through the HA Patient Powered Interactive Engagement Registry (HAPPIER, hydroassoc.org/happier). HANDS is designed to support basic and translational research by directly funding research studies, building shared infrastructure, and convening workshops and conferences. HANDS is also a platform for improving communication between researchers and developing new research collaborations. HAPPIER is a patient reported database. The survey data generated through HAPPIER can be used by researchers. In addition, researchers can work with HA to send out new surveys and also to recruit patients for clinical trials. The HA will continue to develop and modify research programs to best serve the hydrocephalus research community as well as continue advocacy efforts to increase the availability of federal funding for hydrocephalus research.

Conclusions

Intraventricular hemorrhage and posthemorrhagic hydrocephalus is a potentially devastating condition in premature neonates with no effective non-surgical therapies. The Hydrocephalus Association Posthemorrhagic Hydrocephalus Workshop identified many important areas for future research to help produce a pathway for reducing the occurrence and effects of PHH.

Abbreviations

AHCRN: Adult Hydrocephalus Clinical Research Network; BPN: Blueprint Neurotherapeutics Network; CCC: Clinical Coordinating Center; CPC: choroid plexus cauterization; CREATE Bio: Cooperative Research to Enable and Advance Translational Enterprises for Biologics; DCC: Data Coordinating Center; DRIFT: Drainage, Irrigation, and Fibrinolytic Therapy; ELVIS: Early versus Late Ventricular Intervention Study; ETV: endoscopic third ventriculostomy; CPC: choroid plexus cauterization; EVD: external ventricular drain; FDA: Food and Drug Administration; GCP: good clinical practice; HA: Hydrocephalus Association; HANDS: Hydrocephalus Association Network for Discovery Science; HAPPIER: Hydrocephalus Association Patient Powered Interactive Engagement Registry; HCRN: Hydrocephalus Clinical Research Network; ICH: intracerebral hemorrhage; ICP: intracranial pressure; IGNITE: Innovation Grants to Nurture Initial Translational Efforts; IL: interleukin; IND: investigational new drug; IVH: intraventricular hemorrhage; IVT: intraventricular thrombolysis; LPA: lysophosphatidic acid; MIS: minimally invasive surgery; MLSMR: Molecular Libraries Small Molecule Repository; NCATS: National Center for Advancing Translational Sciences; NeuroNext: Network for Excellence in Neuroscience Clinical Trials; NICHD: National Institute of Child Health and Human Development; NIH: National Institutes of Health; NINDS: National Institute of Neurological Disorders and Stroke; PATCH: Pre-hospital Anti-fibrinolytics for Traumatic Coagulopathy and Haemorrhage; PHH: posthemorrhagic hydrocephalus; PHVD: posthemorrhagic ventricular dilation; rtPA: recombinant tissue plasminogen activator; SOPHH: Shunting Outcomes in Post-Hemorrhagic Hydrocephalus; STAIR: Stroke Therapy Academic Industry Roundtable; TGF: transforming growth factor; TNF: tumor necrosis factor; VAD: ventricular access device; VSG: ventriculosubgaleal.

Authors' contributions

JEK wrote the initial manuscript. RFK, DDL, JPM, JAM, JS, and YCY critically revised the document and significantly contributed to the writing of select sections. All authors read and approved the final manuscript.

Author details

[1] Hydrocephalus Association, 4340 East West Highway, Bethesda, MD 20814, USA. [2] University of Michigan, 1500 East Medical Center Drive, Ann Arbor, MI 48109, USA. [3] Washington University in St. Louis School of Medicine, 660 S. Euclid Ave, St. Louis, MO 63110, USA. [4] National Institute of Neurological Disorders and Stroke, National Institutes of Health, Neuroscience Center, 6001 Executive Blvd, NSC Rm 2112, Bethesda, MD 20892, USA. [5] Sanford Burnham Prebys Medical Discovery Institute, 10901 North Torrey Pines Rd., Building 7, La Jolla, CA 92037, USA.

Acknowledgements

We would like to thank everyone who participated in the 2016 Hydrocephalus Association Posthemorrhagic Hydrocephalus Workshop. A special thanks to the National Institutes of Health for providing the venue and Elizabeth Quartey and Lyna Merzoug for providing planning and logistical support.

Workshop Participants:

Stephen Back, MD, PhD, Oregon Health Sciences University, Andrew Baird, PhD, University of California San Diego, Praveen Ballabh, MD, New York Medical College, Christopher Batterman, Hydrocephalus Association, Craig Brown, Hydrocephalus Association, Vicki Brown, Hydrocephalus Association, Adam Chodobski, PhD, Warren Alpert Medical School of Brown University, Joanne Conover, PhD, University of Connecticut, Marc Del Bigio, MD, PhD, University of Manitoba, Amanda Garzon, MA, Hydrocephalus Association, Paul Gross, Hydrocephalus Association (Planning Committee Member), Diana Gray,

MA, Hydrocephalus Association, Carolyn Harris, PhD, Wayne State University, Aisha Heath, MPA, CFRE, Hydrocephalus Association, Terrie Inder, MD, Harvard University (Planning Committee Member), Richard Keep, PhD, University of Michigan (Planning Committee Member), Jenna Koschnitzky, PhD, Hydrocephalus Association (Planning Committee Member), Maria K. Lehtinen, PhD, Boston Children's Hospital, Harvard Medical School, David Limbrick, MD, PhD, Washington University School of Medicine (Planning Committee Member), James P. (Pat) McAllister, II, PhD, Washington University School of Medicine (Planning Committee Member), Lyna Merzoug, Hydrocephalus Association (Planning Committee Member), Laura Ment, MD, Yale School of Medicine, Jill A. Morris, PhD, NIH, NINDS (Planning Committee Member), Shenandoah (Dody) Robinson, MD, Johns Hopkins University, Joseph Scafidi, DO, Children's National, Jennifer Strahle, MD, Washington University School of Medicine, Evan Synder, MD, PhD, Sanford Burnham Prebys Medical Discovery Institute, Joanna Szmydynger-Chodobski, PhD, Warren Alpert Medical School of Brown University, Hudson Taylor, PhD, ABPP/CN, Nationwide Children's Hospital Research Institute, The Ohio State University, Robert Thorne, PhD, University of Wisconsin-Madison School of Pharmacy, Andrew Whitelaw, MD, PhD, University of Bristol, Guohua Xi, MD, University of Michigan, Yun Yung, PhD, Sanford Burnham Prebys Medical Discovery Institute (Planning Committee Member), John Zhang, MD, PhD, Loma Linda University, Wendy Ziai, MD, MPH, Johns Hopkins University.

Competing interests

DDL and JPM receive research funding from Medtronic, Inc., Karl Storz, Inc., and Microbot Medical, Inc. RFK is co-Editor-in-Chief of *Fluids Barriers CNS*.

Funding

The 2016 Hydrocephalus Association (HA) Posthemorrhagic Hydrocephalus Workshop was funded through the HA Network for Discovery Science (HANDS.hydroassoc.org).

References

1. Rodriguez EM, Guerra MM. Neural stem cells and fetal-onset hydrocephalus. Pediatr Neurosurg. 2017;52:446–61.
2. Papile LA, Burstein J, Burstein R, Koffler H. Incidence and evolution of subependymal and intraventricular hemorrhage: a study of infants with birth weights less than 1,500 gm. J Pediatr. 1978;92:529–34.
3. Strahle J, Garton H, Maher C, Muraszko K, Keep R, Xi G. Mechanisms of hydrocephalus after neonatal and adult intraventricular hemorrhage. Transl Stroke Res. 2012;3(Suppl 1):25–38.
4. Kazan S, Gura A, Ucar T, Korkmaz E, Ongun H, Akyuz M. Hydrocephalus after intraventricular hemorrhage in preterm and low-birth weight infants: analysis of associated risk factors for ventriculoperitoneal shunting. Surg Neurol. 2005;64:S77–81.
5. Stoll BJ, Hansen NI, Bell EF, Shankaran S, Laptook AR, Walsh MC, Hale EC, Newman NS, Schibler K, Carlo WA, et al. Neonatal outcomes of extremely preterm infants from the NICHD Neonatal Research Network. Pediatrics. 2010;126:443–56.
6. Limbrick DD Jr, Mathur A, Johnston JM, Munro R, Sagar J, Inder T, Park TS, Leonard JL, Smyth MD. Neurosurgical treatment of progressive posthemorrhagic ventricular dilation in preterm infants: a 10-year single-institution study. J Neurosurg Pediatr. 2010;6:224–30.
7. Radic JA, Vincer M, McNeely PD. Temporal trends of intraventricular hemorrhage of prematurity in Nova Scotia from 1993 to 2012. J Neurosurg Pediatr. 2015;15:573–9.
8. Romero L, Ros B, Arraez MA, Rius F, Gonzalez L, Martin A, Carrasco A, Segura M. Analysis of risk factors for hydrocephalus development in newborn infants with germinal matrix hemorrhage. Minerva Pediatr. 2015;67:401–6.
9. Bassan H. Intracranial hemorrhage in the preterm infant: understanding it, preventing it. Clin Perinatol. 2009;36:737–62.
10. Murphy BP, Inder TE, Rooks V, Taylor GA, Anderson NJ, Mogridge N, Horwood LJ, Volpe JJ. Posthaemorrhagic ventricular dilatation in the premature infant: natural history and predictors of outcome. Arch Dis Child Fetal Neonatal Ed. 2002;87:F37–41.
11. Bhattathiri PS, Gregson B, Prasad KS, Mendelow AD, Investigators S. Intraventricular hemorrhage and hydrocephalus after spontaneous intracerebral hemorrhage: results from the STICH trial. Acta Neurochir Suppl. 2006;96:65–8.
12. Hwang BY, Bruce SS, Appelboom G, Piazza MA, Carpenter AM, Gigante PR, Kellner CP, Ducruet AF, Kellner MA, Deb-Sen R, et al. Evaluation of intraventricular hemorrhage assessment methods for predicting outcome following intracerebral hemorrhage. J Neurosurg. 2012;116:185–92.
13. Christian EA, Jin DL, Attenello F, Wen T, Cen S, Mack WJ, Krieger MD, McComb JG. Trends in hospitalization of preterm infants with intraventricular hemorrhage and hydrocephalus in the United States, 2000–2010. J Neurosurg Pediatr. 2016;17:260–9.
14. Stoll BJ, Hansen NI, Bell EF, Walsh MC, Carlo WA, Shankaran S, Laptook AR, Sanchez PJ, Van Meurs KP, Wyckoff M, et al. Trends in care practices, morbidity, and mortality of extremely preterm neonates, 1993–2012. JAMA. 2015;314:1039–51.
15. Ballabh P. Intraventricular hemorrhage in premature infants—mechanism of disease. Pediatr Res. 2010;67:1–8.
16. Philip AG, Allan WC, Tito AM, Wheeler LR. Intraventricular hemorrhage in preterm infants: declining incidence in the 1980s. Pediatrics. 1989;84:797–801.
17. Jain NJ, Kruse LK, Demissie K, Khandelwal M. Impact of mode of delivery on neonatal complications: trends between 1997 and 2005. J Matern Fetal Neonatal Med. 2009;22:491–500.
18. Wilson-Costello D, Friedman H, Minich N, Fanaroff AA, Hack M. Improved survival rates with increased neurodevelopmental disability for extremely low birth weight infants in the 1990s. Pediatrics. 2005;115:997–1003.
19. Ballabh P. Pathogenesis and prevention of intraventricular hemorrhage. Clin Perinatol. 2014;41:47–67.
20. Sherlock RL, Anderson PJ, Doyle LW, Victorian Infant Collaborative Study G. Neurodevelopmental sequelae of intraventricular haemorrhage at 8 years of age in a regional cohort of ELBW/very preterm infants. Early Hum Dev. 2005;81:909–16.
21. Martin JA, Osterman MJ, Centers for Disease C, Prevention. Preterm births—United States, 2006 and 2010. MMWR Suppl. 2013;62:136–8.
22. Riva-Cambrin J, Kestle JR, Holubkov R, Butler J, Kulkarni AV, Drake J, Whitehead WE, Wellons JC 3rd, Shannon CN, Tamber MS, et al. Risk factors for shunt malfunction in pediatric hydrocephalus: a multicenter prospective cohort study. J Neurosurg Pediatr. 2016;17:382–90.
23. Shankaran S, Lin A, Maller-Kesselman J, Zhang H, O'Shea TM, Bada HS, Kaiser JR, Lifton RP, Bauer CR, Ment LR, Gene Targets for Intraventricular Hemorrhage S. Maternal race, demography, and health care disparities impact risk for intraventricular hemorrhage in preterm neonates. J Pediatr. 2014;164(1005–1011):e1003.
24. McCrea HJ, Ment LR. The diagnosis, management, and postnatal prevention of intraventricular hemorrhage in the preterm neonate. Clin Perinatol. 2008;35:777–92.
25. Gagliardi L, Rusconi F, Da Fre M, Mello G, Carnielli V, Di Lallo D, Macagno F, Miniaci S, Corchia C, Cuttini M. Pregnancy disorders leading to very preterm birth influence neonatal outcomes: results of the population-based ACTION cohort study. Pediatr Res. 2013;73:794–801.
26. Linder N, Haskin O, Levit O, Klinger G, Prince T, Naor N, Turner P, Karmazyn B, Sirota L. Risk factors for intraventricular hemorrhage in very low birth weight premature infants: a retrospective case-control study. Pediatrics. 2003;111:e590–5.
27. Kent AL, Wright IM, Abdel-Latif ME, New South W, Australian Capital Territory Neonatal Intensive Care Units Audit G. Mortality and adverse neurologic outcomes are greater in preterm male infants. Pediatrics. 2012;129:124–31.

28. Volpe JJ. The encephalopathy of prematurity–brain injury and impaired brain development inextricably intertwined. Semin Pediatr Neurol. 2009;16:167–78.
29. Szpecht D, Frydryszak D, Miszczyk N, Szymankiewicz M, Gadzinowski J. The incidence of severe intraventricular hemorrhage based on retrospective analysis of 35939 full-term newborns-report of two cases and review of literature. Childs Nerv Syst. 2016;32:2447–51.
30. Robinson S. Neonatal posthemorrhagic hydrocephalus from prematurity: pathophysiology and current treatment concepts. J Neurosurg Pediatr. 2012;9:242–58.
31. Been JV, Rours IG, Kornelisse RF, Lima Passos V, Kramer BW, Schneider TA, de Krijger RR, Zimmermann LJ. Histologic chorioamnionitis, fetal involvement, and antenatal steroids: effects on neonatal outcome in preterm infants. Am J Obstet Gynecol. 2009;201(587):e581–8.
32. Malaeb S, Dammann O. Fetal inflammatory response and brain injury in the preterm newborn. J Child Neurol. 2009;24:1119–26.
33. Moscuzza F, Belcari F, Nardini V, Bartoli A, Domenici C, Cuttano A, Ghirri P, Boldrini A. Correlation between placental histopathology and fetal/neonatal outcome: chorioamnionitis and funisitis are associated to intraventricular haemorrage and retinopathy of prematurity in preterm newborns. Gynecol Endocrinol. 2011;27:319–23.
34. Shatrov JG, Birch SC, Lam LT, Quinlivan JA, McIntyre S, Mendz GL. Chorioamnionitis and cerebral palsy: a meta-analysis. Obstet Gynecol. 2010;116:387–92.
35. Soraisham AS, Singhal N, McMillan DD, Sauve RS, Lee SK, Canadian Neonatal N. A multicenter study on the clinical outcome of chorioamnionitis in preterm infants. Am J Obstet Gynecol. 2009;200(372):e371–6.
36. Tully HM, Traudt CM, Rue T, Oron AP, Simon TD, Kukull WA, Doherty D. Risk factors for post-hemorrhagic hydrocephalus among infants with intraventricular hemorrhage. Fluids Barriers CNS. 2015;12:O18.
37. du Plessis AJ. Cerebrovascular injury in premature infants: current understanding and challenges for future prevention. Clin Perinatol. 2008;35:609–41.
38. du Plessis AJ. The role of systemic hemodynamic disturbances in prematurity-related brain injury. J Child Neurol. 2009;24:1127–40.
39. Gould SJ, Howard S. Glial differentiation in the germinal layer of fetal and preterm infant brain: an immunocytochemical study. Pediatr Pathol. 1988;8:25–36.
40. Ballabh P, Braun A, Nedergaard M. The blood–brain barrier: an overview: structure, regulation, and clinical implications. Neurobiol Dis. 2004;16:1–13.
41. Del Bigio MR. Cell proliferation in human ganglionic eminence and suppression after prematurity-associated haemorrhage. Brain. 2011;134:1344–61.
42. Braun A, Xu H, Hu F, Kocherlakota P, Siegel D, Chander P, Ungvari Z, Csiszar A, Nedergaard M, Ballabh P. Paucity of pericytes in germinal matrix vasculature of premature infants. J Neurosci. 2007;27:12012–24.
43. Whitelaw A. Intraventricular haemorrhage and posthaemorrhagic hydrocephalus: pathogenesis, prevention and future interventions. Semin Neonatol. 2001;6:135–46.
44. Vela-Huerta MM, Amador-Licona M, Medina-Ovando N, Aldana-Valenzuela C. Factors associated with early severe intraventricular haemorrhage in very low birth weight infants. Neuropediatrics. 2009;40:224–7.
45. Gomez DG, DiBenedetto AT, Pavese AM, Firpo A, Hershan DB, Potts DG. Development of arachnoid villi and granulations in man. Acta Anat. 1982;111:247–58.
46. Iliff JJ, Wang M, Zeppenfeld DM, Venkataraman A, Plog BA, Liao Y, Deane R, Nedergaard M. Cerebral arterial pulsation drives paravascular CSF-interstitial fluid exchange in the murine brain. J Neurosci. 2013;33:18190–9.
47. Ratner V, Gao Y, Lee H, Elkin R, Nedergaard M, Benveniste H, Tannenbaum A. Cerebrospinal and interstitial fluid transport via the glymphatic pathway modeled by optimal mass transport. Neuroimage. 2017;152:530–7.
48. Yang L, Kress BT, Weber HJ, Thiyagarajan M, Wang B, Deane R, Benveniste H, Iliff JJ, Nedergaard M. Evaluating glymphatic pathway function utilizing clinically relevant intrathecal infusion of CSF tracer. J Transl Med. 2013;11:107.
49. Spector R, Keep RF, Robert Snodgrass S, Smith QR, Johanson CE. A balanced view of choroid plexus structure and function: focus on adult humans. Exp Neurol. 2015;267:78–86.
50. Nagra G, Li J, McAllister JP 2nd, Miller J, Wagshul M, Johnston M. Impaired lymphatic cerebrospinal fluid absorption in a rat model of kaolin-induced communicating hydrocephalus. Am J Physiol Regul Integr Comp Physiol. 2008;294:R1752–9.
51. Koh L, Zakharov A, Johnston M. Integration of the subarachnoid space and lymphatics: is it time to embrace a new concept of cerebrospinal fluid absorption? Cerebrospinal Fluid Res. 2005;2:6.
52. Johnston M, Zakharov A, Papaiconomou C, Salmasi G, Armstrong D. Evidence of connections between cerebrospinal fluid and nasal lymphatic vessels in humans, non-human primates and other mammalian species. Cerebrospinal Fluid Res. 2004;1:2.
53. Greitz D. Radiological assessment of hydrocephalus: new theories and implications for therapy. Neuroradiol J. 2006;19:475–95.
54. Greitz D, Greitz T, Hindmarsh T. A new view on the CSF-circulation with the potential for pharmacological treatment of childhood hydrocephalus. Acta Paediatr. 1997;86:125–32.
55. Miyajima M, Arai H. Evaluation of the production and absorption of cerebrospinal fluid. Neurol Med Chir. 2015;55:647–56.
56. Mori E, Yamada S. A hypothesis of cerebrospinal fluid formation and absorption: from the clinical viewpoint of idiopathic normal pressure hydrocephalus. Rinsho Shinkeigaku. 2014;54:1190–2.
57. Hladky SB, Barrand MA. Mechanisms of fluid movement into, through and out of the brain- evaluation of the evidence. Fluids Barriers CNS. 2014;11:26.
58. Del Bigio MR. Cellular damage and prevention in childhood hydrocephalus. Brain Pathol. 2004;14:317–24.
59. McAllister JP 2nd, Williams MA, Walker ML, Kestle JR, Relkin NR, Anderson AM, Gross PH, Browd SR, Hydrocephalus Symposium Expert P. An update on research priorities in hydrocephalus: overview of the third National Institutes of Health-sponsored symposium "Opportunities for Hydrocephalus Research: Pathways to Better Outcomes". J Neurosurg. 2015;123:1163–6.
60. Williams MA, McAllister JP, Walker ML, Kranz DA, Bergsneider M, Del Bigio MR, Fleming L, Frim DM, Gwinn K, Kestle JR, et al. Priorities for hydrocephalus research: report from a National Institutes of Health-sponsored workshop. J Neurosurg. 2007;107:345–57.
61. Hill A, Shackelford GD, Volpe JJ. A potential mechanism of pathogenesis for early posthemorrhagic hydrocephalus in the premature newborn. Pediatrics. 1984;73:19–21.
62. Motohashi O, Suzuki M, Yanai N, Umezawa K, Shida N, Yoshimoto T. Thrombin and TGF-beta promote human leptomeningeal cell proliferation in vitro. Neurosci Lett. 1995;190:105–8.
63. Greitz D. The hydrodynamic hypothesis versus the bulk flow hypothesis. Neurosurg Rev. 2004;27:299–300.
64. Greitz D. Paradigm shift in hydrocephalus research in legacy of Dandy's pioneering work: rationale for third ventriculostomy in communicating hydrocephalus. Childs Nerv Syst. 2007;23:487–9.
65. Xiang J, Routhe LJ, Wilkinson DA, Hua Y, Moos T, Xi G, Keep RF. The choroid plexus as a site of damage in hemorrhagic and ischemic stroke and its role in responding to injury. Fluids Barriers CNS. 2017;14:8.
66. Karimy JK, Zhang J, Kurland DB, Theriault BC, Duran D, Stokum JA, Furey CG, Zhou X, Mansuri MS, Montejo J, et al. Inflammation-dependent cerebrospinal fluid hypersecretion by the choroid plexus epithelium in posthemorrhagic hydrocephalus. Nat Med. 2017;23:997–1003.
67. Yung YC, Mutoh T, Lin ME, Noguchi K, Rivera RR, Choi JW, Kingsbury MA, Chun J. Lysophosphatidic acid signaling may initiate fetal hydrocephalus. Sci Transl Med. 2011;3:99ra87.
68. Guerra M, Henzi R, Ortloff A, Lictin N, Vio K, Jiminez AJ, Dominguez-Pinos MD, Gonzalez C, Bioch MCJ, Hinostroza F, et al. A cell junction pathology of neural stem cells is associated with ventricular zone disruption, hydrocephalus and abnormal neurogenesis. J Neuropathol Exp Neurol. 2015;74:653–71.
69. Rodriguez EM, Guerra MM, Vio K, Gonzalez C, Ortloff A, Batiz LF, Rodriguez S, Jara MC, Munoz RI, Ortega E, et al. A cell junction pathology of neural stem cells leads to abnormal neurogenesis and hydrocephalus. Biol Res. 2012;45:231–42.
70. Jimenez AJ, Garcia-Verdugo JM, Gonzalez CA, Batiz LF, Rodriguez-Perez LM, Paez P, Soriano-Navarro M, Roales-Bujan R, Rivera P, Rodriguez S, et al. Disruption of the neurogenic niche in the subventricular zone of postnatal hydrocephalic hyh mice. J Neuropathol Exp Neurol. 2009;68:1006–20.

71. McAllister JP, Guerra MM, Ruiz LC, Jimenez AJ, Dominguez-Pinos D, Sival D, den Dunnen W, Morales DM, Schmidt RE, Rodriguez EM, Limbrick DD. Ventricular zone disruption in human neonates with intraventricular hemorrhage. J Neuropathol Exp Neurol. 2017;76:358–75.
72. Whitelaw A, Evans D, Carter M, Thoresen M, Wroblewska J, Mandera M, Swietlinski J, Simpson J, Hajivassiliou C, Hunt LP, Pople I. Randomized clinical trial of prevention of hydrocephalus after intraventricular hemorrhage in preterm infants: brain-washing versus tapping fluid. Pediatrics. 2007;119:e1071–8.
73. Whitelaw A, Odd DE. Intraventricular streptokinase after intraventricular hemorrhage in newborn infants. Cochrane Database Syst Rev. 2007;4:CD000498.
74. Whitelaw A, Rivers RP, Creighton L, Gaffney P. Low dose intraventricular fibrinolytic treatment to prevent posthaemorrhagic hydrocephalus. Arch Dis Child. 1992;67:12–4.
75. Yapicioglu H, Narli N, Satar M, Soyupak S, Altunbasak S. Intraventricular streptokinase for the treatment of posthaemorrhagic hydrocephalus of preterm. J Clin Neurosci. 2003;10:297–9.
76. Group IPDT. International randomised controlled trial of acetazolamide and furosemide in posthaemorrhagic ventricular dilatation in infancy. International PHVD Drug Trial Group. Lancet. 1998;352:433–40.
77. Kennedy CR, Ayers S, Campbell MJ, Elbourne D, Hope P, Johnson A. Randomized, controlled trial of acetazolamide and furosemide in posthemorrhagic ventricular dilation in infancy: follow-up at 1 year. Pediatrics. 2001;108:597–607.
78. Mazzola CA, Choudhri AF, Auguste KI, Limbrick DD Jr, Rogido M, Mitchell L, Flannery AM, Pediatric Hydrocephalus Systematic R, Evidence-Based Guidelines Task F. Pediatric hydrocephalus: systematic literature review and evidence-based guidelines. Part 2: management of posthemorrhagic hydrocephalus in premature infants. J Neurosurg Pediatr. 2014;14(Suppl 1):8–23.
79. Perlman JM, Lynch B, Volpe JJ. Late hydrocephalus after arrest and resolution of neonatal post-hemorrhagic hydrocephalus. Dev Med Child Neurol. 1990;32:725–9.
80. Chaplin ER, Goldstein GW, Myerberg DZ, Hunt JV, Tooley WH. Posthemorrhagic hydrocephalus in the preterm infant. Pediatrics. 1980;65:901–9.
81. Schulz M, Buhrer C, Pohl-Schickinger A, Haberl H, Thomale UW. Neuroendoscopic lavage for the treatment of intraventricular hemorrhage and hydrocephalus in neonates. J Neurosurg Pediatr. 2014;13:626–35.
82. Drake JM, Kestle JR, Milner R, Cinalli G, Boop F, Piatt J Jr, Haines S, Schiff SJ, Cochrane DD, Steinbok P, MacNeil N. Randomized trial of cerebrospinal fluid shunt valve design in pediatric hydrocephalus. Neurosurgery. 1998;43:294–303.
83. Kestle JR, Drake JM, Cochrane DD, Milner R, Walker ML, Abbott R III, Boop FA. Lack of benefit of endoscopic ventriculoperitoneal shunt insertion: a multicenter randomized trial. J Neurosurg. 2003;98:284–90.
84. Naftel RP, Safiano NA, Falola MI, Shannon CN, Wellons JC 3rd, Johnston JM Jr. Technology preferences among caregivers of children with hydrocephalus. J Neurosurg Pediatr. 2013;11:26–36.
85. Stone SS, Warf BC. Combined endoscopic third ventriculostomy and choroid plexus cauterization as primary treatment for infant hydrocephalus: a prospective North American series. J Neurosurg Pediatr. 2014;5:439–46.
86. Zandian A, Haffner M, Johnson J, Rozzelle CJ, Tubbs RS, Loukas M. Endoscopic third ventriculostomy with/without choroid plexus cauterization for hydrocephalus due to hemorrhage, infection, Dandy–Walker malformation, and neural tube defect: a meta-analysis. Childs Nerv Syst. 2014;30:571–8.
87. Kulkarni AV, Riva-Cambrin J, Browd SR, Drake JM, Holubkov R, Kestle JR, Limbrick DD, Rozzelle CJ, Simon TD, Tamber MS, et al. Endoscopic third ventriculostomy and choroid plexus cauterization in infants with hydrocephalus: a retrospective Hydrocephalus Clinical Research Network study. J Neurosurg Pediatr. 2014;14:224–9.
88. Wang S, Stone S, Weil AG, Fallah A, Warf BC, Ragheb J, Bhatia S, Kulkarni AV. Comparative effectiveness of flexible versus rigid neuroendoscopy for endoscopic third ventriculostomy and choroid plexus cauterization: a propensity score-matched cohort and survival analysis. J Neurosurg Pediatr. 2017;19:585–91.
89. Chamiraju P, Bhatia S, Sandberg DI, Ragheb J. Endoscopic third ventriculostomy and choroid plexus cauterization in posthemorrhagic hydrocephalus of prematurity. J Neurosurg Pediatr. 2014;13:433–9.
90. Warf BC, Campbell JW, Riddle E. Initial experience with combined endoscopic third ventriculostomy and choroid plexus cauterization for post-hemorrhagic hydrocephalus of prematurity: the importance of prepontine cistern status and the predictive value of FIESTA MRI imaging. Childs Nerv Syst. 2011;27:1063–71.
91. Roberts D, Brown J, Medley N, Dalziel SR. Antenatal corticosteroids for accelerating fetal lung maturation for women at risk of preterm birth. Cochrane Database Syst Rev. 2017;3:CD004454.
92. Deshmukh M, Patole S. Antenatal corticosteroids for neonates born before 25 weeks—a systematic review and meta-analysis. PLoS ONE. 2017;12:e0176090.
93. Chawla S, Natarajan G, Shankaran S, Pappas A, Stoll BJ, Carlo WA, Saha S, Das A, Laptook AR, Higgins RD, et al. Association of neurodevelopmental outcomes and neonatal morbidities of extremely premature infants with differential exposure to antenatal steroids. JAMA Pediatr. 2016;170:1164–72.
94. El-Ganzoury MM, El-Farrash RA, Saad AA, Ali MS, El-Bhbiti AR, Selem AM. Antenatal administration of vitamin K1: relationship to vitamin K-dependent coagulation factors and incidence rate of periventricular-intraventricular hemorrhage in preterm infants; Egyptian randomized controlled trial. J Matern Fetal Neonatal Med. 2014;27:816–20.
95. Crowther CA, Crosby DD, Henderson-Smart DJ. Vitamin K prior to preterm birth for preventing neonatal periventricular haemorrhage. Cochrane Database Syst Rev. 2010;1:CD000229.
96. Zeng X, Xue Y, Tian Q, Sun R, An R. Effects and safety of magnesium sulfate on neuroprotection: a meta-analysis based on PRISMA guidelines. Medicine. 2016;95:e2451.
97. Shankaran S, Papile LA, Wright LL, Ehrenkranz RA, Mele L, Lemons JA, Korones SB, Stevenson DK, Donovan EF, Stoll BJ, et al. The effect of antenatal phenobarbital therapy on neonatal intracranial hemorrhage in preterm infants. N Engl J Med. 1997;337:466–71.
98. Crowther CA, Crosby DD, Henderson-Smart DJ. Phenobarbital prior to preterm birth for preventing neonatal periventricular haemorrhage. Cochrane Database Syst Rev. 2010;1:CD000164.
99. Barzilay E, Gadot Y, Koren G. Safety of vaginal delivery in very low birth-weight vertex singletons: a meta-analysis. J Matern Fetal Neonatal Med. 2016;29:3724–9.
100. Riskin A, Riskin-Mashiah S, Bader D, Kugelman A, Lerner-Geva L, Boyko V, Reichman B. Delivery mode and severe intraventricular hemorrhage in single, very low birth weight, vertex infants. Obstet Gynecol. 2008;112:21–8.
101. Wylie BJ, Davidson LL, Batra M, Reed SD. Method of delivery and neonatal outcome in very low-birthweight vertex-presenting fetuses. Am J Obstet Gynecol. 2008;198:640.e641–7 **(discussion e641–644)**.
102. Humberg A, Hartel C, Paul P, Hanke K, Bossung V, Hartz A, Fasel L, Rausch TK, Rody A, Herting E, et al. Delivery mode and intraventricular hemorrhage risk in very-low-birth-weight infants: observational data of the German Neonatal Network. Eur J Obstet Gynecol Reprod Biol. 2017;212:144–9.
103. Hubner ME, Ramirez R, Burgos J, Dominguez A, Tapia JL. Mode of delivery and antenatal steroids and their association with survival and severe intraventricular hemorrhage in very low birth weight infants. J Perinatol. 2016;36:832–6.
104. Mercer JS, Vohr BR, McGrath MM, Padbury JF, Wallach M, Oh W. Delayed cord clamping in very preterm infants reduces the incidence of intraventricular hemorrhage and late-onset sepsis: a randomized, controlled trial. Pediatrics. 2006;117:1235–42.
105. Rabe H, Diaz-Rossello JL, Duley L, Dowswell T. Effect of timing of umbilical cord clamping and other strategies to influence placental transfusion at preterm birth on maternal and infant outcomes. Cochrane Database Syst Rev. 2012;8:CD003248.
106. Mercer JS, Erickson-Owens DA, Vohr BR, Tucker RJ, Parker AB, Oh W, Padbury JF. Effects of placental transfusion on neonatal and 18 month outcomes in preterm infants: a randomized controlled trial. J Pediatr. 2016;168(50–55):e51.
107. Tarnow-Mordi W, Morris J, Kirby A, Robledo K, Askie L, Brown R, Evans N, Finlayson S, Fogarty M, Gebski V, et al. Delayed versus immediate cord clamping in preterm infants. N Engl J Med. 2017;377:2445–55.
108. Fogarty M, Osborn DA, Askie L, Seidler AL, Hunter K, Lui K, Simes J, Tarnow-Mordi W. Delayed vs early umbilical cord clamping for preterm

infants: a systematic review and meta-analysis. Am J Obstet Gynecol. 2018;218:1–18.
109. Dani C, Poggi C, Bertini G, Pratesi S, Di Tommaso M, Scarselli G, Rubaltelli FF. Method of delivery and intraventricular haemorrhage in extremely preterm infants. J Matern Fetal Neonatal Med. 2010;23:1419–23.
110. Fulkerson DH, Vachhrajani S, Bohnstedt BN, Patel NB, Patel AJ, Fox BD, Jea A, Boaz JC. Analysis of the risk of shunt failure or infection related to cerebrospinal fluid cell count, protein level, and glucose levels in low-birth-weight premature infants with posthemorrhagic hydrocephalus. J Neurosurg Pediatr. 2011;7:147–51.
111. Linder N, Bello R, Hernandez A, Rosen C, Birk E, Sirota L, Pushkov Y, Klinger G. Treatment of patent ductus arteriosus: indomethacin or ibuprofen? Am J Perinatol. 2010;27:399–404.
112. Garay RP, Chiavaroli C, Hannaert P. Therapeutic efficacy and mechanism of action of ethamsylate, a long-standing hemostatic agent. Am J Ther. 2006;13:236–47.
113. Hunt R, Hey E. Ethamsylate for the prevention of morbidity and mortality in preterm or very low birth weight infants. Cochrane Database Syst Rev. 2010;1:CD004343.
114. Liebowitz M, Clyman RI. Antenatal betamethasone: a prolonged time interval from administration to delivery is associated with an increased incidence of severe intraventricular hemorrhage in infants born before 28 weeks gestation. J Pediatr. 2016;177(114–120):e111.
115. Ment LR, Vohr B, Allan W, Westerveld M, Sparrow SS, Schneider KC, Katz KH, Duncan CC, Makuch RW. Outcome of children in the indomethacin intraventricular hemorrhage prevention trial. Pediatrics. 2000;105:485–91.
116. Ment LR, Oh W, Ehrenkranz RA, Philip AG, Vohr B, Allan W, Duncan CC, Scott DT, Taylor KJ, Katz KH, et al. Low-dose indomethacin and prevention of intraventricular hemorrhage: a multicenter randomized trial. Pediatrics. 1994;93:543–50.
117. Luque MJ, Tapia JL, Villarroel L, Marshall G, Musante G, Carlo W, Kattan J, Neocosur Neonatal N. A risk prediction model for severe intraventricular hemorrhage in very low birth weight infants and the effect of prophylactic indomethacin. J Perinatol. 2014;34:43–8.
118. Kalani M, Shariat M, Khalesi N, Farahani Z, Ahmadi S. A comparison of early ibuprofen and indomethacin administration to prevent intraventricular hemorrhage among preterm infants. Acta Med Iran. 2016;54:788–92.
119. Johnston PG, Gillam-Krakauer M, Fuller MP, Reese J. Evidence-based use of indomethacin and ibuprofen in the neonatal intensive care unit. Clin Perinatol. 2012;39:111–36.
120. Schmidt B, Davis P, Moddemann D, Ohlsson A, Roberts RS, Saigal S, Solimano A, Vincer M, Wright LL, Trial of Indomethacin Prophylaxis in Preterms I. Long-term effects of indomethacin prophylaxis in extremely-low-birth-weight infants. N Engl J Med. 2001;344:1966–72.
121. Hallman M, Bry K, Hoppu K, Lappi M, Pohjavuori M. Inositol supplementation in premature infants with respiratory distress syndrome. N Engl J Med. 1992;326:1233–9.
122. Hallman M, Jarvenpaa AL, Pohjavuori M. Respiratory distress syndrome and inositol supplementation in preterm infants. Arch Dis Child. 1986;61:1076–83.
123. Howlett A, Ohlsson A, Plakkal N. Inositol in preterm infants at risk for or having respiratory distress syndrome. Cochrane Database Syst Rev. 2015;2:CD000366.
124. Phelps DL, Ward RM, Williams RL, Nolen TL, Watterberg KL, Oh W, Goedecke M, Ehrenkranz RA, Fennell T, Poindexter BB, et al. Safety and pharmacokinetics of multiple dose myo-inositol in preterm infants. Pediatr Res. 2016;80:209–17.
125. Phelps DL, Ward RM, Williams RL, Watterberg KL, Laptook AR, Wrage LA, Nolen TL, Fennell TR, Ehrenkranz RA, Poindexter BB, et al. Pharmacokinetics and safety of a single intravenous dose of myo-inositol in preterm infants of 23–29 wk. Pediatr Res. 2013;74:721–9.
126. Barrington KJ, Finer N. Inhaled nitric oxide for respiratory failure in preterm infants. Cochrane Database Syst Rev. 2010;12:CD000509.
127. Whitelaw A, Odd D. Postnatal phenobarbital for the prevention of intraventricular hemorrhage in preterm infants. Cochrane Database Syst Rev. 2007;4:CD001691.
128. Soll R, Ozek E. Prophylactic protein free synthetic surfactant for preventing morbidity and mortality in preterm infants. Cochrane Database Syst Rev. 2010;1:CD001079.
129. Halliday HL, Ehrenkranz RA, Doyle LW. Early (< 8 days) postnatal corticosteroids for preventing chronic lung disease in preterm infants. Cochrane Database Syst Rev. 2010;1:CD001146.
130. Baer VL, Lambert DK, Henry E, Snow GL, Butler A, Christensen RD. Among very-low-birth-weight neonates is red blood cell transfusion an independent risk factor for subsequently developing a severe intraventricular hemorrhage? Transfusion. 2011;51:1170–8.
131. Volpe JJ. Neurology of the newborn. Philadelphia: Saunder Elsevier; 2008.
132. Christensen RD, Baer VL, Lambert DK, Ilstrup SJ, Eggert LD, Henry E. Association, among very-low-birthweight neonates, between red blood cell transfusions in the week after birth and severe intraventricular hemorrhage. Transfusion. 2014;54:104–8.
133. Brion LP, Bell EF, Raghuveer TS. Vitamin E supplementation for prevention of morbidity and mortality in preterm infants. Cochrane Database Syst Rev. 2003;4:CD003665.
134. Del Bigio MR, Di Curzio DL. Nonsurgical therapy for hydrocephalus: a comprehensive and critical review. Fluids Barriers CNS. 2016;13:3.
135. Shooman D, Portess H, Sparrow O. A review of the current treatment methods for posthaemorrhagic hydrocephalus of infants. Cerebrospinal Fluid Res. 2009;6:1.
136. Libenson MH, Kaye EM, Rosman NP, Gilmore HE. Acetazolamide and furosemide for posthemorrhagic hydrocephalus of the newborn. Pediatr Neurol. 1999;20:185–91.
137. Whitelaw A, Kennedy CR, Brion LP. Diuretic therapy for newborn infants with posthemorrhagic ventricular dilatation. Cochrane Database Syst Rev. 2001;2:CD002270.
138. Whitelaw A, Saliba E, Fellman V, Mowinckel MC, Acolet D, Marlow N. Phase I study of intraventricular recombinant tissue plasminogen activator for treatment of posthaemorrhagic hydrocephalus. Arch Dis Child Fetal Neonatal Ed. 1996;75:F20–6.
139. Luciano R, Velardi F, Romagnoli C, Papacci P, De Stefano V, Tortorolo G. Failure of fibrinolytic endoventricular treatment to prevent neonatal post-haemorrhagic hydrocephalus. A case-control trial. Childs Nerv Syst. 1997;13:73–6.
140. Hudgins RJ, Boydston WR, Hudgins PA, Morris R, Adler SM, Gilreath CL. Intrathecal urokinase as a treatment for intraventricular hemorrhage in the preterm infant. Pediatr Neurosurg. 1997;26:281–7.
141. Whitelaw A, Jary S, Kmita G, Wroblewska J, Musialik-Swietlinska E, Mandera M, Hunt L, Carter M, Pople I. Randomized trial of drainage, irrigation and fibrinolytic therapy for premature infants with posthemorrhagic ventricular dilatation: developmental outcome at 2 years. Pediatrics. 2010;125:e852–8.
142. Whitelaw A, Pople I, Cherian S, Evans D, Thoresen M. Phase 1 trial of prevention of hydrocephalus after intraventricular hemorrhage in newborn infants by drainage, irrigation, and fibrinolytic therapy. Pediatrics. 2003;111:759–65.
143. Badhiwala JH, Hong CJ, Nassiri F, Hong BY, Riva-Cambrin J, Kulkarni AV. Treatment of posthemorrhagic ventricular dilation in preterm infants: a systematic review and meta-analysis of outcomes and complications. J Neurosurg Pediatr. 2015;16(5):545–55.
144. Whitelaw A, Lee-Kelland R. Repeated lumbar or ventricular punctures in newborns with intraventricular haemorrhage. Cochrane Database Syst Rev. 2017;4:CD000216.
145. Wellons JC 3rd, Shannon CN, Holubkov R, Riva-Cambrin J, Kulkarni AV, Limbrick DD Jr, Whitehead W, Browd S, Rozzelle C, Simon TD, et al. Shunting outcomes in posthemorrhagic hydrocephalus: results of a Hydrocephalus Clinical Research Network prospective cohort study. J Neurosurg Pediatr. 2017;20:19–29.
146. de Vries LS, Liem KD, van Dijk K, Smit BJ, Sie L, Rademaker KJ, Gavilanes AW, Dutch Working Group of Neonatal N. Early versus late treatment of posthaemorrhagic ventricular dilatation: results of a retrospective study from five neonatal intensive care units in The Netherlands. Acta Paediatr. 2002;91:212–7.
147. Hanley DF. Intraventricular hemorrhage: severity factor and treatment target in spontaneous intracerebral hemorrhage. Stroke. 2009;40:1533–8.
148. Gregson BA, Broderick JP, Auer LM, Batjer H, Chen XC, Juvela S, Morgenstern LB, Pantazis GC, Teernstra OP, Wang WZ, et al. Individual patient data subgroup meta-analysis of surgery for spontaneous supratentorial intracerebral hemorrhage. Stroke. 2012;43:1496–504.

149. Tuhrim S, Horowitz DR, Sacher M, Godbold JH. Volume of ventricular blood is an important determinant of outcome in supratentorial intracerebral hemorrhage. Crit Care Med. 1999;27:617–21.
150. Andrews CO, Engelhard HH. Fibrinolytic therapy in intraventricular hemorrhage. Ann Pharmacother. 2001;35:1435–48.
151. Keep RF, Hua Y, Xi G. Intracerebral haemorrhage: mechanisms of injury and therapeutic targets. Lancet Neurol. 2012;11:720–31.
152. Thabet AM, Kottapally M, Hemphill JC 3rd. Management of intracerebral hemorrhage. Handb Clin Neurol. 2017;140:177–94.
153. Mayer SA, Brun NC, Begtrup K, Broderick J, Davis S, Diringer MN, Skolnick BE, Steiner T, Investigators FT. Efficacy and safety of recombinant activated factor VII for acute intracerebral hemorrhage. N Engl J Med. 2008;358:2127–37.
154. Qureshi AI, Palesch YY, Suarez JI. Intensive blood-pressure lowering in cerebral hemorrhage. N Engl J Med. 2016;375:e48.
155. Morotti A, Brouwers HB, Romero JM, Jessel MJ, Vashkevich A, Schwab K, Afzal MR, Cassarly C, Greenberg SM, Martin RH, et al. Intensive blood pressure reduction and spot sign in intracerebral hemorrhage: a secondary analysis of a randomized clinical trial. JAMA Neurol. 2017;74:950–60.
156. Morotti A, Boulouis G, Romero JM, Brouwers HB, Jessel MJ, Vashkevich A, Schwab K, Afzal MR, Cassarly C, Greenberg SM, et al. Blood pressure reduction and noncontrast CT markers of intracerebral hemorrhage expansion. Neurology. 2017;89:548–54.
157. Delcourt C, Sato S, Zhang S, Sandset EC, Zheng D, Chen X, Hackett ML, Arima H, Hata J, Heeley E, et al. Intracerebral hemorrhage location and outcome among INTERACT2 participants. Neurology. 2017;88:1408–14.
158. Delcourt C, Zheng D, Chen X, Hackett M, Arima H, Hata J, Heeley E, Al-Shahi Salman R, Woodward M, Huang Y, et al. Associations with health-related quality of life after intracerebral haemorrhage: pooled analysis of INTERACT studies. J Neurol Neurosurg Psychiatry. 2017;88:70–5.
159. Wang X, Arima H, Al-Shahi Salman R, Woodward M, Heeley E, Stapf C, Lavados PM, Robinson T, Huang Y, Wang J, et al. Rapid blood pressure lowering according to recovery at different time intervals after acute intracerebral hemorrhage: pooled analysis of the INTERACT studies. Cerebrovasc Dis. 2015;39:242–8.
160. Baharoglu MI, Cordonnier C, Al-Shahi Salman R, de Gans K, Koopman MM, Brand A, Majoie CB, Beenen LF, Marquering HA, Vermeulen M, et al. Platelet transfusion versus standard care after acute stroke due to spontaneous cerebral haemorrhage associated with antiplatelet therapy (PATCH): a randomised, open-label, phase 3 trial. Lancet. 2016;387:2605–13.
161. Mendelow AD, Gregson BA, Rowan EN, Murray GD, Gholkar A, Mitchell PM, Investigators SI. Early surgery versus initial conservative treatment in patients with spontaneous supratentorial lobar intracerebral haematomas (STICH II): a randomised trial. Lancet. 2013;382:397–408.
162. Hanley DF, Thompson RE, Muschelli J, Rosenblum M, McBee N, Lane K, Bistran-Hall AJ, Mayo SW, Keyl P, Gandhi D, et al. Safety and efficacy of minimally invasive surgery plus alteplase in intracerebral haemorrhage evacuation (MISTIE): a randomised, controlled, open-label, phase 2 trial. Lancet Neurol. 2016;15:1228–37.
163. Vespa P, Hanley D, Betz J, Hoffer A, Engh J, Carter R, Nakaji P, Ogilvy C, Jallo J, Selman W, et al. ICES (Intraoperative Stereotactic Computed Tomography-Guided Endoscopic Surgery) for brain hemorrhage: a multicenter randomized controlled trial. Stroke. 2016;47:2749–55.
164. Gaberel T, Magheru C, Parienti JJ, Huttner HB, Vivien D, Emery E. Intraventricular fibrinolysis versus external ventricular drainage alone in intraventricular hemorrhage: a meta-analysis. Stroke. 2011;42:2776–81.
165. Khan NR, Tsivgoulis G, Lee SL, Jones GM, Green CS, Katsanos AH, Klimo P Jr, Arthur AS, Elijovich L, Alexandrov AV. Fibrinolysis for intraventricular hemorrhage: an updated meta-analysis and systematic review of the literature. Stroke. 2014;45:2662–9.
166. Hanley DF, Lane K, McBee N, Ziai W, Tuhrim S, Lees KR, Dawson J, Gandhi D, Ullman N, Mould WA, et al. Thrombolytic removal of intraventricular haemorrhage in treatment of severe stroke: results of the randomised, multicentre, multiregion, placebo-controlled CLEAR III trial. Lancet. 2017;389:603–11.
167. Baker AD, Rivera Perla KM, Yu Z, Dlugash R, Avadhani R, Mould WA, Ziai W, Thompson RE, Staykov D, Hanley DF. Fibrinolytic for treatment of intraventricular hemorrhage: a meta-analysis and systematic review. Int J Stroke. 2018;13:11–23.
168. Wang D, Liu J, Norton C, Liu M, Selim M. Local fibrinolytic therapy for intraventricular hemorrhage: a meta-analysis of randomized controlled trials. World Neurosurg. 2017;107(1016–1024):e1011.
169. Staykov D, Kuramatsu JB, Bardutzky J, Volbers B, Gerner ST, Kloska SP, Doerfler A, Schwab S, Huttner HB. Efficacy and safety of combined intraventricular fibrinolysis with lumbar drainage for prevention of permanent shunt dependency after intracerebral hemorrhage with severe ventricular involvement: a randomized trial and individual patient data meta-analysis. Ann Neurol. 2017;81:93–103.
170. Li Y, Zhang H, Wang X, She L, Yan Z, Zhang N, Du R, Yan K, Xu E, Pang L. Neuroendoscopic surgery versus external ventricular drainage alone or with intraventricular fibrinolysis for intraventricular hemorrhage secondary to spontaneous supratentorial hemorrhage: a systematic review and meta-analysis. PLoS ONE. 2013;8:e80599.
171. Ginsberg MD. Neuroprotection for ischemic stroke: past, present and future. Neuropharmacology. 2008;55:363–89.
172. Fouda AY, Newsome AS, Spellicy S, Waller JL, Zhi W, Hess DC, Ergul A, Edwards DJ, Fagan SC, Switzer JA. Minocycline in acute cerebral hemorrhage: an early phase randomized trial. Stroke. 2017;48(10):2885–7.
173. Zhao F, Hua Y, He Y, Keep RF, Xi G. Minocycline-induced attenuation of iron overload and brain injury after experimental intracerebral hemorrhage. Stroke. 2011;42:3587–93.
174. Fu Y, Hao J, Zhang N, Ren L, Sun N, Li YJ, Yan Y, Huang D, Yu C, Shi FD. Fingolimod for the treatment of intracerebral hemorrhage: a 2-arm proof-of-concept study. JAMA Neurol. 2014;71:1092–101.
175. Gonzales NR, Shah J, Sangha N, Sosa L, Martinez R, Shen L, Kasam M, Morales MM, Hossain MM, Barreto AD, et al. Design of a prospective, dose-escalation study evaluating the safety of pioglitazone for hematoma resolution in intracerebral hemorrhage (SHRINC). Int J Stroke. 2013;8:388–96.
176. Galbreath E, Kim SJ, Park K, Brenner M, Messing A. Overexpression of TGF-beta 1 in the central nervous system of transgenic mice results in hydrocephalus. J Neuropathol Exp Neurol. 1995;54:339–49.
177. McAllister JP II. Experimental hydrocephalus. In: Winn HR, editor. Youmans textbook of neurological surgery, vol. 6. New York: Elsevier; 2011. p. 2002–8.
178. Morales DM, Townsend RR, Malone JP, Ewersmann CA, Macy EM, Inder TE, Limbrick DD Jr. Alterations in protein regulators of neurodevelopment in the cerebrospinal fluid of infants with posthemorrhagic hydrocephalus of prematurity. Mol Cell Proteom. 2012;11(M111):011973.
179. Morales DM, Holubkov R, Inder TE, Ahn HC, Mercer D, Rao R, McAllister JP 2nd, Holtzman DM, Limbrick DD Jr. Cerebrospinal fluid levels of amyloid precursor protein are associated with ventricular size in post-hemorrhagic hydrocephalus of prematurity. PLoS ONE. 2015;10:e0115045.
180. Morales DM, Silver SA, Morgan CD, Mercer D, Inder TE, Holtzman DM, Wallendorf MJ, Rao R, McAllister JPI, Limbrick DD Jr. Lumbar cerebrospinal fluid biomarkers of post-hemorrhagic hydrocephalus of prematurity—amyloid precursor protein, soluble APPα, and L1 cell adhesion molecule. Neurosurgery. 2017;80(1):82–90.
181. Yung YC, Stoddard NC, Mirendil H, Chun J. Lysophosphatidic acid signaling in the nervous system. Neuron. 2015;85:669–82.
182. Gao C, Du H, Hua Y, Keep RF, Strahle J, Xi G. Role of red blood cell lysis and iron in hydrocephalus after intraventricular hemorrhage. J Cereb Blood Flow Metab. 2014;34:1070–5.
183. Garton T, Keep RF, Wilkinson DA, Strahle JM, Hua Y, Garton HJ, Xi G. Intraventricular hemorrhage: the role of blood components in secondary injury and hydrocephalus. Transl Stroke Res. 2016;7(6):447–51.
184. Okubo S, Strahle J, Keep RF, Hua Y, Xi G. Subarachnoid hemorrhage-induced hydrocephalus in rats. Stroke. 2013;44:547–50.
185. Strahle JM, Garton T, Bazzi AA, Kilaru H, Garton HJ, Maher CO, Muraszko KM, Keep RF, Xi G. Role of hemoglobin and iron in hydrocephalus after neonatal intraventricular hemorrhage. Neurosurgery. 2014;75:696–705 **(discussion 706)**.
186. Guo J, Chen Q, Tang J, Zhang J, Tao Y, Li L, Zhu G, Feng H, Chen Z. Minocycline-induced attenuation of iron overload and brain injury after experimental germinal matrix hemorrhage. Brain Res. 2015;1594:115–24.
187. Klebe D, Flores JJ, McBride DW, Krafft PR, Rolland WB, Lekic T, Zhang JH. Dabigatran ameliorates post-haemorrhagic hydrocephalus development after germinal matrix haemorrhage in neonatal rat pups. J Cereb Blood Flow Metab. 2017;37:3135–49.

188. Babu R, Bagley JH, Di C, Friedman AH, Adamson C. Thrombin and hemin as central factors in the mechanisms of intracerebral hemorrhage-induced secondary brain injury and as potential targets for intervention. Neurosurg Focus. 2012;32:E8.
189. Crews L, Wyss-Coray T, Masliah E. Insights into the pathogenesis of hydrocephalus from transgenic and experimental animal models. Brain Pathol. 2004;14:312–6.
190. Paul DA, Leef KH, Stefano JL. Increased leukocytes in infants with intraventricular hemorrhage. Pediatr Neurol. 2000;22:194–9.
191. Xue M, Del Bigio MR. Immune pre-activation exacerbates hemorrhagic brain injury in immature mouse brain. J Neuroimmunol. 2005;165:75–82.
192. Ballabh P, Xu H, Hu F, Braun A, Smith K, Rivera A, Lou N, Ungvari Z, Goldman SA, Csiszar A, Nedergaard M. Angiogenic inhibition reduces germinal matrix hemorrhage. Nat Med. 2007;13:477–85.
193. Dummula K, Vinukonda G, Xu H, Hu F, Zia MT, Braun A, Shi Q, Wolk J, Ballabh P. Development of integrins in the vasculature of germinal matrix, cerebral cortex, and white matter of fetuses and premature infants. J Neurosci Res. 2010;88:1193–204.
194. Botfield H, Gonzalez AM, Abdullah O, Skjolding AD, Berry M, McAllister JPI, Logan A. Decorin prevents the development of juvenile communicating hydrocephalus. Brain. 2013;136:2842–58.
195. Chow LC, Soliman A, Zandian M, Danielpour M, Krueger RC Jr. Accumulation of transforming growth factor-beta2 and nitrated chondroitin sulfate proteoglycans in cerebrospinal fluid correlates with poor neurologic outcome in preterm hydrocephalus. Biol Neonate. 2005;88:1–11.
196. Heep A, Stoffel-Wagner B, Bartmann P, Benseler S, Schaller C, Groneck P, Obladen M, Felderhoff-Mueser U. Vascular endothelial growth factor and transforming growth factor-beta1 are highly expressed in the cerebrospinal fluid of premature infants with posthemorrhagic hydrocephalus. Pediatr Res. 2004;56:768–74.
197. Merhar S. Biomarkers in neonatal posthemorrhagic hydrocephalus. Neonatology. 2012;101:1–7.
198. Savman K, Blennow M, Hagberg H, Tarkowski E, Thoresen M, Whitelaw A. Cytokine response in cerebrospinal fluid from preterm infants with posthaemorrhagic ventricular dilatation. Acta Paediatr. 2002;91:1357–63.
199. Schmitz T, Heep A, Groenendaal F, Huseman D, Kie S, Bartmann P, Obladen M, Felderhoff-Muser U. Interleukin-1beta, interleukin-18, and interferon-gamma expression in the cerebrospinal fluid of premature infants with posthemorrhagic hydrocephalus–markers of white matter damage? Pediatr Res. 2007;61:722–6.
200. Limbrick DD Jr, Castaneyra-Ruiz L, Han RH, Berger D, McAllister JP, Morales DM. Cerebrospinal fluid biomarkers of pediatric hydrocephalus. Pediatr Neurosurg. 2017;52(6):426–35.
201. Habiyaremye G, Morales DM, Morgan CD, McAllister JP, CreveCoeur TS, Han RH, Gabir M, Baksh B, Mercer D, Limbrick DD Jr. Chemokine and cytokine levels in the lumbar cerebrospinal fluid of preterm infants with post-hemorrhagic hydrocephalus. Fluids Barriers CNS. 2017;14:35.
202. Garton T, He Y, Garton HJ, Keep RF, Xi G, Strahle JM. Hemoglobin-induced neuronal degeneration in the neonatal hippocampus after intraventricular hemorrhage. Brain Res. 2016;1635:86–94.
203. Aojula A, Botfield H, McAllister JP 2nd, Gonzalez AM, Abdullah O, Logan A, Sinclair A. Diffusion tensor imaging with direct cytopathological validation: characterisation of decorin treatment in experimental juvenile communicating hydrocephalus. Fluids Barriers CNS. 2016;13:9.
204. Klebe D, Krafft PR, Hoffmann C, Lekic T, Flores JJ, Rolland W, Zhang JH. Acute and delayed deferoxamine treatment attenuates long-term sequelae after germinal matrix hemorrhage in neonatal rats. Stroke. 2014;45:2475–9.
205. McAllister JP, Miller JM. Minocycline inhibits glial proliferation in the H-Tx rat model of congenital hydrocephalus. Cerebrospinal Fluid Res. 2010;7:7.
206. Di Curzio DL, Turner-Brannen E, Mao X, Del Bigio MR. Magnesium sulfate treatment for juvenile ferrets following induction of hydrocephalus with kaolin. Fluids Barriers CNS. 2016;13:7.
207. Khan OH, McPhee LC, Moddemann LN, Del Bigio MR. Calcium antagonism in neonatal rats with kaolin-induced hydrocephalus. J Child Neurol. 2007;22:1161–6.
208. Del Bigio MR. Neuropathology and structural changes in hydrocephalus. Dev Disabil Res Rev. 2010;16:16–22.
209. Del Bigio MR, Khan OH, da Silva Lopes L, Juliet PA. Cerebral white matter oxidation and nitrosylation in young rodents with kaolin-induced hydrocephalus. J Neuropathol Exp Neurol. 2012;71:274–88.
210. Del Bigio MR, Wilson MJ, Enno T. Chronic hydrocephalus in rats and humans: white matter loss and behavior changes. Ann Neurol. 2003;53:337–46.
211. Di Curzio DL, Buist RJ, Del Bigio MR. Reduced subventricular zone proliferation and white matter damage in juvenile ferrets with kaolin-induced hydrocephalus. Exp Neurol. 2013;248C:112–28.
212. McAllister JP 2nd. Pathophysiology of congenital and neonatal hydrocephalus. Semin Fetal Neonatal Med. 2012;17:285–94.
213. McAllister JP 2nd, Chovan P. Neonatal hydrocephalus. Mechanisms and consequences. Neurosurg Clin N Am. 1998;9:73–93.
214. Yuan W, McKinstry RC, Shimony JS, Altaye M, Powell SK, Phillips JM, Limbrick DD Jr, Holland SK, Jones BV, Rajagopal A, et al. Diffusion tensor imaging properties and neurobehavioral outcomes in children with hydrocephalus. AJNR Am J Neuroradiol. 2013;34:439–45.
215. Yuan W, Air E, Altaye M, Holland S, Jones B, Bierbrauer K, Mangano F. Abnormal fractional anisotropy in hydrocephalic children: a DTI study. Cerebrospinal Fluid Res. 2009;6:S14.
216. Eskandari R, Abdullah O, Mason C, Lloyd KE, Oeschle AN, McAllister JP 2nd. Differential vulnerability of white matter structures to experimental infantile hydrocephalus detected by diffusion tensor imaging. Childs Nerv Syst. 2014;30:1651–61.
217. Eskandari R, McAllister JP 2nd, Miller JM, Ding Y, Ham SD, Shearer DM, Way JS. Effects of hydrocephalus and ventriculoperitoneal shunt therapy on afferent and efferent connections in the feline sensorimotor cortex. J Neurosurg. 2004;101:196–210.
218. Yuan W, Deren KE, McAllister JP 2nd, Holland SK, Lindquist DM, Cancelliere A, Mason M, Shereen A, Hertzler DA, Altaye M, Mangano FT. Diffusion tensor imaging correlates with cytopathology in a rat model of neonatal hydrocephalus. Cerebrospinal Fluid Res. 2010;7:19.
219. Yuan W, Holland SK, Shimony JS, Altaye M, Mangano FT, Limbrick DD, Jones BV, Nash T, Rajagopal A, Simpson S, et al. Abnormal structural connectivity in the brain networks of children with hydrocephalus. Neuroimage Clin. 2015;8:483–92.
220. Yuan W, McAllister JP 2nd, Lindquist DM, Gill N, Holland SK, Henkel D, Rajagopal A, Mangano FT. Diffusion tensor imaging of white matter injury in a rat model of infantile hydrocephalus. Childs Nerv Syst. 2012;28:47–54.
221. Yuan W, McAllister JPI, Mangano FT. Neuroimaging of white matter abnormalities in pediatric hydrocephalus. J Pediatr Neuroradiol. 2013;2:119–28.
222. Karimy JK, Duran D, Hu JK, Gavankar C, Gaillard JR, Bayri Y, Rice H, DiLuna ML, Gerzanich V, Marc Simard J, Kahle KT. Cerebrospinal fluid hypersecretion in pediatric hydrocephalus. Neurosurg Focus. 2016;41:E10.
223. Uldall M, Botfield H, Jansen-Olesen I, Sinclair A, Jensen R. Acetazolamide lowers intracranial pressure and modulates the cerebrospinal fluid secretion pathway in healthy rats. Neurosci Lett. 2017;645:33–9.
224. Schmidt MJ, Rummel C, Hauer J, Kolecka M, Ondreka N, McClure V, Roth J. Increased CSF aquaporin-4, and interleukin-6 levels in dogs with idiopathic communicating internal hydrocephalus and a decrease after ventriculo-peritoneal shunting. Fluids Barriers CNS. 2016;13:12.
225. Castaneyra-Ruiz L, Gonzalez-Marrero I, Castaneyra-Ruiz A, Gonzalez-Toledo JM, Castaneyra-Ruiz M, Perez-Molto FJ, Carmona-Calero EM, Castaneyra-Perdomo A. The neuroepithelium disruption could generate autoantibodies against AQP4 and cause neuromyelitis optica and hydrocephalus. Int Sch Res Notices. 2014;2014:580572.
226. Sveinsdottir S, Gram M, Cinthio M, Sveinsdottir K, Morgelin M, Ley D. Altered expression of aquaporin 1 and 5 in the choroid plexus following preterm intraventricular hemorrhage. Dev Neurosci. 2014;36:542–51.
227. Kim H, Moore SA, Johnston MG. Potential for intranasal drug delivery to alter CSF outflow via the nasa turbinate lymphatics. Fluids Barriers CNS. 2014;11:4.
228. Ballabh P, Hu F, Kumarasiri M, Braun A, Nedergaard M. Development of tight junction molecules in blood vessels of germinal matrix, cerebral cortex, and white matter. Pediatr Res. 2005;58:791–8.
229. Iliff JJ, Wang M, Liao Y, Plogg BA, Peng W, Gundersen GA, Benveniste H, Vates GE, Deane R, Goldman SA, et al. A paravascular pathway facilitates

CSF flow through the brain parenchyma and the clearance of interstitial solutes, including amyloid beta. Sci Transl Med. 2012;4:147ra111.
230. Mukerji A, Shah V, Shah PS. Periventricular/intraventricular hemorrhage and neurodevelopmental outcomes: a meta-analysis. Pediatrics. 2015;136:1132–43.
231. Koschnitzky JEW, Wright JM, White M, Garzon A, Bechard J, Unguru Y, Walker M, Williams MA. Incorporating the patient voice in hydrocephalus research: translation to transform project. Hydroceph Assoc. 2017;1:1–22.
232. Riva-Cambrin J, Shannon CN, Holubkov R, Whitehead WE, Kulkarni AV, Drake J, Simon TD, Browd SR, Kestle JR, Wellons JC 3rd, Hydrocephalus Clinical Research N. Center effect and other factors influencing temporization and shunting of cerebrospinal fluid in preterm infants with intraventricular hemorrhage. J Neurosurg Pediatr. 2012;9:473–81.
233. Del Bigio MR. Future directions for therapy of childhood hydrocephalus: a view from the laboratory. Pediatr Neurosurg. 2001;34:172–81.
234. Balasubramaniam J, Del Bigio MR. Animal models of germinal matrix hemorrhage. J Child Neurol. 2006;21:365–71.
235. Zhu W, Gao Y, Chang CF, Wan JR, Zhu SS, Wang J. Mouse models of intracerebral hemorrhage in ventricle, cortex, and hippocampus by injections of autologous blood or collagenase. PLoS ONE. 2014;9:e97423.
236. Xue M, Del Bigio MR. Comparison of brain cell death and inflammatory reaction in three models of intracerebral hemorrhage in adult rats. J Stroke Cerebrovasc Dis. 2003;12:152–9.
237. Lodhia KR, Shakui P, Keep RF. Hydrocephalus in a rat model of intraventricular hemorrhage. Acta Neurochir Suppl. 2006;96:207–11.
238. Balasubramaniam J, Xue M, Buist RJ, Ivanco TL, Natuik S, Del Bigio MR. Persistent motor deficit following infusion of autologous blood into the periventricular region of neonatal rats. Exp Neurol. 2006;197:122–32.
239. Aquilina K, Chakkarapani E, Love S, Thoresen M. Neonatal rat model of intraventricular haemorrhage and post-haemorrhagic ventricular dilatation with long-term survival into adulthood. Neuropathol Appl Neurobiol. 2011;37:156–65.
240. Chen Z, Zhang J, Chen Q, Guo J, Zhu G, Feng H. Neuroprotective effects of edaravone after intraventricular hemorrhage in rats. Neuroreport. 2014;25:635–40.
241. Marinkovic I, Strbian D, Mattila OS, Abo-Ramadan U, Tatlisumak T. A novel combined model of intracerebral and intraventricular hemorrhage using autologous blood-injection in rats. Neuroscience. 2014;272:286–94.
242. Chen Q, Zhang J, Guo J, Tang J, Tao Y, Li L, Feng H, Chen Z. Chronic hydrocephalus and perihematomal tissue injury developed in a rat model of intracerebral hemorrhage with ventricular extension. Transl Stroke Res. 2015;6:125–32.
243. Gu W, Li F, Zhang W, Jia P. Expression and significance of aquaporin protein in Sprague–Dawley rats after experimental intraventricular hemorrhage. Cell Mol Biol. 2016;62:59–62.
244. Sugimoto T, Yasuhara A, Matsumura T. Intracranial hemorrhage following administration of sodium bicarbonate in rabbits. Brain Dev. 1981;3:297–303.
245. Lorenzo AV, Welch K, Conner S. Spontaneous germinal matrix and intraventricular hemorrhage in prematurely born rabbits. J Neurosurg. 1982;56:404–10.
246. Karwacki Z, Kowianski P, Morys J, Dziewiatkowski J, Suchorzewska J. The influence of the intraventricular hemorrhage on the intracranial pressure and hemodynamic changes in the experimental intracerebral hemorrhage in the rabbits. Folia Neuropathol. 2000;38:55–9.
247. Georgiadis P, Xu H, Chua C, Hu F, Collins L, Huynh C, Lagamma EF, Ballabh P. Characterization of acute brain injuries and neurobehavioral profiles in a rabbit model of germinal matrix hemorrhage. Stroke. 2008;39:3378–88.
248. Chua CO, Chahboune H, Braun A, Dummula K, Chua CE, Yu J, Ungvari Z, Sherbany AA, Hyder F, Ballabh P. Consequences of intraventricular hemorrhage in a rabbit pup model. Stroke. 2009;40:3369–77.
249. Vinukonda G, Zia MT, Bhimavarapu BB, Hu F, Feinberg M, Bokhari A, Ungvari Z, Fried VA, Ballabh P. Intraventricular hemorrhage induces deposition of proteoglycans in premature rabbits, but their in vivo degradation with chondroitinase does not restore myelination, ventricle size and neurological recovery. Exp Neurol. 2013;247:630–44.
250. Dohare P, Zia MT, Ahmed E, Ahmed A, Yadala V, Schober AL, Ortega JA, Kayton R, Ungvari Z, Mongin AA, Ballabh P. AMPA-kainate receptor inhibition promotes neurologic recovery in premature rabbits with intraventricular hemorrhage. J Neurosci. 2016;36:3363–77.
251. Rudy TA, Westergaard JL, Yaksh TL. Hyperthermia produced by simulated intraventricular hemorrhage in the cat. Exp Neurol. 1978;58:296–310.
252. Ment LR, Stewart WB, Duncan CC. Local cerebral glucose utilization in the beagle puppy model of intraventricular hemorrhage. J Neurosurg. 1982;57:384–9.
253. Johnson DL, Getson P, Shaer C, O'Donnell R. Intraventricular hemorrhage in the newborn beagle puppy. A limited model of intraventricular hemorrhage in the premature infant. Pediatr Neurosci. 1987;13:78–83.
254. Reynolds ML, Evans CA, Reynolds EO, Saunders NR, Durbin GM, Wigglesworth JS. Intracranial haemorrhage in the preterm sheep fetus. Early Hum Dev. 1979;3:163–86.
255. Farstad T, Odden JP, Bratlid D. Effect of intraventricular hemorrhage on pulmonary function in newborn piglets. Biol Neonate. 1994;66:238–46.
256. Mayfrank L, Kim Y, Kissler J, Delsing P, Gilsbach JM, Schroder JM, Weis J. Morphological changes following experimental intraventricular haemorrhage and intraventricular fibrinolytic treatment with recombinant tissue plasminogen activator. Acta Neuropathol. 2000;100:561–7.
257. Aquilina K, Hobbs C, Cherian S, Tucker A, Porter H, Whitelaw A, Thoresen M. A neonatal piglet model of intraventricular hemorrhage and posthemorrhagic ventricular dilation. J Neurosurg. 2007;107:126–36.
258. Tang T, Weiss MD, Borum P, Turovets S, Tucker D, Sadleir R. In vivo quantification of intraventricular hemorrhage in a neonatal piglet model using an EEG-layout based electrical impedance tomography array. Physiol Meas. 2016;37:751–64.
259. Alles YCJ, Greggio S, Alles RM, Azevedo PN, Xavier LL, DaCosta JC. A novel preclinical rodent model of collagenase-induced germinal matrix/intraventricular hemorrhage. Brain Res. 2010;1356:130–8.
260. Goddard J, Lewis RM, Alcala H, Zeller RS. Intraventricular hemorrhage—an animal model. Biol Neonate. 1980;37:39–52.
261. Ment LR, Stewart WB, Duncan CC, Pitt BR, Cole JS. Beagle puppy model of perinatal cerebral infarction. J Neurosurg. 1986;65:851–5.
262. Juliet PA, Frost EE, Balasubramaniam J, Del Bigio MR. Toxic effect of blood components on perinatal rat subventricular zone cells and oligodendrocyte precursor cell proliferation, differentiation and migration in culture. J Neurochem. 2009;109:1285–99.
263. Juliet PA, Mao X, Del Bigio MR. Proinflammatory cytokine production by cultured neonatal rat microglia after exposure to blood products. Brain Res. 2008;19(1210):230–9 **(Epub 2008 Mar 18)**.
264. Gamo NJ, Birknow MR, Sullivan D, Kondo MA, Horiuchi Y, Sakurai T, Slusher BS, Sawa A. Valley of death: a proposal to build a "translational bridge" for the next generation. Neurosci Res. 2017;115:1–4.
265. Yu HW. Bridging the translational gap: collaborative drug development and dispelling the stigma of commercialization. Drug Discov Today. 2016;21:299–305.
266. Kochanek PM, Bramlett HM, Dixon CE, Shear DA, Dietrich WD, Schmid KE, Mondello S, Wang KK, Hayes RL, Povlishock JT, Tortella FC. Approach to modeling, therapy evaluation, drug selection, and biomarker assessments for a multicenter pre-clinical drug screening consortium for acute therapies in severe traumatic brain injury: operation brain trauma therapy. J Neurotrauma. 2016;33:513–22.
267. Fisher M, Feuerstein G, Howells DW, Hurn PD, Kent TA, Savitz SI, Lo EH, Group S. Update of the stroke therapy academic industry roundtable preclinical recommendations. Stroke. 2009;40:2244–50.
268. Stroke Therapy Academic Industry R. Recommendations for standards regarding preclinical neuroprotective and restorative drug development. Stroke. 1999;30:2752–8.
269. Lapchak PA, Zhang JH, Noble-Haeusslein LJ. RIGOR guidelines: escalating STAIR and STEPS for effective translational research. Transl Stroke Res. 2013;4:279–85.
270. Vinukonda G, Dummula K, Malik S, Hu F, Thompson CI, Csiszar A, Ungvari Z, Ballabh P. Effect of prenatal glucocorticoids on cerebral vasculature of the developing brain. Stroke. 2010;41:1766–73.
271. Schmitz T. Prevention of preterm birth complications by antenatal corticosteroid administration. J Gynecol Obstet Biol Reprod. 2016;45:1399–417.

272. Romejko-Wolniewicz E, Oleszczuk L, Zareba-Szczudlik J, Czajkowski K. Dosage regimen of antenatal steroids prior to preterm delivery and effects on maternal and neonatal outcomes. J Matern Fetal Neonatal Med. 2013;26:237–41.
273. Wei JC, Catalano R, Profit J, Gould JB, Lee HC. Impact of antenatal steroids on intraventricular hemorrhage in very-low-birth weight infants. J Perinatol. 2016;36:352–6.
274. Wapner RJ. Antenatal corticosteroids for periviable birth. Semin Perinatol. 2013;37:410–3.
275. Ment LR, Vohr BR, Makuch RW, Westerveld M, Katz KH, Schneider KC, Duncan CC, Ehrenkranz R, Oh W, Philip AG, et al. Prevention of intraventricular hemorrhage by indomethacin in male preterm infants. J Pediatr. 2004;145:832–4.
276. Ment LR, Oh W, Ehrenkranz RA, Phillip AG, Vohr B, Allan W, Makuch RW, Taylor KJ, Schneider KC, Katz KH, et al. Low-dose indomethacin therapy and extension of intraventricular hemorrhage: a multicenter randomized trial. J Pediatr. 1994;124:951–5.
277. Dani C, Bertini G, Pezzati M, Poggi C, Guerrini P, Martano C, Rubaltelli FF, IntraVentricular Ibuprofen Study G. Prophylactic ibuprofen for the prevention of intraventricular hemorrhage among preterm infants: a multicenter, randomized study. Pediatrics. 2005;115:1529–35.
278. Schulte J, Osborne J, Benson JW, Cooke R, Drayton M, Murphy J, Rennie J, Speidel B. Developmental outcome of the use of etamsylate for prevention of periventricular haemorrhage in a randomised controlled trial. Arch Dis Child Fetal Neonatal Ed. 2005;90:F31–5.
279. Benson JW, Drayton MR, Hayward C, Murphy JF, Osborne JP, Rennie JM, Schulte JF, Speidel BD, Cooke RW. Multicentre trial of ethamsylate for prevention of periventricular haemorrhage in very low birthweight infants. Lancet. 1986;2:1297–300.
280. Hasan SU, Potenziano J, Konduri GG, Perez JA, Van Meurs KP, Walker MW, Yoder BA, Newborns Treated With Nitric Oxide Trial G. Effect of inhaled nitric oxide on survival without bronchopulmonary dysplasia in preterm infants: a randomized clinical trial. JAMA Pediatr. 2017;171:1081–9.
281. Barrington KJ, Finer N, Pennaforte T, Altit G. Nitric oxide for respiratory failure in infants born at or near term. Cochrane Database Syst Rev. 2017;1:CD000399.
282. Smit E, Odd D, Whitelaw A. Postnatal phenobarbital for the prevention of intraventricular haemorrhage in preterm infants. Cochrane Database Syst Rev. 2013;8:CD001691.
283. Ma CC, Ma S. The role of surfactant in respiratory distress syndrome. Open Respir Med J. 2012;6:44–53.
284. Polin RA, Carlo WA, Committee on F, Newborn, American Academy of P. Surfactant replacement therapy for preterm and term neonates with respiratory distress. Pediatrics. 2014;133:156–63.
285. McCord FB, Curstedt T, Halliday HL, McClure G, Reid MM, Robertson B. Surfactant treatment and incidence of intraventricular haemorrhage in severe respiratory distress syndrome. Arch Dis Child. 1988;63:10–6.
286. Doyle LW, Ehrenkranz RA, Halliday HL. Early (< 8 days) postnatal corticosteroids for preventing chronic lung disease in preterm infants. Cochrane Database Syst Rev. 2014;5:CD001146.
287. Doyle LW, Ehrenkranz RA, Halliday HL. Late (> 7 days) postnatal corticosteroids for chronic lung disease in preterm infants. Cochrane Database Syst Rev. 2014;5:CD001145.
288. Jelin AC, Salmeen K, Gano D, Burd I, Thiet MP. Perinatal neuroprotection update. F1000Res. 2016;5(F1000 Faculty Rev):1939.
289. Crowther CA, Middleton PF, Voysey M, Askie L, Duley L, Pryde PG, Marret S, Doyle LW, Group A. Assessing the neuroprotective benefits for babies of antenatal magnesium sulphate: an individual participant data meta-analysis. PLoS Med. 2017;14:e1002398.
290. Horton AL, Lai Y, Rouse DJ, Spong CY, Leveno KJ, Varner MW, Mercer BM, Iams JD, Wapner RJ, Sorokin Y, et al. Effect of magnesium sulfate administration for neuroprotection on latency in women with preterm premature rupture of membranes. Am J Perinatol. 2015;32:387–92.
291. Petrova A, Mehta R. Magnesium sulfate tocolysis and intraventricular hemorrhage in very preterm infants. Indian J Pediatr. 2012;79:43–7.
292. Szpecht D, Szymankiewicz M, Nowak I, Gadzinowski J. Intraventricular hemorrhage in neonates born before 32 weeks of gestation-retrospective analysis of risk factors. Childs Nerv Syst. 2016;32:1399–404.
293. Andersson O, Lindquist B, Lindgren M, Stjernqvist K, Domellof M, Hellstrom-Westas L. Effect of delayed cord clamping on neurodevelopment at 4 years of age: a randomized clinical trial. JAMA Pediatr. 2015;169:631–8.
294. Committee on Obstetric P. Committee Opinion No. 684: delayed umbilical cord clamping after birth. Obstet Gynecol. 2017;129:e5–10.
295. Committee on Obstetric Practice ACoO, Gynecologists. Committee Opinion No.543: timing of umbilical cord clamping after birth. Obstet Gynecol. 2012;120:1522–6.

22

Paradigm-shift: radiological changes in the asymptomatic iNPH-patient to be

D. C. Engel[1*], S. D. Adib[1], M. U. Schuhmann[1] and C. Brendle[2]

Abstract

Background: Many radiological signs are known for the diagnosis of idiopathic normal pressure hydrocephalus (iNPH). However, there is little information about these signs in the pre-symptomatic phase. For pathophysiological investigative purposes we conducted a descriptive image analysis study on pre-symptomatic patients.

Methods: Patients that had contact with either the neurological or neurosurgical department of the university hospital Tuebingen from 2010 through 2016 with magnetic resonance images > 3 years before onset of symptoms, were included. The date of onset and severity of symptoms, date of first imaging and birth date were recorded. Evan's index (EI), width of the third ventricle (3VW), tight high convexity (THC), Sylvian fissure, extent of white matter hyperintensities and aqueductal flow were assessed in images before and around symptom onset.

Results: Ten patients were included. In all ten patients the first symptom was gait disturbance. Nine of ten pre-symptomatic images showed classic signs for iNPH. EI showed a significant increase between the pre-symptomatic and symptomatic phase. 3VW showed a trend for increase without significance. THC changed back and forth over time within some patients.

Conclusions: In accordance with the scarce literature available, radiological changes are present at least 3 years before onset of iNPH-symptoms. EI seems to be a robust measure for pre-symptomatic radiological changes. Extrapolating the data, the development of iNPH typical changes might be an insidious process and the development of THC might be a variable and non-linear process. Further studies with larger sample sizes are necessary to put these findings into the pathophysiological perspective for the development of iNPH.

Keywords: Etiology, Pathophysiology, Idiopathic normal pressure hydrocephalus, Tight high convexity, Ventriculomegaly, Evan's index

Background

The etiology of idiopathic normal pressure hydrocephalus (iNPH) has been a research focus since its first description in 1965 [1]. The overall prevalence is estimated to be 10.2–31.4/100,000, and might even be 5900/100,000 in the > 80 year olds [2–4]. Better understanding of the pathophysiology and better treatment possibilities are needed for our aging populations.

The pathophysiology of iNPH is not completely understood currently. Studies indicate that a prolonged, possibly lifelong process underlies the development of what we know as iNPH [5–7]. Known changes in pathophysiological parameters measured at the time of symptomatic iNPH include decreased subcortical cerebral blood flow (CBF) [8], decreased flow in the internal carotid artery [9], reduced flow velocity in the superior sagittal sinus [10], a higher incidence of retrograde jugular flow during the Valsalva maneuver [11], increased aqueductal cerebrospinal fluid (CSF) flow velocity [12–14], decreased cervical CSF stroke volume [9], decreased elastance of the intradural compartment and increased CSF pulsatility

*Correspondence: doortje.engel@med.uni-tuebingen.de
[1] Department of Neurosurgery, University Hospital of Tuebingen, Hoppe-Seyler-Strasse 3, 72076 Tuebingen, Germany

and outflow resistance [15, 16], increased lactate concentrations in the lateral ventricles [17], deep and (partially reversible) periventricular white matter hyperintensities (WMH) [18–20] and increased neurofilament light chain protein in CSF as a sign of neurodegeneration [21, 22].

The hydraulic press hypothesis of Hakim and Adams explains the development of iNPH by disturbance of CSF-resorption leading to an increased outflow resistance, which in turn leads to an initial increase of ICP. The authors postulate that due to the increased ICP the ventriculomegaly occurs from the indirect linearity of pressure and surface at constant pressure according to Pascal's Law [23]. However, it lacks an explanation for the asymptomatic phase of increased ICP. Furthermore, a transmantle pulsatile gradient within the CSF of the cerebral ventricles in symptomatic iNPH patients could not be proven [24].

Another theory exists called the two-hit hypothesis, comprised of the occurrence of a benign external hydrocephalus during infancy followed by ischaemic insults leading to deep and periventricular WMH [7]. The first hit results in a larger intracranial volume in iNPH patients [7]. The second hit, ischemic insults, could be induced by worsening of periventricular ischemia [25, 26], softening of the brain [27], or decreased CSF resorption [28, 29] leading to the beginning of symptoms [7].

A third, hydrodynamic, hypothesis of Greitz is explained as "restricted arterial pulsation hydrocephalus" or "increased capillary pulsation hydrocephalus" [30]. An increasing rigidity of the cerebral arteries by arteriosclerosis could lead to the inability to attenuate the pulsations of CBF into the brain parenchyma, causing a reduction of the periventricular metabolism and degeneration of the periventricular parenchyma [30–32].

In addition to the above-mentioned mechanical hypotheses, genetic predispositions such as homozygous apolipoprotein E allele on chromosome 19, play an important role in familial iNPH [33–35].

The above-mentioned pathophysiological parameters cannot prove any of the stated hypotheses, because all data have been logically derived in patients who already had symptomatic iNPH. Therefore we aimed to investigate the presence of iNPH-typical changes in diagnostic images in the pre-symptomatic phase of iNPH.

Methods

Patient inclusion

The diagnosis of iNPH was screened as either probable or possible and secured according to international guidelines by an objective improvement of gait in the 10 m walking test after either (repetitive) CSF tap-test(s) or lumbar drainage for 3 days [36–39]. Those patients with imaging available 3 or more years before symptom-onset, that had contact with the neurological or neurosurgical department of the university hospital Tuebingen for the diagnosis of iNPH from 2010 thru 2016 were included. Time of symptom-onset was extracted from the medical history. The 3-year cut-off was chosen because of the insidious onset of iNPH. Patients with an unclear hydrocephalus-type, possibly due to neurotrauma, meningitis or intracranial bleeding or with an unclear symptom-onset or origin, i.e. due to simultaneous high-grade cervical spinal stenosis were excluded. Age, time of symptom onset, time of first imaging and first presenting symptoms were assessed. All of the imaging data (MRI and CT) were included in this retrospective analysis.

Image analysis

Imaging data were acquired on CT and MRI scanners approved for clinical routine use. Data were reconstructed according to clinical standard orientated at the corpus callosum in the axial slices and at the brain stem in the coronal slices. For image analysis in CT, the axial slices and where available the coronal slices were assessed. For image analysis in MRI, the axial fluid attenuated inversion recovery (FLAIR) sequence and where available the axial, coronal or sagittal T2-weighted images were assessed. Images after treatment by ventriculoperitoneal shunt implantation (VPS) were not included.

A neuroradiologist (CB) scored the imaging data being blinded for the hypotheses of this project and the clinical data. The following measurements were obtained:

1. Evan's index (EI) was determined as the ratio of the maximum transverse diameter of the frontal horns of the lateral ventricles and the diameter of the inner skull [40].
2. The width of the third ventricle (3VW) was measured in the axial plane in the mid-portion of the third ventricle.
3. Tight high convexity (THC) of the subarachnoid space was measured following the method of Narita et al. [41] in both transverse and coronal sections and rated as: 0, normal; 1, mild tightness; 2, moderate tightness; 3, severe tightness.
4. Width of the Sylvian fissure was assessed only on transverse sections as: 0, narrowed, 1, normal; 2, mildly dilated; 3, severely dilated [41].
5. Periventricular and deep WMH were scored according to Fazekas [42].
6. The existence of aqueductal flow voids/jets was documented if appropriate MR-sequences were available.

The callosal angle was not included due to missing coronal sections in many of examinations.

Statistics

Normal distribution of the data was denied by the Shapiro–Wilk test. Wilcoxon text was performed to compare EI and 3VW before and after onset of symptoms in patients with available imaging data at both time points.

Results

From 2010 through 2016, 382 patients suspected of having NPH had contact with either the neurological or neurosurgical department. Ten patients met inclusion criteria and were finally included in the study with a male-to-female ratio of 1:1 and a mean age at symptom-onset of 77.4 years (range 70.9–88.7).

Clinical data

Seven patients were treated by VPS and improved long-term (> 1 year); the other 3 either refused treatment or received repetitive lumbar punctures. Gait disturbance was the first reported symptom in all cases. Nine patients suffered all three symptoms of the Hakim triad at the time of diagnosis. Only one patient reported no cognitive deficits and had a Mini Mental State Examination (MMSE) score at time of diagnosis 30/30. The other patients did indicate cognitive deficits. In this group MMSE ranged from 12 to 29/30. Nine patients were diagnosed with hypertension before symptom-onset.

Imaging data

On average the first imaging examination (CT or MRI) was conducted − 6.2 years to symptom onset (range 3.1–10.3). In 2 cases 3 MRIs were available at − 6.1, − 2.8 and 0.2 and − 10.3, − 4.1 and 0.5 years to symptom onset respectively. All time points are relative to symptom onset. Details of the available imaging data are shown in Table 1. An illustrative case (patient 7) with increasing radiological changes from the pre-symptomatic to symptomatic phase is shown in Fig. 1.

Evan's index and width of 3rd ventricle

EI was $\geq$ 0.3 in all cases at all imaging times. Figure 2 shows EI over time. The values most prior to and closest to symptom onset were included. The same was done for 3VW (see Fig. 3). One patient suffered from bithalamic ischemia 4 years before symptom onset. This patient was not excluded because EI and 3VW had already been enlarged before the occurrence of the ischemic event. Six patients had available imaging data at time points before and after onset of symptoms. In the remaining four patients, the second examination was performed shortly before symptom onset. In these six patients, the mean value of EI was significantly higher after symptom onset than at the pre-symptomatic time point (mean value 0.39 $\pm$ 0.02 and 0.35 $\pm$ 0.03, respectively, $p = 0.0354$). 3VW did not show a significant difference between both time points (mean value 18.3 $\pm$ 3.0 and 15.8 $\pm$ 3.4, respectively).

Tight high convexity

Data on THC were available on the first image in nine patients. Seven of nine had a positive THC-score of 1, 2 or 3. The 2 patients who had no THC score of 0 in the first image at − 10 and − 6 years, did have mild score of 1 at − 4 years or a moderate score of 2, at − 1 year on the second available image. Two patients had mild THC of score 1 before symptom onset at − 5 and − 7 years, scored 0 after symptom onset at + 1.5 and 0 years. In the remaining 5 patients, THC score increased over time. All patients are depicted in Fig. 4.

Table 1 Images available per patient

Patnr	Imaging 1		Imaging 2		Imaging 3		Imaging 4	
	Timepoint	Modality	Timepoint	Modality	Timepoint	Modality	Timepoint	Modality
1	− 4.7	CT	− 3.3	CT	− 0.9	MRI	2.1	CT
2	− 5.4	CT	− 0.1	CT	0.2	MRI		
3	− 6.1	MRI	− 2.8	MRI	0.2	CT	1.9	CT
4	− 3.1	CT	0.9	CT				
5	− 3.6	CT	− 0.1	MRI				
6	− 7.8	MRI	1.5	MRI	1.9	CT		
7	− 10.3	MRI	− 4.1	MRI	− 1.4	CT	0.5	MRI
8	− 6.1	MRI	0.7	MRI	2.0	CT		
9	− 9.2	CT	0.8	MRI				
10	− 5.8	CT	2.0	MRI				

Available imaging according to time-to-symptom-onset including first image available around symptom-onset, either CT or MRI. Patnr: patient number; timepoint: interval between imaging and onset of symptoms in years

In 2 cases 3 MRIs were available at − 6.1, − 2.8 and 0.2 and − 10.3, − 4.1 and 0.5 years to symptom onset respectively

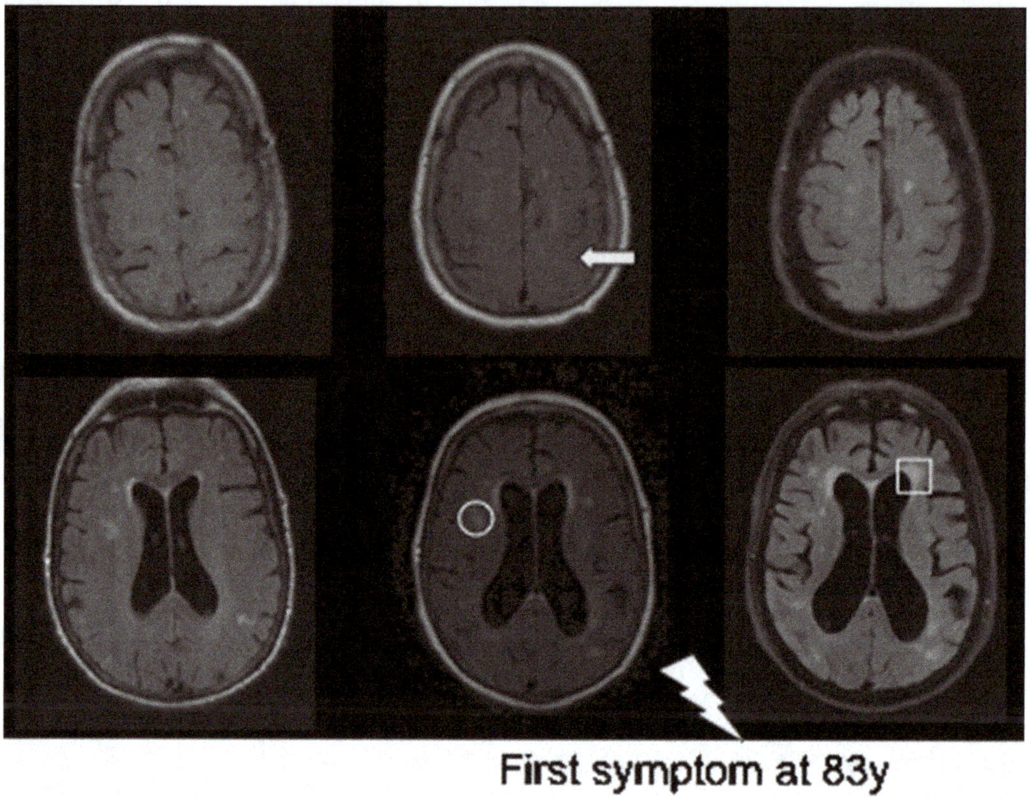

Fig. 1 Pre- and post-symptomatic magnetic resonance images of a patient that developed symptoms after 10 years. The MRI images show the changes in ventricle width, deterioration of white matter hyperintensities (circle: deep; square: periventricular) and tight high convexity (arrow) all before onset of symptoms (thunderbolt) of a typical case. Left: 10 years before symptom onset. Middle: 4 years before symptom onset. Right: 6 months after symptom onset

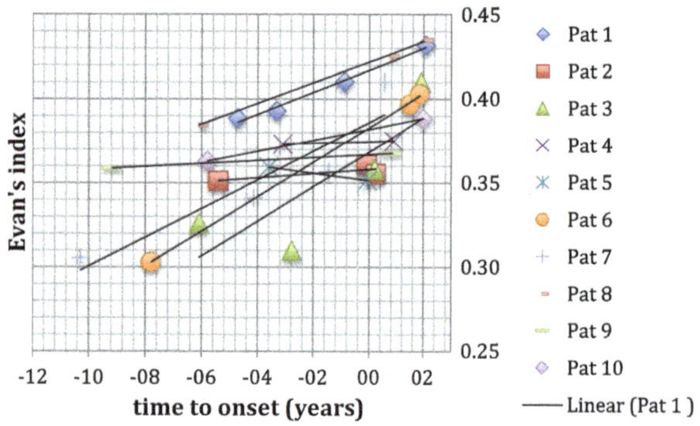

Fig. 2 Change in Evan's Index over time. Each patient is depicted separately. EI was above 0.3 in all patients and increased over time significantly. Time 0 is time of symptom onset

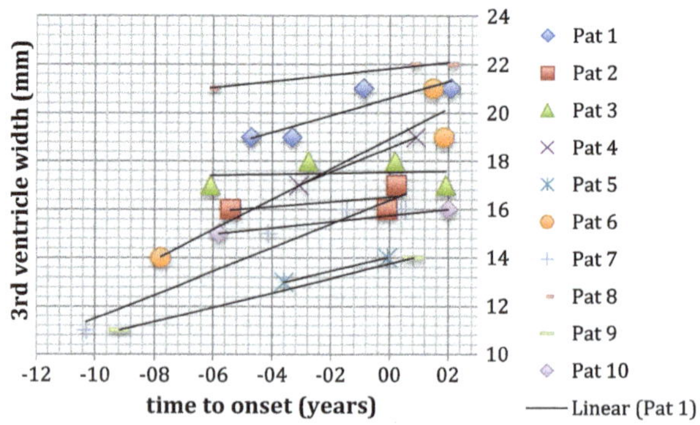

Fig. 3 Change in third ventricle width over time. Each patient is depicted separately. Third ventricle width (in mm) was above 9 mm in all patients and increased over time. Time 0 is time of symptom onset

Other imaging findings

All patients with the relevant MRI (n = 7) showed periventricular and deep WMH. Only in 4 patients was MRI-data available at least 3 years before symptom-onset. The Fazekas score for both deep and periventricular WMH ranged from mild to severe (score 1–3) [42]. Aqueductal flow voids could be determined in 7 patients with T2-weighted sagittal MRI images and was present in all 7 cases. No major Sylvian fissure atrophy was seen.

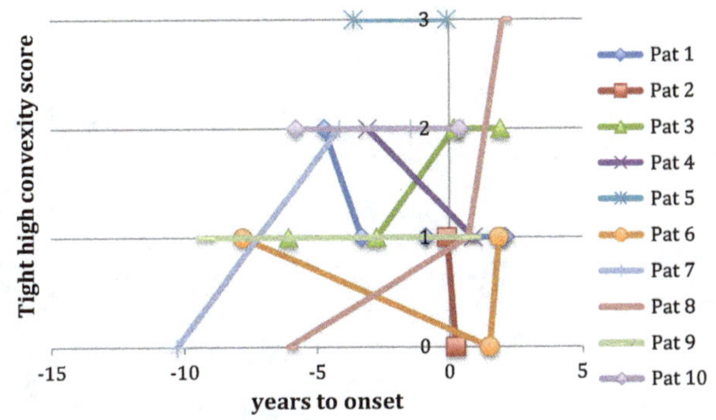

Fig. 4 Change in tight high convexity over time. Each patient is depicted separately. THC varied through time within patients. Time 0 is time of symptom onset

Discussion

This study shows that increased ventricular width, aqueductal flow void, deep and periventricular WMH and fluctuating THC precede symptom-onset of iNPH by at least 3 years. The presence or absence of THC seems to be a dynamic process varying in a non-linear fashion. This gives new insights into the pathogenesis of iNPH.

EI seems to be a robust measure for pre-symptomatic radiological changes in iNPH. EI increased significantly from the pre-symptomatic images to the time point of iNPH diagnosis. Extrapolation of the obtained data, assuming that EI change is linear over time, implies that the pathophysiological start of iNPH could be around 10–15 years before symptom onset. An on-going change in ventricular width might contradict the two-hit hypothesis on iNPH pathogenesis of the presence of benign external hydrocephalus in infancy followed by deep white matter ischemia later on as proposed by Bradley et al. [7, 43]. However, no proof of either theory exists to date. Further pre-symptomatic and long-term investigations are necessary. Moreover, it is conceivable that different subtypes of iNPH exist with different pathophysiological pathways.

Unlike Iseki et al. [5], our data show ventriculomegaly in almost all patients with only mild to moderate THC. A selection bias logically exists in the current study due to the retrospective nature and its inclusion criteria. The imaging studies at the pre-symptomatic time points were performed because of different neurological indications not connected to iNPH, whereas Iseki et al. have investigated a population-based cohort. Nevertheless, our data show a certain dynamic trend of THC in both increasing and decreasing throughout the years. These data suggest rather a variable than linear development of THC over time, possibly due to build up of internal CSF pressure followed by pressure decline after widening of the ventricles due to cell loss. Although the hypothesis of a transmantle gradient in pulsatile ICP in the lateral ventricles was disproven in 2010 [44], pressure was measured only in symptomatic patients. As CSF pulsatility index and CSF outflow resistance are increased in iNPH patients in the symptomatic phase [15, 16], increased ICP in the pre-symptomatic phase cannot be ruled out completely.

The presence of deep WMH together with the high prevalence of hypertension in our patients supports aspects of the hydrodynamic hypothesis of Greitz [45]. Approximately 50–60% of the 70–79 year old general population had hypertension according to a health survey 1988–1991 [46]. A more recent German survey showed that 60% of 50–59 year olds and 75% of 70–79 year olds suffer from hypertension [47]. Also signs of cerebrovascular disease were found in post-mortem and biopsy studies in iNPH patients [48–50]. Next to increasing blood pressure with age, there is a reduction of the dampening effect in cerebral arteries during aging due to stiffening of the arteries. This would further support the hydrodynamic theory [51]. In contrast, Qvarlander et al. did not find a significant difference in total cerebral artery inflow pulsatility index between healthy and iNPH patients [9]. It is thus unclear, if the extracranial arterial pulsatility reflects intracranial pulsatility, since the extracranial compartment is highly compliant as opposed to the intracranial compartment.

Transependymal edema or microangiopathic ischemia presenting as periventricular WMH was seen in all of our patients and existed in at least four patients before symptom onset. Previous data show that acetazolamide can reduce periventricular WMH with or without corresponding gait improvement in some but not all patients [19]. Acetazolamide inhibits CSF production in the choroid plexus, inhibits aquaporin-mediated water transport and normally leads to a CBF increase by vasodilation [52]. iNPH patients have an impaired cerebrovascular reactivity as shown before [53, 54]. The cerebrovascular reactivity was improved by acetazolamide in patients that showed clinical improvement after shunt surgery but not in the so-called non-responders [54]. All of our patients showed improved gait after shunt surgery or multiple lumbar punctures, while having had periventricular WMH for several years. Even years after symptom onset patients can improve after shunt surgery [55]. It remains unclear when the point of no return kicks in, where transependymal edema turns into ischemic tissue. To date no asymptomatic patient has received therapy for dilated lateral ventricles with typical iNPH imaging signs, as surgery has risks. Our data suggest that due to long-term progression a follow up of these asymptomatic patients with ventriculomegaly is necessary. These patients should be informed about the risk of developing iNPH symptoms in order to offer treatment at an early stage and preserve quality of life for as long as possible.

Limitations of this study include the retrospective nature of the investigation as well as the non-standardized documentation of clinical data, partially due to the fact that the patients were examined in two different departments. Furthermore, only low numbers of patients could be included due to the cut-off of available imaging at 3 years before symptom onset. The 3-year cutoff was set arbitrarily. Many patients already had symptoms 1–2 years before seeking medical advice. As symptoms start insidiously, imaging conducted at least 3 years before implied symptom-onset was considered to be realistically pre-symptomatic. The available imaging data was inconsistent, in some cases only CTs were available and not all parameters could be derived. This might have introduced biased assessments of the imaging data. However, length measurements as used in the EI and width of the third ventricle should be comparable between both modalities, and other measurements were based on rough scoring systems. Confounding is the fact that only iNPH-patients were investigated and not a population-dwelling cohort. However, it is likely that these changes are linked to iNPH, as patients in a previous study all developed iNPH-symptoms and very few asymptomatic participants were found after 10 years of scanning [5]. Due to the limited patient number, the statistical analysis can only give a preliminary overview. More longitudinal prospective research needs to be conducted similar to the work of Iseki et al. combining large cohort MRI data with clinical and neuropsychological data [5].

Conclusions

In accordance with scarcely available literature radiological changes are present at least 3 years before onset of iNPH-symptoms. Evan's index seems to be a robust measure for pre-symptomatic radiological changes. Extrapolating the data, the development of iNPH typical changes might be an insidious process and the development of tight high convexity might be a variable and non-linear process. Further studies with larger sample sizes are necessary to put these findings into the pathophysiological perspective of the development of iNPH.

Authors' contributions

DCE was responsible for conception and design, conducted acquisition, analysis and interpretation of data; drafting of manuscript and gave final approval of the version to be published. SDA has been involved in critical revision of the manuscript. MUS has been involved in critical revision of the manuscript. CB made substantial contributions to acquisition and analysis of data; critical revision of the manuscript. All authors read and approved the final manuscript.

Author details

[1] Department of Neurosurgery, University Hospital of Tuebingen, Hoppe-Seyler-Strasse 3, 72076 Tuebingen, Germany. [2] Department of Neuroradiology, University Hospital of Tuebingen, Hoppe-Seyler-Strasse 3, 72076 Tuebingen, Germany.

Competing interests

The authors declare that they have no competing interests.

Funding

Author DE was funded by the Tübingen Program for the promotion of Women in Research.

References

1. Adams RD, Fisher CM, Hakim S, Ojemann RG, Sweet WH. Symptomatic occult hydrocephalus normal cerebrospinal-fluid pressure. A treatable syndrome. N Engl J Med. 1965;273:117–26.
2. Kuriyama N, Miyajima M, Nakajima M, Kurosawa M, Fukushima W, Watanabe Y, et al. Nationwide hospital-based survey of idiopathic normal pressure hydrocephalus in Japan: epidemiological and clinical characteristics. Brain Behav. 2017;7:e00635.
3. Brean A, Eide PK. Prevalence of probable idiopathic normal pressure hydrocephalus in a Norwegian population. Acta Neurol Scand. 2008;118:48–53.
4. Jaraj D, Rabiei K, Marlow T, Jensen C, Skoog I, Wikkelsö C. Prevalence of idiopathic normal-pressure hydrocephalus. Neurology. 2014;82:1449–54.
5. Iseki C, Takahashi Y, Wada M, Kawanami T, Adachi M, Kato T. Incidence of idiopathic normal pressure hydrocephalus (iNPH): a 10-year follow-up study of a rural community in Japan. J Neurol Sci. 2014;339:108–12.
6. Wilson RK, Williams MA. Evidence that congenital hydrocephalus is a precursor to idiopathic normal pressure hydrocephalus in only a subset of patients. J Neurol Neurosurg Psychiatry. 2007;78:508–11.
7. Bradley WG, Safar FG, Hurtado C, Ord J, Alksne JF. Increased intracranial volume: a clue to the etiology of idiopathic normal-pressure hydrocephalus? Am J Neuroradiol. 2004;25:1479–84.
8. Nakano H, Bandoh K, Miyaoka M, Sato K. Evaluation of hydrocephalic periventricular radiolucency by dynamic computed tomography and xenon-computed tomography. Neurosurgery. 1996;39:758–63.
9. Qvarlander S, Ambarki K, Wåhlin A, Jacobsson J, Birgander R, Malm J, et al. Cerebrospinal fluid and blood flow patterns in idiopathic normal pressure hydrocephalus. Acta Neurol Scand. 2017;135:576–84.
10. Kuriyama N, Tokuda T, Yamada K, Akazawa K, Hosoda M, Sakai K, et al. Flow velocity of the superior sagittal sinus is reduced in patients with idiopathic normal pressure hydrocephalus. J Neuroimaging. 2011;21:365–9.
11. Kuriyama N, Tokuda T, Miyamoto J, Takayasu N, Kondo M, Nakagawa M. Retrograde jugular flow associated with idiopathic normal pressure hydrocephalus. Ann Neurol. 2008;64:217–21.
12. El Sankari S, Fichten A, Gondry-Jouet C, Czosnyka M, Legars D, Deramond H, et al. Correlation between tap test and CSF aqueductal stroke volume in idiopathic normal pressure hydrocephalus. Acta Neurochir Suppl. 2012;113:43–6.
13. Ringstad G, Emblem KE, Eide PK. Phase-contrast magnetic resonance imaging reveals net retrograde aqueductal flow in idiopathic normal pressure hydrocephalus. J Neurosurg. 2015;1–8.
14. Eklund A, Smielewski P, Chambers I, Alperin N, Malm J, Czosnyka M, et al. Assessment of cerebrospinal fluid outflow resistance. Med Biol Eng Comput. 2007;45:719–35.
15. Qvarlander S, Lundkvist B, Koskinen L-OD, Malm J, Eklund A. Pulsatility in CSF dynamics: pathophysiology of idiopathic normal pressure hydrocephalus. J Neurol Neurosurg Psychiatry. 2013;84:735–41.
16. Wikkelsø C, Hellström P, Klinge PM, Tans JTJ. The European iNPH Multicentre Study on the predictive values of resistance to CSF outflow and the CSF Tap Test in patients with idiopathic normal pressure hydrocephalus. J Neurol Neurosurg Psychiatry. 2013;84:562–8.
17. Kizu O, Yamada K, Nishimura T. Proton chemical shift imaging in normal pressure hydrocephalus. AJNR Am J Neuroradiol. 2001;22:1659–64.
18. Relkin N, Marmarou A, Klinge P, Bergsneider M, Black PM. Diagnosing idiopathic normal-pressure hydrocephalus. Neurosurgery. 2005;57(3 Suppl):S4–16 **(discussion ii–v)**

19. Alperin N, Oliu CJ, Bagci AM, Lee SH, Kovanlikaya I, Adams D, et al. Low-dose acetazolamide reverses periventricular white matter hyperintensities in iNPH. Neurology. 2014;82:1347–51.
20. Shinoda N, Hirai O, Hori S, Mikami K, Bando T, Shimo D, et al. Utility of MRI-based disproportionately enlarged subarachnoid space hydrocephalus scoring for predicting prognosis after surgery for idiopathic normal pressure hydrocephalus: clinical research. J Neurosurg. 2017;1–7.
21. Pyykkö OT, Lumela M, Rummukainen J, Nerg O, Seppälä TT, Herukka S-K, et al. Cerebrospinal fluid biomarker and brain biopsy findings in idiopathic normal pressure hydrocephalus. PLoS ONE. 2014;9:e91974.
22. Tullberg M, Rosengren L, Blomsterwall E, Karlsson JE, Wikkelsö C. CSF neurofilament and glial fibrillary acidic protein in normal pressure hydrocephalus. Neurology. 1998;50:1122–7.
23. Hakim S, Adams RD. The special clinical problem of symptomatic hydrocephalus with normal cerebrospinal fluid pressure. Observations on cerebrospinal fluid hydrodynamics. J Neurol Sci. 1965;2:307–27.
24. Eide PK, Sorteberg W. Diagnostic intracranial pressure monitoring and surgical management in idiopathic normal pressure hydrocephalus: a 6-Year review of 214 patients. Neurosurgery. 2010;66:80–90.
25. Miyake H, Ohta T, Kajimoto Y, Deguchi J. Diamox® challenge test to decide indications for cerebrospinal fluid shunting in normal pressure hydrocephalus. Acta Neurochir (Wien). 1999;141:1187–93.
26. Tanaka A, Kimura M, Nakayama Y, Yoshinaga S, Tomonaga M. Cerebral blood flow and autoregulation in normal pressure hydrocephalus. Neurosurgery. 1997;40:1165–7.
27. Rekate HL, Brodkey JA, Chizeck HJ, el Sakka W, Ko WH. Ventricular volume regulation: a mathematical model and computer simulation. Pediatr Neurosci. 1988;14:77–84.
28. Bradley WG. Diagnostic tools in hydrocephalus. Neurosurg Clin N Am. 2001;12:661–84 **(viii)**.
29. Bradley WG. Cerebrospinal fluid dynamics and shunt responsiveness in patients with normal-pressure hydrocephalus. Mayo Clin Proc. 2002;77:507–8.
30. Greitz D. Radiological assessment of hydrocephalus: new theories and implications for therapy. Neurosurg Rev. 2004;27:145–65.
31. Greitz D. Cerebrospinal fluid circulation and associated intracranial dynamics. A radiologic investigation using MR imaging and radionuclide cisternography. Acta Radiol Suppl. 1993;386:1–23.
32. Jeppsson A, Zetterberg H, Blennow K, Wikkelsø C. Idiopathic normal-pressure hydrocephalus: pathophysiology and diagnosis by CSF biomarkers. Neurology. 2013;80:1385–92.
33. Cusimano MD, Rewilak D, Stuss DT, Barrera-Martinez JC, Salehi F, Freedman M. Normal-pressure hydrocephalus: is there a genetic predisposition? Can J Neurol Sci. 2011;38:274–81.
34. Huovinen J, Kastinen S, Komulainen S, Oinas M, Avellan C, Frantzen J, et al. Familial idiopathic normal pressure hydrocephalus. J Neurol Sci. 2016;368:11–8.
35. Takahashi Y, Kawanami T, Nagasawa H, Iseki C, Hanyu H, Kato T. Familial normal pressure hydrocephalus (NPH) with an autosomal-dominant inheritance: a novel subgroup of NPH. J Neurol Sci. 2011;308:149–51.
36. Stolze H, Kuhtz-Buschbeck JP, Drücke H, Jöhnk K, Diercks C, Palmié S, et al. Gait analysis in idiopathic normal pressure hydrocephalus—which parameters respond to the CSF tap test? Clin Neurophysiol. 2000;111:1678–86.
37. Jaraj D, Rabiei K, Marlow T, Jensen C, Skoog I, Wikkelsö C. Prevalence of idiopathic normal-pressure hydrocephalus. Neurology. 2014;82:1449–54.
38. Tolze H, Kuhtz-Buschbeck JP, Drücke H, Jöhnk K, Illert M, Deuschl G. Comparative analysis of the gait disorder of normal pressure hydrocephalus and Parkinson's disease. J Neurol Neurosurg Psychiatry. 2001;70:289–97.
39. Relkin N, Marmarou A, Klinge P, Bergsneider M, Black PM. INPH guidelines, part II: diagnosing idio-pathic normal-pressure hydrocephalus. Neurosurgery. 2005;57(3 SUPPL):S2–17.
40. Evans WA, Davidoff LM, Dyke CG, King GC. An encephalographic ratio for estimating ventricular enlargement and cerebral atrophy. Arch Neurol Psychiatry. 1942;47:931.
41. Narita W, Nishio Y, Baba T, Iizuka O, Ishihara T, Matsuda M, et al. High-convexity tightness predicts the shunt response in idiopathic normal pressure hydrocephalus. Am J Neuroradiol. 2016;37:1831–7.
42. Fazekas F, Chawluk JB, Alavi A. MR signal abnormalities at 1.5 T in alzheimer's dementia and normal aging. Am J Neuroradiol. 1987;8:421–6.
43. Bradley WG. CSF Flow in the brain in the context of normal pressure hydrocephalus. AJNR Am J Neuroradiol. 2015;36:831–8.
44. Eide PK, Saehle T. Is ventriculomegaly in idiopathic normal pressure hydrocephalus associated with a transmantle gradient in pulsatile intracranial pressure? Acta Neurochir (Wien). 2010;152:989–95.
45. Greitz D. New view on the CSF circulation: CSF is produced and absorbed by brain capillaries. Neuroradiol J. 2010;23:94–5.
46. Burt VL, Whelton P, Roccella EJ, Brown C, Cutler JA, Higgins M, et al. Prevalence of hypertension in the US adult population. Results from the Third National Health and Nutrition Examination Survey, 1988–1991. Hypertension. 1995;25:305–13.
47. Neuhauser HK, Adler C, Rosario AS, Diederichs C, Ellert U. Hypertension prevalence, awareness, treatment and control in Germany 1998 and 2008–11. J Hum Hypertens. 2015; August:1–7.
48. Akai K, Uchigasaki S, Tanaka U, Komatsu A. Normal pressure hydrocephalus, neuropathological study. Acta Pathol Jpn. 1987;37:97–110.
49. Newton H, Pickard JD, Weller RO. Normal pressure hydrocephalus and cerebrovascular disease: findings of postmortem. J Neurol Neurosurg Psychiatry. 1989;52:804.
50. Bech RA, Waldemar G, Gjerris F, Klinken L, Juhler M. Shunting effects in patients with idiopathic normal pressure hydrocephalus; correlation with cerebral and leptomeningeal biopsy findings. Acta Neurochir (Wien). 1999;141:633–9.
51. Zarrinkoob L, Ambarki K, Wåhlin A, Birgander R, Carlberg B, Eklund A, et al. Aging alters the dampening of pulsatile blood flow in cerebral arteries. J Cereb Blood Flow Metab. 2016;36:1519–27.
52. Swenson ER. Pharmacology of acute mountain sickness: old drugs and newer thinking. J Appl Physiol. 2016;120:204–15.
53. Czosnyka Z, van den Boogaard F, Czosnyka M, Momjian S, Gelling L, Pickard JD. The relationship between CSF circulation and cerebrovascular pressure-reactivity in normal pressure hydrocephalus. Acta Neurochir Suppl. 2005;95:207–11.
54. Yamada SM, Masahira N, Kawanishi Y, Fujimoto Y, Shimizu K. Preoperative acetazolamide SPECT is useful for predicting outcome of shunt operation in idiopathic normal pressure hydrocephalus patients. Clin Nucl Med. 2013;38:671–6.
55. Vakili S, Moran D, Hung A, Elder BD, Jeon L, Fialho H, et al. Timing of surgical treatment for idiopathic normal pressure hydrocephalus: association between treatment delay and reduced short-term benefit. Neurosurg Focus. 2016;41:E2.

Patient-specific cranio-spinal compliance distribution using lumped-parameter model: its relation with ICP over a wide age range

Ritambhar Burman[1], Noam Alperin[2*], Sang H. Lee[2] and Brigit Ertl-Wagner[3]

Abstract

Background: The distribution of cranio-spinal compliance (CSC) in the brain and spinal cord is a fundamental question, as it would determine the overall role of the compartments in modulating ICP in healthy and diseased states. Invasive methods for measurement of CSC using infusion-based techniques provide overall CSC estimate, but not the individual sub-compartmental contribution. Additionally, the outcome of the infusion-based method depends on the infusion site and dynamics. This article presents a method to determine compliance distribution between the cranium and spinal canal non-invasively using data obtained from patients. We hypothesize that this CSC distribution is indicative of the ICP.

Methods: We propose a lumped-parameter model representing the hydro and hemodynamics of the cranio-spinal system. The input and output to the model are phase-contrast MRI derived volumetric transcranial blood flow measured in vivo, and CSF flow at the spinal cervical level, respectively. The novelty of the method lies in the model mathematics that predicts CSC distribution (that obeys the physical laws) from the system dc gain of the discrete-domain transfer function. 104 healthy individuals (48 males, 56 females, age 25.4 ± 14.9 years, range 3–60 years) without any history of neurological diseases, were used in the study. Non-invasive MR assisted estimate of ICP was calculated and compared with the cranial compliance to prove our hypothesis.

Results: A significant negative correlation was found between model-predicted cranial contribution to CSC and MR-ICP. The spinal canal provided majority of the compliance in all the age groups up to 40 years. However, no single sub-compartment provided majority of the compliance in 41–60 years age group. The cranial contribution to CSC and MR-ICP were significantly correlated with age, with gender not affecting the compliance distribution. Spinal contribution to CSC significantly positively correlated with CSF stroke volume.

Conclusions: This paper describes MRI-based non-invasive way to determine the cranio-spinal compliance distribution in the brain and spinal canal sub-compartments. The proposed mathematics makes the model always stable and within the physiological range. The model-derived cranial compliance was strongly negatively correlated to non-invasive MR-ICP data from 104 patients, indicating that compliance distribution plays a major role in modulating ICP.

Keywords: Cerebrospinal fluid dynamics, Cranio-spinal compliance distribution, Intracranial pressure

*Correspondence: nalperin@med.miami.edu
[2] Radiology Department, University of Miami, Miami, FL 33136, USA
Full list of author information is available at the end of the article

Background

Compliance of a distensible chamber is defined as the ratio of the change in volume and the corresponding change in pressure. A compartment that can accommodate additional volume without a large increase in pressure has large compliance. The brain and the spinal cord are contained within the cranium and the spinal canal, respectively. The cranio-spinal (CS) compartment is filled with the cerebrospinal fluid (CSF) and sealed by the thick dura mater. The individual compliances of the cranium and the spinal canal sub-compartments add up to determine the overall compliance of the CS system [1]. This CS compliance (CSC) governs the relationship between intracranial fluid volume and the intracranial pressure (ICP).

There is a disagreement among investigators regarding which sub-compartment, the cranial or the spinal canal, contributes more to the overall CSC in the supine posture. This is a fundamental question, as it would determine the overall role of the compartments in modulation of ICP in the healthy and diseased states. This overall CSC and relative contributions of each sub-compartment changes with a change in body posture [2]. By combining MRI CSF flow measurement and infusion techniques, Wahlin et al. [3] assumed a constant venous outflow, and concluded that the cranial compartment provides nearly two-thirds of the overall CSC. A follow-up publication by Tain et al. [4] showed that when venous drainage dynamics are accounted for, the compliance of the spinal canal dominates the overall cranio-spinal compliance and hydrodynamics. A larger spinal compliance is consistent with fact that the dura mater in the spinal canal, particularly in the lumbar region and spinal sac, is less confined by bony structures than the cranial dura matter in the cranium and upper spine.

Infusion-based methods to calculate CSC have significant limitations. In addition to risks of intracranial infection [5], the measured compliances depend on the location and dynamics of the infusion [3]. The infused amount is often large in order to overwhelm the pulsatility of CSF pressure waves [6], thereby often changing the initial state of the system. The infusion methods also do not provide the relative contributions of the cranium and spinal canal to the overall CSC.

Both generic and subject-specific lumped parameter models have been proposed to assess the CSC distribution. Gehlen et al. developed a generic lumped-parameter biomechanical model of the CSF and cardiovascular system [7] that uses arterial blood inflow to explain the hydrodynamic physiology in supine and upright position. The model assumed a lower spinal compliance contribution (35%) in supine position and showed that it further reduced in upright posture. This generic model assumes literature values of physiological parameters like elastance index, pressure offset and exponential parameter of Marmarou model [8] along with relative spinal compliance ratio for the model mechanical components to try to explain data obtained from individual subjects. Yallapragada [9] and later Tain et al. [4] used a subject-specific lumped-parameter model based on a bond-graph representation of the CS system [10], with the MRI derived net transcranial blood flow as input and the cranio-spinal CSF flow as output. The model not only predicted a higher spinal canal compliance in healthy individuals (78%), but also showed that spinal compliance contribution is lower in idiopathic intracranial hypertension patients (60%) than in control and therefore the IIH patients have a lower buffer for increased ICP. Recently, Atsumi et al. [11] modelled the bilateral carotid and vertebral arteries, and CSF flows by a transformer-coupled electrical circuit, to calculate the brain compliance index.

In this paper, we propose a new mathematical approach for the previously developed subject-specific lumped-parameter CS model of Tain et al. [4] to compute the CSC distribution in the cranium and the spinal canal. The previous model mathematics required conversion of data from discrete to continuous domain, a conversion that is not unique. The previous model also did not account for a physically viable solution where compliances are positive and have real values. The discrete transfer function predicts a set of CSC distributions (solutions for the model) by searching within a set of responses to the input parameters that yield a stable system. Each steady state response to a step function is equivalent to the dc gain of the system. The final spinal canal to cranio-spinal compliance ratio is chosen from the compliance histogram, which always provides a stable and physically realizable model, with a percentage contribution that is a real number between 0 and 100%. The cranio-spinal model utilizes the momentary transcranial blood flow (arterial minus venous) as input to predict the system transfer function that best matches the CSF flow into the spinal canal, and derives the cranio-spinal compliance distribution in the process. We hypothesize that CSC distribution is related to the cranial CSF pressure or ICP. We evaluated the relationship of the CS system to a previously developed MRI-derived ICP (MRICP) using a data from large cohort of healthy subjects over a wide age range.

Methods

Subjects

Following institutional review board approval, written informed consent was obtained from all subjects. In case of children, informed consent was obtained from their parents. Data from 104 out of 129 healthy individuals (48 males, 56 females, age 25.4 ± 14.9 years, range 3–60 years) were used in the study. The study population included 17 subjects in age range 3–10 years, 31 subjects in age range 11–20 years, 36 in age range 21–40 years and 20 in 41–60 age group. Seventeen cases were excluded because of data inconsistency between the arterial and venous flow where venous outflow preceded arterial inflow. This suggests active venous drainage, which the current model does not account for. Seven additional cases were excluded due to poor image quality due to subject motion during the scan. All subjects were without any history of neurological diseases, determined by self-reported and/or assessed by means of conventional MR imaging.

MR imaging acquisition

MRI scans were acquired using a 3T scanner (Magnetom Verio; Siemens Healthcare, Erlangen, Germany) with subjects in supine position, with legs slightly elevated to improve comfort. An ECG-gated high velocity encoding cine phase-contrast scan was used to measure the arterial inflow and venous outflow to and from the cranium, with the following parameters: VENC = 70–90 cm/s, FOV = 14 × 11.4 cm, slice thickness = 6 mm, flip angle = 20°, TR/TE = 40/4.05 ms, acquisition matrix = 256 × 143, and 32 cardiac phases. A second ECG-gated low velocity encoding cine phase-contrast scan was used to measure the CSF flow at the cranio-cervical region, with the following parameters: VENC = 7–9 cm/s, FOV = 14 × 11.4 cm, slice thickness = 6 mm, flip angle = 20°, TR/TE = 53.7/7.48 ms, acquisition matrix = 256 × 143, and 32 cardiac phases. MR scan time per cine sequence was about 1.5 to 2 min (specific scan time is heartrate dependent). One average and two views per segment were used to keep acquisition time short. Imaging planes to measure blood and CSF flow were placed at the dens axis perpendicular to internal carotid and vertebral arteries, and at the mid C2 level where the spinal walls are parallel, respectively.

MR-ICP

The calculation of non-invasive ICP with the help of phase-contrast MRI (MR-ICP) has been described previously [12]. Briefly, basis of the method is the mono-exponential relationship between volume and pressure, which makes the pressure inversely related to compliance. The compliance is defined as the ratio of intracranial volume and pressure changes during the cardiac cycle, obtained from the difference in transcranial blood and CSF volumetric flow rates, and change in CSF pressure gradient, using Navier–Stokes equation.

Cranio-spinal lumped-parameter model

The lumped-parameter model of the CS system [4] is used to determine the compliance distribution between the cranium and spinal canal. The model and its electrical equivalent are shown in Fig. 1. With each heartbeat, intracranial blood volume increases during systole. The temporary increase in the net intracranial blood volume, i.e. the difference between arterial inflow and venous outflow drives the CSF to the spinal canal. The MR derived net transcranial blood flow Q_{A-V} and CSF flow Q_{CSF} are used as input and output to the model, respectively. Volumetric flow rate through blood and CSF lumens were obtained by PUBS method [13] which utilize velocity dynamic information to differentiate lumen voxels from background. Arterial inflow and venous outflow rates are obtained by summing the flow velocities inside the respective lumens (left and right internal carotid arteries, and left and right vertebral arteries, and left and right internal jugular veins and secondary venous pathways for veins). The lumped mechanical dampers or flow resistances in the cranial and spinal compartment are denoted by R_C and R_S respectively. The compliances of the cranium and spinal canal are denoted by C_C and C_S respectively. The inertial component of the CSF flow from the cranium into the spinal canal is denoted by L_S. The frequency response of the transfer function of the system, $H(s)$ in the Laplace domain is given by Eq. (1), where s denotes the Laplace variable.

$$H(s) = \frac{Q_{CSF}(s)}{Q_{A-V}(s)} = \frac{s\frac{R_C}{L_S} + \frac{1}{C_C L_S}}{s^2 + s\frac{R_C + R_S}{L_S} + \frac{\frac{1}{C_C} + \frac{1}{C_S}}{L_S}} \quad (1)$$

Derivation of cranial and spinal compliance distribution from transfer function

The phase contrast MRI provides 32 discrete-time samples of Q_{CSF} and Q_{A-V} per cardiac cycle. Discrete to continuous-time domain conversion does not provide a unique solution as some information may be lost while sampling the transcranial flow and CSF flow from continuous to the discrete time domain [14]. Transfer function $H(s)$ however is only valid in the continuous-time domain system. The structure of $H(s)$ lets us calculate the compliance ratio without having to calculate the R_C, R_S, L_S, C_C and C_S individually. The zero frequency gain or dc gain of the system, obtained by substituting $s = 0$ in Eq. (1), gives the spinal compliance to total CSC, $C_S/(C_C + C_S)$. This dc gain is the amplitude ratio of the system steady state response to a step input. The discrete-time domain transfer function $H(z)$ is given by Eq. (2), where z is the z-transform variable for discrete model. Continuous-time transfer function and its discrete-time domain equivalent have the same form and same dc gain in pole-zero matched method [15]. Thus $H(z)$ is represented by

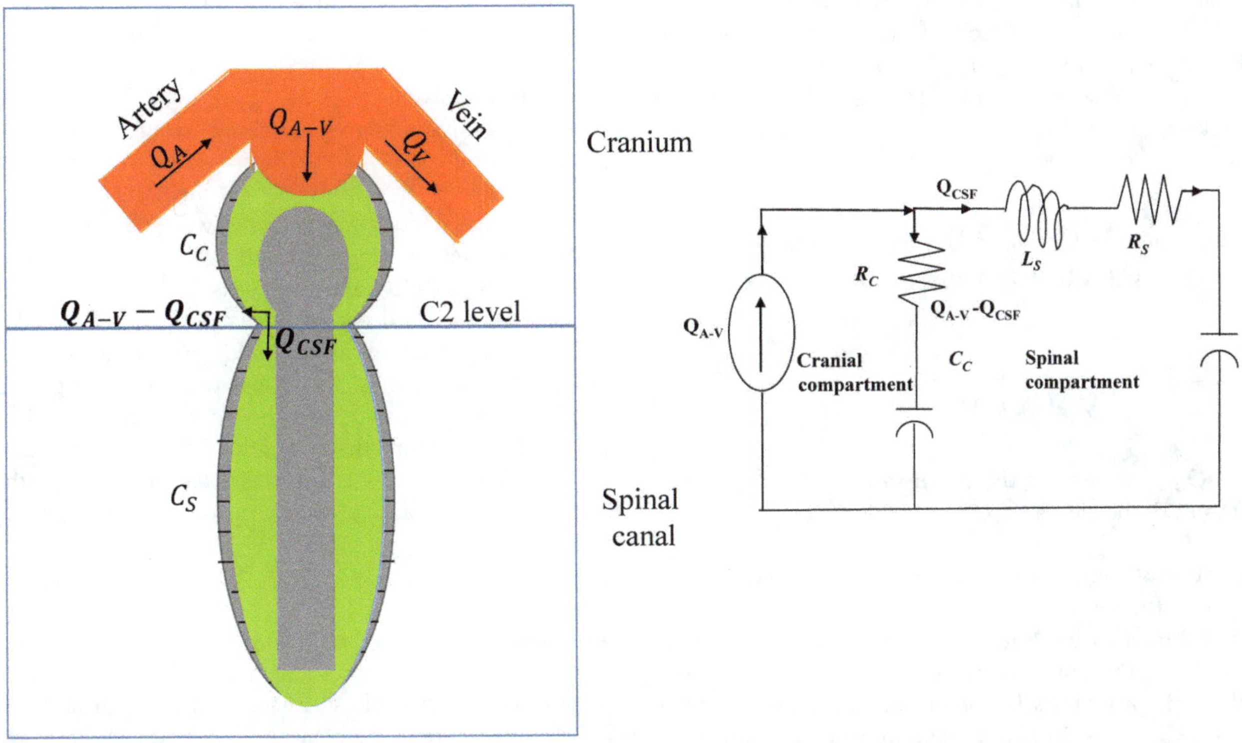

Fig. 1 Cranio-spinal model and its electrical analogous circuit. The cranio-spinal model is divided into two compartments, cranium and spinal canal. The MR derived net transcranial blood flow Q_{A-V} and CSF flow Q_{CSF} are used as input and output to the model, respectively. The lumped mechanical dampers or flow resistances in the cranial and spinal compartment are denoted by R_C and R_S respectively. The compliances of the cranium and spinal canal are denoted by C_C and C_S respectively. The inertial component of the CSF flow from the cranium into the spinal canal is denoted by L_S

the quartet (p_1, p_2, q_1, q_2), which are real numbers which makes the form of $H(z)$ correspond to $H(s)$. The corresponding dc gain, obtained by substituting $z = 1$ in $H(z)$, estimates the compliance distribution in the cranium and the spinal canal as it is equivalent to H (s = 0).

$$H(z) = \frac{Q_{CSF}(z)}{Q_{A-V}(z)} = \frac{p_1 z + p_2}{z^2 + q_1 z + q_2} \quad (2)$$

Procedure to estimate accuracy and dc gain of second order stable model

Roots Z_p of the second order transfer function $H(z)$ in Eq. (2) follow the form given by Eq. (3). The discrete system, and subsequently its continuous counterpart, are stable if both poles of $H(z)$, Z_p, lie within unit circle from the origin, given by (4). The modulus of sum ($|q_1|$) and product ($|q_2|$) of poles of such a second order transfer function is less than 2 and 1 respectively, given by Eq. (5) and Eq. (6) respectively. The fourth constraint, given by Eq. (7), is real domain of coefficients q_1 and q_2 due to presence of complex conjugate poles in second order transfer function. While Eq. (3) and Eq. (4) are sufficient, Eq. (5–7) are necessary, but not sufficient to achieve a stable system.

$$Z_p = \frac{-q_1 \pm \sqrt{q_1^2 - 4q_2}}{2} \quad (3)$$

$$|Z_p| < 1 \quad (4)$$

$$|q_1| < 2 \quad (5)$$

$$|q_2| < 1 \quad (6)$$

$$q_1, q_2 \in R \quad (7)$$

Equations (4–7) can be used to draw the $q_1 - q_2$ mesh-grid domain in steps of 0.001 along each axis, which always gives a stable second order system. For a fixed (q_1, q_2) pair and known values of input $Q_{A-V}(n)$ and output $Q_{CSF}(n)$, ordinary least squared estimate can be used to estimate (p_1, p_2) in Eq. (8) that minimizes the right-hand side for all 32 frames of the cardiac cycle. For a given quartet (q_1, q_2, p_1, p_2), $\hat{Q}_{CSF}(n)$ can be estimated for all 32 frames of the cardiac cycle using Eq. (2). Each quartet in CS model gives a different dc gain and hence a different compliance distribution, obtained by substituting $z=1$ in Eq. (3). The power of the model is how well the predicted CSF flow matches the observed flow, and is represented by Nash–Sutcliffe coefficient E [16], given by Eq. (9). E can take values between $-\infty$ and 1, with better model accuracy indicated by a larger E.

$$Q_{CSF}(n) + q_1 Q_{CSF}(n-1) + q_2 Q_{CSF}(n-2) = p_1 Q_{A-V}(n-1) + p_2 Q_{A-V}(n-2) \tag{8}$$

$$\mathrm{E} = 1 - \frac{\sum_{n=1}^{32}\left(Q_{CSF}(\mathrm{n}) - \hat{Q}_{CSF}(n)\right)^2}{\sum_{n=1}^{32}\left(Q_{CSF}(\mathrm{n}) - \bar{Q}_{CSF}(\mathrm{n})\right)^2} \tag{9}$$

where $\bar{Q}_{CSF}(n)$ denotes the mean value of the Q_{CSF} over 32 frames of the cardiac cycle.

Calculation of compliance distribution in the CS system

Among all the stable systems with $E > 0.7$, $C_S/(C_C + C_S)$ is constrained to be in a range between 0 and 100% in steps of 1%, thereby making the model physically realizable. This provides a histogram of solutions. The final solution $C_S/(C_C+C_S)$ is the maximum of the histogram, representing the most commonly occurring compliance ratio. The cranial compliance counterpart is obtained by subtracting the spinal contribution from 100%.

Statistical analysis

Statistical analyses were performed using Excel (Windows Version 2016). All data were presented as mean ± standard deviation or as median and interquartile range. Univariate analyses were performed for analyzing the effect of gender and age on cranial contribution to CSC. Multi-variate analysis was used to analyze the effect of age and gender on cranial contribution to CSC. Ordinary least squared estimate was used wherever relevant and smoothing spline was used in some graphs for illustrative purposes. Pearson correlation coefficient was used to measure the strength of linear regressions. A two-sided Student's t-test was used throughout the analysis, and a p of < 0.05 was considered as statistically significant.

Results

Overview

An example of cine images which include the magnitude images and the two phase images with a high and low VENC for a 21 year-old healthy female subject is shown in Fig. 2a–c. MRI derived Q_{A-V} and Q_{CSF} flow waveforms

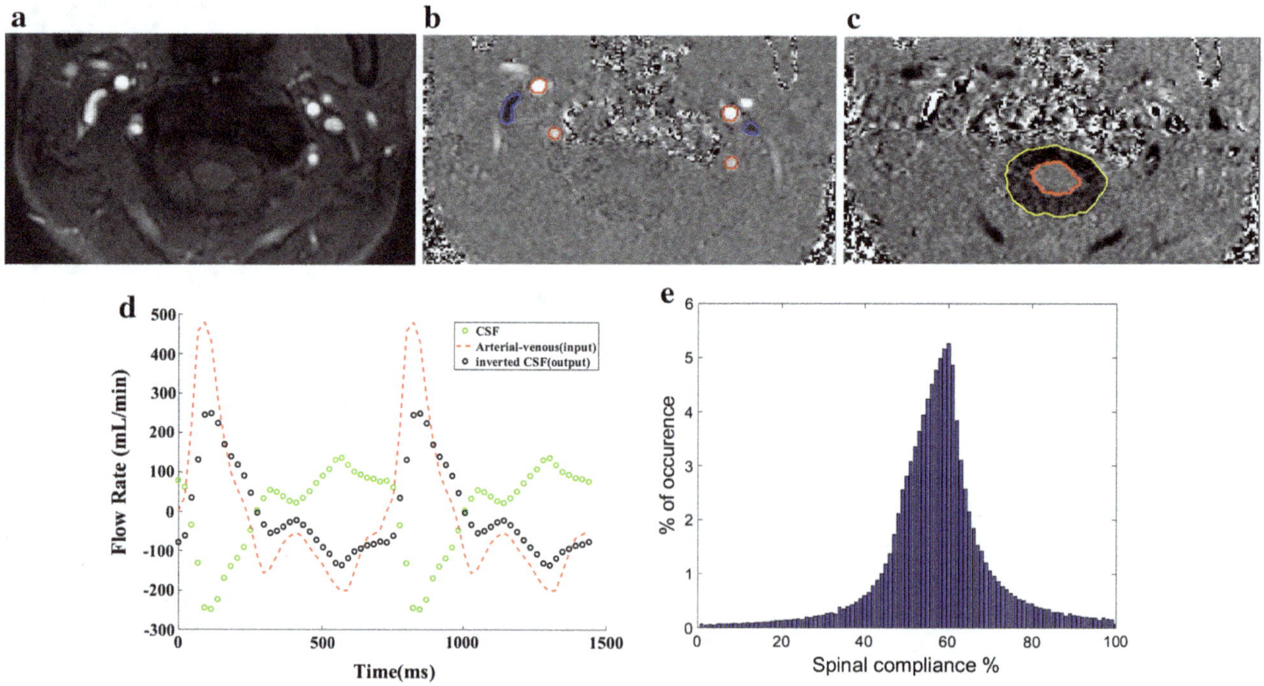

Fig. 2 Example of determination of cranial contribution to cranio-spinal compliance from sample input and output waveforms. **a** Flow compensated magnitude image showing bright signal from blood vessels. **b** High-velocity encoding images used for measurements of arterial inflow and venous outflow. **c** Low-velocity encoding images used for measurements of CSF flow. **d** Phase contrast MRI derived cardiac cycle of Q_{A-V} (red) and Q_{CSF} (green) in an 21-year-old healthy female subject is plotted. Q_{A-V} is used as input to the model, which predicts the inverted Q_{CSF} (black) waveform. **e** Histogram corresponding to model-derived spinal contribution to cranio-spinal compliance, $C_S/(C_C+C_S)$, is plotted for all the model parameters that give $E > 0.7$. The final spinal contribution to CSC is chosen from the mode of the histogram (60%)

are shown in Fig. 2d. In Fig. 2e, the solutions histogram is plotted for all quartets (q_1, q_2, p_1, p_2) which gives $E > 0.7$, with the vertical axis indicating the frequency of occurrence of the 100 possible compliance percentages (along the horizontal axis). The spinal compliance to CSC ratio is 60% in this case.

Compliance distribution in the CS system and its relation with ICP

Linear regression of cranial contribution to CSC and MR-ICP with age (Fig. 3a, b) showed significant positive ($p < 0.001$, $R = 0.33$) and negative correlations ($p < 0.001$, $R = -0.55$), respectively. The cranial contribution to CSC in 104 subjects, stratified by age and sex, respectively are shown in Fig. 4a, b. The age was stratified into 3–10 years, 11–20 years, 21–40 years and 41–60 years. When analyzed over different age groups (Fig. 4a), median cranial contribution to CSC was found to be the highest in the older population of 41–60 years (median = 49.5%, IQR 44%–57%), with the lowest median cranial contribution to CSC of 38% occurring in the age range of 11–20 years (IQR 32%–46%). Spinal compliance was significantly greater than the cranial compliance for the age groups 3–10 years ($p = 0.008$), 11–20 years ($p < 0.001$), and 21–40 years ($p < 0.001$). However, no significant difference was found in the compliance contribution of the two compartments in the older population of age 41–60 years ($p = 0.75$).

The median cranial compliance was equal in both males (median = 42%, IQR 36%–47%) and females (median = 42%, IQR 35%–49%) (Fig. 4b) with no significant statistical difference ($p = 0.88$). Multivariate regression analysis of cranial contribution to CSC with both age and gender, showed that only age has a significant influence on the compliance distribution (p for age < 0.001, p for gender = 0.54).

Scatterplot of model-derived cranial contribution to CSC and MR-ICP is shown in Fig. 5. Least squared regression showed a significant negative correlation of the cranial compliance contribution with the MR-ICP ($p < 0.001$, $R = -0.69$).

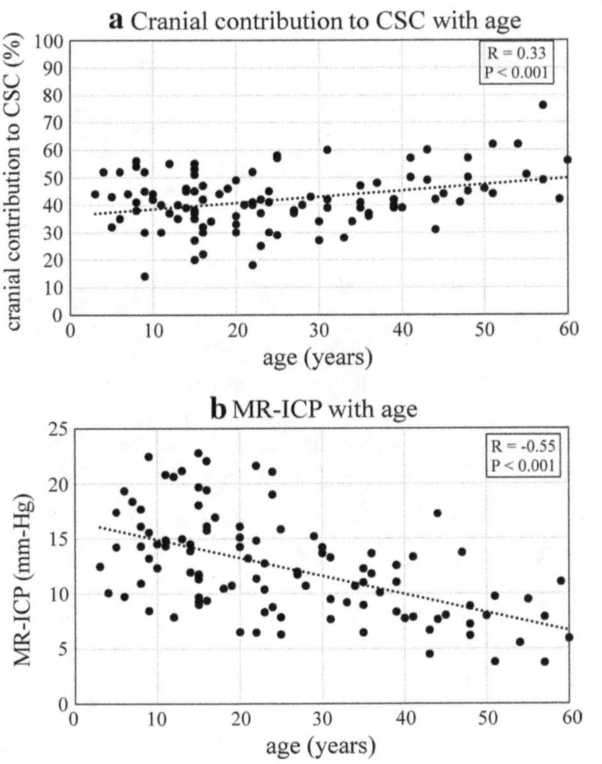

Fig. 3 Effect of age on cranial contribution to cranio-spinal compliance distribution and MR-ICP. **a** The plot shows significant positive correlation ($p < 0.001$, $R = 0.33$) between cranial contribution to CSC and age. **b** The plot shows significant negative correlation ($p < 0.001$, $R = -0.55$) between non-invasively determined MR-ICP and age

Spinal compliance, CSF stroke volume and total cranial blood flow

Linear regression of CS CSF stroke volume with respect to spinal compliance (Fig. 6) showed a significant positive correlation ($p = 0.001$, $R = 0.32$). The dependence of CS CSF stroke volume with Linear regressions of CSF stroke volume and mean cranial blood flow with age showed significant negative correlations ($p < 0.001$, $R = -0.74$, Fig. 7a; $p < 0.001$, $R = -0.82$, Fig. 7b, respectively).

Sensitivity of the parameters

The reproducibility of the compliance contribution for a given data set can be affected by the Nash–Sutcliffe coefficient E. It provides a measure of how accurate the model parameters describe the output of the system when compared to its original waveform. For the cases studied, the least squared estimated best-fit case has an E value between 0.76 and 0.96, except one case which had an E equal to 0.69. For the compliance estimation, the value of 0.7 was empirically decided to be the threshold for E. To calculate the goodness of the threshold, we also recalculated the compliance contribution from each of the two models with a lower threshold of $E = 0.6$. The absolute difference of compliance predicted by $E = 0.7$ and $E = 0.6$ in the two models was 2.2% ± 1.7% (0%–5%), with two out of 104 cases having a compliance difference of more than 10% and excluded from this analysis.

The step-size in $q_1 - q_2$ domain is chosen to be 10^{-2} in this study. It was found that a finer step size of 10^{-3} converged the system to the same compliance value. A finer step size however is computationally inefficient.

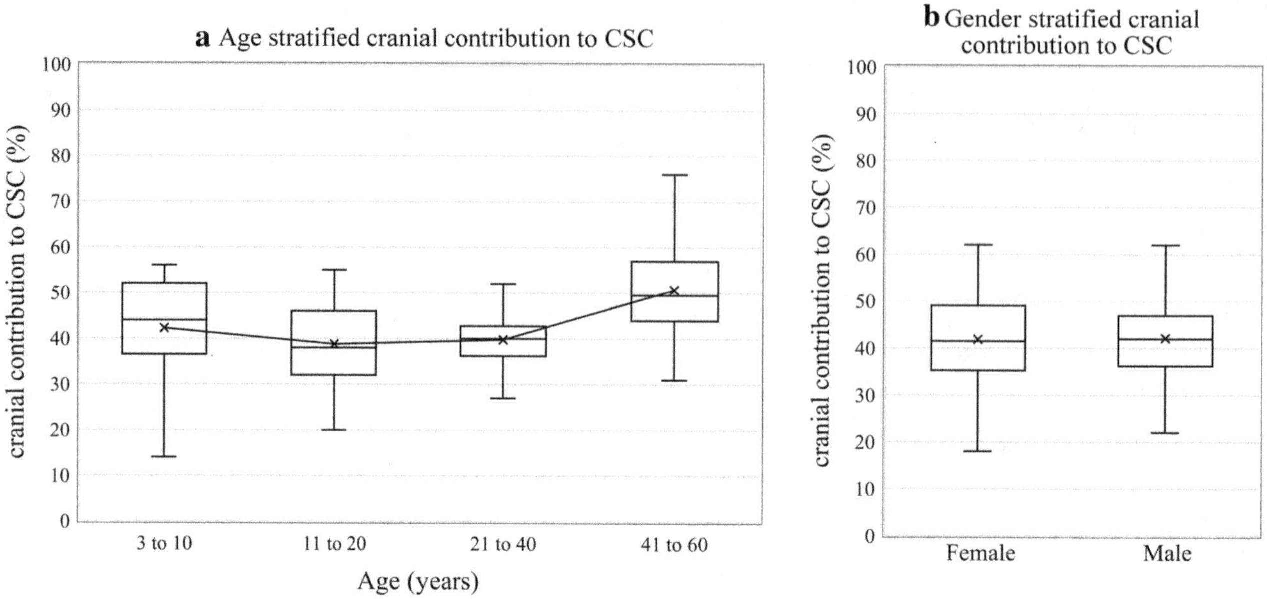

Fig. 4 Effect of age and gender on cranial contribution to cranio-spinal compliance distribution. **a** Boxplot of cranial contribution to CSC and stratified age shows the cranial compliance contribution decreases slightly in the younger population before increasing in the 20+ population. **b** Boxplot of cranial contribution to CSC does not vary significantly with gender ($p = 0.88$)

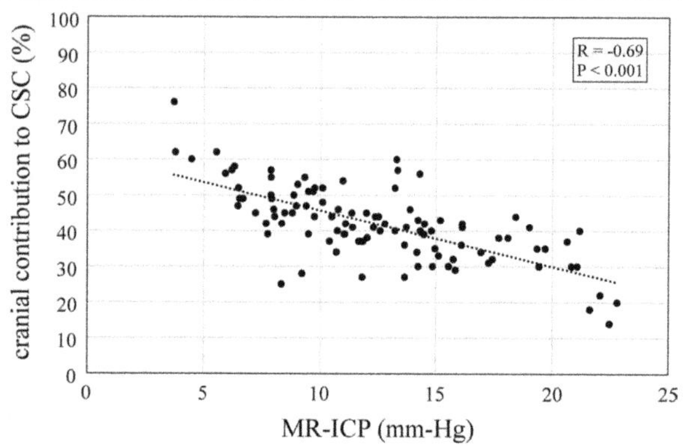

Fig. 5 Relationship between cranial contribution to cranio-spinal compliance distribution and MR-ICP. Significant negative correlation is shown between cranial contribution to CSC on MR-ICP ($p < 0.001$, $R = -0.69$)

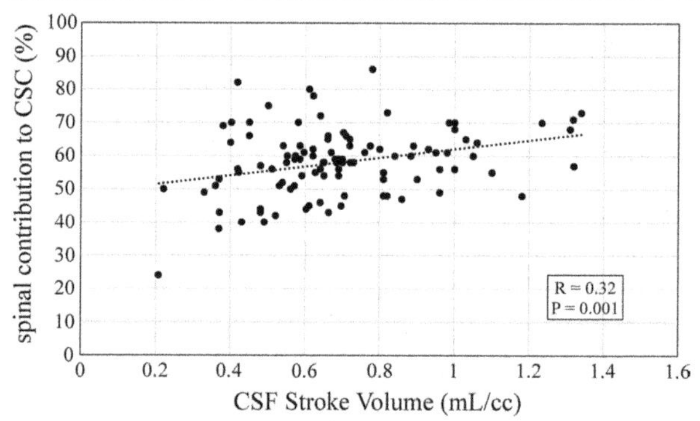

Fig. 6 Effect of CSF stroke volume on spinal contribution to cranio-spinal compliance distribution. The plot shows a significant positive regression of spinal contribution to CSC on CSF stroke volume ($p = 0.001$, $R = 0.32$)

Discussion

Overview

This paper describes a modular patient-specific lumped-parameter model to non-invasively determine the distribution of the total CS compliance between the cranium and the spinal canal. The measurement of CSF flow by MRI in the upper spine provided us means to separate the CS system to two sub compartments, which infusion based method are incapable. The patient-specific model utilizes the measurements of blood and CSF flows to and from the two sub-compartments. The model further demonstrates that the cranial contribution to total cranio-spinal compliance distribution is significantly negatively correlated with the non-invasively derived MR-ICP. This inverse relationship is expected and can be explained by the inverse relation of absolute ICP with compliance. The inverse relationship between ICP and compliance is due to the mono-exponential relationship between ICP and intracranial volume [8].

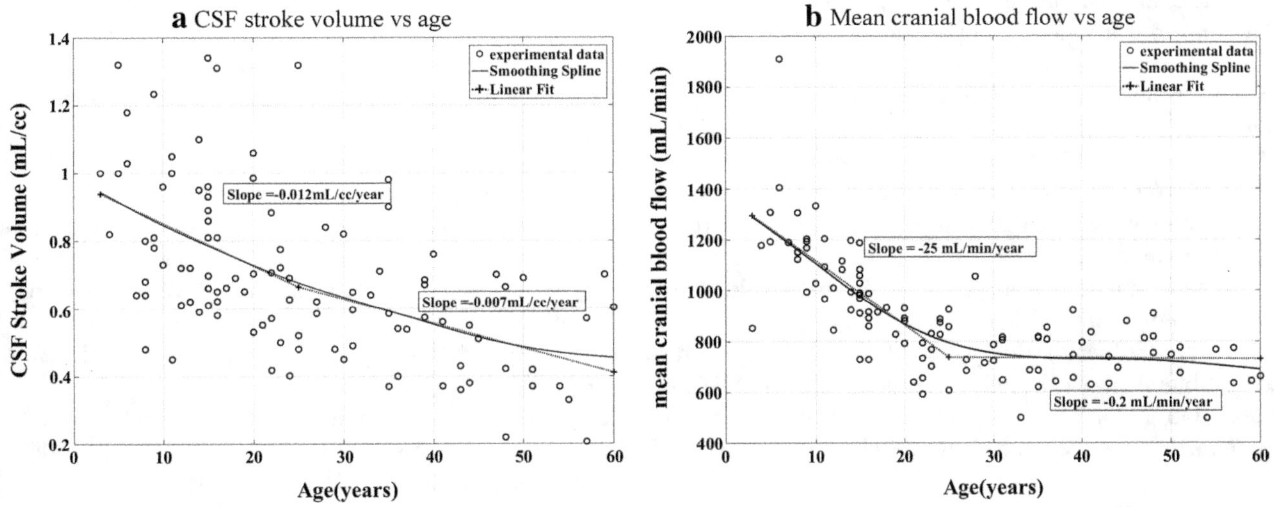

Fig. 7 Effect of age on CSF stroke volume and mean cranial blood flow. **a** Significant negative correlation is shown between CSF stroke volume (mL per cardiac cycle) at C2 level and age (Spline fit $p<0.001$, $R=-0.74$). **b** Significant negative correlation is shown between transcranial blood flow and age (Spline fit $p<0.001$, $R=0.82$)

The model-predicted spinal compliance over total compliance is significantly higher than the cranial contribution in population of age less than 40 years. This may be attributed to the less-confined dura matter in the spinal canal relative to that in the cranium. A higher spinal compartment compliance is in accord with previous results which used invasive techniques (70% [1] and 63% [17]). Lofgren and Zwetnow [1] infused artificial CSF in the cisterna magna in six dogs after isolating the cranial and spinal compartments using a block at the C1 level, and found that the spinal section contributed to 70% of volume change. The finding of a larger spinal compliance is consistent with a much earlier report by Magnaes [17], who used bolus infusion separately into the cranium and the spinal canal in human patients with CSF block at cervical level. These results contrast with recent studies suggesting that the cranium contribution is a dominant source of CSC in supine position [3, 7, 8] accounting for almost two-thirds of the total CSC. Wahlin [3] assumed constant relative pulse pressure coefficient in the cranio-spinal compliance to quantify 65% compliance coming from the intracranial compartment in thirty-seven healthy elderly subject. Marmarou et al. [8] determined that nearly two-third of the compliance came from the cranial compartment in anaesthetized adult cats with cranio-spinal compartment isolated at c6 level.

When looked at the effect of age on the compliance distribution, our study found significantly higher contribution of spinal canal to CSC in young subjects (age less than 40 years), and non-significantly lower spinal contribution to CSC on an average in the 41–60 age group. Wahlin [3] reported 35% spinal contribution to CSC in 37 healthy adults (60–82 years of age), while unpublished data from our group showed 61.9% spinal compliance in ten healthy adults (60–79 years of age). This anomaly may be due to lack of Body Mass Index data of the subjects in [3] that makes the study group population incomparable. Body Mass Index is significantly negatively correlated with cranial compliance, which in turn is significantly positively correlated with ICP (Ritambhar Burman, Ashish Shah, Ronald Benveniste, George Jimsheleishvili, Sang Lee, David Loewenstein, Noam Alperin). Literature suggests that in obese patients, the intra-thoracic pressure is greater than normal [18], which causes a significant increase in ICP by causing a functional obstruction to cerebral venous outflow via jugular venous system [19].

In addition to the cardiac pulsation, respiration also influences the CSF dynamics [20]. The respiration effect is superimposed on the cardiac pulsation. During exhalation, the intrathoracic pressure increase results in lower venous drainage and therefore increased ICP and CSF is pushed to the spinal canal, while during inspiration, the reverse occurs [21]. The derived images from the cine scan represent an average cardiac cycle over more than a minute and therefore respiratory effect is averaged out. Only the cardiac related components are considered by the model.

Relationship of cranial compliance contribution with ICP

The strong negative correlation between cranial compliance contribution and the non-invasively determined MR-ICP supports our hypothesis that the CS distribution plays a major role in regulating the ICP. Small increases in intracranial volume can result in exponential rise in ICP once the compensatory reserve volume is exhausted [22]. Cranium with a higher compensatory reserve (compliance) can accommodate larger capacity of fluid without an appreciable increase in ICP, which supports the strong negative correlation between the cranial contribution to CSC and MR-ICP. The cranial contribution to CSC was also negatively correlated to MR-ICP and lumbar puncture opening pressure in 10 healthy volunteers and External Ventricular Drain measurements in six brain trauma patients (Ritambhar Burman, Ashish Shah, Ronald Benveniste, George Jimsheleishvili, Sang Lee, David Loewenstein, Noam Alperin). The MR-ICP calculation is done using a biomechanical model [12], while the compliance calculation is done using a lumped parameter electrical model, which are not equivalent to each other.

Relationship of cranial compliance contribution with CSF stroke volume

Strong linear correlation between CSF stroke volume at C2 level (the amount of CSF going back and forth between the cranium and spinal canal) and spinal contribution to CSC proves that a spinal canal chamber with higher contribution to CSC can accommodate higher volume of CSF outflow from a less compliant cranium. A less compliant cranium in turn has higher ICP to drive the CSF out of the cranium.

Relationship of cranial compliance contribution with age

In our study, we observed a significant and continuous increase of cranial contribution to the total cranio-spinal compliance in the groups with age range of 20 years and above, while it showed a non-significant decrease in the younger cohorts. To our knowledge, this is one of the first papers to report the effect of age on the compliance distribution in the CS system. The mechanism of this compliance distribution in the cranium and spinal canal is affected by the complex response of these two CS compartments to aging. In patients of age 50 years or older, degenerative spinal stenosis [23], resulting from decrease in canal diameter and thicker ligamentum flavum, and calcification of the spinal canal dura result in lowered spinal canal compliance. On the other hand, the brain tissue becomes more rigid [24] with reduced CSF absorption [25], which in turn reduces the intracranial compliance [26, 27]. For the study population with age greater than 3 years, the net cranial blood flow and CSF stroke volume were also found to decrease with age, which support existing literature [28]. Both net cranial blood flow and CSF stroke volume however, increases during the first 2–3 years after birth [29]. For our study population, decreasing CSF stroke volume at C2 level with age is indicative of increasing CSF outflow resistance, which supports previous literature [25]. With the absolute values of both the cranial and spinal compliances decreasing due to age, it is difficult to ascertain the effect of age on cranio-spinal compliance ratio.

With cranial contribution to CSC negatively correlated to ICP and positively correlated to age, ICP is expected to correlate to age negatively and matches our findings. This phenomenon can be attributed to the decrease in mean cranial blood inflow with age. Fleischman et al. [30] found similar evidence, with enough power for a conclusive evidence in 12,118 patients. Several older studies with smaller sample size however have failed to find a significant relationship between ICP and age [31, 32].

Compliance calculation and Nash–Sutcliffe coefficient *E*

In the proposed methodology, the compliance ratio is estimated from the dc gain of the system, which is estimated from the least squared estimate parameters. Thus, the dc gain estimated from only the best-fit least squared estimate parameters can be below zero or above one, implying compliance contribution of sub-compartments to be below 0% or greater than 100%. For the control model to be robust, the compliance of sub-compartments should be same over various parameter values as well, and should not rely on the best-fit case. Thus the compliance contribution is not only restricted to the physiological range of (0%, 100%), but also provides a better estimate from a pool of solutions with the guidance of Nash–Sutcliffe coefficient E. E helps to segregate the parameters that give a high fit from the ones that give poor fits. A low threshold of E will include a large number of cases including poor ones, which may not be a precise representative of the actual system. Again, the number of cases for a very high value of E will not be large enough to describe the system accurately. Thus, it is a trade-off problem. The 2.2% average deviation in compliance value when E was changed from 0.7 to 0.6 shows that the model is insensitive to threshold of E. The convergence to the same compliance value with different step sizes of $q_1 - q_2$ grid shows that the model is very robust to the step-size as well.

CS compliance ratio cannot be calculated from the ratio of the average values of the output signal Q_{A-V} and input signal Q_{CSF} as both signals are periodic, that follow the Kellie-Monroe doctrine of conservation of CS and blood volumes in the brain over the whole cardiac cycle.

Limitations

Several limitations of the study need to be considered when interpreting the data. The number of volunteers for each age range are limited. Our study population did not include enough volunteers to make a 60+ age group. The model-derived compliances are not absolute values, but percentages relative to the total cranio-spinal compliance.

Obtained values were not compared against the invasive gold standard technique. Such study can be done only when patients in whom invasive measurements are justified by standard clinical care. Furthermore, the lack of Body Mass Index information in the other studies we are comparing our study with, pose a challenge for comparison.

This study was done using a snapshot in time for a single subject, and hence a prospective study is needed to confirm the age related findings. The proposed model also cannot deal with active systems with pulsatile jugular flow having an onset before the arterial blood inflow. The model assumes that the arterial blood is pumped into the cranium pushing the venous blood of the cranium, which in turn drives the CSF out of the cranium.

Conclusion

This paper describes MRI-based non-invasive way to determine the cranio-spinal compliance distribution in the brain and spinal canal sub-compartments. The proposed mathematics makes the model always stable and within the physical range, and is robust to step-size and Nash–Sutcliffe coefficient. The model-derived cranial compliance was strongly negatively correlated to non-invasive MR-ICP data in 104 subjects, indicating that compliance distribution plays a major role in modulating ICP. Consistent with the anatomical considerations, we found that the model-estimated spinal compliance contribution is greater than the cranial compliance in young subjects (age $\leq$ 40 years), but could not attribute either of the compartments with major source of CSC contribution in the older subjects (age > 40 years). The cranial contribution to CSC was positively correlated with age, particularly in the population of age > 20 years. MR-ICP was negatively correlated with age. Gender was not a significant factor for CSC distribution. Spinal canal contribution to CSC was strongly correlated to CSF stroke volume at the C2 level.

Abbreviations

CS: cranio-spinal; CSF: cerebrospinal fluid; CSC: cranio-spinal compliance; ICP: intracranial pressure; IQR: interquartile range; MRI: magnetic resonance imaging; MR-ICP: magnetic resonance-based intracranial pressure.

Authors' contributions

RB: made substantial contributions to conception and design, analysis and interpretation of data; has been involved in drafting the manuscript or revising it critically for important intellectual content; NA: made substantial contributions to conception and design, acquisition of data, and interpretation of data; has been involved in drafting the manuscript; agreed to be accountable for all aspects of the work in ensuring that questions related to the accuracy or integrity of any part of the work are appropriately investigated and resolved. SL and BEW contributed to the acquisition of the data and to the drafting of the manuscript. All authors read and approved the final manuscript.

Author details

[1] Biomedical Engineering Department, University of Miami, Coral Gables, FL 33146, USA. [2] Radiology Department, University of Miami, Miami, FL 33136, USA. [3] Department of Radiology, Ludwig-Maximilians University, 80539 Munich, Germany.

Competing interests

Noam Alperin is a shareholder in Alperin noninvasive Diagnostic. The authors declare that they have no competing interests.

References

1. Lofgren J, von Essen C, Zwetnow NN. The pressure-volume curve of the cerebrospinal fluid space in dogs. Acta Neurol Scand. 1973;49:557–74.
2. Alperin N, Lee SH, Sivaramakrishnan A, Hushek SG. Quantifying the effect of posture on intracranial physiology in humans by MRI flow studies. J Magn Reson Imaging. 2005;22:591–6.
3. Wahlin A, Ambarki K, Birgander R, Alperin N, Malm J, Eklund A. Assessment of craniospinal pressure-volume indices. AJNR Am J Neuroradiol. 2010;31:1645–50.
4. Tain RW, Bagci AM, Lam BL, Sklar EM, Ertl-Wagner B, Alperin N. Determination of cranio-spinal canal compliance distribution by MRI: methodology and early application in idiopathic intracranial hypertension. J Magn Reson Imaging. 2011;34:1397–404.
5. Avezaat CJ, van Eijndhoven JH. Clinical observations on the relationship between cerebrospinal fluid pulse pressure and intracranial pressure. Acta Neurochir (Wien). 1986;79:13–29.
6. Crockard HA, Hanlon K, Ganz E, Duda EE. Intracranial pressure gradients in a patient with a thalamic tumor. Surg Neurol. 1976;5:151–5.
7. Gehlen M, Kurtcuoglu V, Schmid Daners M. Is posture-related craniospinal compliance shift caused by jugular vein collapse? A theoretical analysis. Fluids Barriers CNS. 2017;14:5.
8. Marmarou A, Shulman K, LaMorgese J. Compartmental analysis of compliance and outflow resistance of the cerebrospinal fluid system. J Neurosurg. 1975;43:523–34.
9. Yallapragada N. A model based description of the cerebrospinal fluid dynamics in the craniospinal system. Champaign: M. S. University of Illinois, Department of BioEngineering; 2003.
10. Alperin N, Vikingstad EM, Gomez-Anson B, Levin DN. Hemodynamically independent analysis of cerebrospinal fluid and brain motion observed with dynamic phase contrast MRI. Magn Reson Med. 1996;35:741–54.
11. Atsumi H, Matsumae M, Hirayama A, Kuroda K. Measurements of intracranial pressure and compliance index using 1.5-T clinical MRI machine. Tokai J Exp Clin Med. 2014;39:34–43.
12. Alperin NJ, Lee SH, Loth F, Raksin PB, Lichtor T. MR-Intracranial pressure (ICP): a method to measure intracranial elastance and pressure noninvasively by means of MR imaging: baboon and human study. Radiology. 2000;217:877–85.
13. Alperin N, Lee SH. PUBS: pulsatility-based segmentation of lumens conducting non-steady flow. Magn Reson Med. 2003;49:934–44.
14. Seborg D, Edgar TF, Mellichamp DA. Process dynamics and control. Hoboken: Wiley; 1989.
15. Mutambara AGO. Design and analysis of control systems. London: Taylor & Francis; 1999.
16. Nash JE, Sutcliffe JV. River flow forecasting through conceptual models part I—a discussion of principles. J Hydrol. 1970;10:282–90.
17. Magnaes B. Clinical studies of cranial and spinal compliance and the craniospinal flow of cerebrospinal fluid. Br J Neurosurg. 1989;3:659–68.
18. Behazin N, Jones SB, Cohen RI, Loring SH. Respiratory restriction and elevated pleural and esophageal pressures in morbid obesity. J Appl Physiol. 1985;2010(108):212–8.
19. Bloomfield GL, Ridings PC, Blocher CR, Marmarou A, Sugerman HJ. A proposed relationship between increased intra-abdominal, intrathoracic, and intracranial pressure. Crit Care Med. 1997;25:496–503.
20. Czosnyka M, Pickard JD. Monitoring and interpretation of intracranial pressure. J Neurol Neurosurg Psychiatry. 2004;75:813–21.
21. Yamada S, Miyazaki M, Yamashita Y, Ouyang C, Yui M, Nakahashi M, Shimizu S, Aoki I, Morohoshi Y, McComb JG. Influence of respiration on cerebrospinal fluid movement using magnetic resonance spin labeling. Fluids Barriers CNS. 2013;10:36.
22. Sullivan HG, Miller JD, Becker DP, Flora RE, Allen GA. The physiological basis of intracranial pressure change with progressive epidural brain compression. An experimental evaluation in cats. J Neurosurg. 1977;47:532–50.

23. Genevay S, Atlas SJ. Lumbar spinal stenosis. Best Pract Res Clin Rheumatol. 2010;24:253–65.
24. Uftring SJ, Chu D, Alperin N, Levin DN. The mechanical state of intracranial tissues in elderly subjects studied by imaging CSF and brain pulsations. Magn Reson Imaging. 2000;18:991–6.
25. Albeck MJ, Skak C, Nielsen PR, Olsen KS, Borgesen SE, Gjerris F. Age dependency of resistance to cerebrospinal fluid outflow. J Neurosurg. 1998;89:275–8.
26. Czosnyka M, Czosnyka ZH, Whitfield PC, Donovan T, Pickard JD. Age dependence of cerebrospinal pressure-volume compensation in patients with hydrocephalus. J Neurosurg. 2001;94:482–6.
27. Hayashi N, Matsumae M, Yatsushiro S, Hirayama A, Abdullah A, Kuroda K. Quantitative analysis of cerebrospinal fluid pressure gradients in healthy volunteers and patients with normal pressure hydrocephalus. Neurol Med Chir (Tokyo). 2015;55:657–62.
28. Stoquart-ElSankari S, Baledent O, Gondry-Jouet C, Makki M, Godefroy O, Meyer ME. Aging effects on cerebral blood and cerebrospinal fluid flows. J Cereb Blood Flow Metab. 2007;27:1563–72.
29. Capel C, Makki M, Gondry-Jouet C, Bouzerar R, Courtois V, Krejpowicz B, Baledent O. Insights into cerebrospinal fluid and cerebral blood flows in infants and young children. J Child Neurol. 2014;29:1608–15.
30. Fleischman D, Berdahl JP, Zaydlarova J, Stinnett S, Fautsch MP, Allingham RR. Cerebrospinal fluid pressure decreases with older age. PLoS ONE. 2012;7:e52664.
31. Ekstedt J. CSF hydrodynamic studies in man. 2. Normal hydrodynamic variables related to CSF pressure and flow. J Neurol Neurosurg Psychiatry. 1978;41:345–53.
32. Malm J, Jacobsson J, Birgander R, Eklund A. Reference values for CSF outflow resistance and intracranial pressure in healthy elderly. Neurology. 2011;76:903–9.

Permissions

All chapters in this book were first published in F&BTCNS, by BioMed Central; hereby published with permission under the Creative Commons Attribution License or equivalent. Every chapter published in this book has been scrutinized by our experts. Their significance has been extensively debated. The topics covered herein carry significant findings which will fuel the growth of the discipline. They may even be implemented as practical applications or may be referred to as a beginning point for another development.

The contributors of this book come from diverse backgrounds, making this book a truly international effort. This book will bring forth new frontiers with its revolutionizing research information and detailed analysis of the nascent developments around the world.

We would like to thank all the contributing authors for lending their expertise to make the book truly unique. They have played a crucial role in the development of this book. Without their invaluable contributions this book wouldn't have been possible. They have made vital efforts to compile up to date information on the varied aspects of this subject to make this book a valuable addition to the collection of many professionals and students.

This book was conceptualized with the vision of imparting up-to-date information and advanced data in this field. To ensure the same, a matchless editorial board was set up. Every individual on the board went through rigorous rounds of assessment to prove their worth. After which they invested a large part of their time researching and compiling the most relevant data for our readers.

The editorial board has been involved in producing this book since its inception. They have spent rigorous hours researching and exploring the diverse topics which have resulted in the successful publishing of this book. They have passed on their knowledge of decades through this book. To expedite this challenging task, the publisher supported the team at every step. A small team of assistant editors was also appointed to further simplify the editing procedure and attain best results for the readers.

Apart from the editorial board, the designing team has also invested a significant amount of their time in understanding the subject and creating the most relevant covers. They scrutinized every image to scout for the most suitable representation of the subject and create an appropriate cover for the book.

The publishing team has been an ardent support to the editorial, designing and production team. Their endless efforts to recruit the best for this project, has resulted in the accomplishment of this book. They are a veteran in the field of academics and their pool of knowledge is as vast as their experience in printing. Their expertise and guidance has proved useful at every step. Their uncompromising quality standards have made this book an exceptional effort. Their encouragement from time to time has been an inspiration for everyone.

The publisher and the editorial board hope that this book will prove to be a valuable piece of knowledge for researchers, students, practitioners and scholars across the globe.

List of Contributors

Gakwaya Habiyaremye, Diego M. Morales, James P. McAllister, Travis S. CreveCoeur, Rowland H. Han, Mohamed Gabir, Brandon Baksh and Deanna Mercer
Department of Neurological Surgery, Washington University in St. Louis School of Medicine, One Children's Way, 4S20, St. Louis, MO 63110, USA

Clinton D. Morgan
Barrow Neurological Institute, 350 West Thomas Road, Phoenix, AZ 85013, USA

David D. Limbrick Jr.
Department of Neurological Surgery and Pediatrics, Washington University in St. Louis School of Medicine, One Children's Way, 4S20, St. Louis, MO 63110, USA

Emma K. Hollmann, Amanda K. Bailey, Archit V. Potharazu and Ethan S. Lippmann
Department of Chemical and Biomolecular Engineering, Vanderbilt University, 2201 West End Ave, Nashville, TN 37235, USA

Aaron B. Bowman
Department of Biochemistry, Vanderbilt University, 2201 West End Ave, Nashville, TN 37235, USA
Department of Pediatrics, Vanderbilt University Medical Center, 1211 Medical Center Dr, Nashville, TN 37232, USA
Department of Neurology, Vanderbilt University Medical Center, 1211 Medical Center Dr, Nashville, TN 37232, USA

M. Diana Neely
Department of Pediatrics, Vanderbilt University Medical Center, 1211 Medical Center Dr, Nashville, TN 37232, USA

A. Jeppsson, C. Wikkelsø and Mats Tullberg
Hydrocephalus Research Unit, Institute of Neuroscience and Physiology, The Sahlgrenska Academy, University of Gothenburg, 413 45 Gothenburg, Sweden

Mikko Höltta
Department of Psychiatry and Neurochemistry, Institute of Neuroscience and Physiology, the Sahlgrenska Academy, University of Gothenburg, Gothenburg, Sweden

K. Blennow
Department of Psychiatry and Neurochemistry, Institute of Neuroscience and Physiology, the Sahlgrenska Academy, University of Gothenburg, Gothenburg, Sweden
Clinical Neurochemistry Laboratory, Sahlgrenska University Hospital, Molndal, Sweden

H. Zetterberg
Department of Psychiatry and Neurochemistry, Institute of Neuroscience and Physiology, the Sahlgrenska Academy, University of Gothenburg, Gothenburg, Sweden
Clinical Neurochemistry Laboratory, Sahlgrenska University Hospital, Molndal, Sweden
Department of Molecular Neuroscience, UCL Institute of Neurology, Queen Square, London, UK

Tilman Hottenrott, Rick Dersch, Benjamin Berger and Oliver Stich
Department of Neurology and Neurophysiology, University Medical Center Freiburg, Breisacher Strasse 64, 79106 Freiburg, Germany

Sebastian Rauer
Department of Neurology and Neurophysiology, University Medical Center Freiburg, Breisacher Strasse 64, 79106 Freiburg, Germany
Ravo Diagnostika GmbH, Oltmannsstrasse 5, 79100 Freiburg, Germany

Daniela Huzly
University Medical Center Freiburg, Institute of Virology, Hermann-Herder-Strasse 11, 79104 Freiburg, Germany

Jianming Xiang, D. Andrew Wilkinson, Ya Hua and Guohua Xi
Department of Neurosurgery, University of Michigan, R5018 BSRB, 109 Zina Pitcher Place, Ann Arbor, MI 48109-2200, USA

Lisa J. Routhe and Torben Moos
Department of Health Science and Technology, Aalborg University, Aalborg, Denmark

Richard F. Keep
Department of Neurosurgery, University of Michigan, R5018 BSRB, 109 Zina Pitcher Place, Ann Arbor, MI 48109-2200, USA
Department of Molecular & Integrative Physiology, University of Michigan, Ann Arbor, USA

David Bueno and Jordi Garcia-Fernàndez
Department of Genetics, Microbiology and Statistics, Unit of Biomedical, Evolutionary and Developmental Genetics, Faculty of Biological Sciences, University of Barcelona, Av. Diagonal 643, 08028 Barcelona, Catalonia, Spain

Margaret J. Ochocinska
National Heart, Lung, and Blood Institute, National Institutes of Health, 6701 Rockledge Dr., Room 9149, Bethesda, MD 20892-7950, USA

Berislav V. Zlokovic
Zilkha Neurogenetic Institute, Los Angeles, CA, USA

Peter C. Searson
Johns Hopkins School of Medicine, Baltimore, MD, USA

A. Tamara Crowder
Combat Casualty Care Research Program, Fort Detrick, MD, USA

Richard P. Kraig
University of Chicago Medical Center, Chicago, IL, USA

Julia Y. Ljubimova
Cedars-Sinai Medical Center, Los Angeles, CA, USA

Todd G. Mainprize
Sunnybrook Health Science Centre, Toronto, ON, Canada

William A. Banks
University of Washington, Seattle, WA, USA

Ronald Q. Warren and Andrei Kindzelski
National Heart, Lung, and Blood Institute, National Institutes of Health, Bethesda, MD, USA

William Timmer and Christina H. Liu
National Cancer Institute, National Institutes of Health, Bethesda, MD, USA

Manuel Gehlen
Institute for Dynamic Systems and Control, Department of Mechanical and Process Engineering, ETH Zurich, Zurich, Switzerland
The Interface Group, Institute of Physiology, University of Zurich, Zurich, Switzerland

Vartan Kurtcuoglu
The Interface Group, Institute of Physiology, University of Zurich, Zurich, Switzerland
Neuroscience Center Zurich, and the Zurich Center for Integrative Human Physiology, University of Zurich, Zurich, Switzerland

Marianne Schmid Daners
Product Development Group Zurich, Department of Mechanical and Process Engineering, ETH Zurich, Zurich, Switzerland

Francesco Tuniz, Maria Caterina Vescovi and Miran Skrap
Department of Neurosurgery, AOU-UD "Santa Maria della Misericordia", Piazzale S.M. della Misericordia, 33100 Udine, Italy

Daniele Bagatto and Maria Cristina De Colle
Department of Neuroradiology, AOU-UD "Santa Maria della Misericordia", Udine, Italy

Daniela Drigo
Institute of Epidemiology, AOU-UD "Santa Maria della Misericordia", Udine, Italy

Marta Maieron
Department of Physics, AOU-UD "Santa Maria della Misericordia", Udine, Italy

B. Shackleton, F. Crawford and C. Bachmeier
The Roskamp Institute, Sarasota, FL 34243, USA
The Open University, Milton Keynes, Buckinghamshire MK7 6AA, UK

Marc R. Del Bigio
Department of Pathology, University of Manitoba; Children's Hospital Research Institute of Manitoba, Diagnostic Services Manitoba, 401 Brodie Centre, 715 McDermot Avenue, Winnipeg, MB R3E 3P5, Canada

Domenico L. Di Curzio
Department of Human Anatomy and Cell Science, University of Manitoba, Winnipeg, Canada

Ken Takizawa, Mitsunori Matsumae, Naokazu Hayashi and Akihiro Hirayama
Department of Neurosurgery, Tokai University School of Medicine, 143 Shimokasuya, Isehara, Kanagawa 2591193, Japan

Satoshi Yatsushiro and Kagayaki Kuroda
Course of Science and Technology, Graduate School of Science and Technology, Tokai University, 4-1-1 Kitakaname, Hiratsuka, Kanagawa 2591292, Japan
Department of Biological Engineering, Tokai University, School of Biological Engineering, 4-1-1 Kitakaname, Hiratsuka, Kanagawa 2591292, Japan

Shyanne Page, Alli Munsell and Abraham J. Al-Ahmad
Department of Pharmaceutical Sciences, School of Pharmacy, Texas Tech University Health Sciences Center, 1300 South Coulter Street, Amarillo, TX, USA

Ronak Patel and Abraham J. Alahmad
Department of Pharmaceutical Sciences, School of Pharmacy, Texas Tech University Health Sciences Center, 1300 South Coulter Street, Amarillo, TX 79106, USA

Stephanie M. Patton and James R. Connor
Department of Neurosurgery, Penn State Hershey Medical Center, 500 University Drive, Mailbox H110, Hershey, PA 17033, USA

Quan Wang
Department of Biomedical Informatics, Vanderbilt University School of Medicine, Nashville, TN, USA

Todd Hulgan
Department of Medicine, Vanderbilt University School of Medicine, Nashville, TN, USA

Peilin Jia and Zhongming Zhao
School of Biomedical Informatics, The University of Texas Health Science Center at Houston, Houston, TX, USA

Scott L. Letendre and Donald R. Franklin
Department of Medicine, University of California-San Diego, San Diego, CA, USA

Ronald J. Ellis
Department of Neurology, University of California-San Diego, San Diego, CA, USA

William S. Bush
Department of Epidemiology and Biostatistics, Case Western Reserve University School of Medicine, Cleveland, OH, USA

David C. Samuels
Department of Molecular Physiology and Biophysics, Vanderbilt University, Nashville, TN, USA

Harpreet Kaur
Genomic Medicine Institute, Cleveland Clinic/ Lerner Research Institute, Cleveland, OH, USA

Asha R. Kallianpur
Genomic Medicine Institute, Cleveland Clinic/ Lerner Research Institute, Cleveland, OH, USA
Department of Molecular Medicine, Cleveland Clinic Lerner College of Medicine of Case Western Reserve University, Cleveland, OH, USA

Jennifer Iudicello and Igor Grant
Department of Psychiatry, University of California-San Diego, San Diego, CA, USA

Domenico L. Di Curzio
Department of Human Anatomy & Cell Science, University of Manitoba, Winnipeg, MB, Canada
Children's Hospital Research Institute of Manitoba, Winnipeg, MB, Canada

Emily Turner-Brannen and Xiaoyan Mao
Children's Hospital Research Institute of Manitoba, Winnipeg, MB, Canada

Marc R. Del Bigio
Children's Hospital Research Institute of Manitoba, Winnipeg, MB, Canada
Department of Pathology, University of Manitoba Brodie 401-727 McDermot Avenue, Winnipeg, MB R3E 3P5, Canada

Shin-ichi Akanuma, Yuhei Yamazaki, Yoshiyuki Kubo and Ken-ichi Hosoya
Department of Pharmaceutics, Graduate School of Medicine and Pharmaceutical Sciences, University of Toyama, 2630 Sugitani, Toyama 930-0194, Japan

Shinuo Liu, Magdalena A. Lam, Alisha Sial, Sarah J. Hemley and Marcus A. Stoodley
Department of Clinical Medicine, Faculty of Medicine and Health Sciences, Macquarie University, Suite 407, Clinic Building, 2 Technology Place, Sydney, NSW 2109, Australia

Lynne E. Bilston
Neuroscience Research Australia, Prince of Wales Clinical School, University of New South Wales, Margarete Ainsworth Building, Barker Street, Randwick, Sydney, NSW 2031, Australia

Moriah E. Katt, Lakyn N. Mayo and Peter C. Searson
Institute for Nanobiotechnology, Johns Hopkins University, Baltimore, MD, USA
Department of Materials Science and Engineering, Johns Hopkins University, Baltimore, MD, USA

Raleigh M. Linville and Zinnia S. Xu
Institute for Nanobiotechnology, Johns Hopkins University, Baltimore, MD, USA
Department of Biomedical Engineering, Johns Hopkins University, Baltimore, MD, USA

Qin Wang, Luisette Delva, Paul H. Weinreb, Robert B. Pepinsky, Danielle Graham, Elvana Veizaj, Weiping Chen, Ivan Nestorov and Tonika Bohnert
Biogen, Inc., 250 Binney Street, Cambridge, MA 02142, USA

Anne E. Cheung
Biogen, Inc., 250 Binney Street, Cambridge, MA 02142, USA
Ribon Therapeutic, 99 Hayden Ave #100, Lexington, MA 02421, USA

Ellen Rohde
Biogen, Inc., 250 Binney Street, Cambridge, MA 02142, USA
Present Address: Intellia Therapeutics, 40 Erie St, Cambridge, MA 02139, USA

Robin Caputo
Biogen, Inc., 250 Binney Street, Cambridge, MA 02142, USA
Present Address: Thermo Fisher Scientific Inc, 790 Memorial Dr, Cambridge, MA 02139, USA

Geoffrey M. Kuesters
Biogen, Inc., 250 Binney Street, Cambridge, MA 02142, USA
Present Address: Merrimack pharmaceuticals, 1 Kendall Square, Cambridge, MA 02139, USA

Liang-Shang Gan
Biogen, Inc., 250 Binney Street, Cambridge, MA 02142, USA
Foresee pharmaceuticals, 1 Innovation Way, Suite 100, Newark, DE 19711, USA

Jenna E. Koschnitzky
Hydrocephalus Association, 4340 East West Highway, Bethesda, MD 20814, USA

Richard F. Keep
University of Michigan, 1500 East Medical Center Drive, Ann Arbor, MI 48109, USA

David D. Limbrick Jr., James P. McAllister II and Jennifer Strahle
Washington University in St. Louis School of Medicine, 660 S. Euclid Ave, St. Louis, MO 63110, USA

Jill A. Morris
National Institute of Neurological Disorders and Stroke, National Institutes of Health, Neuroscience Center, 6001 Executive Blvd, NSC Rm 2112, Bethesda, MD 20892, USA

Yun C. Yung
Sanford Burnham Prebys Medical Discovery Institute, 10901 North Torrey Pines Rd., Building 7, La Jolla, CA 92037, USA

D. C. Engel, S. D. Adib and M. U. Schuhmann
Department of Neurosurgery, University Hospital of Tuebingen, Hoppe-Seyler-Strasse 3, 72076 Tuebingen, Germany

C. Brendle
Department of Neuroradiology, University Hospital of Tuebingen, Hoppe-Seyle-Strasse 3, 72076 Tuebingen, Germany

Ritambhar Burman
Biomedical Engineering Department, University of Miami, Coral Gables, FL 33146, USA

Noam Alperin and Sang H. Lee
Radiology Department, University of Miami, Miami, FL 33136, USA

Brigit Ertl-Wagner
Department of Radiology, Ludwig-Maximilians University, 80539 Munich, Germany

Index

M

N

O

P

R

S

T

V

www.ingramcontent.com/pod-product-compliance
Lightning Source LLC
LaVergne TN
LVHW080922210926
848485LV00004B/712
* 9 7 8 1 6 3 9 2 7 3 3 2 4 *